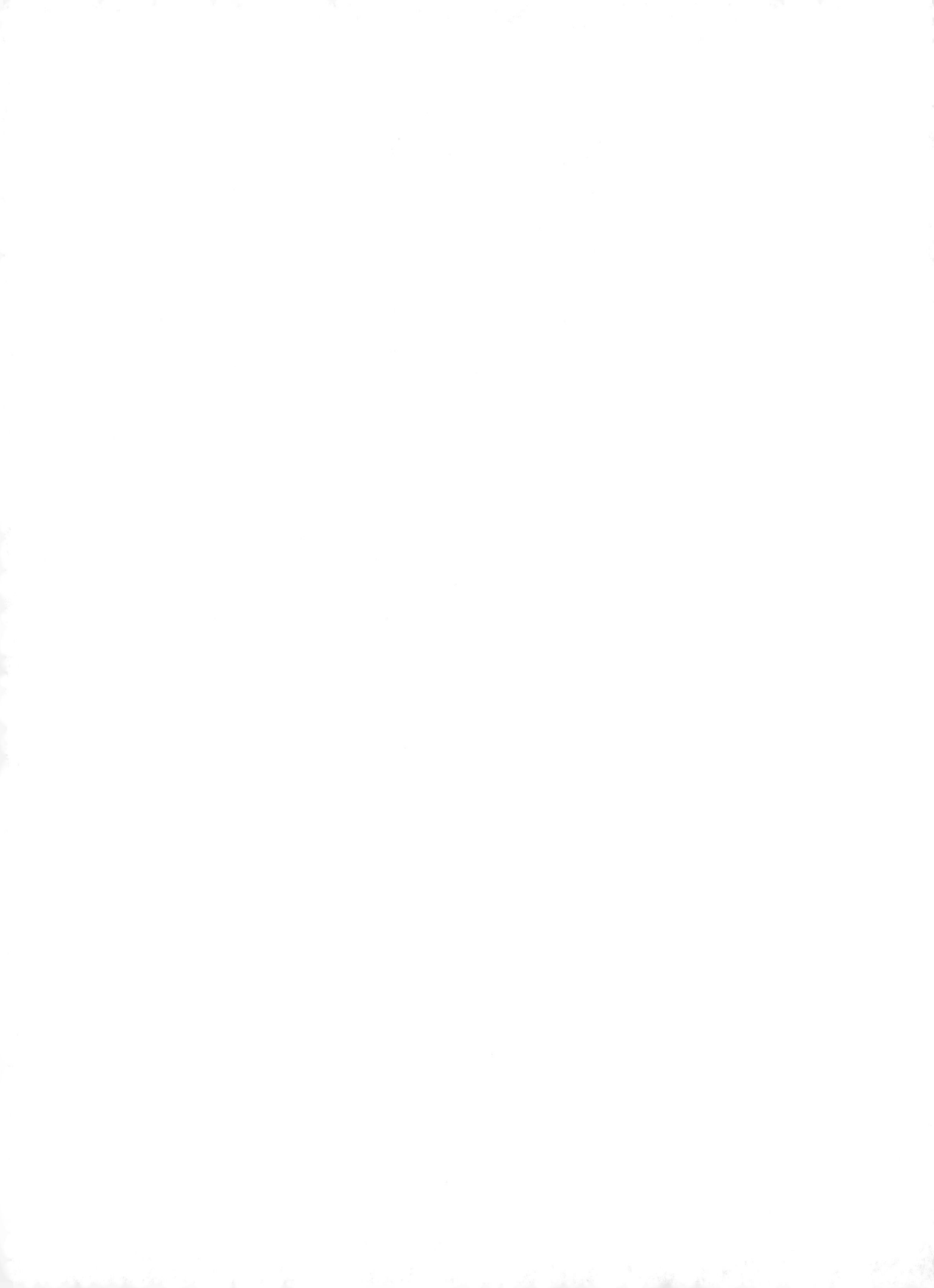

THE UNIQUE HERBAL

NEW INSIGHTS INTO ANCIENT MEDICINES

VOLUME ONE (A-C)

ROBERT DALE ROGERS (RH) AHG

CONTENTS

INTRODUCTION

Over the years, I have accumulated some information, a bit of knowledge and even a little wisdom about medicinal plants.

Many of the healing herbs in this volume set are relatively unknown; and some are little used in day-to-day clinical practice. Some are well known, but not utilized to their full extent of possibilities.

It is my hope that these pages may lead to a new and expanded materia medica, and a wider appreciation of many, often neglected, overlooked, and useful medicinal plants.

North American herbals tend to repeat, with increasingly useful additions, the same hundred or so plant medicines. The purpose of this book is to expand that awareness and hope that other herbalists will begin to look at the plants in their backyard and explore, observe and experience for themselves.

In turn, we could reconnect and continue the work begun in past centuries by the Eclectics and other plant people.

Like some of my previous publications, this book records indigenous use of medicinal herbs, garnered respectfully from the oral tradition, as well as work by various cultures around the world, the Eclectic physicians, modern herbalists, and recent scientific findings on various plant constituents.

It also includes homeopathic usage, essential oils, hydrosols, gemmotherapy, flower essences, personality traits, spiritual properties and astrological correspondences.

Please contact me if you wish to contribute; I am always learning.

Some Other Books by Robert Dale Rogers - www.amazon.com/author/robertdalerogers

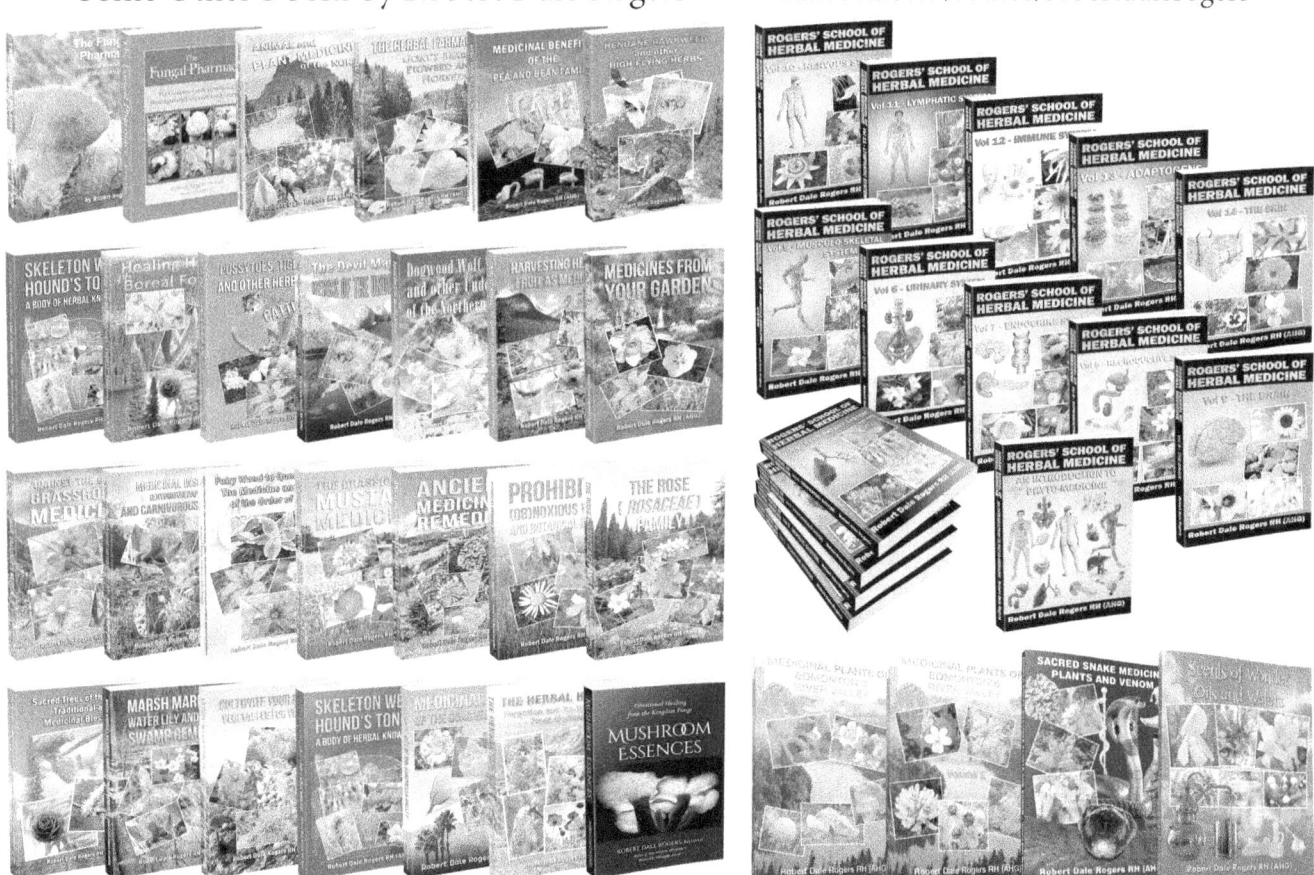

www.selfhealdistributing.com or www.scentsofwonder.ca - email: scents@telusplanet.net - Fax: 1 780-439-9540

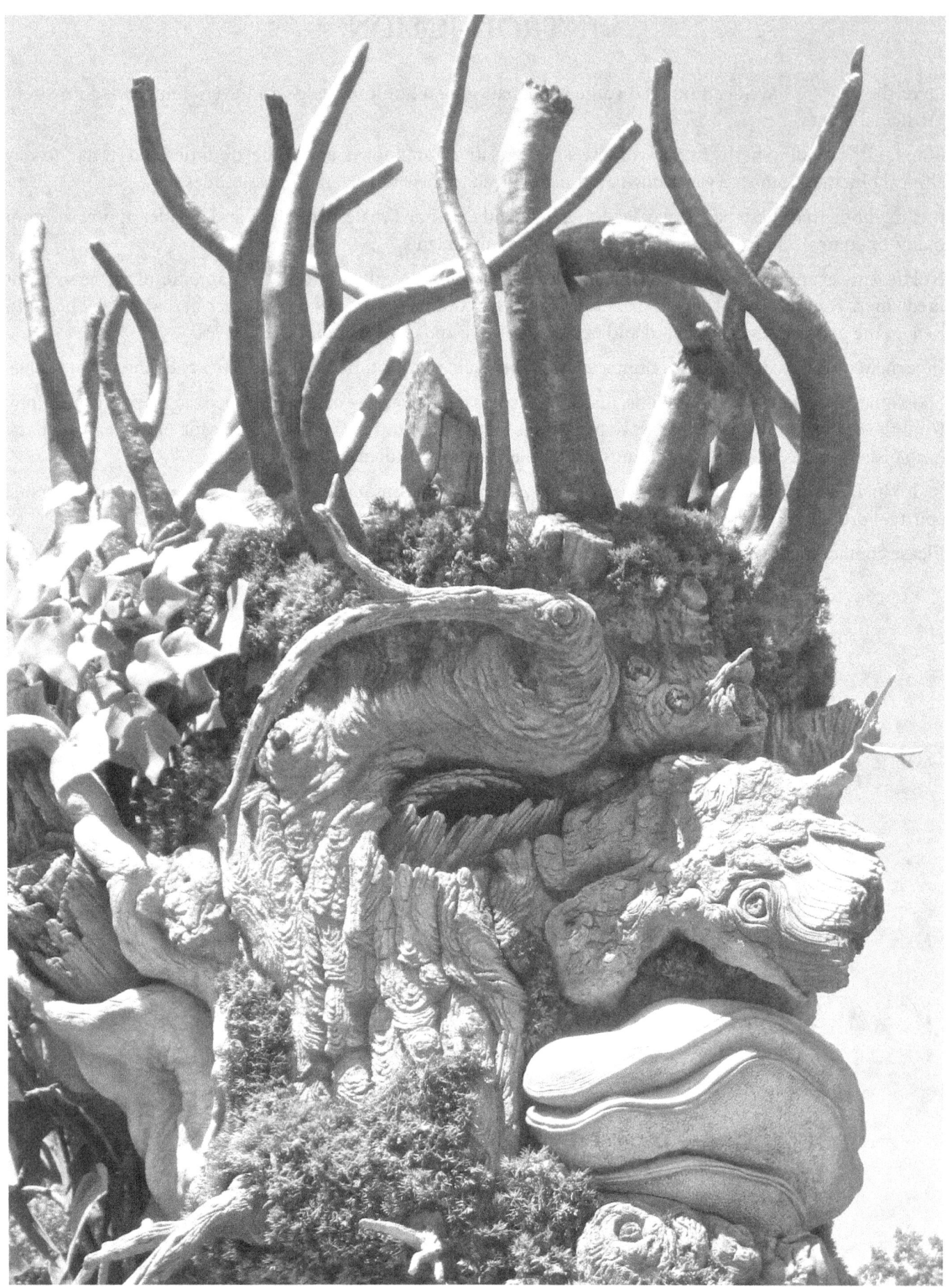

GREEN ALDER
(*Alnus crispa* [Ait.] Pursh) not accepted
(*A. viridis* **ssp.** *crispa* [Ait] Turrill)
SIBERIAN ALDER
(*A. viridis* **ssp.** *fruticosa*)
SITKA ALDER
(*A. sinuata* [Regal] Rydb.) not accepted
(*A. viridis* **ssp.** *sinuata* [Regel] A. Löve & D. Löve)
RIVER ALDER
MOUNTAIN ALDER
THIN LEAF ALDER
(*A. incana* **ssp.** *tenuifolia* [Nutt.] Breitung)
(*A. tenuifolia* Nutt.) not accepted
SPECKLED ALDER
SMOOTH ALDER
GRAY ALDER
(*A. incana* **ssp.** *rugosa* [Du Roi] R. T. Clausen)
(*A. rugosa* [Du Roi] Spreng.) not accepted
PARTS USED- catkins, leaf, bark

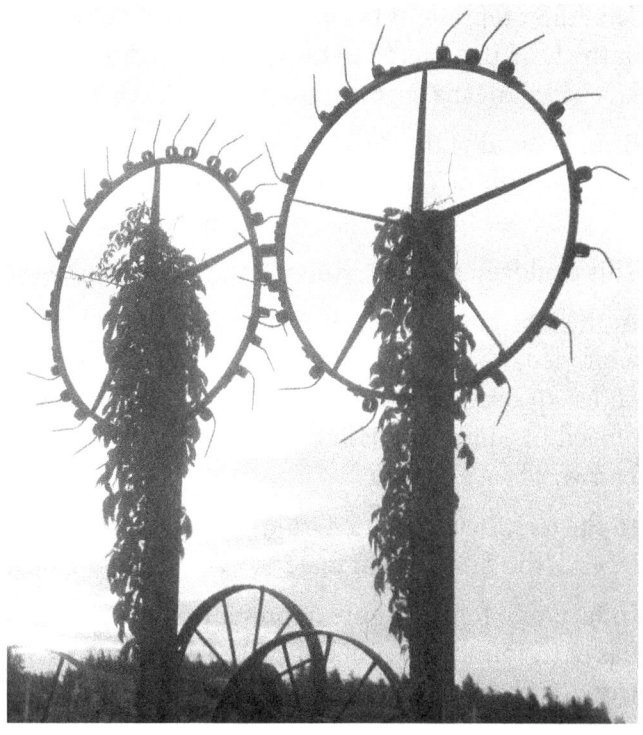

"The Alder, whose fat shadow nourisheth
Each plant set neere to him flourisheth."

WILLIAM BROWNE

"The meadows were veiled in a low creeping haze, through which tufts of Alders peered out like puffs of dark smoke."

POLISH SAYING

"I thought the sparrow's note from heaven
Singing at dawn in the alder bough.
I brought him home in his nest at even,
He signs the song, but it cheers not now,
For I did not bring home the river and sky."

EMERSON

Alnus is from the Anglo Saxon **ALR**, the Old English **ALOR** and in turn from the Old German **ELAWER** or **ELO** meaning, "reddish-yellow". It progressed to **ALER**, then **ALLER**, and from **ALDIR** to present spelling.

The German term **ALUZA** may be from Indo-European **ALISA**. Alys was the name of the goddess of the burial island. It is possible the Elysian fields or "islands of souls" were originally found in similar rivers.

The color is from the characteristic of wood to change color after felling. **INCANA** is from Latin meaning light gray, in reference to the white under leaf. **CRISPUS** meaning curled, and **TENUFOLIA** means, thin leaves.

At one time it was considered unlucky to fell an alder, most interesting considering that the city of Venice is built on alder and larch posts. The wood hardens like iron under water, and makes long lasting bridges, jetties, sluices and pumps.

The ancient Greeks considered alder sacred to Cronos, the God of Time. Its Greek name **KLETHRA** derives from kleio meaning, "to surround or enclose". The tree was considered the transformed sister of Phaeton, son of Helios and brother of Circe.

In Scotland, the wood was valued for construction and known as Scottish Mahogany, due in part to the rust colour of the new cut wood and sap.

The Alder represents the letter F (fearn) in the Druidic tree alphabet. It was known in medieval legend as the tree of the Erl King, sacred to the Celtic God Bran, the brother of Branwen, who kept the cauldron of Regeneration. His name means crow or raven.

Bran is a god of the dead, who carries a cauldron that brings the dead back to life. The cult of Bran was melded with the cult of Teutates, who drowned humans in alder groves. Later, both were transformed into the Fisher King to accommodate Christian myth.

This cauldron was the womb of the Great Goddess of paleolithic times, and thus is the fountain of youth.

In the famous *Battle of the Trees*, from a 10th century Welsh poem, followers of Bran wore alder sprigs. Fatally wounded, he had them cut off his head and carry it to a secret island (Avalon?) where for 80 years he told stories and sang songs. Other versions tell of his head remaining alive for 80 years on the way to London before being buried in the White Hill beneath the Tower of London. The purple of the buds is associated with Bran, and known as royal purple.

In the territory of Celtic Druids there was at one time a tribe known as Averni, or People of the Alder. In Irish legend, the first human male was created from alder, and the first female human from mountain ash.

In fact, one female figure, representing Alder Woman, carved from alder and dated between 728 and 524 BC, has been found in a peat bog on the west coast of Scotland. Across the sea, in Ireland, the wood was carved into wooden clogs for dry, warm footwear.

Alder is associated with the God Neptune, planet Venus, and the astrological signs of Cancer and Pisces (water).

In Norse legends, the month of March was associated with the waking Alder, and known as Lenet. This was a time of enforced fasting due to lack of food, and became the origin of the Christian festival of Lent. Alder is also associated with the 11th Norse Rune, IS.

Alder is our only broad-leaved tree to produce cones. These ripe, green cones were decocted in water in parts of England and drunk daily to alleviate gout.

The alder of Northern Alberta would be considered a tall, spreading shrub rather than a tree. The branches have a somewhat sticky surface that can be used as natural flypaper.

Alders are natural nitrogen fixers, like clover, and change atmospheric nitrogen into a form plants can use as fertilizer. They are valuable for restoring and regenerating mined and oil sand sites, checking erosion, and building up organic content.

These pioneer trees add the equivalent of ten bags of high nitrogen fertilizer to every hectare per year. It has been estimated that the leaves, when shed, provide another 160 kilos of nitrogen per hectare of soil. Inter-planting with hybrid poplar increases growth.

Green Alder is a very protein rich source of food that is virtually never browsed by moose or mice. This may be due to the presence of pinosylvan methyl ether, a strong herbivore repellant and abortifacient. In fact, this same compound extracted from tropical plants, is used as a wood preservative at low concentrations, protecting wood from termites for over two years.

Metal binding, histidine-rich proteins have been isolated from the root nodules of alder, suggesting some potential in bioremediation. Gupta RK et al, *Journal Protein Chem* 2002 21:8.

Experiments in Holland have shown growing alders in an apple orchard raise fruit yields by 36%.

It is much prized for smoking fish or game due to the mild flavor and slow burning properties of the wood. When well dried it produces a hot fire that doesn't throw sparks and leaves little ash. It is not as rich in BTUs as birch, but much better than aspen or pine.

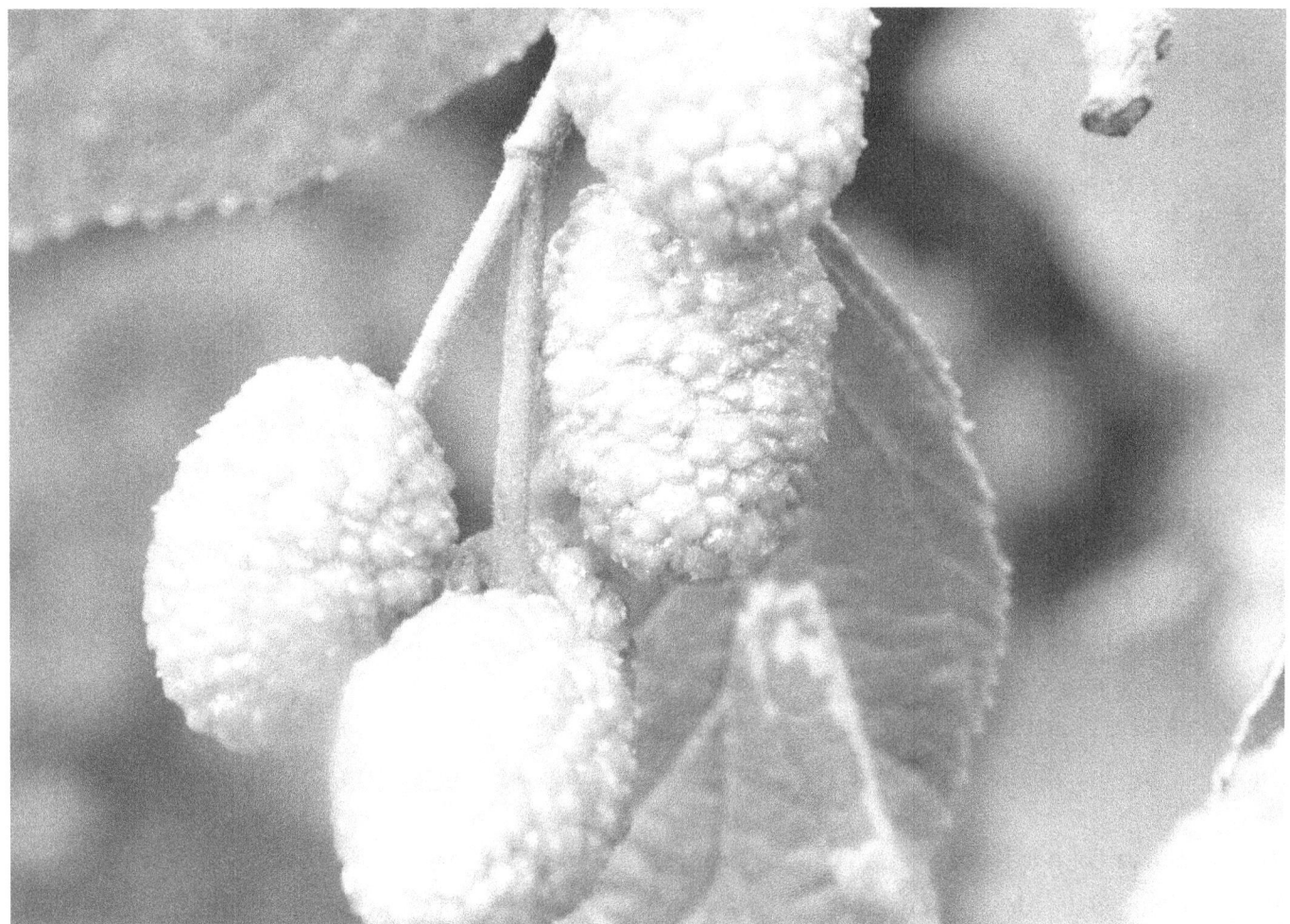

GREEN ALDER UNRIPE CONES

The Cree call it **ATOSPI** or **MISKWATOSPI** and use the plant in a variety of ways. The dormant bark was stripped and dried for dying hides used for clothing and moccasins. The bark was mixed with animal fats for body paint in traditional dances.

The Flathead boiled the bark for a bright red dye. They sometimes used this to produce odd-looking bright orange hair. Alder contributes a number of dye colors. The flowers give a green dye, the bark a fiery red, the young shoots cinnamon, and with copper mordant a pure yellow.

The Eastern Cree call Green Alder, **NEPATIHE**, and used bark decoctions to treat dropsy.

Speckled Alder is known, to Potawatomi as **ATOB**, meaning bitter. The inner bark was used for itchy skin and a bark tea for vaginal infections and as enema for hemorrhoids.

The wood can be carved into pipes, form the framework of birch bark baskets, or bent into small bows for hunting squirrels or birds.

A pipe stem can be made by sealing a grub into one end of an alder stem, forcing the insect to burrow its way out the other end.

The natural curve commonly found at the base of the shrub can be carved and fire hardened to peel bark from other trees. The wood was traditionally used to make the bottom and lid of birch bark containers, including one for beaver castors.

Work at the University of Maine in the 1960s, showed alder makes good kraft pulp, or can be chipped for hardwood composite board.

The rotten wood makes a good smudge, a smoke for tanning hides, or smoking fish. This dry rot was traditionally mixed with powdered willow bark for burns, in the form of a poultice.

Alder walking sticks, made from rotting branches, were lit and smoldered as a traveling mosquito repellant. The drifting smoke kept them away, and the periodic waving of the stick kept the fire slowly smoldering.

The fresh leaves were crushed and used as a poultice by nursing mothers with sore or swollen breasts. If the fresh leaves are ground and combined with small amount of warm milk, a suitable cheesecloth poultice can be used. The crushed leaves will relieve pain and decoctions of the leaves will quickly relieve sore feet when soaked in a warm footbath.

Leaves, with the morning dew still clinging, are placed in areas of the home having problems with fleas. They are attracted to the resins and can then be gathered and removed.

Various western tribes injected cool alder enemas to soothe bleeding hemorrhoids.

The Blackfoot used hot bark decoctions internally to heal tuberculosis of lymph glands in the neck. They call it **A-MUCK-KO-IYSTIS**, or red mouth bush, caused by chewing the bark.

The Dene people used the dried green cones, finely chopped, in smoking mixtures.

Both Dene and Cree of northern Saskatchewan boiled the green female catkins to treat venereal disease in men. The stems were boiled as an emetic for upset stomach.

The roots are dug up and decocted to relieve menstrual cramps or used as part of a steam/sweat to bring on menstruation.

The Chipewyan of northern Alberta know green alder as **K'AI LISEN**, or "willow that smells".

Further north on the Mackenzie delta, the Gwich'in call the plant red willow, or **K'OH**. Sophie Thomas, a Sai'Kuz healer, used bark shavings of **K'US** for cancers and ulcers, and sores in baby's mouth. It was combined with raspberry and chokecherry as a wash for skin ulcer and cancers including leukemia.

They used the inner bark to dye hides, skins, snowshoe frames and fish nets. Animal hides, for example, were soaked in a cool bark solution for 24 hours.

The inner bark was pounded and rolled up in beaver and wolverine skins to make them softer. This same decoction was used to revive worn moccasins, or at least restore and re-condition them.

For various human skin conditions, the bark was peeled from the stem, boiled, and cooled. The liquid, including the oily film on surface, was bathed on skin sores, scabs, eczema, sunburn and rashes. Stiff, arthritic joints were likewise treated.

The small green cones were chewed and the juice swallowed to relieve colds.

The Dena'ina of Alaska call this species fire willow or **QENQ'EYA**. It is used for fish traps and net-like drags, and digging sticks. The inner bark is boiled and taken for gas and to relieve fever. Like others, the bark was used to dye skin, and wooden objects, the latter preserved by rubbing animal fat over the newly dyed wood.

Alder roots can be split and used as twine if spruce or tamarack roots are not available.

The Nlaka'pamux used the fragrant stems of mountain alder as a perfume, and the small twigs for basket ornamentation. The Okanogan people made a string from the bark of young alder, as well as coiled baskets from the peeled, split and soaked roots.

The Gitksan name is **AMLUUX**, meaning neck ring, in reference to a special neck ring worn by chiefs and shamans composed of red cedar inner bark dyed red from alder bark decoctions.

In British Columbia, the red alder (*A. rubra*) is used for rabbit's dental care.

Thin-leaf Alder (*A. incana*) was used, by the Dena'ina, for a similar purpose. Some say it should not be used for cooking as the red juice looks like blood when it is burning. The red juice from tea is taken to treat tuberculosis.

This same dye was used for woven maple baskets and wool. After the bark is cut in small pieces and boiled, it is removed and chewed and chewed until all the dye is removed and spit into a container. It is believed the saliva acts as a mordant to set the color.

Green Alder is known as **GIIST**, by Gitksan. The root and bark is decocted six hours for cough medicine. The pistillate catkins are a physic made by crushing the catkins and eating them when one is sleepy and thin.

For gonorrhea, both pistillate catkins and bark shavings were boiled and taken three times daily, working as a strong diuretic.

Natives of New Brunswick boiled stems until the bark came off, then chewed and swallowed the juice for lung hemorrhage, and to promote healing of fractures, and wounds.

The Mohawk used a decoction of alder twigs and couch grass root for "thick" urine.

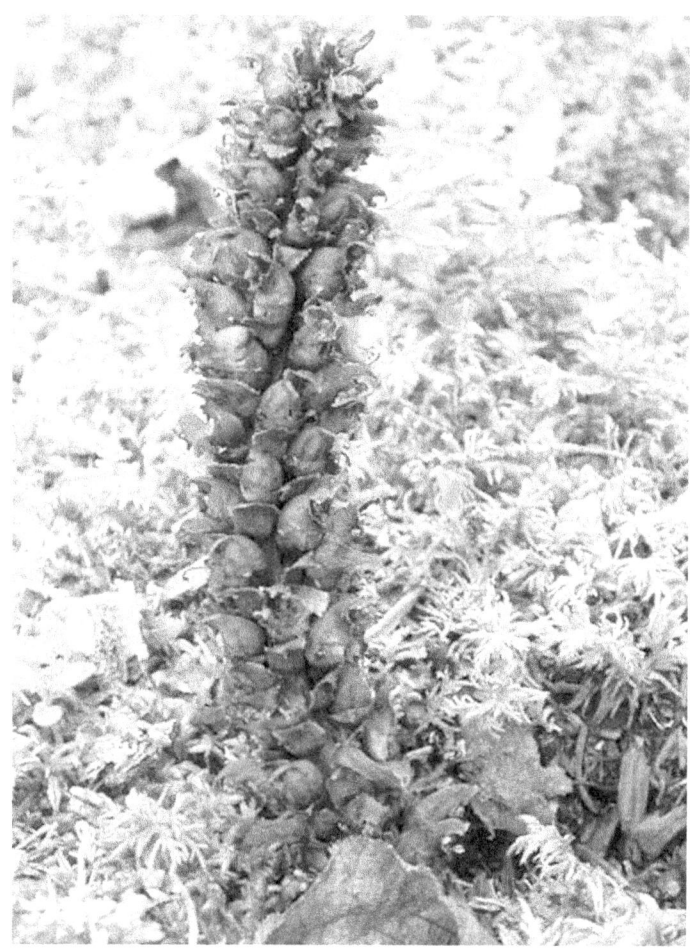

POQUE - PHOTO COURTESY OF LYNDSEY LARSON

Gray alder green cones were decocted to treat venereal disease in men, and as a wash for sore eyes. A root decoction was used by Seneca to treat burns, scalds and menstrual cramps.

Strong root decoctions were painted on traps for various animals, helping disguise the scent of humans.

Another interesting use was adding four dried, powdered bees to a root decoction for eye disease.

The early Acadian settlers brewed a reddish-brown tonic from the bark, to prevent anemia, and to treat kidney and skin complaints. Bark decoctions give a natural looking brown rinse to white or gray hair. In parts of Newfoundland, bark infusions are used for skin itching and rheumatism, or oil infused salves are applied to burns.

Herbal books of the 1600s suggested the use of fresh leaves for dissolving tumours. In 1973, a study into the properties of *Alnus oregona* verified that the stem bark contains lupeol and betulin, two compounds that suppress tumor activity. Sheth K et al, *Journal Pharm Sci* 62:1.

Charcoal made from alder was used in Europe for making gunpowder. It makes a charcoal highly prized by artists. River alder charcoal was mixed with pitch by boreal natives to seal canoe seams. Bark decoctions were used to soak toboggan boards to soften them for bending and shaping.

A parasitic plant that grows near the root of Green Alder, or Spruce shows strong free radical scavenging activity. Poque, or Northern Ground Cone (*Boschniakia rossica*) contains various iridoid glucosides, and several other compounds of interest. It is occasionally found near birch, willow, and even leather leaf. Grizzly bears sometimes like to gorge on the thick, fleshy plants, which can be abundant in the floodplain cottonwood forests of northern valleys. In Alberta, it is most commonly found in the northern Caribou Mountains; but is somewhat rare.

The plants can grow for 4-5 years as an underground tuber, before flowering.

The name Poque probably originates from **P'UKW'ES**, the name given to the parasitic plant by the Kwakwaka'wakw.

The Slave tribe drank decoctions of the thick base stem for stomach aches.

The Gwich'in call this plant **DU'IINAHSHEE**, meaning "uncle's plant". They took the white core at the base of the plant and ground it into a powder, or simply chewed it for medicine. The powder could be combined with fat for skin rashes. The white middle part was boiled and eaten to increase appetite or relieve stomachaches.

It was called "pipe", as the wet, bulb-like underground portion was dried and a hole cut in to make a pipe. This was filled with dried willow leaves. Or the ground cone roots were dried, pounded and mixed with tobacco.

Studies in Poland show pollen extracts from alder increased survival rate of mice injected with acetaminophen.

Speckled or smooth alder is identified by its distinct visible triangular pith in a cross section of the stem. The leaf tea was used as a skin wash for pimples and a tonic, according to Seton. The bark and cones were used by the Inuit to dye reindeer and caribou skins.

River Alder is distributed from Alaska to western Saskatchewan; where the nearly identical Speckled Alder continues onto Atlantic Canada. River Alder may be simply a regional variation.

Sitka Alder is found in the extreme southwestern part of Alberta, near Waterton National Park, but throughout British Columbia and north. Its uses are similar to above.

MEDICINAL

CONSTITUENTS – *A. crispa* bark- tannins, oils, resins, emodin, alnulin, protoalnulin, beta sitosterol, pinocembrin and phlobaphenes; nine diarylheptanoids, catechin.
A. crispa- resins from buds and catkins (30-60%), pinosylvin and its methyl ether, pinostrobin and 2-phenethyl cinnamate, alpha and beta amyrin, betulin, lupeol, sterols.
A. incana bark- triterpenoids alnin-canone,taraxerol, salicin, and taraxerone.
Buds- betuletol, mikanin, quercitin, iso-rhamnetin, and 4'-6-7trimethyl-pectolinarigenin scutellarein.
Buds- ayanin, 3'-4'-5-trihydroxy-3-7-dimethoxy flavone, and 4'-5-dihydroxy-3-7-dimethoxy flavone, and genkwanin, quercitin, benzenoid 4'-5'-dihydroxy-3'-methoxy stilbene.
A. viridis ssp. *viridis*- bark- various 27-hydroxyalphitolic acid derivatives, a 27-hydroxybetulinic acid derivative, 3-epi-maslinic acid derivative.

Both the leaves and dried inner bark of alder are bitter, helping stimulate digestion. Decoctions of the dried bark are astringent and hemostatic, reducing inflammations and even stopping internal hemorrhage. The powdered bark is a good hemostat for external bleeding. The fresh bark is emetic, and may cause cramping and vomiting.

Decoctions make an effective gargle for sore throats, pharyngitis, and toothaches. Milder dilutions cleanse teeth but also help to tighten and strengthen abscessed gums.

Work by Ritch-Krc et al, at College of New Caledonia in Prince George, BC found Mountain Alder (*A. incana*) possesses anti-cancer activity against mouse mastocytoma cells, with an IC50 value of only 6 ug/ml. *J Ethnopharm* 1996 52 151-6.

He mentions the case of an 11 year-old boy diagnosed with leukemia by a medical doctor in town of Vanderhoof. Sophie Thomas kept the boy at her home for a month and successfully treated him with *Alnus incana*. She also treated a young native woman with cervical cancer using alder and willow species.

Nine diarylhetanoids, derived from the bark, exert pronounced effect on decreasing DNA damage of human lymphocytes, in a stronger manner than amifostine. One of the best known diarylheptanoids is curcumin, derived from tumeric. Novakovic M et al, *Chem Biodivers* 2004 11:872.

The diarylhetanoids from the bark significantly reduced activity of the Pseudomonas aeruginosa, a drug-resistant, hospital acquired, pathogenic bacteria. Ilic-Tomic T et al, *Planta Medica* 2017 83(1-2):117-25.

Earlier studies found *A. crispa* extracts possess activity against gram-positive bacteria.

The inner bark of *A. incana ssp. rugosa* is a partial agonist of PPAR gamma activity, suggesting use in obesity and metabolic disease. Martineau et al, *Planta Med* 2010 13. Oregonin was identified as an inhibitor of adipogenesis in volume 14 of same journal.

Pinocembrin, found in poplar and scullcap species, is active against *Bacillus subtilis, Candida albicans, Saccharcervisine species* and *Cryptococcus neoformans.*

Work in Poland by Gryzbek et al, found water extracts of *A. incana* cones have an inhibiting effect on HIV-1 reverse transcriptase. Both the stipes and cones, when extracted with ethyl acetate were found to exhibit weak activity against the D6 and W2 clones of *Plasmodium falciparum,* implicated in malaria.

Janice Schofield gives a recipe for diarrhea, using the unripe, green cones in decoction internally. (See below)

Externally, a useful wash can be made for various skin conditions including eczema, impetigo, poison ivy, bee stings, and various itching rashes.

Work by Webster et al, *J Ethnopharm* 2008 115:1 found mild anti-fungal activity from alder and giant goldenrod, and significant activity from strawberry, fireweed and *Potentilla simplex.*

David Winston, RH (AHG) writes, "Alder bark is considered a specific for skin conditions where the eruptions (pimples) are red, raised, and never come to a head. It can be used orally, and topically for boils, carbuncles, staph infections, and large painful pimples on back, buttocks, face or neck".

Ellingwood noted similar benefits, as well as improvement in gastric secretions and improved digestion.

A good combination for pustular psoriasis is equal parts of alder bark, Oregon grape root and yellow dock root.

When available fresh, the slimy cambium layer can be rubbed over skin conditions, for even better effect.

Alder's primary use is to improve nutrition, by increasing digestion and the rate of waste excretion. Like poplar and willow, the bark of alder contains salicin, but in lesser amounts. Lupeol, is found in both alder and birch.

Catkins, from Red Alder (*A. rubra*), common throughout British Columbia, showed significant anti-fungal activity against all nine species studied; the catkins more so than the bark. McCutcheon et al, *Journal Ethnopharm* 1994 44:3.

Anti-microbial activity was found by same authors for bark and catkins, with nine of nine species showing some degree of inhibition. *J Ethnopharm* 1992 37.

Both *A. incana* and *A. viridis* bark are cytotoxic to HeLa cancer cells. A dry extract of the cones is anti-microbial. Stevic et al, *J Med Food* 2010 13:3.

Alnus incana bark has been found, *in vitro*, to inhibit CYP3A4 enzyme activity in the liver and hence delay breakdown of various prescription drugs; at least in theory. Tam et al, *Can J Physio Pharmacol* 2011 89:1.

Altan, obtained from cones of Black Alder (*A. glutinosa*) exhibits hepatoprotective activity at 1 mg/kg, which is about ten times less than traditional flavonoid-based medicines.

The green cones may be tinctured and used for allergies, as well as bacteria, fungal and amoebic infections. The freshly dried green cones, catkins, leaves and twigs can be tinctured for moving blood and lymph.

Kiva Rose, noted herbalist, writes: "Alder is a staple of my clinical work and one of my most beloved herbal allies. Its consistent and powerful ability to act as a profound alterative and lymphatic while addressing even the most severe microbial infections makes it truly invaluable to almost any practitioner."

She notes alder does not add to fluids or move or contain them, but transforms their quality.

She continues. "I have repeatedly seen cases of staph (including several confirmed cases of MRSA) infection manifesting as repeated outbreaks of boils clear up with the consistent use of Alder tincture."

Combine with Oregon grape root for constipation with poor fat digestion and skin problems.

Boggy congested conditions call for alder and bogbean, or perhaps Spanish Needles (*Bidens tripartita*) if the pattern suits.

Small amounts of tincture in ice-cold water will help move congested lymph, swollen glands and chronic sore throats.

Combine with redroot for severe lymphatic congestion, or with wild bergamot or calendula when a warming stimulant for circulation is needed.

Alnus viridus ssp. *viridus* bark contains derives of pentacyclic acids that show cytotoxicity against various cancer cell lines. Novakovic M et al, *J Nat Prod* 2017 April 3. Some pentacylic triterpenoids were selected as potential inhibitors of topoisomerases I and IIalpha.

Tag Alder (*A. serrulata*) is used for chronic skin conditions, lymphatic stagnation, dyspepsia in the elderly, and external hemorrhoids.

The leaves are a suitable substitute for plantain in cases of insect bites, bee stings, and assorted thorns, splinters and wilderness nicks and scrapes.

The leaf of the related *A. hirsuta* contains hirsutanonol, a compound that blocks LPS- and IFN-γ-induced macrophage iNOS expression.

Alnustic acid, derived from leaves of related *A. firma* inhibits HIV. Yu et al, *Arch Pharm Res* 30:7.

The leaves of *A. japonica* possess anti-inflammatory compounds. Han et al, *J Ag Food Chem* 2008 56:1.

NOTE- The fresh bark is griping and can be emetic or cathartic. Use dried bark. Fresh green cones can be tinctured as soon as possible. Chop well.

HOMEOPATHY

Red Alder is a close relative used as a remedy for skin afflictions, sub-maxillary glandular enlargements, and poor digestion due to insufficient secretion of gastric juices.

It stimulates nutrition and soothes ulcerated membranes of throat and mouth.

In the female, it may be used for vaginal discharge, cervical dysplasia, or where there is easy bleeding. It will help bring on delayed menstruation when the pain is from the back towards the pubic area.

In chronic herpes infection of the skin, or poison ivy it may be used locally.

DOSE- Tincture to the third potency.

GEMMOTHERAPY

EUROPEAN ALDER
(*A. glutinosa*)

This is the remedy for all chronic, inflammatory conditions. It is for all patients with coronary conditions, arthritis, pleuro-pneumonia, peritonitis, osteomyelitis, and staph infections. It is also for the early stages of acute articular rheumatism, coronary thrombosis, mitral stenosis, Paget's disease, osteoporosis, Consequently this is a global hypo coagulant, hypo-viscosant and anti-thrombosis bud therapy.

Use in resolution stage after infarction or other vascular spasms, phlebitis, acute or chronic migraines associated with cerebral circulation.

Take at first stage of flu, sinusitis, tracheitis. Use for colitis, peritonitis and cholecystitis. Use in cases of chronic urticaria, as well as kidney issues such as cystitis and pyelitis.

MOUNTAIN/RIVER ALDER
(*A. incana*)

The action is similar to the European species but is stronger and shorter acting in nature. It has the ability to reduce severe inflammatory and thrombosis conditions, but must be used more often in smaller doses.

DOSE- 15-20 drops in water three times daily. European Alder once daily. Both are 1 DH glycerine macerates. *Alnus incana* buds contain quinic and ferulic acid.

NORTHERN GROUNDCONE
POQUE
(*Boschniakia rossica* [Cham & Schltdl] B. Fedtsch)
(*B. glabra* CA Mey ex Bong)

Boschniakia is named after the Russian amateur botanist A. K. Boschniak.

Boschniakia is a brown to yellow to red parasitic plant found near the Green Alder (*A. crispa*) and other *Alnus* species. It is commonly found at the foot of trees looking like an upright pinecone, about 20 cm long, with dense dark flowers and a dark scale-like leaf below it. At first glance they appear dead, but are fresh and resilient when touched. It belongs to the Broomrape family. It is widely distributed from North America to northeastern Asia.

The Tlingit of Alaska use *B. glabra* root as part of a treatment for sores. The Dena'ina of Alaska call it **QINAZ'IN**, or "that which sticks up". A piece of the plant was tied around the neck of puppies or babies to help them grow correctly. It is said to be a favourite food source of bears.

The holoparasitic plant is found on Alnus species in Asia, but is over-harvested and becoming increasingly rare.

MEDICINAL

CONSTITUENTS- Two iridoid glucosides, boschnaloside and boschnaside, an oligosaccaride (+)-pinoresinol-beta-D-glucopyranoside, and rossicaside, an phenylpropanoid glycoside, have been isolated. Orobanin of an iridoid glucoside and the pyridine alkaloids of boschniaside, boschnilactone and boschniakine have been identified amongst the more than 100 compounds. These include thirty terpenoids, 49 phenylpropanoids, six alkaloids, four sterols.
Aerial parts- roschinialactones, C_9, C_{10} and C_{11} terpene lactones, salidrosides, rossaicasides A-K. Monosaccharides in leaves and flowers (?) measure 41.83%; polysaccharides in latter are 32.43%.
Rhizomes- mannitol, alkaloids. For full analysis see Zhang Le et al, *J Ethnopharm* 2016 194:987-1004.

In Japan, Russia, Korea and China, the dried herb, or stem is used as a tonic, or invigorating medicine for kidney function and erectile dysfunction.

The latter may be due, in part, to its phallic growth appearance.

In Jilin province, China, *B. rossica* is used as an anti-senile agent. Ethanol extracts were administered to rats whose cholinergic nucleus had been destroyed by ibotenic acid. Rats treated with the extract showed significant improvement in learning ability, and it was concluded *B. rossica* would be therapeutic in the treatment of senility. Not a very rigorous trial, but certainly compelling. Zhou LS et al, *J Trad Chin Med* 2008 10: 1431-4.

Another study found alcohol extracts induced improvement on learning ability, memory and free radical scavenging action. Tsuda T et al, *J Ethnopharm* 1994 41:67-71 & 85-90.

In Traditional Chinese Medicine, the herb is known as **JOU-TSUNG-JUNG**. It possesses nutritious but no harsh qualities, as well as providing ease and smoothness. It is sometimes referred to as **JINSIN**, **DIJING** or Bulao herb. In traditional Mongolian medicine is called **BAORI GAO YAO**.

The earliest records appear in the Tang Materia Medica, revised by Su Gong in 659 A.D.

Later, it was found in *Herbal Medicine of Rihuazi* (935-960 A.D.) and *Ben Cao Tu Jing* (1020-1101 A.D.).

It is sometimes substituted for *Cistanche deserticola*, used as a stamina tonic herb.

It is considered a sweet, salty flavour with warming properties, affecting the kidney and large intestine. It nourishes the kidneys and sperm, supplements yang, and moistens the intestines. It has been used for impotence, infertility in women, and cold obstructions of the loins and knees.

Pharmacological studies show toning and laxative effect. It increases saliva secretions in laboratory mice and shows hypotensive effect from both water and alcohol soluble extracts.

Work by Piao et al, *Zhong Xi Yi He Xue Bao* 2003 1:2 found extracts clear free radicals for D-galactose-induced senile rats.

Anti-tumor activity, by tinctures of whole plants was found by Jin AH et al, *Chinese J Public Health* 2011 27(11): 1433-4.

Iridoid glucosides prevented lung carcinoma cell proliferation and induced apoptosis. Yin XZ et al, *J Food Sci* 2015 15: 173-8.

The same compounds were found to inhibit the growth of H_{22} tumors in mice. Jin AH et al, *Chin Trad Herb Drugs* 2012 43(2): 332-5.

Wu et al, *World J Gastroenterol* 2005 11:1 found extracts prevent pig serum induced liver rat fibrosis, by inhibiting activation of hepatic stellate cells and synthesizing collagen.

The herb has been found to protect ECly hepatic cells by reducing oxidative stress, suppressing inflammation and improved CYP2E1 detoxification of liver. Quan et al, *Biosci Biotech Biochem* 2009 73:4.

Another study found polysaccharides reduced free radical and lipid peroxide damage in early to middle life stages of liver cancer. Xue Y et al, *Heilongjiang Med Pharm* 2011 34(5): 1-2.

Ethanol extracts alleviated induced hepatic fibrosis in a triple arm rat study. Piao XX et al, *World Chin J Dig* 2005 3(18): 2205-9.

One mouse study looked at normal control, one group with silymarin (Milk thistle), and high and low doses of butanol and water fractions of herb.

Serum liver levels confirmed the benefit of the latter to protect from acute liver injury, via anti-oxidant activity. Li D et al, *J Med Sci Yanbian University* 2012 35(2): 98-100.

Water extracts are anti-inflammatory, anti-fatigue and strengthen oxygen resistance ability and improve brain blood circulation. Yu QH et al, *Trad Chin Med Mater* 1993 7: 32-4.

Ethanol extracts increase the antibody secreting cells of mice spleen cells. Jiang YN et al, *J Yanbian Med Coll* 1992 3:170-2.

The holoparasite contains three compounds that induce the excitable catnip response in cats. These are boschniakine, boschnialactone, and onikulactone. It is very likely the plant was smeared on trap lures to attract larger cats, by native hunters of west coast.

Boschniakine is found in various species of *Pedicularis*, the semi-parasitic lousewort.

BARK LEAF/OIL

Combine one part of freshly dried bark and leaves to five parts canola oil in a low temperature crockpot for six hours. Strain and use as part of anti-inflammatory salves or ointments, or indolent slow-healing skin ulcers. It combines well with goldenrod and Artemisia plant oils for strained or injured tissue, with arnica and St. John's wort for nerve and muscle pain, and with wild bergamot or cleaver oil for inflamed, swollen glands.

HYDROSOL

Upon distillation of the green leaves, catkins and twigs of alder, a hydrosol is obtained. Dr. Ayer recommended the use of *Alnus* water for periodic hyperasthetic rhinitis (hay-fever). The hydrosol is combined with an equal amount of water and snuffed up the nostrils 5-6 times, or atomized at full strength into the nose.

At night the water is combined with un-petroleum jelly and smeared into the nose; while the distillate is taken internally, one teaspoon three times daily one hour before or after meals to improve digestion.

Dr. Ayer also recommended this as a cure in the acute stage of gonorrhea, or as an antidote to poison ivy skin rashes.

The hydrosol is produced when catkins are forming, using bark and catkins.

WAX

Psylla wax is secreted by an aphid (*Prociphilus alni*), living on leaves of River Alder (*Alnus incana*). It is obtained by extracting it from the insects first in hot ether, in order to remove the glycerides, and then with hot chloroform.

The wax is insoluble in hot ether, and only poorly soluble in cold chloroform. It crystallizes in needles with a silky luster; and melts at 96 degrees Celsius.

Psylla wax is the psyllostearylic acid of psyllostearyl alcohol.

No commercial use at present time.

The aphids cover themselves with wax, secreted by their bodies. They have an interesting relationship with the Green Lacewing (*Chrysopa spp.*)

Their larvae are the same size and shape as aphids, which they love to puncture and suck dry.

The aphids produce honey nectar for ants that protect them like milk cows. Lacewing larvae protect themselves by stripping the wax off their prey and piling it on themselves.

It adheres very well to their bristly hooked bodies, fooling ants into thinking they are aphids. When stripped of the wax, it takes them only about twenty minutes to go back into disguise.

FLOWER ESSENCES

Green alder flower essence helps to open our hearts and minds to aspects of light which are beyond normal perception. This relaxation and expansion of our sensory awareness allows us to access subtle levels of information from our surroundings. It helps us integrate this level so that we may see beyond our current habits and belief systems.
                                                                                                        ALASKA

Alder flower essence is for acceptance of our destiny, and the anger and blame, including self-blame, and lack of energy and joy that comes from acceptance of self. With the essence, we learn to forgive ourselves and learn about spiritual protection in disputes.
                                                                                                          OGAM

Essence of Alder is associated with the principle of release. It reduces stress, anxiety, and nervousness and increases life energy.
                                                                                                       GIFFORD

Speckled Alder (*A. incana*) essence is for stepping out of habitual patterns, enabling on to listen to instinct and take responsibility. It helps release energy deficiency, victim mentality and not learning from mistakes.
                                                                                                      ICELANDIC

River Alder (*A. incana*) essence helps relax groups and work with colleagues.
                                                                                                        MIRIAM

Alder essence is for taking life at surface value; being unable to see what one senses to be true; helps us to integrate seeing with knowing so that we can recognize our highest truth in each life experience.

DARCY WILLIAMSON

Poque is the remedy for claustrophobia—enables us to survive in close quarters, to maintain self in closed area, cities, apartments. Also assists when feeling too much going on around us. Feeling closed in by demands.

FREEMAN & MONGEAU

SPIRITUAL PROPERTIES

Red Alder energy has a quality of innocent, child-like enthusiasm that is both stimulating and cheerful. It offers an outpouring of energy that insists that you get on with life and open your eyes to the beauty around you. Seek out red alder when you feel depressed, overly serious, or find yourself dwelling on the past. Red Alder turns up the music, sets your toes to tapping, and before you know it, you are dancing into the future.

CHASE/PAWLIK

The alder reminds us of the need to blend strength and courage with generosity of spirit and compassion. There is a time to challenge things and a time to hold our peace. The alder teaches us this discrimination and the need to see beneath the surface of things.

GIFFORD

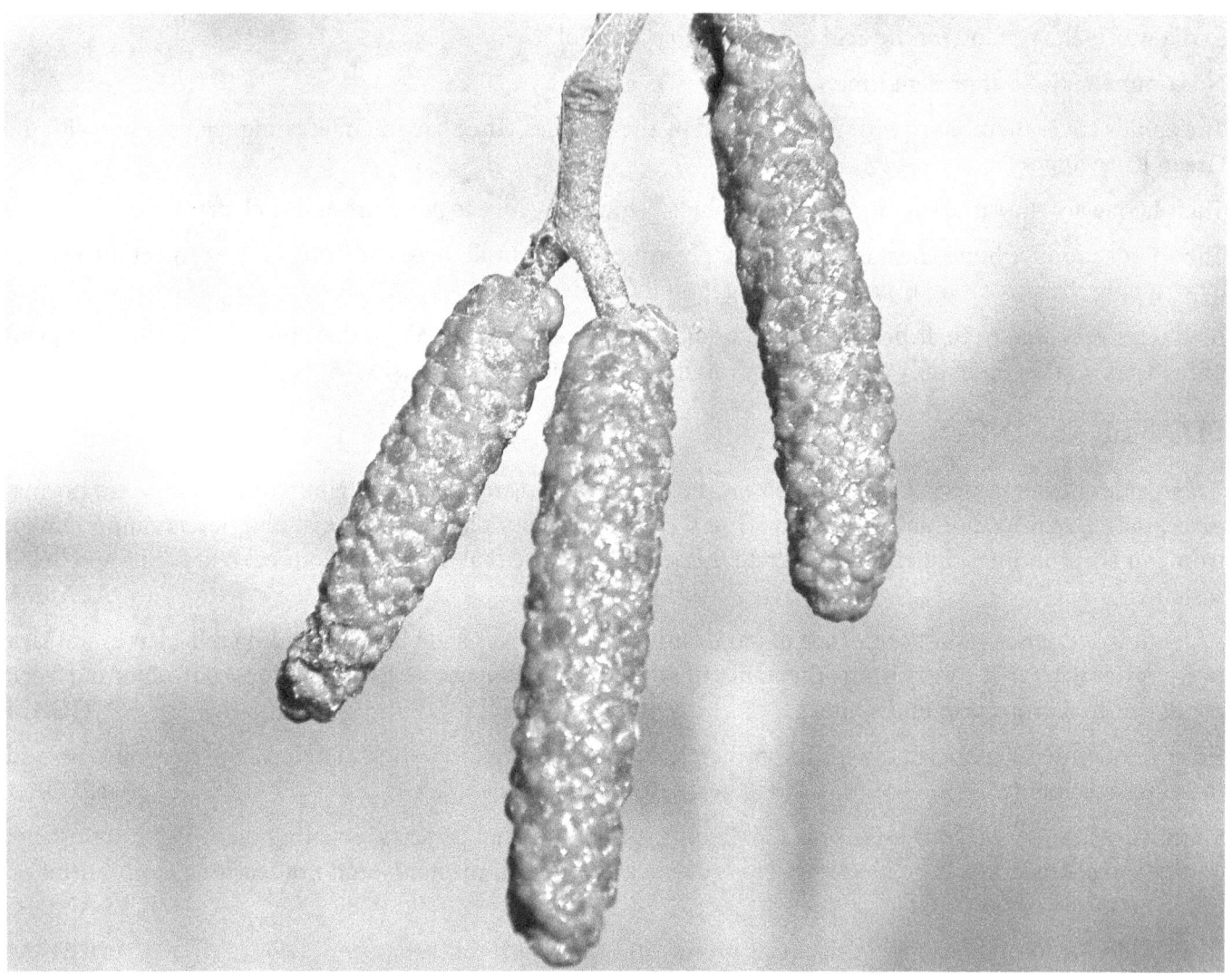

GREEN ALDER CATKINS

12

PERSONALITY TRAITS

The flames of Alder are green, but its blood is red. Alder is the bleeding mother and the wounded healer who understands; it is the listener, who can listen to your sorrow and weave your tears into her life-giving carpet. Master of the elements, Alder can heal with water, fire, earth and air.   **HAGENEDER**

Alder is an excellent magical name for one who is secretive, changeable, a fire sign; one who loves color; a seamstress or an artist; one who loves incense, aftershave lotion or perfume; a down-to-earth person who is a forest lover and a wise experienced Witch. This is the sort of person who loves the drams of ritual, who likes to dance skyclad in the shadows of the forest. Alder will bring out the hidden sensitivity and sentimentality lurking within you.   **MCFARLAND**

If the patient is healthy on the emotional level, the only characteristic personality trait may be his tendency to generosity. One would not normally consider "having a kind heart" to be a symptom, but in the case of Alnus it is something that is at the centre of the patient's being.

He or she is willing to make sacrifices for others and to do favours, which, for most other people, would not be possible. As this type of behaviour often brings its own day-to-day rewards, there may not be a noticeable loss of vitality in the patient.

Many remedies have the feeling of being isolated and alone. Alnus is unique in their reaction to this feeling of isolation in that, in order to overcome it, they may tell the practitioner: "I try harder and work harder as I easily feel guilt. Also, I have a tremendous natural sympathy for others, especially for those people who have less or who are suffering in some way."

They deny that they have needs; therefore, they postpone gratification and then eventually they suffer from not having their emotional and physical nourishment needs met. They can become resentful, bitter and empty; then later, in theory, they might "gorge" themselves emotionally, taking more than they need from life.

In the third stage, depression becomes constant and then, finally, they start to become apathetic, as if all the previous caring had been "burned" out of them. Eventually they develop a complete indifference to life. At the end of this stage, when they hate life, they hate other people for being so selfish.   **OLSEN**

MYTHS AND LEGENDS

According to legend, at the time of Creation, there was a rivalry between God and the devil. The wolf was shaped by God, but the devil tried to intervene and bring it to life.

However, the wolf refused to breathe and live. It was only when infused with the power of God that the wolf sprang to life and began to attack the devil. The devil hid in an alder tree but the wolf caught hold of his heal (sic) and blood ran down the trunk. From that time forward, the alder has had its reddish bark   **KNAB**

According to one such tale, mink-man, a primordial human-animal figure of the Distant Time, approached a group of human-plant figures known as tree-women…His solemn duty was to inform the tree-women that Raven, the sacred transformer spirit who happened to also be husband to each of the tree-women, had just died. Upon hearing this sad news, each of the tree-women expressed her profound sorrow by inflicting a superficial flesh wound to her body…One of the grieving tree-women was transformed into an alder [and] she cried and pinched herself until she bled…her distinctively colored bark oozed a blood red juice, which the Koyukon traditionally used as a red dye.   **KNUDTSON/SUZUKI**

The medieval Wulfdietrich Saga gives a strong idea of Alder Woman. In various German legends she appears to wanderers as a seductive woman teaching wanton males a lesson by turning into a hairy or bark-like creature once in their embrace. Her different German names—Else, Elsa, Elise—are derived from the Anglo-Saxon Alor, or the Gothic Alisa…

13

In the second song of the Wulfdietrich, Saga the Rough Else, a wild-looking woman of the woods who is covered in hair, puts a spell on the hero eventually making him made. He runs wildly through the woods, living on herbs for six months. Then she takes him on a ship over the sea to another land where she is queen.

She bathes in a magical well that washes away her rough skin, and is transformed into the most beautiful of women and has a new name—Sigeminne (victory of love).   **HAGENEDER**

An old European legend about the origin of alders is related to April 21st, the festival day of the goddess Pales. She was the Roman goddess of shepherds and herdsmen.

Two men decided to spend the holiday fishing, instead of attending the required ceremonies. In punishment, the goddess turned them both into trees destined forever to haunt the banks of streams, watching for fish.

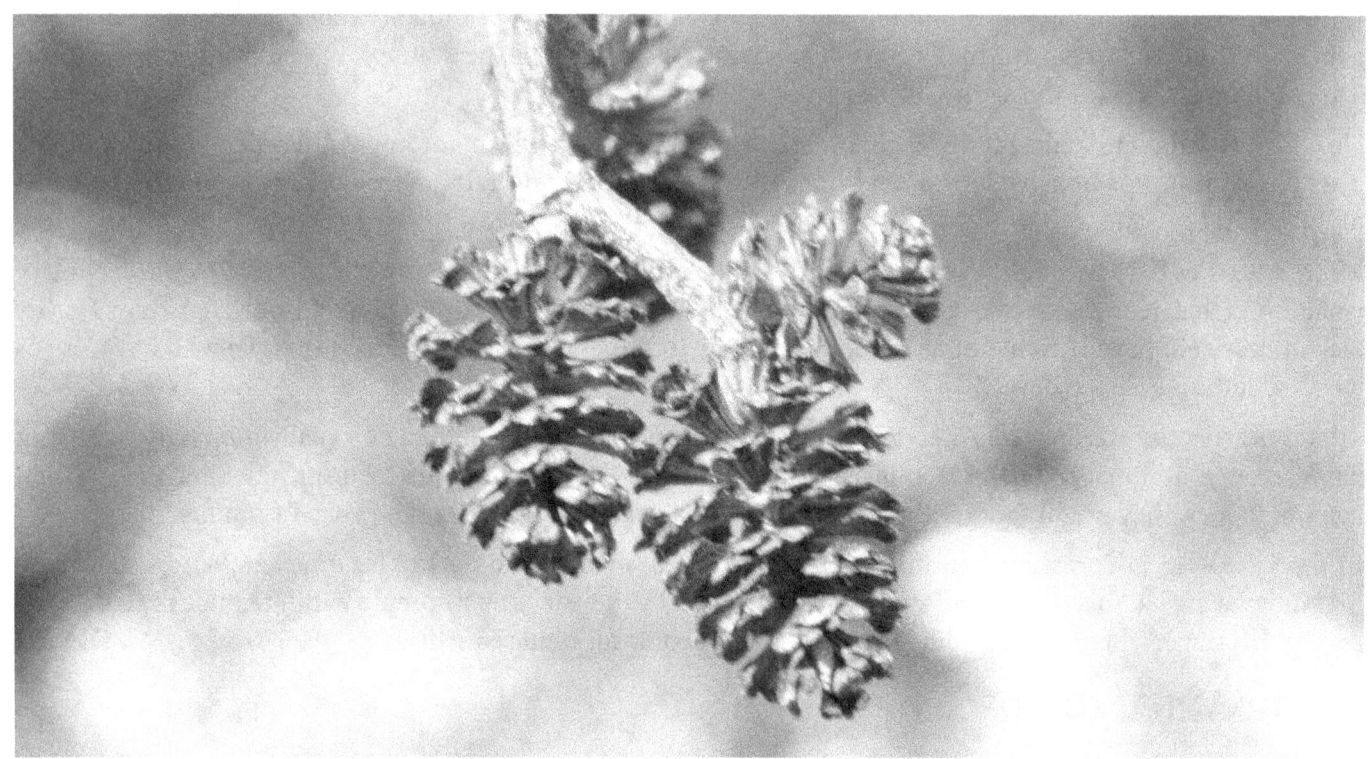

DRY BROWN ALDER CONE

RECIPES

INFUSION- To one ounce of fresh or dried bark add one pint of boiling water. Let steep 20 minutes. Take 1-2 tablespoons as needed.

DECOCTION- Take one ounce of green, unripe female cones and simmer in one pint of water for twenty minutes. Drink as needed. (Janice Schofield)

Decoct the dried bark (1:20) for improving food absorption and fat metabolism. Take one to two ounces before meals. Also good for throat gargles, gum weakness, etc.

TINCTURE- 5-20 drops, as needed. For pustular psoriasis, as noted above, 25 drops three times daily in cool water for 4-6 months. A tincture is made from the dried, green cones, and twigs at 1:5 and 40% alcohol. Use for intestinal inflammation.

SALVE- Cover one part fresh-stripped alder bark with five parts coconut oil in a glass jar. Let sit in sun for two weeks, shaking daily. Strain. If inclement weather, use low temperature crockpot. Strain and use for skin conditions such as eczema and psoriasis.

SYRUP- Macerate three pounds of crushed dry bark in cold water for six hours. Put into percolator and add water until five pints have passed over. Put on low heat and stir in eight pounds of honey or sugar. When cold, add a pint of whiskey or vodka.

B. rossica- 6-18 grams. For treating constipation, 12-18 grams dry powder.

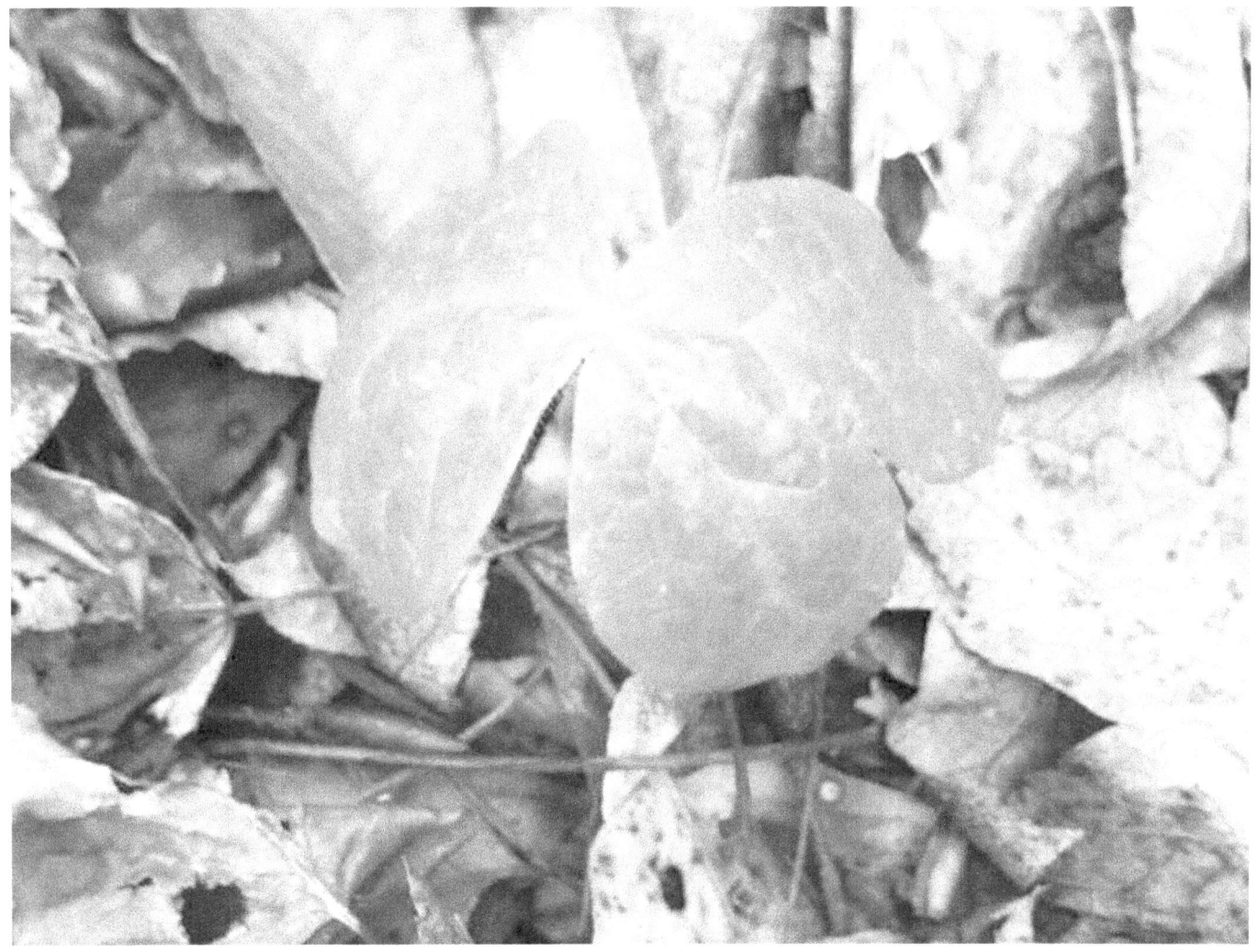

AMERICAN TWINLEAF

AMERICAN TWINLEAF
RHEUMATISM ROOT
(***Jeffersonia diphylla*** [L.] Pers.)
PARTS USED–root

Jeffersonia is named after the popular US president Thomas Jefferson. He was deeply interested in botany, and agriculture.

Diphylla means two-leafed. The single leaf is deeply divided into two lobes, giving the appearance of separate foliage.

Twinleaf is a popular perennial for the shaded garden, or wooded areas of an acreage. The pale lavender to white, eight-petal flowers are a popular spring-time treat that complements the violet tinted leaves. The flowers look very similar to bloodroot.

It is common from southern Ontario to New York and west to Wisconsin and south to Virginia and Alabama. It is hardy to zone 5, and yet here it was growing in the Devonian Botanical Garden near Edmonton, Alberta; considered zone 3. I really did not know much about the plant, but was somewhat fascinated at first sight.

I quickly came to realize this was an important plant that fit a number of categories for a newly evolved *Northern Materia Medica*.

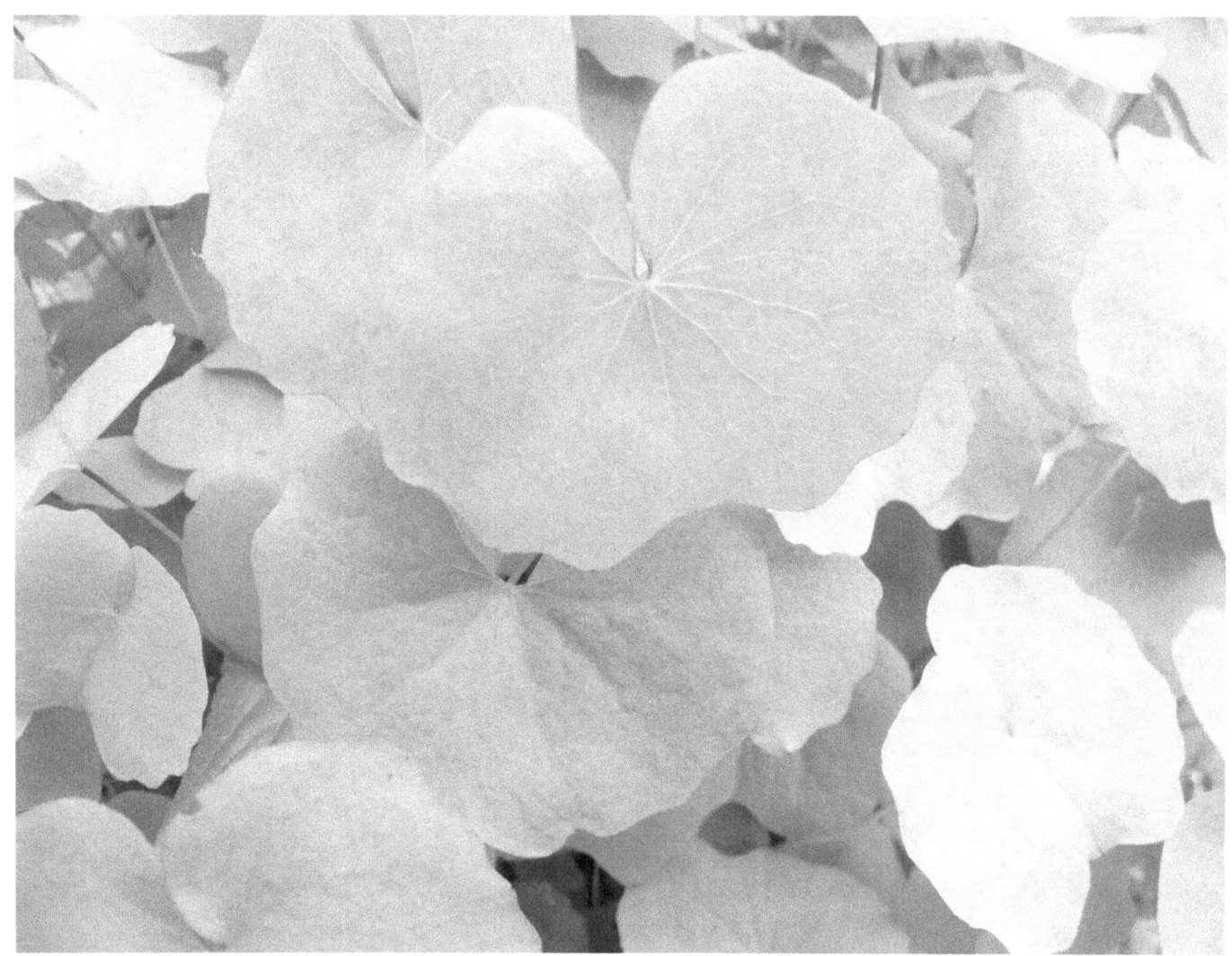

TWINLEAF

Arthur Osol and George Farrar Jr., wrote in the *Dispensatory of the United States of America*: "The root is said to be emetic in large doses, and expectorant in smaller doses and not unlike senega, as a substitute for which it has sometimes been used". Senega refers, of course, *Polygala senega*.

It can be used as a gargle for sore throat, for rheumatic and muscular spasms, to increase urine flow, treat syphilis, cramps, ulcers, and scarlet fever.

The Cherokee used Twinleaf poultices on skin sores, ulcers and other inflamed parts. An infusion was used for dropsy, gravel and other urinary problems.

The Iroquois decocted the whole plant for diarrhea in adults and children. It was considered a useful herb for gall bladder problems.

In China, the related *J. dubia* (*Plagiorhegma dubium*) is valued for its rhizome that contains some of the berberine-like compounds and other bitter constituents common to the barberry family.

In fact the name **HSIEN HUANG LIEN**, by which it is known in Northeast China is interesting. It is sometimes known as **HUANG LIAN**, or **XIAN HUANG LIAN**.

Huang Lian is the common name for Goldthread (*Coptis chinensis* or *C. teetoides*).

Huang means yellow, and refers to the root color. It is prized for its bitter properties.

In past years, twinleaf root was frequently used to adulterate goldenseal root.

The roots show strong anti-feedant activity against a variety of insects. It is worthy of a trial on prairie pests.

MEDICINAL

CONSTITUENTS – root- jatrorrhizine (a tetra-hydro-isoquinolone alkaloid) also known as neprotin, and the lignan glucosides: dehydrodiconiferyl-alcohol-4-beta-D-glucoside, and its isomer dehydroiconiferyl-alcohol-y-beta-D-glucoside; magnoflorine (aporphine alkaloid).

Jethro Kloss considered Twinleaf, "very useful in chronic rheumatism, nervous and spasmodic affections. Very successful in neuralgia, cramps and syphilis. Splendid gargle for throat troubles. Fine in scarlet fever, scarletina (sic), and indolent ulcers. Applied as a poultice, or a hot fomentation wrung out of the strong tea, [it] will relieve pain, anywhere in the body.

It can be used in dropsy, and in various conditions of nervous excitability even during pregnancy. In severe pains, take hot internally. Steep a teaspoonful of root in a cup of boiling water thirty minutes, simmer ten minutes, strain, drink one cupful, and follow with small frequent doses."

Dr. Cook, in his *Physio Medical Dispensatory* of 1869, suggested the plant is suited, "only to sluggish conditions, and states of laxity and enfeebled action. It promotes expectoration in chronic coughs and hepatization; a warm infusion will elevate capillary circulation, increase the secretion of the skin, and promote the menstrual function.

It is much used in depressed forms of chronic rheumatism... and atonic forms of amenorrhea."

He rates it a pungent and bitter stimulant, with relaxing properties. "It acts with moderate promptness upon the mucous membranes; and afterwards influences the stomach, kidneys, circulation, and glandular system more slowly and permanently."

Cook recommended a moderate portion be used with tulip poplar bark and partridge berry (*Mitchella repens*) for uterine pains; a cooled infusion used as a gargle for mild ulcerations of the throat.

He mentions the use in syrups for secondary syphilis, an opinion shared by King, who suggested a combination with equal parts of corydalis.

Twinleaf possesses some very interesting pharmacological compounds.

Arens et al, *Offentl Gesundheitswes* 1984 46(9):475-80 found twinleaf contains various anti-inflammatory compounds.

The compound jatrorrhizine is also found in Goldtread (Coptis), Barberry (Berberis) and Goldenseal (Hydrastis) species. But twinleaf does not contain palmatine, berberine and other related compounds, suggesting an herb with benefit in certain conditions, without the downside, sometimes associated with long-term use of berberine-rich herbs.

It plays a critical role in neuro-protection, albeit a rat study, and may be useful in Alzheimer's disease, due to its high bioavailability. Luo T et al, *CNS Neurol Disord Drug Targets* 2016 July 10.

Earlier work suggests jatrorrhizine provides neuroprotection against cytotoxicity and apoptosis in HT22 hippocampal neuron cells. Jiang W et al, *CNS Neurol Disord Drug Targets* 2015 14(10):1334-42.

The compound lowers blood sugar, cholesterol and triglyceride levels in diabetic mice. Ma H et al, *Drug Dev Res* 2016 77(4):163-70. Magnoflorine, also present in herb, is an alpha glucosidase inhibitor, which limits the amount of starch and sugar broken down in small intestine, thereby reducing insulin need and response. Xiong Y et al, *J Chromatogr B Analyt Technol Biomed Life Sci* 2016 1022:75-80.

Magnoflorine exerts anti-adipogenic activity by down-regulating proliferator activated receptor gamma (PPAR-y), suggestive of benefit in treating obesity. Choi JS et al, *Fitoterapia* 2014 98:199-208.

I believe this is a great choice for syndrome X scenarios, with high blood pressure, blood sugar, and total cholesterol, associated with obesity and pre-diabetic symptoms.

Magnoflorine possesses sedative and anxiolytic effects, probably via GABAergic mechanisms. De la Pena JB et al, *J Nat Med* 2013 67(4):814-21.

Magnoflorine, also found in magnolia leaves, is cytotoxic to HEPG2 (liver) and U251 (brain) cancer cell lines, and more potent than doxorubicin against the former. Mohamed SM et al, *Nat Prod Res* 2010 24(15):1395-402.

Work by Wu H et al, *Phytomedicine* 2014 21(11):1373-81 suggests jatrorrhizine is a safe anti-hypercholesterolemic compound. The LD_{50} in mice is more than 5500 mg/kg in a three-month trial. It appears to improve utilization and excretion of cholesterol by up-regulating the mRNA and protein expression of LDLR (low density lipoprotein receptor) and CYP7A1. It also slowed the rate of weight gain.

It helps protect liver cells and may be useful in treating jaundice. Wang S et al, *J Sep Sci* 2016 39(19): 3690-99.

Jatrorrhizine inhibited colon cancer cell line SW480, showing complete reduction in vitro. Singh S et al, *Pharm Biol* 2016 54(4):740-5.

It shows activity against KB (human oral squamous carcinoma) and CHOK-1 (hamster ovary) cells lines. Bala M et al, *J Ethnopharm* 2015 175:131-7.

It also reversed multidrug resistance for vincristine on KBv200 cell lines. Zhang H et al, *Zhong Yao Cai* 2001 24(9): 655-7.

Both jatrorrhizine and magnoflorine demonstrate cardioprotective benefit. Tan HL et al, *Front Pharmacol* 2016 7:362.

Specific indications are a pain in the head with dizziness and the sensation of tension.

Early studies by Hale suggested there was no plant as efficacious as Goldenseal for sore eyes, except perhaps *Jeffersonia*.

The herb suppresses LPS-induced nitric oxide production. Kim JM et al, *Arch Pharm Research* 2010 33(8):1149-57; suggesting anti-oxidant activity.

RECIPES

COLD INFUSION- 2-6 ounces three times daily. Use one part root to twenty parts of water and let sit overnight. In morning gently bring up to a simmer and remove from heat.

TINCTURE- 10-30 drops up to three times daily. The fresh root is tinctured at 75% alcohol, at 1:4 ratio. The dried root is also effective at 40% alcohol and 1:5 ratio.

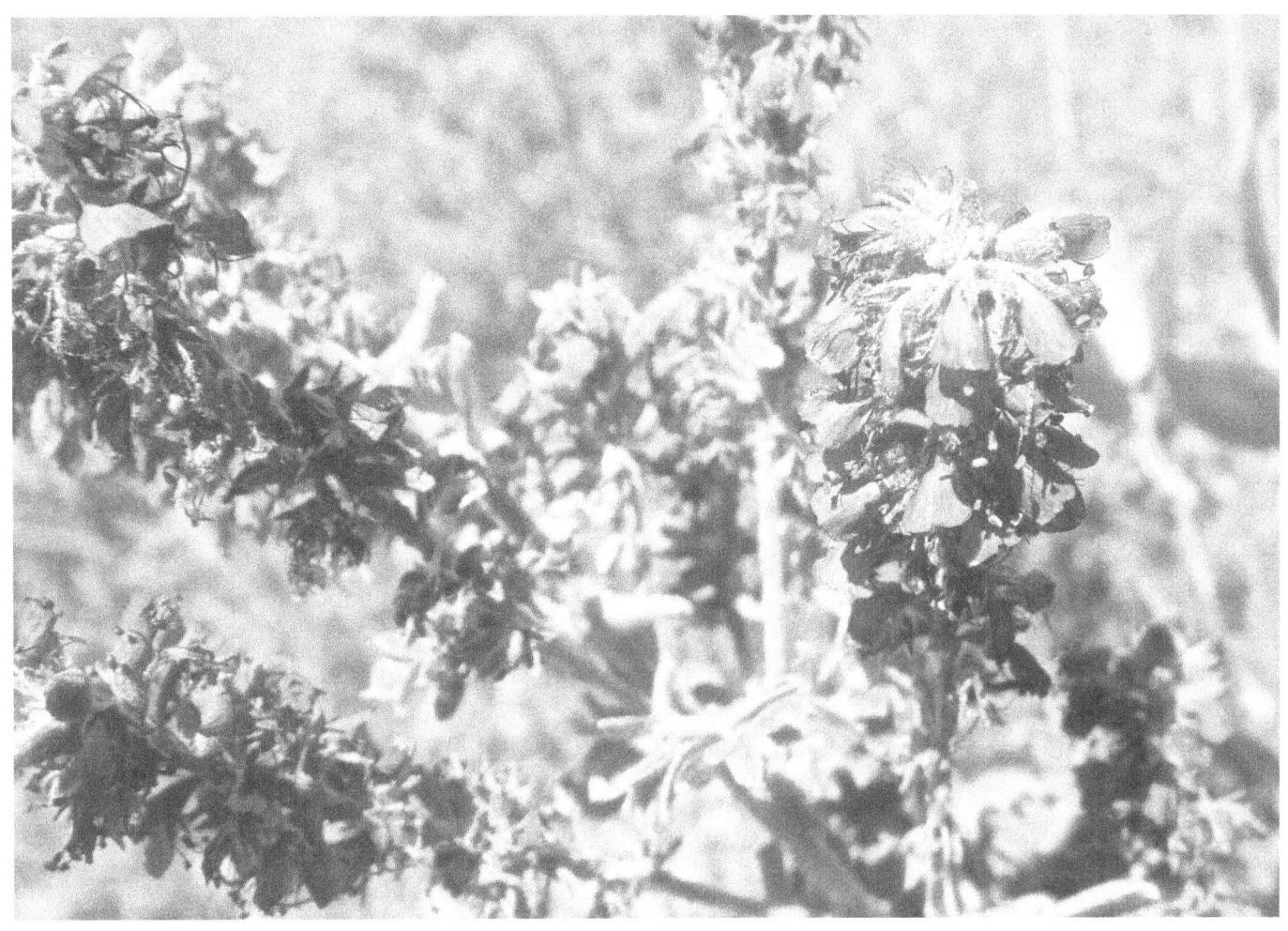

AMORPHA FRUTICOSA

AMORPHA
FALSE INDIGO
(*Amorpha fruticosa* L.)
LEADPLANT
PRAIRIE SHOESTRING
(*A. canescens* Pursh)
DWARF FALSE INDIGO
(*A. nana* Nutt.)
PARTS USED- flower, root, bark, fruit

The Amorpha in full bloom was remarkable for its large and luxuriant purple clusters.

JOHN FREMONT 1842

Amorpha is from the Greek *AMORPHOS* meaning deformed, formless or shapeless, and refers to the absence of four of the five petals.

Amorpha from the Latin and Greek refers to an elongated, bulbous shaped earthenware vessel with two handles and a pointed or flat bottom. These were used for storing wine or olive oil.

Amphoteric is a term used in herbal medicine to indicate bi-directional activity associated with normalizing function. For example, the same herb can increase or decrease blood pressure in two different individuals.

Canescens means, becoming gray. False Indigo refers to its use as an indigo substitute, and Leadplant due to its presence indicating lead deposits in the soil beneath its roots, or its gray, leaden, dead looking leaves.

Prairie Shoestring refers to the long, stringy roots, that when plowed, pop up like a shoestring snapping. Nana means, "dwarf".

False Indigo is a small shrub or bush that seems to be slowly moving north and west on the Canadian prairies. I'm glad.

It's beautiful purple and yellow flowers are distinct. The shrub is fume, drought, and saline resistant, and yet not carried by many nurseries. This is probably due to its sprawling nature and weak stems. I have photographed its beautiful flowers in Manitoba, Saskatchewan, Idaho and down into northern Colorado. It is considered a non-native invasive in Washington state, but native from New Jersey to Minnesota and Wyoming, and south to Florida, Texas and into Mexico. The plant is a nitrogen-fixer, and able to tolerate nutrient poor and saline soil. It does contain indigo pigment, but in amounts too small for commercial use.

It is a nectar plant for butterflies, releasing a vanilla scented perfume.

Leadplant is a small shrub with grey leaves, and blue to violet flowers.

It is restricted in Canada, to south-central Manitoba, and is usually considered indicative of a well-managed natural pasture, or native prairie.

Leadplant was known to the Omaha-Ponca as **TE-HUNTONHI,** "buffalo bellow plant", as the blooming of the plant was synchronous with the rutting season of buffalo. The plant has pleasant-scented lavender flowers in summer. This plant was considered female, and the round-headed *Lespedeza capitata* was called "male buffalo bellow plant".

The Lakota call it bird's wood or tree, **ZITKA'TACAN'**, because, well, where else do birds perch on the open prairie?

The small, end stems were used by First Nation peoples for moxibustion, to treat neuralgia and rheumatism. The pieces of stem were attached to the skin by moistening one end with the tongue. They were then allowed to burn down to the skin. The leaves were made into a pleasant yellow-brown hot tea.

The leaves were mixed with buffalo fat and sometimes used as smoking material. The powdered leaves were blown into wounds and cuts, the astringency helping promote granulation.

The Mesquakie used leaf infusions to kill pinworms and other intestinal parasites. The infusion was also applied externally to skin eczemas. The Ojibwa used root decoctions for analgesic effect in stomach pains.

Both the Mesquakie and Potawatomi had very similar names for the plant, meaning "something to wipe the buttocks."

Both the Sioux and Assiniboine pounded the roots with Bee Plant (*Cleome species*) to attract buffalo. The mixture was rubbed on clothing and had the power to both attract and kill buffalo as the hunter desired.

Amorphigenin, derived from seeds of False Indigo, inhibits the mitochondrial complex of mosquitoes, in a manner similar to rotenone. Ji M et al, *Int J Mol Sci* 2015 16(8):19713-27. The crushed seeds are decocted and resultant water, with small addition of liquid soap is poured on top of the waters, home to the larvae. The seeds of shepherd's purse are a potent addition.

Dwarf Indigo bush (*A. nana*) was traditionally dried and powdered as a snuff for catarrh.

False Indigo has been studied for phyto-remediation of lead, zinc and copper mine tailings. Work by Shi X et al, *Int J Phytoremediation* 2016 18(11): 1155-63 found the plant had the highest tolerance and biomass production, of plants tested.

MEDICINAL

CONSTITUENTS – *A. fruticosa*- bark- three prenyl-flavanones, amooranin, amoradin, amoradicin, amoratin and amoradinin root bark-prenylated chromeno-flavonones including amoricin, isoamoricin, amoridon, isoamoridin, amorin, and isoamorin, amoradicin, amorisin, isoamoritin, and rotenoids amorphigeni, dalbinol and 6-ketodehydroamorphigenin.
leaves- polyphenols (780 mg/g dry extract); flavonoids (32 mg/g dry extract), amorphispironone, tephrosin, 11-hydroxytephrosin, deguelin, amorphigenin; isoflavone afrormosin, dalpanol, 12a-hydroxyamorphigenin, 12a-hdyroxydalpanol, 12a-betahydroxy-amorphigenin; 6'-O-D-glucopyranosyldalpanol (6-ODGPSP); 8-methyl-retusin; amorphastilbol (a phenolic stilbene terpenoid); 9-demethyl-munduserine; 5,7-dihydroxy-6-geranylflavanone.
seed- hydroxycinnamic derivatives (153 mg/g dry extract) fruticine (rotenone) and a flavanone with as isoprenoid C10 side chain; frutitsin, amorphigenin, dihydro-, dalpanol, amorhigenol, dalbinol, 11-hydroxy tephrosin, amorfrutin A and B; 5,7-dihydroxy-8-geranylflavanone; amorphaside A-D.
fruit- amorfrutin A (0.54-3.52%), B (0.64-4.63%) & D, rotenoids, 7, 2', 4', 5'-tetramethoxyisoflavone, tephrosin, the rotenoids 6-hydroxy-6a,12a-dehydro-alpha-toxicarol; 3-O-demethylamorphigenin; dehydro-degnellin, 11-hydroxy-tephrosin, dehydrosermundone, 6a,12a-dehydroamorphin; 6'-O-beta-D:-glucopyranosyl-12a-hydroxydalpanol, amorphispironones B & C,
A. canescens- pinitol

Both False Indigo and Leadplant are useful internally and externally for skin cancer, eczema, cuts and wounds. Qu X et al, *Afr J Trad Complement Altern Med* 2013 10(3) foun d several compounds in fresh fruit pulp enhanced fibroblasts proliferation, leading to promotion of wound healing.

Japanese studies reveal amorphispironone and tephrosin, in leaves, are inhibitors of Epstein-Barr virus early antigen activation; and show inhibitory effect in two stage carcinogenesis tests on mouse skin tumors. Konoshima T et al, *J Nat Prod* 1993 56(6):843-8.

Amorphispironone is a spirorotenoid that is extremely rare in nature.

The same year, at the University of North Carolina, studies were conducted with rotenoid, 12a beta-hydroxyamphigenin. This compound proved to be highly toxic against neo-plastic cell lines; and 6-ODGPSP showed activity against 5 human cancer cell lines. Li et al, *Journal of Natural Products* 56:5.

Work by Wang et al, *Fitoterapia* 2015 100:75-80 showed isoflavones from *A. fruticosa* to be cytotoxic. Selective toxicity against human breast cancer MCF-7 cells lines was noted in work, with two compounds more toxic than cisplatin.

Amorphigenin and afrormosin exhibit strong anti-proliferative activity in MDA-MB-231 breast cancer cell lines, and the latter compound showed additive effect with epirubicin against drug resistant cancer cells. Gyemant N et al, *In Vivo* 2005 19(2): 367-74.

The flavonoid amoradicin has been found to inhibit tumour necrosis factor, or TNF, in lipo-polysaccharide stimulated RAW264.7 cells. The IC 50 value is 28.5 microM, compared to genistein at 24.9 and silybin from milk thistle seed at 140.3 microM. Cho JY et al, *Journal of Ethnopharmacology* 2000 70(2): 127-33.

Amorpha rotenoids and isoflavonoids from the fruit showed inhibition of rat heart phosphodiesterase. Petkov et al, *Planta Medica* 1983 47:4.

This has led to the development of the drug glirofam, approved as an agent for the treatment of atherosclerosis.

Tephrosin, 11-hydroxytephrosin and dequelin, derived from leaves, inhibit NFkappaB activation, with extremely low IC$_{50}$ of 0.1-0.22 mM. Dat et al, *J Nat Prod* 2008 71:10.

Deguelin potentiates apoptosis activity of an EGFR tyrosine kinase inhibitor on head and neck squamous cell carcinoma. Normally EGFR (epidermal growth factor receptor) inhibitors have poor clinical outcome. Baba Y et al, *Int J Mol Sci* 2017 18(2).

The compound suppresses the hedgehog signaling pathway, as well as matrix metalloproteinases 2 and 9 in two pancreatic cancer cell lines. Zheng W et al, *Oncol Lett* 2016 12(4): 2761-65. It induces apoptosis of lung squamous cancer cells by regulating the expression of galectin-1. Yan B et al, *Int J Biol Sci* 2016 12(7):850-60. Deguelin also shows selective activity against MDA-MB-453 and SUM-185PE, suggesting benefit in triple negative breast cancers. Robles AJ et al, *Breast Cancer Res Treat* 2016 157(3): 475-88.

Animal studies suggest it may have benefit in treating B-cell lymphocytic leukemia, which has poor prognosis and outcomes at present. Rebolleda N et al, *PLoS One* 2016 11(4):e0154159. It may inhibit a mutant form of nucleophosmin, which is present in up to one third of patient with acute myeloid leukemia. Yi S et al, *Ann Hematol* 2015 94(2):201-10.

Deguelin, along with berberine, pterostibene, andrographolide and resveratrol, may be potent compounds for oral cancer treatment, with minimal side effects compared to synthetic drugs. Bundela S et al, *PLoS One* 2015 10(11):e0141719.

Low dose deguelin suppressed invasion and migration of oral cancer by down-regulating TNF-alpha induced NF-kappaB signaling. Liu YP et al, *Head Neck* 2016 38 (Suppl 1).

Deguelin has been shown to inhibit ocular neovascularization in several disease models.

This may be useful as ocular angiogenesis underlies retinopathy of premature babies, diabetic retinopathy, and macular degeneration in adults. Sulaiman RS et al, *Exp Eye Research* 2014 129:161-71.

It may be a useful adjunct with cisplatin in the treatment of gastric cancer. Li Z et al, *Oncol Lett* 2014 8(4): 1603-7.

It inhibits surviving, suggesting synergy and increased efficacy with doxetaxel and vinblastine. By using lower doses of chemotherapy, less side effects and damage to normal tissue could be realized. Ghanbari P et al, *Appl Biochem Biotechnol* 2014 174(2): 667-81.

Deguelin selectively induced apoptosis of Raji cells associated with Burkitt's lymphoma. The anti-tumor effects are due to down regulation of cyclin D1, P21 and pRb proteins. Xiong JR et al, *J Huazhong Univ Sci Technol Med Sci* 2013 22(4): 491-5.

Amorfrutin A and B, from the fruit and seed are both anti-microbial. Mitscher et al *Phytochemistry* 1981 20:4. Amorfrutin A potentiates TNFalpha induced apoptosis, and reduces inflammation of major inflammatory cytokines. Shi H et al, *Int Immunopharmacol* 2014 21(1): 56-62.

Isoflavones from False Indigo protected the liver from damage caused by acetominophen in work by Diao et al, *Chin Chem Letters* 2009 20:8.

Afrormosin, from the leaves, is anti-oxidant and anti-inflammatory, and is a potent inhibitor of the protein kinase C activity. De Araujo Lopes A et al, *Basic Clinic Pharmacol Toxicol* 2013 113(6):363-9.

Amorfrutins have been found to reduce blood sugar and inflammation, as well as prevent fatty liver. Sascha Sauer at the Max Planck Institute for Molecular Genetics in Berlin found amorfrutin molecules dock directly onto receptors in cells called peroxisome proliferator-activated receptor gamma, or PPARy. These compounds are also found in licorice root (*G. foetida*). *Proc Natl Acad Sci U S A.* 2012 109(19):7257-62.

Amorfrutins significantly reduce inflammatory disorders, such as chronic bowel conditions. Fuhr L et al, *Journal Nat Products* 2015 78(5):1160-4.

Recent work isolated 5,7-dihydroxy-6-geranylflavanone, a PPARalpha/gamma dual agonist that improves insulin sensitivity and lipid metabolism. Lee W et al, *Int J Mol Med* 2016 37(5):1397-1404.

Amorfrutin B is a selective PPARgamma modulator. Lavecchia A et al, *Expert Opin Ther Pat* 2015 25(11):1341-7. Some in vivo studies suggest amorfrutin B and amorphastilbol improve metabolic patterns in diabetic animals, with reduced side effects in comparison to full thiazolidinedione agonist drugs. Wang L et al, *Biochem Pharmacol* 2014 92(1):73-89. One study with insulin-resistant mice, found amorfrutin B improved insulin sensitivity,

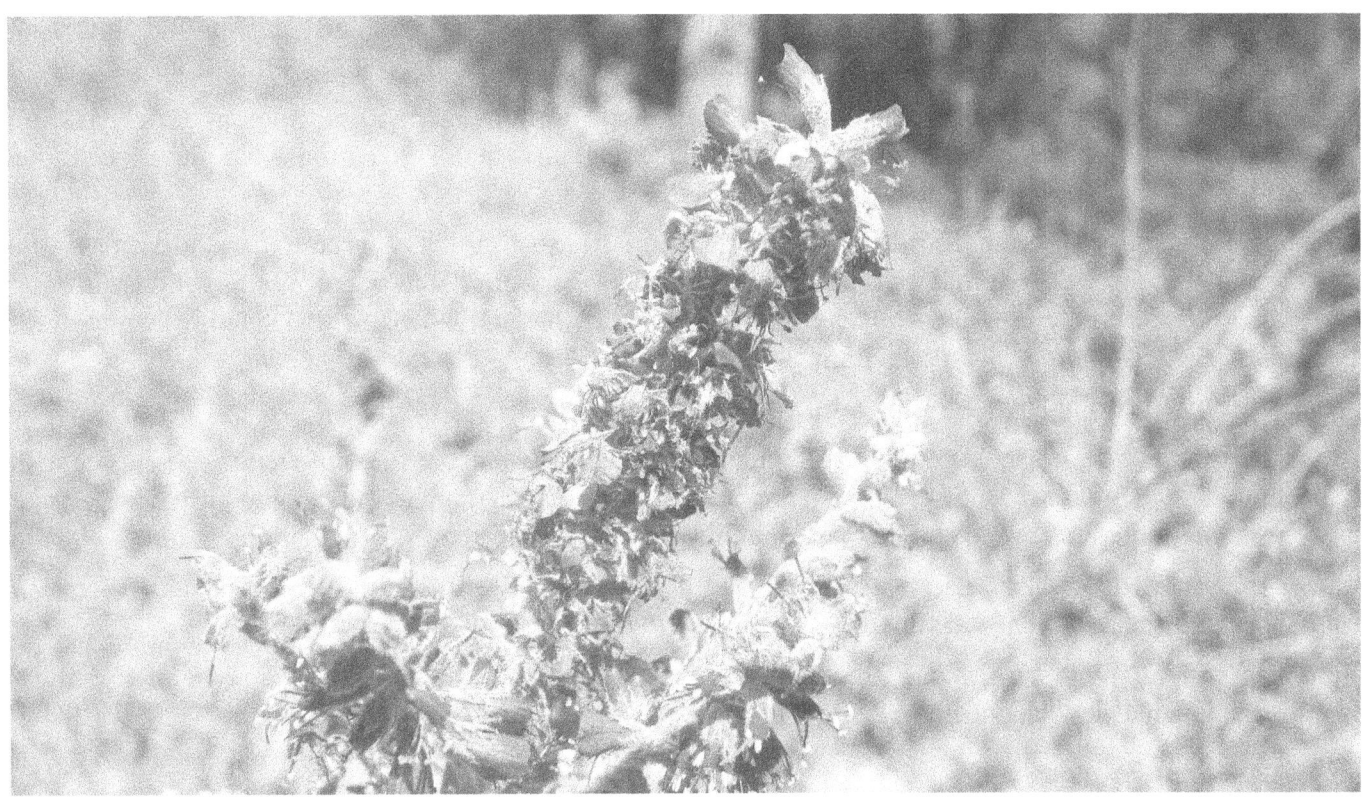

FALSE INDIGO

glucose tolerance and blood lipid variables within a few days, but did not induce weight gain and showed liver protecting properties. It also had not adverse effect on osteoblastogeneis and fluid retention. Weidner C et al, *Diabetologia* 2013 56(8).

Amorphastilbol and herb extracts show benefit in glucose and lipid metabolism in studies by Lee W et al, *Int J Mol Med* 2015 36(2):527-33. Both the compound and herb improve insulin sensitivity through inhibition of protein tyrosine phosphatase 1B.

Amorphigenin, from seed, inhibits proliferation and induces apoptosis in A549/DDP cancer cell lines. It is synergistic with cisplatin in drug-resistant human lung adenocarcinoma, by down-regulating expression of lung resistance protein. Zhong H et al, *Zhongguo Fei Ai Za Zhi* 2016 19(12):805-12.

The compound synergistically enhanced epirubicin on multi-drug resistant cancer cell lines. Gyémánt N et al, *In Vivo* 2005 19(2):367-74.

In fact, amorphigenin, chrysin, epigallocatechin, formononetin and rotenone may be useful for inhibition of P-gp (as anti-multidrug resistance agents), via the NBD2 blocking mechanism. Wongrattanakamon et al, *Toxicol Mech Methods* 2016 Dec 20:1-38.

Lee HJ et al, *Cytotechnology* 2006 52(3)219-26 found fruit extracts increased cell growth of human T cells by 15%.

Frutitsin, isolated from the seed of *A. fruticosa* is recommended in the former USSR as a sedative in vegetative neuroses, neuroses of the cardiovascular system and paroxysmal tachycardia.

The seeds inhibit acetylcholinesterase activity, suggestive of use in neurodegenerative disorders. Zheleva-Dimitrova DZh, *Pharmacogn Mag* 2013 9(34):109-13.

Fruticine, from the seed, exhibits anti-tachycardia activity.

Fruticine (rotenone) is an insecticidal agent with accumulative toxicity to humans, as is 9-demethyl munduserine. It is a sedative compound.

The seed, fruit and leaf all contain compounds that inhibit NFkappaB, related to immune function and prevention of cancer and tumor formation. Dat et al, *J Nat Prod* 2008 71:10.

The fruit contains a number of compounds with moderate activity against gram positive bacteria, and amorphispironone B, that exhibits significant cytotoxicity against the L5178Y mouse lymphoma cell line. Muharini R bet al, *J Nat Prod* 2017 80(1):169-80.

The roots contain flavanones and rotenoids including amorisin 2 that inhibits neuraminidase thirty fold more potent than quercitin. Neuraminidase is implication in biofilm formation and is a proven target for anti-viral and anti-bacterial activity. Work by Kim YS et al, *Food Chem Toxicol* 2011 49(8):1849-56 identified compounds that inhibit *Pseudomonas aeruginosa* biofilm.

A decoction of the root helps clear pinworms and other minor intestinal parasites.

Amorphastilbol is a cannabinoid compound found in *A. fruiticosa*, *A. nana* and *A. canescens*. When tested with Fast Blue B salt, often used to quick test for cannabinoids in marijuana, it gives the same reddish orange color and chromatograph. A smart defense lawyer could make use of this in a courtroom demonstration.

This is the first case of stilbene derivatives in a legume; and the first indication of a possible link between cannabinoids and other plant constituents.

Lead plant contains pinitol, which has shown some promise in insulin production. This compound is also found in stressed pine needles, legume herbage and other plants.

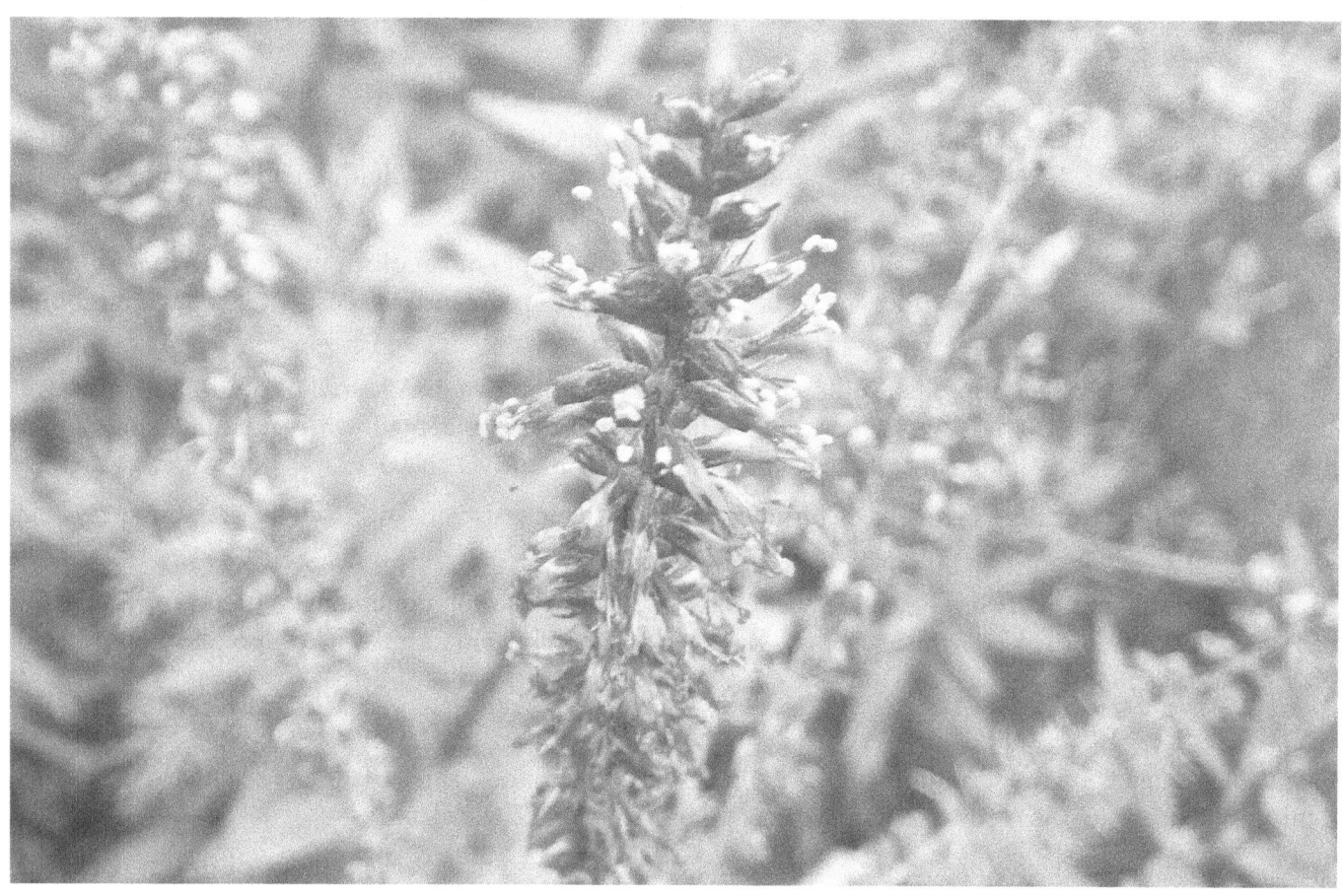

LEAD PLANT (*A. canescens*)

Lead Plant (*A. canescens*) leaves and flowers, and seed from *A. fruticosa* exhibit activity against *Staphylococcus aureus*. Borchardt et al, *J Med Plants Research* 2008 2:4-5. The seeds possess significant anti-oxidant activity, nearly 10 times blueberries.

ESSENTIAL OIL

CONSTITUENTS – *A. fruticosa* fruit- gamma amorphene and gamma-muurolene have been identified.
leaf- cadinene, and amorphene, a sesquiterpene.
The essential oil is very effective against a variety of plant pests and fungi.
The fruit yields from 0.15-0.35% essential oil, from either fresh or dried; while the leaf gives 0.05-0.08% of light yellow oil with a slight bitter taste.
A. canescens- fruit- germacrene D (43%), germacrene D-4-ol (8.3%)
Flowers- beta-elemol (29.4%), germacrene D (14.6%)
Leaf- germacrene D (30%), germacrene D-4-ol (11%), beta-elemol (10%)

Amorpha leaf oil has an unusual scent, sort of a lemon/cumin cross, that lends itself to unusual perfume possibilities.

Work at the Oklahoma Agricultural Experiment Station looked at the insecticidal properties of *Amorpha* oil.

Tests on 29 species of insects and mites showed amorpha was repellent to house flies and horn flies for more than 12 hours when sprayed on cattle. Other insects including chinch bugs, cotton aphids, pea aphids, chrysanthemum aphids and spotted cucumber beetles are very susceptible to the plant extracts and oils.

Honey from *A. fruticosa* shows radical scavenging activity and contains from 38-58% of 2 phenyl ethanol in volatiles.

FLOWER ESSENCES

Indigo Bush (*A. fruticosa*) helps anchor one's spiritually achieved ideas into daily life. It warms the heart, and brings the light of clear seeing or inner sight to an area that needs it.   **DESERT**

False Indigo (*A. fruticosa*) flower essence is associated with the concept and understanding of inner health. To often, there is a lack of understanding the concept of "the human terrain"; and that a virus, bacteria, or other microbe cannot infiltrate a strong defense system. This flower essence works, not only on the psychological aspects of this concept, but actually, on a physical level, exerting immune stimulation and modulation.
PRAIRIE DEVA

RECIPES

LEAF INFUSION- One heaping ounce of dried leaf to one quartt of water. Let steep ten minutes. One half cup as needed.

TINCTURE- 10-20 drops three times daily, as needed. Aerial or root tincture is made fresh at ratio of 1:4 and 60% alcohol. Crushed, dried seed tincture is prepared the same.

Do not combine with fireweed. Do not use during pregnancy or lactation.

FRUTITSIN- Chloroform and ethanol extract in the ratios of 1:1 and 2:1. After three changes of solvent, about 95% of the frutitsin in the raw material has passed into the extract. Greater detail for those interested can be obtained from work conducted by Khodzhaev et al, *Journal of Natural Compounds* 1983.

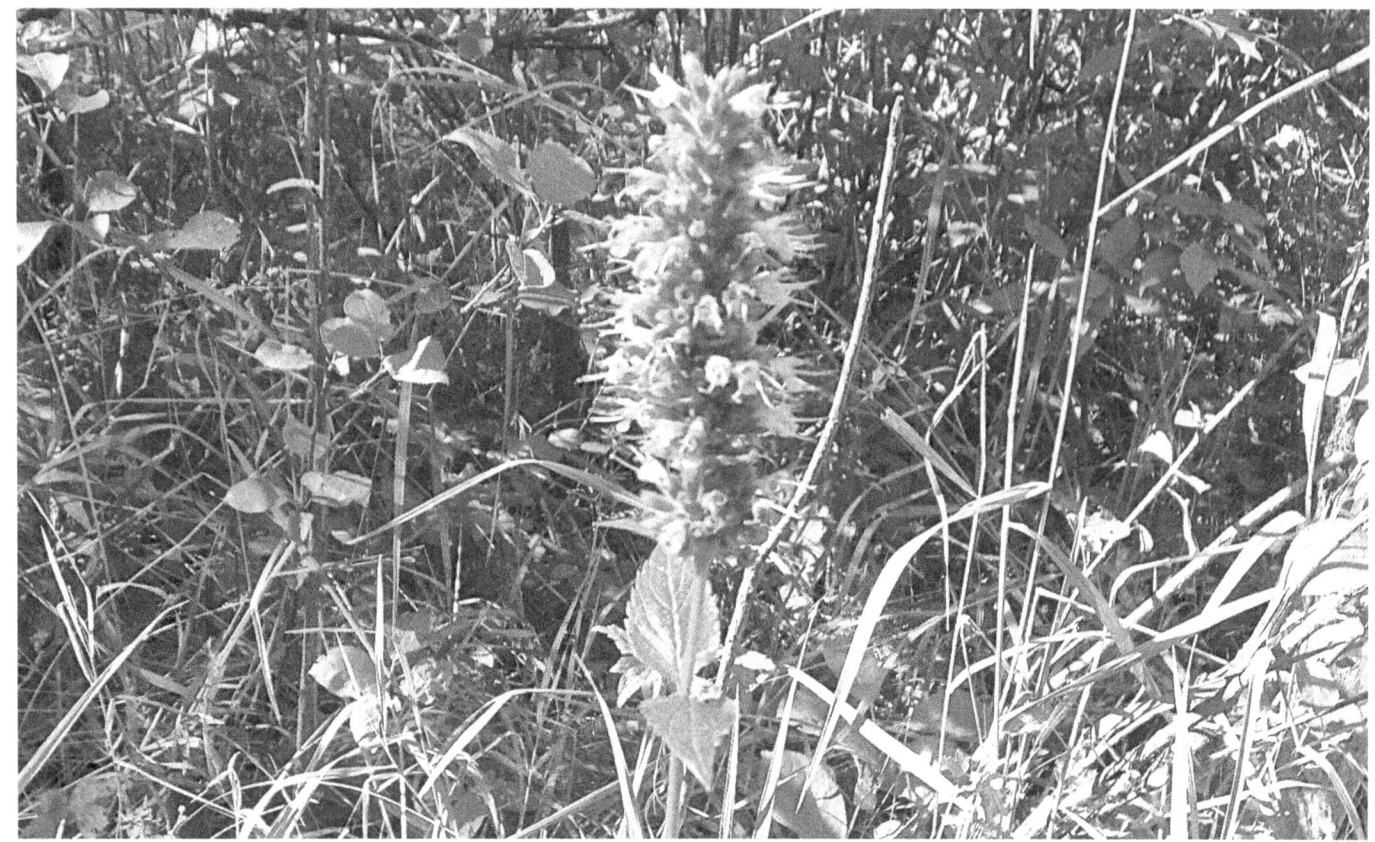

GIANT ANISE HYSSOP

GIANT ANISE HYSSOP
LAVENDER HYSSOP
(***Agastache foeniculum*** [Pursh] Kuntze)
NETTLE LEAVED GIANT HYSSOP
HORSEMINT
HORSE NETTLE
MOUNTAIN MINT
(***A. urticifolia*** [Benth.] Kuntze)
PART USED–leaf, flower

Agastache comes from the Greek *AGAN* meaning, very much, and *STACHYS* a spike or ear of wheat; alluding to the appearance of numerous tiny blossoms of the flower.

Foeniculum is from the Latin **FENUM**, or hay, and alluding to the finely divided leaves.

Urticifolia means leaves like nettle, due to their shape.

Anise Hyssop does not resemble anise in looks, growing up to a metre tall, with bluish to lilac flowers, and felt like hairs on the lighter colored under leaf. Anise comes from the smell and taste of the leaves, hyssop from the square stems of the mint family.

Giant Anise hyssop is a common perennial to the moist meadows and aspen parkland of the prairie. It's pleasant licorice-mint scent is obvious by brushing the plant.

It is plentiful in the ravine near my home, so picking enough for winter tea is not a problem.

Nettle Leaved Giant Hyssop is found in the foothills and sub-alpine montane regions of Alberta, Montana, British Columbia and southward to the Great Basin and beyond. The flowers are rose to purplish, the leaves green on both sides, with no hairs.

Mosquitoes however, do not appreciate the smell, so it can be used as a natural repellent. Bees love it, however, and it is cultivated as a honey plant in the United States. Some tests by Kublick, published in 1990 found they even prefer it to white clover. Butterflies also love the plant.

The Cree traditionally use Giant Anise Hyssop or **KA-WIKIPAKAHK** to improve and sweeten the flavor of store bought tea; and medicinally for those coughing up blood, or in combination for stomach aches. The flower heads are chewed as a breath freshener.

The flowers were often included in Cree medicine bundles.

Other native tribes used the plant to induce sweat in steam baths.

The Chippewa tribe used root infusions for colds, chest pain and coughs. It is known as It Sticks Up, or **BE'DUKADAK'IGISIN**.

For burns, they would moisten the dried powdered leaves, along with Echinacea and Goldenrod, and apply to the affected area. It was worn as a protective charm.

The Lakota name is **WAHPE' YATA'PI**, or leaf that is chewed.

The Cheyenne drank the cooled tea for chest pains or when lungs were sore from coughing. They call it Elk Mint or perfume, **MO?EHE-MOXESHENE**. It is one of ten plants of a special perfume made with the castor gland from beaver. One member of the Montana Cheyenne said it was taken for dispirited heart.

Related species were used by the Navaho for protection from witchcraft.

Nettle-leaved Giant Hyssop was used by Paiute as a cold-water infusion to treat indigestion and intestinal pain, and for colds. As a poultice, the fresh leaves were applied to swellings.

Other native healers placed the leaves in baby's blankets to reduce fevers.

Related species from China and Japan are used for their stomachic and carminative properties. Anti-tumor and cytotoxic activity has been reported. The leaf is used for chest congestion, headache, nausea, and spleen inflammations. The stem and leaf are used together in decoction for angina pains.

Giant Anise Hyssop leaves are used as a poultice for sore hands and feet.

The dried plant is particularly suitable for spicing chicken, fish and lamb; and the flowers are one of the tastiest edible flowers. Add the chopped flower to dough for shortbread, add to fruit dishes like raspberry, strawberry, blackberry, apricot, peach and plums.

The seeds, or nutlets, can be eaten raw or cooked into a gruel.

Dried in the shade, giant anise hyssop retains its aroma for 8-10 months similar to other herbs. They are a lovely addition of color and scent in potpourri.

Nettle leaved Giant Hyssop can be used in a similar manner.

Anise Hyssop, when grown commercially, needs revitalization of roots after about three years, including root division. Research in Brooks found dry plant yields of 5252 kilograms per hectare. Fresh plant yields of 10-20,000 kg/ha are usual.

The related Mosquito Plant (*A. cana*) is a rare perennial with a fragrance similar to bubble gum. It is easily propagated from seed, or cuttings, and helps attract hummingbirds. Mosquito Plant is said to repel mosquitoes by rubbing the leaves on skin or clothing.

MEDICINAL

CONSTITUENTS – *A. foeniculum*-methyl chavicol (estragole), anisaldehyde, methone, mycrene, pulegone, limonene, alpha & beta-pinene (essential oils), z-ocimene, acacetin (5,7-dihydroxy-4'-methoxyflavone), cosmosiin, cynaroside, 4-cadenen-ol, apigenin 1.62 mg/g, quercetin 1.97 mg/g, hydroxycinnamic acid; alpha and beta amyrin, campesterol, campestanol, sitosterol, stigmasterol, stigmastanol, various carotenoids including lutein, zeaxanthin, violaxanthin and antheraxanthin.
A. urticifolia- germacrene, isomethone, limonene, menthone, mycrene, cis-ocimene, trans-ocimene, 3-octanol, 1-octen-3-ol, alpha pinene, beta pinene, pulgeone.

Giant anise hyssop is similar in action to other mints; having diaphoretic action like field mint and wild bergamot.

It is used to dispel hot and damp conditions that give oppressed feelings in the chest, abdominal pains, vomiting and diarrhea. An herbal syrup made from fresh Giant Anise Hyssop can be very soothing.

It relieves fevers, chills and the nausea that accompanies the flu. Anise Hyssop makes a good mouthwash and gargle; and a footbath for athlete's foot.

The plant remedies various arthritic conditions that are exaggerated by damp and cold weather. A cool fomentation relieves headaches and fevers.

It would be fair to generalize that giant anise hyssop is a cardiovascular tonic.

Giant Anise Hyssop contains acacetin that targets COX, inhibits histamine release and is anti-inflammatory. It is a multi-drug resistance transporter, and aldose reductase inhibitor, suggesting use in eye health related to diabetes.

Experiments have shown the plant to stimulate gastric secretion, increase digestion and relax blood capillaries. It shows strong anti-fungal effect, in various studies.

Acacetin inhibits the activity of Sortase A, suggesting benefit in the treatment of multi-drug resistant *Staphylococcus aureus*. Bi C et al, *Molecules* 2016 21(10).

Acacetin has been found to relieve anxiety-like effects in mice. Avila-Villarreal GM et al, *Planta Med* 2016 81 (S01):S1-381.

Acacetin is a potent inhibitor of human MAO A and B, more to the latter. This suggests benefit in various neurological and psychological disorders. Chaurasiya ND et al *J Nat Prod* 2016 79(10).

Acacetin is antispasmodic and helps relieve abdominal pain, via various pathways. The compound is a vaso-relaxant, helping reduce hypertension. In Mexican herbal medicine, the related *A. mexicana* is used to lower blood pressure. Flores-Flores A et al, *Pharm Biol* 2016 54(12):2807-13.

Acacetin enhances the differentiation and proliferation of osteoblasts. Li J et al, *Evid Based Comple Altern Med* 2016: 2587201. This suggest use in osteoporosis conditions.

Intravenous injection of water-soluble acacetin inhibits cardiomyocytes apoptosis and prevent ischemia/reperfusion injury. Liu H et al, *Sci Rep* 2016 6:36435. Acacetin is normally soluble in alcohol, suggesting a tincture is best.

Acacetin induces apoptosis and cytoprotective autophagy in human acute leukemia Jurkat T cells, simultaneously. Lee JY et al, *J Microbiol Biotechnol* 2016 Nov 4.

Acacetin accumulates and kills chronic lymphocytic leukemia B-lymphocytes in a selective manner. Salimi A et al, *Nutr Cancer* 2016 68(8).

Other studies suggest acacetin induces apoptosis in oral squamous cell carcinoma, breast cancer MCF-7 cells, human gastric carcinoma and human prostate cancer cell lines. Kim CD et al, *Arch Oral Biol* 2015 60(9);

Shim HY et al, *Mol Cells* 2007 24(1); Pan MH et al, *J Agric Food Chem* 2005 53(3); and Kim HR et al, *Int J Mol Med* 2014 33(2).

Cosmosiin (apigetrin) may be useful in lowering blood sugar levels. Nguyen Vo TH et al, *Springerplus* 2016 5(1):1359. The flavone glycoside shows weaker, but similar effects as insulin on adiponectin secretion. Rao YK et al, *Evid Based Complement Altern Med* 2011 24375.

Apigetrin may induce cancer cell differentiation on K562 chronic leukemia cells. Tsoimon S et al, *Mol Nutr Food Res* 2011 55 (Suppl 1):93-102.

The compound, also known as apigenin 7-glucoside, exhibits anxiety relief similar to diazepam. Kumar D et al, *Phytomedicine* 2014 21(7):1010-4.

It may also inhibit neuro-inflammation and protect against neuronal injury. Lim HS et al, *J Med Food* 2016 19(11):1032-40. It may help increase melanin production and have possibly application in natural tanning products, or treatment of vitiligo.

Nettle leaved Giant Hyssop, or Mountain Mint as it is sometimes called, has an odor reminiscent of turpentine, honey and skunk.

Brian Weissbuch, in the November 1994 *Herbalist*, had this to say:

"*Agastache (urticifolia)* is the finest herb in the treatment of stomach flu, a common insult of warm spring days. It allays nausea, improves appetite and digestion, stops vomiting and diarrhea, and relieves the surface to expel the pathogen, along with attendant fever, chills and headache. It counters fatigue and is effective for chronic nausea, lethargy, flatulence, fatigue after meals, and sticky stools.

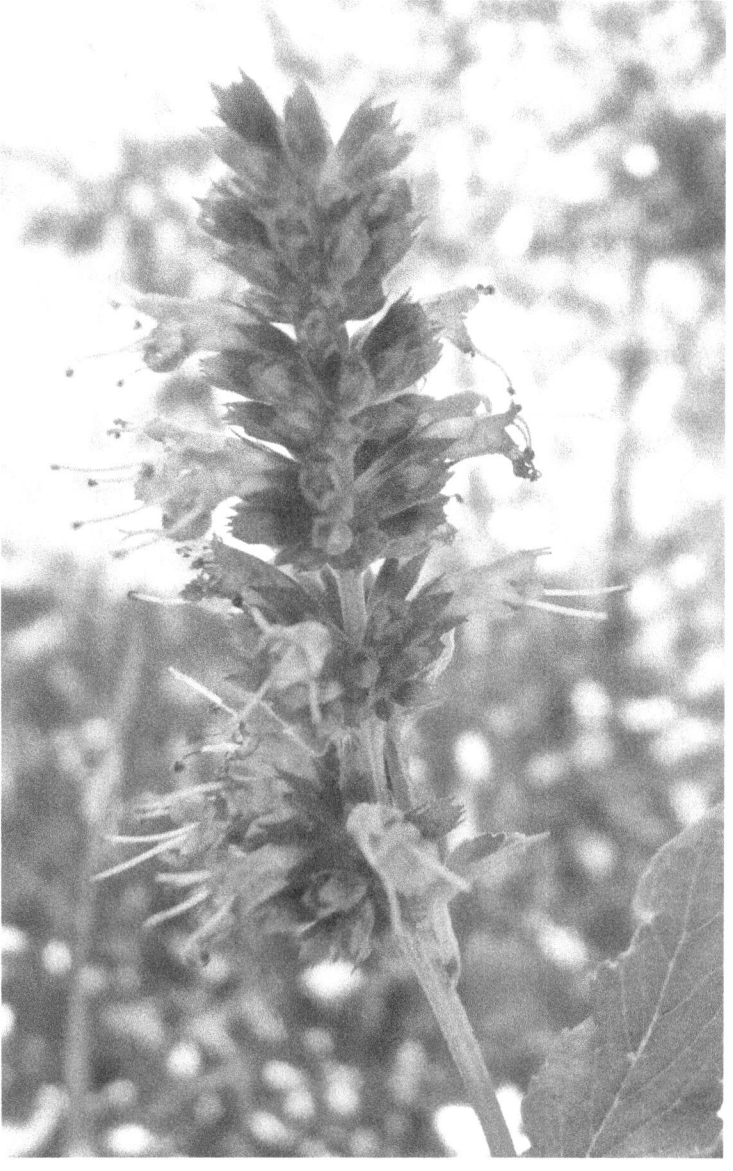

GIANT ANISE HYSSOP

Mountain mint is an effective remedy in formulas for arthritic conditions exacerbated by damp and cold weather. Patients responding favorably to this herb will exhibit the classic signs of dampness, including a rolling pulse, thick sticky tongue coating, and a general sense of lethargy or sluggishness."

Both Giant Hyssops are contra-indicated in inflamed or painful conditions of the stomach; and because of their drying and warming nature are not suitable for weak individuals with high fever, strong thirst, and general dryness. As a strong diaphoretic, it should be avoided, during excessive perspiration, or by individuals with weak constitutions. In TCM terms, avoid in yin deficiency with heat.

Use with caution in cases of constipation due to high tannin content. Pulegone is a uterine stimulant and caution must be observed during pregnancy or menstruation.

ESSENTIAL OIL

CONSTITUENTS – *A. foeniculum*- methyl chavicol (2-85%), germacrene D (13-20%), anisaldehyde, menthone, p-methoxy-cinnamaldehyde, limonene (0-48%), cadinene, pulegone, bornyl acetate, linalool, (E)-ocimene (8-9%) and 50 other constituents. Anise hyssop sometimes contains spathulenol, and in plants low in methyl chavicol, it tends to be higher (10-49%). This chemotype has a more balsamic odor, and contains various amounts of bornyl acetate.
Plants grown in northern Alberta exhibit up to 20% caryophyllene oxide content and less than 5% estragole.
Essential oil content is approximately 0.07-0.245% in leaf and slightly higher in flowers (0.1-0.3%). Plants infected with cucumber mosaic virus decrease estragole and pulegone content and increases limonene and isomenthone.
A. urticifolia- yield- 0.89%.

Optimal yields from both species are obtained during flowering stage. High heat yields optimal levels of essential oil.

Properties of the oil are anti-spasmodic, anti-inflammatory, analgesic, anti-fungal, and nervine.

The oil is used medicinally for gastritis, hepatitis, stomach and intestinal cramping, nerve pain, anxiety, congestive prostate inflammation, varicose veins and other venous circulatory disturbances and poly-arthritis.

The essential oil is not produced commercially on the prairies at the present time, but available from Oregon producers.

Methyl chavicol (estragole), with its anise-like odor, is in demand from many industries, however, and marketing the fractionated product would not be a problem. It is used in the manufacture of perfumes, liqueurs, foods and root beer.

It can be chemically modified to anethole and anisaldehyde, which are used in colour photography, soaps, dentifrices, etc.

Significant aromatic variation is found within the species. Methyl chavicol is highly prized for further use as noted above. One variety containing 29% gamma cadinene, 16% alpha cadinol, 12% beta caryophyllene, and 11% spathulenol is more woody and floral. When spathulenol is present at 50% with 18% bornyl acetate, the oil is more balsamic in nature. Another variation is 37% isomenthone, 23% pulegone and 2% estragole; and as expected has a peppermint, pennyroyal, tarragon scent.

Work at Brooks CDC in 1990 found essential oil yield of 343.7 litres per hectare, or 0.66% yield.

HYDROSOL

Anise Hyssop water is very refreshing to overheated skin. Put it into a spritzer bottle, and use during hot weather, and those suffering heatstroke, sunburn, etc.

FLOWER ESSENCES

Horsemint flower essence is for those who change for change sake, moving all the time.   **ROCKY MTN**

The *shen* is seen as residing in the heart and following shock or trauma it must be restored to the heart in order for healing to occur. The earth-spirit medicine of Anise Hyssop does exactly this, and its flower essence is said to bring back sweetness after the weight of guilt and shame, which is always unwarranted in the case of early childhood sexual abuse. Its flower essence is also used for body-soul integration of pain and suffering. It is a post-trauma stabilizer aiding the ability to forgive and to accept forgiveness.
THEA SUMMER DEER

SPIRITUAL PROPERTIES

The key to the spiritual use of this ubiquitous and beautiful wild plant lies in the purple color of the flower.

It is to be used, as with most plant that have higher or non-physical qualities. The blooming upper spike can be cut just below the lowest flowering portion, baked in a 250 F oven to drive off all moisture and dry the flower, then mixed with pure olive oil and left to stand for three days.

The oil is then ready to use. Place on the third eye location of the forehead, between and slightly above the eyebrow line, it has an excellent ability to clear the lower mind of continuous sexual fixations, habits of lecherous thought and tendencies to allow sexual pictures to obscure the thought patterns.

A similar though less potent effect can be had by boiling the flowers for two minutes to make a tea for internal consumption. This should be drunk three times a day. For the tea, cut the flowers from the main stem and use only the purple petals.   **HILARION**

RECIPES

TINCTURE- 10-20 drops up to six times daily in acute conditions, up to four times in chronic. Make fresh tincture at 1:4 and 50% alcohol.

OIL- Use externally, diluted as needed.

MOUTHWASH- Pour one cup of boiling water over two tsp. of dried herb and leave for ten minutes.

SYRUP- Take four ounces of fresh plant leaf and flower, and add to one quart of boiling water. Simmer down to one pint. Then add one-half cup of honey and pour into sterilized jars. Use 1/4 tsp as needed for sore throats, bronchitis, etc. Dry herb is also acceptable.

AUTUMN OLIVE
(*Elaeagnus umbellata* Thunb.)
WOLF WILLOW
SILVER BERRY
(*E. commutata* Bernh. Ex Rydb.)
(*E. argentea* Pursh.) no longer accepted
RUSSIAN OLIVE
SPINY OLEASTER
(*E. angustifolia* L.)
PARTS USED- flowers, berries, bark

If you live among wolves you have to act like a wolf.   **NIKITA KRUSCHEV**

Elaeagnus is derived from the Greek **ELAION** meaning oil or olive oil, and **HAGNOS** meaning pure, chaste, holy or sacred, or **AGNOS**, Greek for the Chaste Tree. It is pronounced el-ee-AG-nus. The leaves look similar in a remote sort of way.

Another possibility is from the Greek **ELAIA**, meaning Olive Tree, and **AGNOS**, meaning sacred.

Or, just as likely it is from **HELODES**, meaning marshy. **AGNOS** means lamb, and **HAGNOS** means pure or white. Commutata is from Latin **COMMUTARE** meaning "to change", in reference to the upper green and under silver sides of the leaves.

The small, yellow flowers of Wolf Willow and Russian Olive are amazingly fragrant, a musky blend of grape and jonquil, with a note of cestrum.

The silver fruit of wolf willow are edible and peeled and used in soup by the Blackfoot in times of famine, but mostly they were strung for decorative beadwork. Wolf willow is known as **MISS-IS-A-MISOI**. The bark was boiled with grease and applied to sunburn and frostbite.

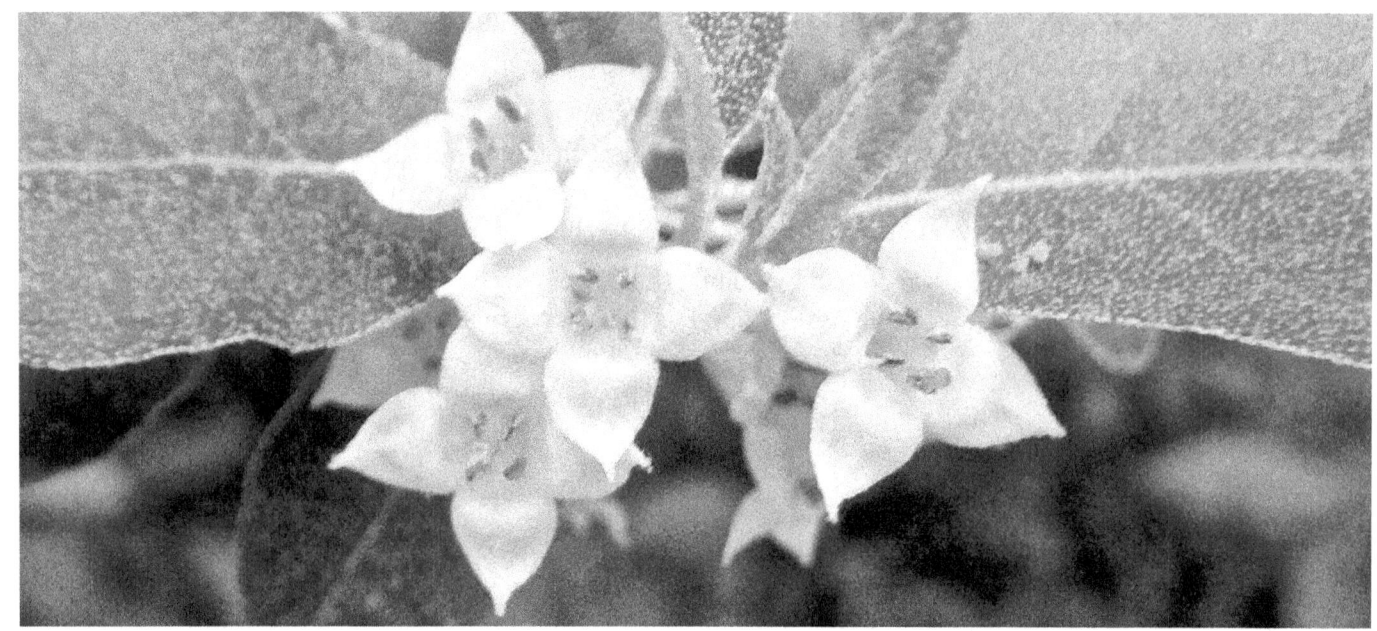

AUTUMN OLIVE FLOWERS

The Cree used the fruit and beads in a similar manner and know the plant as either **WAPI-WUSKWA-MEPISE** or **SONIYAWNIYIPSI**.

To make the seeds usable, they were first boiled and holes drilled. They were then threaded, dried, oiled and polished. After cast iron pans were available, the seeds were cooked to give darker coloration.

The Blood tribe brewed the fruit with Meadow Rue to cure hemorrhoids, and inner bark tea was decocted and drunk by children for chest colds.

Tribes in BC and the northern Cree used the tough inner bark for weaving baskets, and rope for nets, fishing line, and even clothing. The root bark is stronger than the trunk bark, but both remain flexible after drying. The inner bark could be dried for future use and when needed, soaked in water and spun into a strong two ply twine, or larger.

The Thompson, as part of bereavement ceremonies for widows and widowers, traditionally wore a narrow headband of the bark.

For syphilis, a root decoction of Wolf Willow and *Rhus glabra* was taken internally, but said to be poisonous or at least emetic, in large amounts.

The Dena'ina of Alaska refer to the plant as elevated berry, or **DEH GEGA**.

A favorite campfire practical joke is to secretly add a twig of wolf willow to the blaze and watch everyone's reactions to the excrement-scented smoke.

Russian olive is an introduced shelter and ornamental tree that is similar to wolf willow, but a large tree, as opposed to a shrub. The leaves are narrower, and the berries more yellow than silver. The wood makes suitable fence posts and fuel. Russian Olive was planted near the Milk River of southern Alberta and northern Montana in 1950, and now out numbers Cottonwood Poplars throughout the floodplain. In Portugal it is known as the Tree of Paradise.

In the Mediterranean region, the fruits of *E. angustifolia var. orientalis* are dried and powdered into an Arabian pastry. The red skinned fruit is also fermented as a wine beverage; and in Yarkland, western China, a spirit is further distilled from the fermented fruit. The flowers are used in the perfume and production of liqueurs, and were at one time used to treat tetanus. Wang Y et al, *Adv Mat Res* 2013 756:16-20.

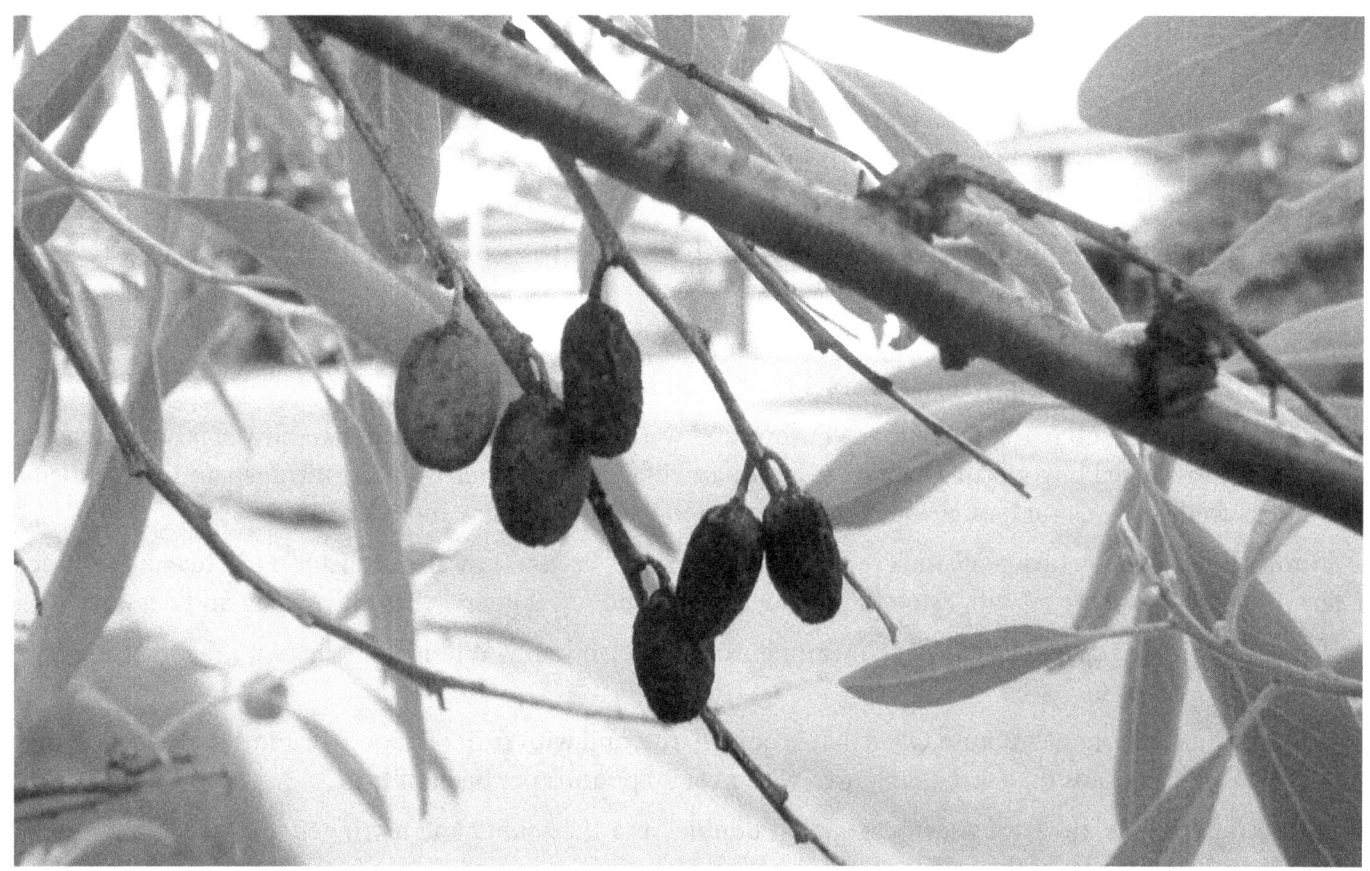

RUSSIAN OLIVE DRIED FRUIT

When dry, the loose skin of **IGDE**, as the fruit is called in Turkey, peels away easily to reveal a cream-colored dusty pulp that practically dissolves in the mouth. It is often eaten an hour before meals as an appetizer.

Mears and Hillman are less charitable in the book, *Wild Foods*. "The fruits are occasionally on sale in London and have pits like elongated olives, skin like polythene, and flesh like sugar-flavored polystyrene, but after six summers living in Turkey in a remote village surrounded by them, I have to admit that I have grown rather fond of them."

Jelly and sherbet treats are made as well. In some areas, the seed oil is pressed and used like olive oil, in bronchitis, burns, wound healing, excessive mucous, and constipation.

In China, the Russian olive is known as Sand Date, or **SHA ZAO**.

It is also known as **HONG DOU**, red bean or love pea. The fruit is used to regulate the menstrual cycle, treat insomnia and promote strength.

In Iran, the fruit is used for dysentery, diarrhea, joint pain and rheumatoid arthritis. The flour has been added to cookies for wound healing. Sahan Y et al, *J Agr Sci* 2013 5:160.

In Turkey, the fruit is taken orally for kidney stones. In Pakistan, the whole plant is used for headache, heart burn and skin infections.

The flowers are made into a tea for nausea, flatulence, vomiting, asthma and jaundice.

The raw or boiled fruit has been used traditionally for sore throat, coughs, flu, colds, and fevers.

One red-fruited cultivar of Russian olive is called King Red. It is nearly thorn-less, with large red fruits up to an inch long, and yielding up to twenty pounds of fruit per tree.

There is no rush to harvest Russian olive, for the fruit hangs on the tree throughout the winter. In Syria, a compound herbal tea known as **ZAHRAA** contains Russian olive fruit.

Wolf Willow is a useful plant for reclamation of strip-mined lands in Western Canada. Studies by Morgensen show that the seed germination rate (96%) is best after stratification at 40 degrees Celsius for 60 to 90 days. Water soaking was the least effective.

The wood has been used in woodwork, including musical instruments. The fresh branches are decocted in hot water in Turkey, and water is applied externally to warts.

Leaf extracts are combined with willow ash to treat external abscess.

The root bark is decocted for dysuria. Fujita T et al, *Econ Botany* 1995(49): 406-22.

Autumn olive is a shrub native to southern Europe and west central Asia. Like Russian olive it is hardy to zone 3, and was introduced into North America as an ornamental, to prevent erosion, fix nitrogen and shelter belts. It is not as well known, and though shrubby, can grow to twenty feet high and wide.

Autumn Olive has a profusion of small red berries, with silver flecks. They are almost too tart to eat. I produce a tart orange-red syrup each fall, using the ripe berries and honey. It goes well with venison and desserts.

In Japan the shrub is called **AKI-GUMI**, meaning Autumn Silverberry. Whole branches with the fruit attached are sold in the streets.

Redwing is one cultivar of Autumn Olive that is quite hardy, and with fruit of good size and sweetness. It grows to 12 feet and is perhaps the most cold hardy, with over 30 pounds per bush of fruit.

If left until dead ripe, the fruit sweetness almost doubles and the acidity and astringency are reduced. Left as long as possible, the size of the fruit, but not the seed, also doubles in size.

The fruit can be used for preserves, condiments, fruit rolls, juice, flavoring, and such. It may well become the next wolfberry/lycium berry nutraceutical health offering.

It has been studied for functionality in flours as well as ice cream. Cakmakci S et al, *Int Journal Food Sci Technol* 2015 (50):472-81.

Work on Autumn Olive plantations by Chow et al, *Can J of Botany* 1999 77 showed the shrub is a good source for fuel, with a relatively high heat value.

Furfural production from pentosan and turpentine production from extractives are good possibilities. Plantation-grown autumn olive juvenile wood could be a suitable material for ethanol and its derivatives due to its high holocellulose content.

Both Russian and Autumn Olive were mentioned in the USDA 1937 *Yearbook of Agriculture* as "plants that await the breeder's attention." Eighty years later, little work has been done. As they all have the ability to reclaim strip-mined land, and grow in nitrogen poor soils, perhaps their time has come.

The province of Alberta does not agree and has placed Autumn Olive on the noxious weeds list. Are you kidding me? On a recent trip to Georgia, I spotted the shrubs in bloom and when I mentioned to some herbal friends the great uses of the plant, they looked at me as if I were making it up. It is a major invasive weed of the US southeast.

While Russian olive requires a pH of 6 or higher, the Autumn Olive tolerates soil ranging from pH 4-8. Work at Morden Research Station in Manitoba shows Autumn Olive has a hardiness rating of 9.6.

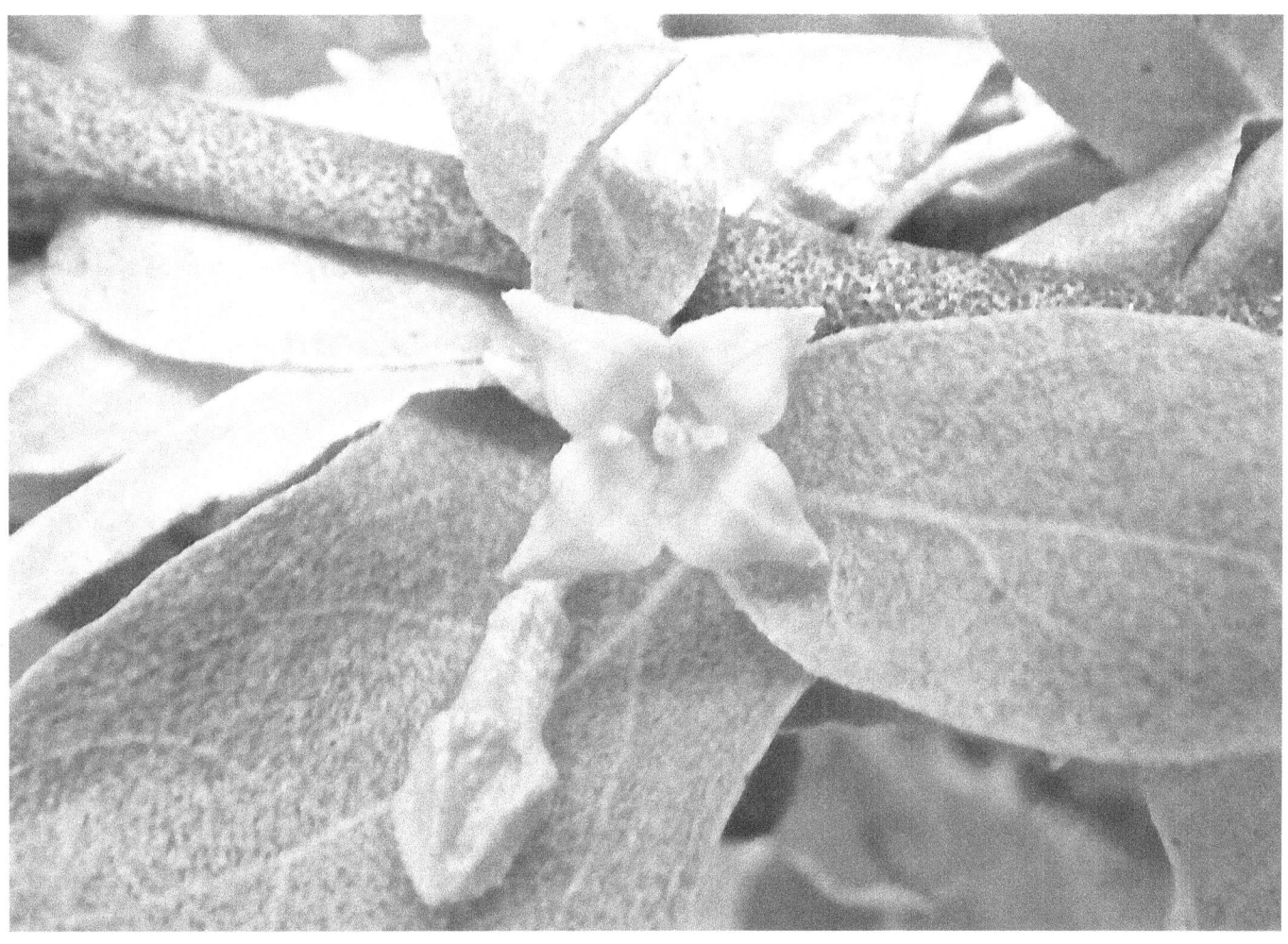

WOLF WILLOW IN FLOWER

MEDICINAL

CONSTITUENTS- Russian olive leaf -harmane, eleagnine, elaeagnoside A-D, oleanolic acid, tetrahydroharman; isorhamnetin, isorhamnetin-3-0-beta-D-galacto-pyranoside, catechin, epicatechin, gallocatechin, epigallocatechin, kaempferol, quercetin, luteolin, isorhamnetin and other flavonoids; caffeic acid; eleagnine, chlorogenic acid; alpha and beta amyrins, fatty alcohols, cycloartenol, triterpene aldehydes, quebrachitol and citrostadienol. Early autumn is optimal time for harvest.

bark- calligonine, tetrahydroharmol, N-methyl tetra-hydroharmol, harman, dihydroharman, harmine, harmol, catechin, beta-carboline, pyrimidines, steroids, epicatechin.

From the root bark has been derived 1-isobutyl, and 2-methyl-1, 2, 3, 4-tetrahydro-beta carboline.

Branch bark- 64% phospholipids, condensed tannins, sinapic and gentisic acid, gitoxigenin (cardiac glycoside), thymine (ketone derivative of pyrimidine).

Analysis of the amino acid content of the berry seeds were found between the proline and glycine peak in samples, but the amino acid remains unidentified.

The seeds contain 42% protein, triacylglycerol with linoleic (49%) and palmitic acid, beta sitosterol, chrysin.

35

The Russian olive fruit ripens in the fall, and is sweet to acidic in nature, with a single seed of a neutral energy. They contain between 43-59% sugar, of which 27% is fructose and 22% glucose; with flavonoids, terpenoids and cardiac glycosides, terpenoids, coumarins, carboxylic acids, tannins, vitamins and minerals. Potassium is abundant in fruit (8504 mg/kg), as is sodium (1731 mg/kg) and phosphorus (635 mg/kg).

Phenolics include 4-hydroxybenzoic acid, caffeic acid. Ripe fruit contain little sucrose, cleaving into fructose and glucose. Amino acids include aspartic acid, theronine, serine, glutamine, proline, glycine, valine.

Fatty acids including 34% palmitic acid, 26% oleic acid, and 17% linolenic acid. Fruit skin contains palmitoleic acid.

Flowers- vitamin B, calcium, vitamins A & K, elaeagnosides A-G (acylated flavonol glycosides), isorhamnetin and kaempferol glycosides.

E. commutata- root bark- 1-isobutyl-1,2,3,4-tetrahydro-beta-carboline, and 6-hydroxy-2'(2-methylpropyl)-3,3'spirotetrahydropyrrolidineohydroxyindole.

E. umbellata fruit- lycopene (15-54 mg/100 grams fresh fruit), alpha and beta cryptoxanthin, beta carotene, lutein, phytoene and phytofluene. The fruit contains 12-21% total sugars, glucose and fructose, and malic acid, as well as 21 accumulated proteins. The fruit content of ascorbic acid decreases from 10mg% to 3mg% from beginning to ripening. This is most unusual for fruit.

leaves- serotonin (5-hydroxytryptamine), chlorogenic acid, p-coumaric acid, sinapic acid, ferulic acid, fumaric acid, syringic acid, ellagic acid, protocatechoic acid, gentisinic acid, 4-hydroxybenzoic acid, rutin, neohesperidin, hesperidin and querctin-3-beta-D-glucoside.

The fresh Russian olive fruit can be used for indigestion where the stomach is swollen and painful; or for coughing and burning sensation in the lungs.

For diarrhea in young children, a soup can be prepared. For chronic enteritis, and stomach inflammation a decoction can be prepared from the dry or fresh fruit. The same tonic can be spread on boils, festering wounds, chilblains, and leg ulcers.

For women suffering from excessive menstruation leading to dizziness, soreness, abdominal pains and lack of vigor; combine with hawthorn berries. The berries are tonifying and sedative.

It combines well with goji berry for loss of memory, insomnia and weakened vision.

A study by Ahmadiani et al in conducted in Tehran, Iran, found that the berries contain anti-inflammatory and analgesic properties not associated with the opioid system. The full study is available in the *Journal of Ethnopharmacology* 2000 72:1-2.

Follow up work by Hosseinzadeh et al, *J Ethnopharm* 2003 84:2-3 found muscle relaxing effect in both ethanol and water extracts of the seeds, as effective as diazepam. This may be due to flavanoids or flavones, such as chrysin.

Ramezani et al, *Fitoterapia* 2001 72:3 found anti-nociceptive effect from seed extracts, suggestive of pain relief and analgesic properties.

The berries encourage production of hydroxyproline. Application of the fruit extract to skin wounds, increased content in of this compound, and collagen in tissue.

Rat studies found the fruit accelerated wound healing, as well as reduction of pain and inflammation. Natanzi MM et al, *Acta Medica Iran* 2012 50:589-96.

A product called Pshatin, produced from the fruit, has been used for colitis and other gastrointestinal inflammation in Armenia. Abizov EA et al, *Pharm Chem Journal* 2009 42:696-98. An earlier study looked at fruit extracts and the inhibiting effect on vascular and respiratory smooth muscles. Mohammed FI et al, *Sci Pharm* 2006 74:21.

The fruit pulp is rich in polysaccharides that exhibit anti-oxidant activity. Chen Q et al, *Int J Mol Sci* 2014 15:11446-55.

Fruit extracts appear to inhibit COX-1 and COX-2 enzymes. Farahbakhsh S et al, *Basic Clin Neurosci* 2011 2:31-37. The action is similar to indomethacin.

Oral lichen planus is a chronic inflammation with rash-like symptoms often treated with oral or local corticosteroids. A topical 19% gel shows great promise for this condition. Taheri JB et al, *J Dent Res Dent Clin Dent Prospects* 2010 4:29.

Fruit extracts, combined with ginger root have shown symptom relief of knee osteoarthritis. Rabiei K et al, *Zahedan J Med Sci* 2015:29-33. Patients took 200 mg extracts for eight weeks, and showed significant improvement in pain intensity and occurrence.

Other studies of powder and whole fruit (15g/kg) for eight weeks showed improvement in pain and inflammation in knee osteoarthritis in women. Nikniaz Z et al, *Complement Ther Med* 2014(22):864-9. This study involved obese women with chronic pain. A more recent randomized, double-blind, placebo-controlled trial found significant reductions in total cholestrol and atherogenic indices, as well as pain relief in mild to moderate osteoporosis in 90 female patients. Nikniaz Z et al, *J Diet Suppl* 2016 13(6):595-606.

Earlier work found water extracts of fruit helped heal skin wounds, including increased collagen and re-epithelialization. Natanzi MM et al, *Acta Med Iranica* 2012 50:589-96.

Two other randomized, double blind studies compared water extracts (0.21% kaempferol) with ibuprofen 800mg/kg, in women with knee osteoarthritis. Ebrahimi A et al, *Int J Rheum Disease* 2015(18):79-80; Panahi Y et al, *EXCLI* 2016 (15):203-10.

A seven week randomized DB, PC trial of fruit on patients with osteoarthritis improved considerably. Alishiri G et al, *Kowsar Med Journal* 2007 12:49-57.

Water extracts of fruit improved memory and spatial learning, in rats given scopolamine injections. Tamtaji OR et al, *Zanjan Univ Med Sci J ZUMS J* 2014(22):101-111.

Fruit extracts inhibit proliferation of HeLa cancer cell lines. Ya W et al, *Adv J Food Sci Technol* 2014(6):707-10.

A tincture of the flowers inhibit angiogenesis of human umbilical endothelial cells, suggesting it may be useful for preventing and treating angiogenesis disorders. Badrhadad A et al, *J Med Plant Res* 2012(6):4633-39. It should be explored for possible benefit in diabetes, retinopathy, rheumatoid arthritis and psoriasis, in addition to cancer.

The fruit shows activity against human hepatoma cells (HepG2). Wang Y et al, *Journal of Chinese Institute of Food Science and Technology* 2013 13:26-31.

The fruit extract is strongly anti-bacteria against *Escherichia coli*. Dehghan MH et al, *Int J Enteric Pathog* 2014 (2):e20157. The fruit was used traditionally for gall bladder problems, which are sometimes related to *E. coli* invasion.

Russian olive flowers are used medicinally, for fevers, neuralgia, and aching pains. It is said that the flowers (perhaps the scent) can bring people back from their deathbeds.

A tincture of flowers showed activity against Walker 256 carcinoma cells, *in vivo*. Bucur L et al, *Archives of the Balkan Medical Union* 2008 43:107-12.

The flower extract was compared with sildenafil citrate in a randomized, clinical trial of women with orgasmic dysfunction. The former was given as 4.5 grams daily in two doses, and the drug at 50 mg, one hour before intercourse. Female sexual function, levels of prolactin and TSH were measured after four weeks treatment. These did not change.

The flower extract was less functional, but was effective in reducing the frequencies of orgasmic disorder. The mechanism is not certain but it may be the result of nitric oxide increase and subsequent cGMP increase in cells, as well as vaginal smooth muscle relaxation, artery vasodilation and swelling of genital area including clitoris. Akbarzadeh M et al, *Journal Reprod Infertil* 2014 15:190-8. Maybe there is truth behind the saying to lock your women up when the flowers bloom. Just kidding!

A recent study of 125 women, with hypoactive sexual desire, were divided into three groups: flower extract, sildeafil citrate and control. Although the drug was more effective than flowers, both showed benefit over control. Zeinalzadeh S et al, *J Evid Based Complement Altern Med* 2016 21(3):186-93.

The flowers and leaves, especially the latter, are rich in phenolics that possess anti-oxidant activity. Saboonchian F et al, *Avicenna Journal Phytomed* 2014 4:231.

Water/alcohol extracts from leaves (50%) give the most potent anti-oxidant activity.

The leaves have value, as an astringent in fever and enteritis. The powdered leaves are used to control bleeding and accelerate wound healing. One study found the leaf extract increased the number of capillary buds and fibroblasts in treated group, compared to control. Fibroblasts are adhering cells in skin connective tissue.

The leaves contain quebrachitol, also found in maple syrup, and a potential sweetening agent. Ethanol extract of flowers and leaves show anti-spasmodic activity on small intestine tissue. Mohammed FI et al, *Sci Pharm* 2006 74:21-30.

Work by Olinda et al, *Phytomed* 2008 15:5 found the compound reduced gastric damage from aspirin, ethanol and other toxins. L-quebrachitol is a building block for the synthesis of biologically active chiral inositol phosphates.

Isorhamnetin attenuates Staphylococcus aureus-induced lung cell damage by inhibitn alpha hemolysin, a secreted pore-forming cytotoxin. Jiang L et al, *J Microbiol Biotechnol* 2016 26(3):596-602.

Calligonine, derived from Russian olive trees, lowers blood pressure, in a manner similar to resperine. Leaf extracts relax smooth muscle. See Mohammed above.

Heart attack, or myocardial infarction is one of the major causes of death. The quick return of blood to the tissue can cause injury, and this may be abated by anti-oxidants including vitamin E, catalaose, melatonin and SOD.

Water extract of leaves showed improved restoration of cardiac function and myocardial values towards normal, suggesting a protective effect. Wang B et al, *J Chem* 2014 69357316.

A four-week administration of fruit oil to healthy people markedly improved lipid profiles, including reduction of triglycerides, total cholesterol and LDL. Belarbi M et al, *J Agric Food Chem* 2011 59:8667-69.

Quercitin is one of the main flavonoids in leaves, helping control chronic pain via several pathways.

Harman and harmaline inhibit MAO (monoamine oxidase) and increase serotonin and noradrenaline (like tricyclic anti-depressants) at the synaptic sites, also contributing to analgesic effect. Karimi G et al, *Iran J Basic Med Sci* 2010(13):97-101.

Alcohol extracts of the leaves inhibit *Bacillus subtilis, Staphylococcus aureus, Salmonella typhimurium* and *Yersinia enterocolitica.* Taamtaji OR et al (see above).

Elaeagnin binds to the human MAO-A sites and lowers blood pressure. Its structure is similar to reserpine, and may work in a similar manner.

The leaves of various Elaeagnus species may be useful in the treatment of asthma and chronic bronchitis. Water extracts are anti-tussive and expectorant, and decrease cough frequency in animal studies. Ge Y et al, *Evid Based Complement Alternat Med* 2015:428208.

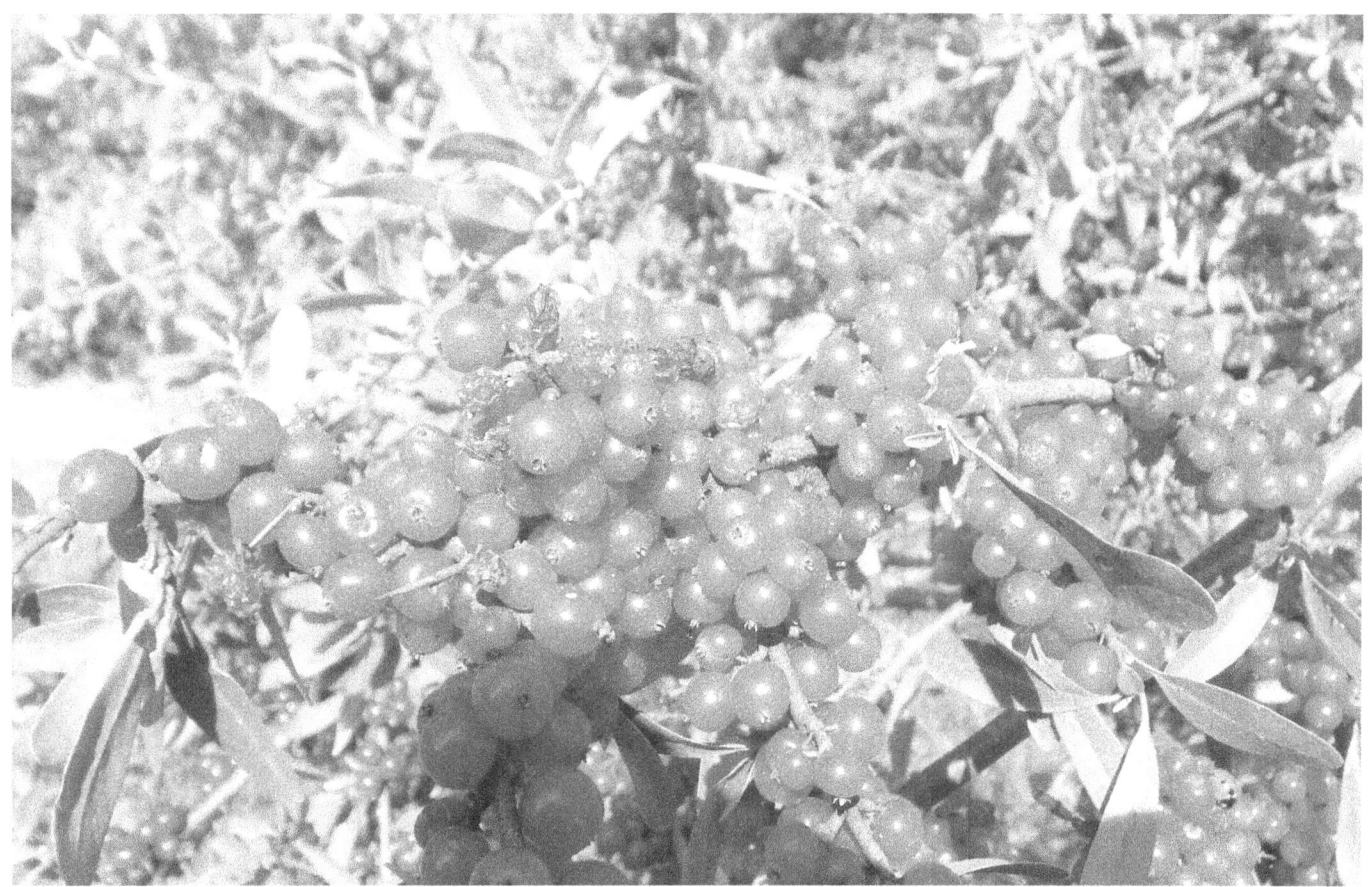

AUTUMN OLIVE FRUIT

Autumn Olive is a particularly rich source of lycopene, a carotenoid protective of myocardial function and various forms of cancer, including prostate.

In the red berries, lycopene accounts for 72-82% of the total carotenoids, and at up to 54 milligrams per 100 grams, compared to the fresh tomato at only about 3 mg, and cooked tomato paste at 29 mg/100 grams. The fully ripened fruit is rich in glucose and fructose.

Plus, the beta cryptoxanthin content is ten times higher than oranges and tangerine. Wang et al, *Planta Medica* 2007 73 5:468-77 found the fruits inhibit human leukemia (HL-60) cancer cells and induced apoptosis. It showed activity against lung epithelial A549 cancer cell lines.

Ether extracts of the flowers show activity against gram-negative *E. coli* and *Pseudomonas aeruginosa* and gram-positive *Staphylococcus aureus* and *Bacillus subtilis*. Alcohol extracts of the leaves are active against both, and a water extract of the berry is active against *E. coli* and *S. aureus*. Sabir MS et al *Saudi Med Journal* 2007 28(2):259-63. Acetone extract of berries is active against *P. aeruginosa*.

Similar findings were found in work by Aziz S et al, *Pak J Pharm Sci* 2015 28(1):65-70.

More exciting is that in the future, lycopene content of the fruits could be enhanced by selecting cultivars or hybridizing selected parent plants. *HortScience* 2001 36:6.

Both fruit and leaf water extracts show anti-proliferative and anti-oxidant properties, with the leaf more effective against HeLa and HT29 cancer cell lines.

The closely related *E. glabra* from Japan contains epigallocatechins shown to inhibit DNA synthesis in the bacteria *Proteus vulgaris*, and RNA synthesis in *Staphylococcus aureus*. More study is needed.

ESSENTIAL OIL

CONSTITUENTS-_E. commutata-_ 0.1% yield of an oil containing 79% ethyl cinnamate, and other unknown constituents.

The yellow green flowers of the silver leaved wolf willow open in June, and exude the most erotic, narcotic and musky sweet smell; reminiscent of a star gazer lily.

The flowers of _E. angustifolia_ yield 0.1% essential oil containing some 85 components; with 53 identified so far. The principal component is trans-ethyl cinnamate that comprises nearly 59%, as well as hexahydrofarnesyl acetone (10%), palmitic acid (5.2%), and phytol (3.3%). Also present are 2-phenyl-ethyl benzoate, 2-phenyl-ethyl isovalerate and anethole.

The leaf essential oil contains 85 components including trans-ethyl cinnamate (37%), phytol (12%), nonanal (107%) and Z-3-hexenyl benzoate (7.65%).

Both show toxicity in brine shrimp tests. Torbati M et al, _Adv Pharm Bull_ 2016 6(2):164-9.

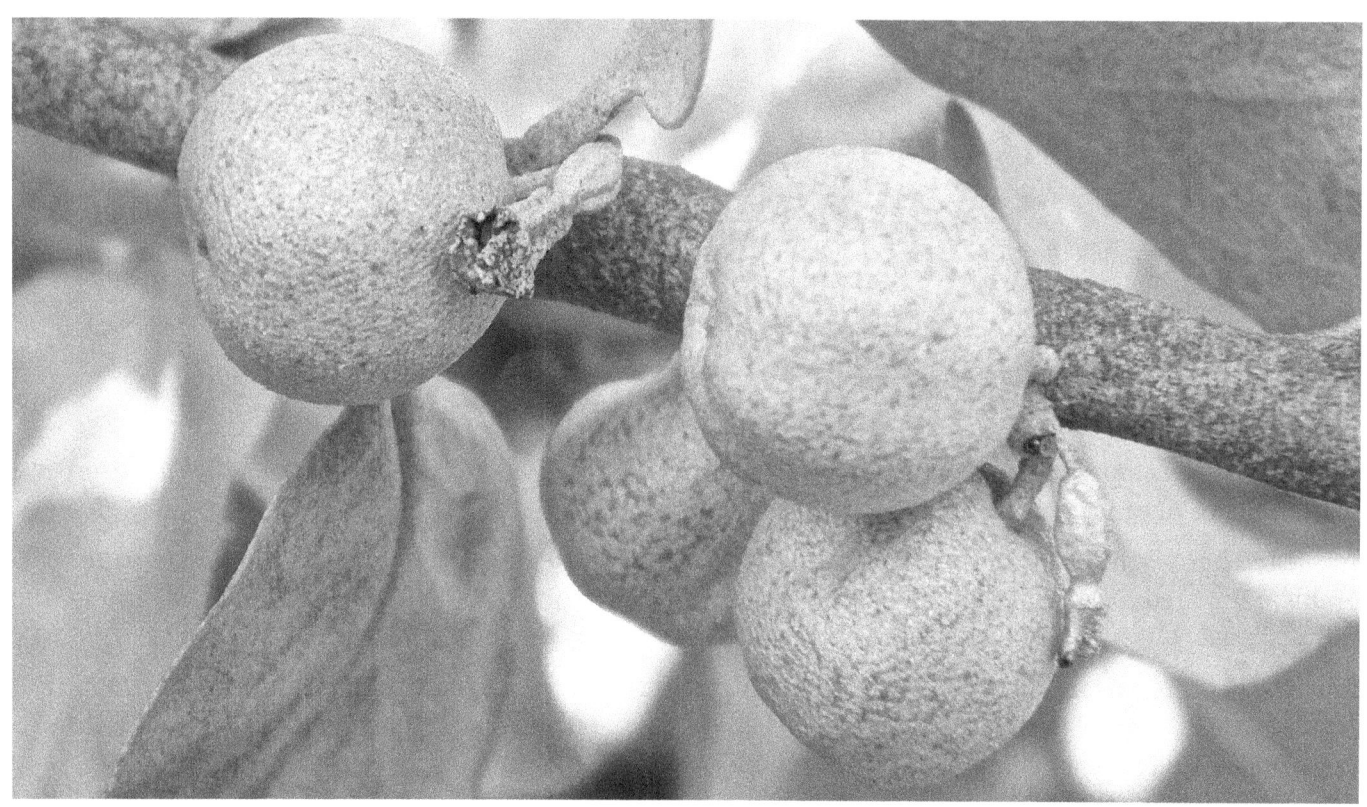

WOLF WILLOW BERRIES

FLOWER OIL

The flowers of Wolf Willow may be sun infused in canola oil to retain their heady and pungent aroma.

This can be a sun infusion for 14 days, using a 1:5 ratio of flowers by weight to oil by volume. You can also use a low temperature crock pot no higher than 120 degrees Fahrenheit for several hours, with lid off.

It shares this scented flower with Russian olive, an imported ornamental tree.

The flowers are certainly more abundant on the imported tree, but they lack some of the deep, musky strength of the wolf willow. In old Persia, the delicious perfume of the _Elaeagnus_ blossoms was said to have a powerful effect on a woman's emotions; and it is said that husbands were told to lock up their wives while the trees were in bloom.

Many years ago, my wife Laurie developed Prairie Essence perfume, utilizing some two dozen essential and scented carrier oils from local prairie and boreal forest plants.

It was beautifully offered in a 7ml cut glass pink perfume bottle shaped like the wild rose of Alberta. Wolf willow flower oil was the deep, base note needed to complete this project.

A 6% soft extract in a water washable cream base exhibited wound-healing effects on skin, superior to control. Bucur L et al, *Rev Med Chir Soc Med Nat Iasi* 2008 112(4):1098-1103.

SEED OIL

The seed oil of Russian olive yields up to 26% and composed of nearly 59% octadecadienoic acid; 23% octadecenoic acid, and lesser amounts of stearic, palmitic and palmitoleic acids.

The seeds yield nine glycolipids and seven phospholipids-the main ones being phosphatidyl choline, phosphatidyl-ethanolamines, and phosphatidyl-inositol.

The oil has an iodine number of 113-155, and saponification of 184-197. Specific gravity is 0.9260. The un-saponifiable parts of the fruit oil contain 9.8 mg% carotenoids and 36.5 mg% tocopherols; with at least 50 identified components including C16-C34 alkanes, steroids, and tocopherols.

Work by Jiang et al, *Zhong Yao Chi* 2001 24:12 found the fat oil of seeds can be extracted more efficiently by ultrasonic technology. See above for study on seed oil in humans.

The pericarp contains 0.8-1.2% lipids, the flowers, 3%, and the leaves from 1.4-9.5%.

The leaf oil consists of 19% palmitic acid, 30-44% linolenic acid, 10% oleic acid, and minor amounts of 22.0 and 22.0 fatty acids.

FLOWER ESSENCES

Wolf willow flower essence speeds up the dilation of the cosmic cervix allowing new birth. It is useful when people are going through transitions and re-birthing or re-making themselves. After the re-birth new boundaries of who they have become are still fragile. Wolf Willow helps establish and guard those boundaries allowing the process to complete itself.   **PRAIRIE DEVA**

Russian Olive is for reawakening and expanding the memory. Russian Olive calms and renews your energy for the journey. Nervous Nelly describes who is best helped with this remedy—timid, hyper, anxious, jumpy, easily startled and generally fearful.   **RAVENWORKS**

PERSONALITY TRAITS

I pick up a handful of mud and sniff it. I step over the little girls and bend my nose to the wet rail of the bridge. I stand above the water and sniff. On the other side I strip leaves off wild rose and dogwood. Nothing doing.

And yet all around me is that odor that I have not smelled since I was eleven, but have never forgotten-have dreamed, more than once. Then I pull myself up the bank by a gray-leafed bush, and I have it. The tantalizing and ambiguous and wholly native smell is not more than the shrub we called Wolf Willow, now blooming with small yellow flowers.

It is Wolf Willow, and not the town or anyone in it that brings me home.   **WALLACE STEGNER**

MYTHS AND LEGENDS

Old Man lay down to sleep after telling Little Brown Eye (his anus) to keep watch over some uneaten toasted gophers.

Soon Little Brown Eye sounded a warning (flatus) but there was only a crow on a nearby tree. Then a lynx came along and again Little Brown Eye sounded a warning. But Old Man was sound asleep and although Little Brown Eye roared away, he refused to wake up. The lynx ate all the gophers.

When Old Man awoke, he was angry with Little Brown Eye because it had let a lynx eat all the meat and had not awakened him.

So Old Man took a stick of a kind of willow and rubbed it into Little Brown Eye and, ever since, this willow has smelled like human excrement and has been known as Stink-Wood.   **WISSLER 1910**

In the Blackfoot language, the Milky Way is called **MAKOI-YOHSOKOYI**, the Wolf Trail, and these stars are a constant reminder for people of how they should live together.   **NANCY TURNER 2005**

RECIPES

RUSSIAN OLIVE TONIC- Take one kilo of part-ripe fruit or one half kilo of dry fruit. Cover with water and simmer for two hours. Strain. Simmer until a thick consistency and serve three times daily.

AUTUMN OLIVE- the ripe fruit makes a delicious preserve with heat and honey.

LEAF TINCTURE- 20-40 drops three times daily. Prepare 1:5 at 50% alcohol.

CHILDREN'S DIARRHEA- Take one-half ounce of dry fruit and stir-fry until surface is golden. Add water and simmer for some time. Serve as soup up to three times daily.

MENSTRUAL- Use equal parts of Russian olive and hawthorn berries. Prepare as above and serve before going to sleep every evening.

BOOK- *Wolf Willow* by Wallace Stegner, which won a Pulitzer Prize, is a hardship story of homesteading in Saskatchewan, and its toll on the human soul.

CAUTION- do not use in pregnancy or breastfeeding. Talaei-Khozani T et al, *Tokai J Exp Clin Med* 2011 36:63-70.

The pollen is a major allergen with up to 30% of people reacting.

AVENS
YELLOW AVENS
(*Geum aleppicum* Jacq.)
LARGE LEAVED AVENS
(*G. macrophyllum* Willd.)
PURPLE/WATER AVENS
(*G. rivale* L.)
OLD MAN'S WHISKERS
THREE FLOWERED AVENS
PRAIRIE SMOKE
TORCH FLOWER
(*G. triflorum* Pursh)
WOOD AVENS
HERB BENNET
(*G. urbanum* L.)
PARTS USED- leaf, flower, root

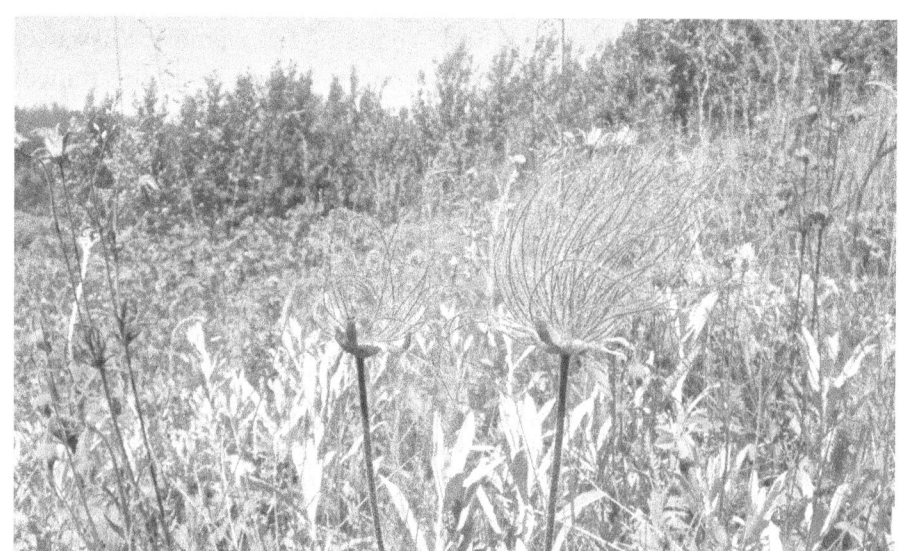

OLD MAN'S WHISKERS

Geum is from the Latin and used by Pliny to describe the plant. It probably originates from the Greek *GENO*, to yield an agreeable perfume or fragrance; due to the clove-like aroma of the roots; from the Greek *GEUEIN* to taste; or from the Greek *GEYO*, to stimulate. **GAIA,** or **GAIOS** meaning the land or earth, is a more remote possibility.

Avens is from the Old French **AVENCE,** or Medieval Latin **AVENCIA**, a type of clover. This signifies an antidote, as it was previously thought to fend off evil by wearing an amulet of the root.

It was believed that people who held avens leaves could communicate telepathically, with each other. Its trefoiled leaf and five petals symbolized the trinity and the five wounds of Christ, and were sculptured into 13th century Church architecture.

St. Benedict is said to have neutralized venomous poison through prayer, leading to name of Herb Bennet.

Rivale is from the Latin **RIVUS** meaning brook or stream. The English word Rival was originally a friendly word for neighbors who were RIVALES that is, living across the river from each other. Neighborly tiffs and spats then led to its more modern sense of rivalry. Urbanum is derived from Latin for city, **URBIS**.

Macrophyllum means big leaved. Aleppicum means "of Aleppo", a now well-known, recently, devastated city in war-torn Syria.

Yellow Avens (*G. aleppicum*) root was used traditionally by Iroquois, and other indigenous healers, to treat diarrhea, high fever, and convulsions.

The Mik'maq used the root in a variety of compounds to treat coughs and croup.

The Woods Cree of Saskatchewan decocted the root alone or in combination to treat sickness associated with teething and to induce sweating. Decoctions were used for sore teeth, or for sore throats.

Both Yellow and Large-leaved Yellow Avens were traditionally known as **KAKWITHITAMOWASK** or "Jealousy plant". This is due to the achenes hooking onto the clothing of passers-by; just like when a person is walking by and someone is jealous of them. It is also called **SAW GEE TOO WUSK**, or **SAKOHTOWASK** meaning Jealous or Love Root, suggesting use as a love charm. The latter is the name used by noted Cree healer, Russell Willier. He uses it for sexual prowess. It is ground up and added to other herbs, or used as a smudge under a blanket.

Yellow Avens (*G. aleppicum*) is used in Traditional Chinese Medicine to treat bleeding, insect bites, fevers, convulsions, fevers and skin disorders. It is known as **SHUI YANG MEI**.

Large-leaved Yellow Avens root was used in traditional medicine, by Bella Coola healers, for a variety of stomach troubles and pain. The leaves were used as poultices by many tribes for boils, cuts, and bruises, either mashed raw or boiled before application.

Some tribes, including the Quinault, chewed the leaves as a universal remedy "good for everything", including labor.

The Thompson men used the plant as a love charm, or for good luck in general. Root decoctions were taken hot to bring out and resolve measles, chicken pox and other eruptive skin diseases. It was noted, by Steedman, a 1930s anthropologist, that none who used the root, died during the last smallpox epidemic.

The Nuxalk name is "lice", for the small, hooked fruit that catches to clothing and hair. They made a tea from the roots for stomach pain, and the leaves were poulticed on boils.

The Salish of south Vancouver Island ate the leaves before visiting a dying person to protect them from harmful germs.

Chehalis tribe women drank a leaf infusion to avoid conception, but only after a woman had previously given birth. They called the plant **T'SIT'SIALK'UM**, meaning "a prairie that sings."

The Quileute chew the leaves during labor, as they were found at the site of the birth of seal pups, and hence the name **XATALITCIXL**, Hair Seal Leaves.

Cowichan men chewed the leaves and fed them to their wives during pregnancy to straighten out the womb (breech?), and aid delivery.

The Squamish used the leaf tea as a diuretic, and eyewash.

The Haida boiled the roots in steam baths for rheumatism.

Further east, the Ojibwa used it as an unspecified female remedy.

A very useful, and versatile herb.

Purple or Water Avens, or Chocolate root, as it is sometimes known, was used for fevers and diarrhea as well. A cocoa substitute was made from the root, hence the name, and use as a tonic.

The root was used in the past by the Cree, and called **KINIPAGWASK** or **KINIPAGWUSKHAS**, meaning "Snake root", to cause miscarriage. It is still used today to help facilitate birthing, or increase sexual potency.

The root was decocted, by Mi'kmaq, for coughs and colds, especially in children. The Eastern Cree used the decocted roots to treat spitting blood.

Root decoctions were used as gargles for sore throats. South American natives used Geum for intermittent fevers, esteeming it like Peruvian bark.

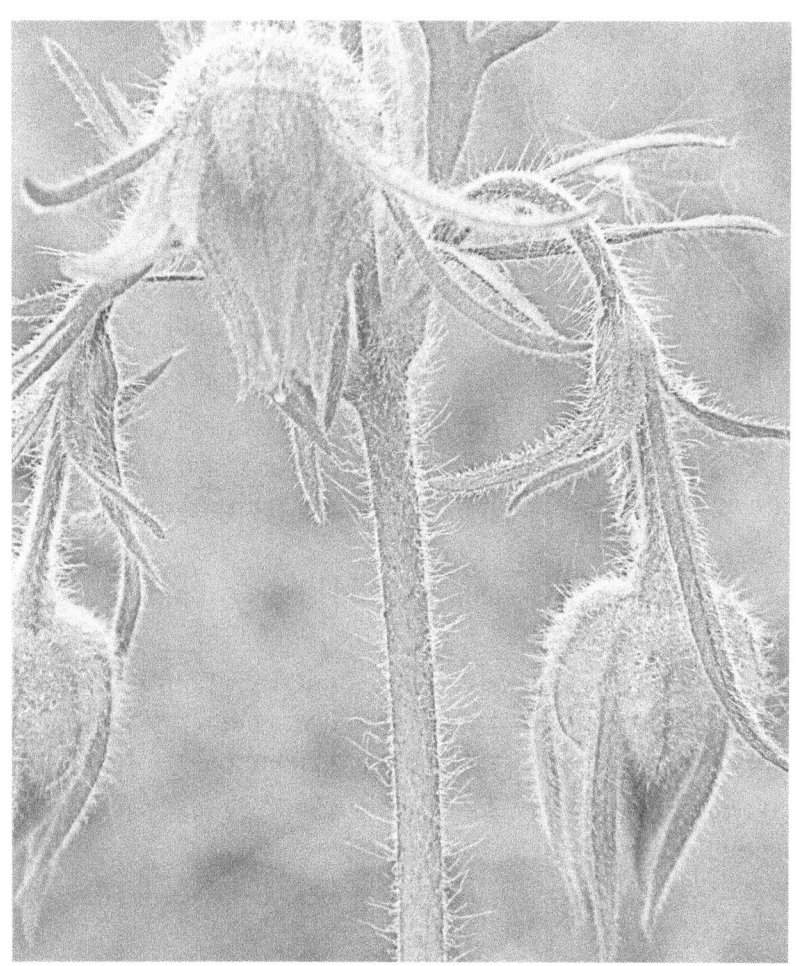

OLD MAN WHISKERS

Monks of the Middle Ages picked the root on March 25th in honor of St. Benedict; and it is found, of course, in the famous Benedictine liqueur. The root was traditionally gathered 3-4 days after Ostara (Easter).

Father Kunzle, a Swiss Abbot, and herbalist wrote, "God gave to avens the virtue of chasing out from the eyes, nose, teeth, brain and even the heart, all that should not be there." The Swiss herbalist believed *G. urbanum* roots, when fresh, could be applied externally to heal infantile paralysis and spinal meningitis.

The flowers taste similar to Porcini or King Bolete (*Boletus edulis*) mushrooms, and can be added to salads.

G. rivale root was official in the US Pharmacopoeia, from 1820-82, as an astringent.

Lucinda Haynes Lombard, writing for the *American Botanist* in November, 1918 noted a peculiar superstition that friends, when provided with *G. rivale* leaves, are able to converse with one another though many miles apart and speaking in whispers, suggestive of telepathy.

The Blackfeet used Old Man's Whiskers (*G. triflorum*) root or seed decoctions for washing sore and inflamed mouth. The leaves were dried, crushed and mixed with other medicines as a tonic.

The ripe seed pods, known as *SO-YA ITS* were crushed and added to fat for perfume.

The whole plant was called Torch Plant. The roots were eaten whole, but a beverage from the roots, obtained by boiling was most sought after. It taste similar to a weak sassafras tea. The boiled roots were applied to swollen or sore eyes, as well as swollen glands in the form of a poultice. If the root is boiled down, it forms a thick gel that can be used as an ointment for skin sores.

Matthew Wood writes. "The leaves and flowers of the beautiful little prairie avens are used by Native American people for inflammation and torsion of the ovary…One can hardly look at the mature red flower hanging down without thinking of an inflamed ovary!"

I find this interesting as early Ukrainian settlers to Alberta used root decoctions for severe internal uterine hemorrhaging. If less severe, nettle leaf infusion would suffice.

The Blood tribe prized Prairie Smoke root for sore throats, sore nipples (while nursing), coughs, and saddle sores on their horses.

It is known as **SO YIA AHTSI**, or **SOOYAIAIIHTSI** (Lies on its Belly). They brewed the roots with melted kidney fat to apply to children's cankers, chapped lips, and sore nipples from nursing and chicken pox. This same mixture was taken internally for stomach ulcers and other digestive disturbance.

The root was scraped and mixed with tobacco, and smoked in a pipe to "clear the head."

The Wood Cree use the plant for similar conditions and know it as **KAM MIST KA SHAWIK.**

Decoctions were used for diarrhea, and as an eyewash for snow blindness.

Leaf infusions were given anyone spitting up blood.

When their horses were losing weight, avens root was boiled with balsam root and the inner bark of willow, strained and given to their prized animals.

The powdered root makes a good styptic, to stop bleeding, and is also a tonic to invigorate and strengthen after illness.

The Thompson tribe used the root decoctions as an analgesic and tonic for stiff and sore muscles and joints. They steamed the above ground plants in their sweats for rheumatism and associated body pain.

The Thompson decocted the roots to help treat smallpox, measles, and chicken pox, like large leaved Avens, and a stronger decoction as a bath for stiffness and pain in the body. They call it **SOPOPKE'KEN** meaning "little hairy or bushy flower".

The Chippewa combined the root with Alum root for indigestion; or chewed on the raw, dried root as a stimulant.

The fresh root smells like celery, but if decocted in water with a little vinegar, it will exhibit the smell of oil of cloves.

Siberian Avens (*Geum urbanum ssp. siberica)* is often planted as a hardy perennial on the prairies. It produces bright orange red flowers.

Avens (*G. urbanum*) is a European herb, also known as The Blessed Herb or Herb Bennett from St. Benedict's Herb. This name was probably assigned in allusion to a legend respecting the saint.

It is said that on one occasion, a monk presented him a goblet of poisoned wine. When the saint blessed it, the poison, being a sort of devil, flew out of it with such force that the glass was shivered to atoms, the crime of the monk being thus exposed.

Hildegard de Bingen wrote that whomever "takes herb bennet in drink…will burn with desire and love."

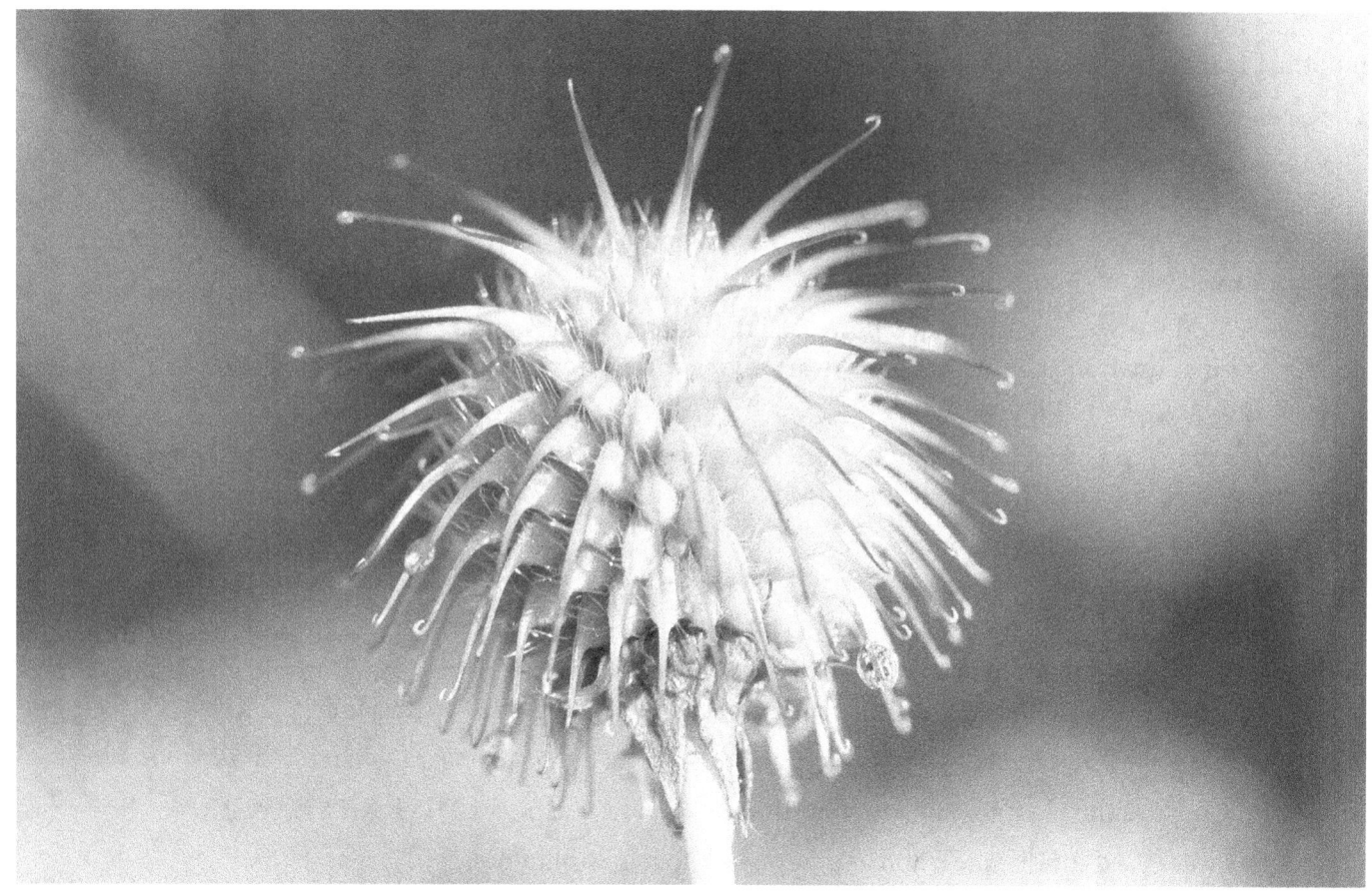

WOOD AVENS (HERB BENNET)

The herb was hung above doors to prevent the devil from entering.

In medieval times, the upper leaves with three leaflets and five gold petals, symbolizing the Holy Trinity and the five wounds of Christ on the cross were displayed in paintings and architecture.

The root is believed to give Augsburg Ale its distinctive flavor. Used fresh it gives a clove flavour, and preserves the brew from spoilage. See recipes below.

The roots were used to tan leather and give a dark yellow dye to wool. The dried roots were used to repel moths from eating clothes.

It is an old febrifuge and dysentery remedy.

Culpepper wrote the herb "dissolves inward congealed blood occasioned by falls and bruises and the spitting of blood."

Old Man's Whiskers (*G. triflorum*) is recommended by the Alberta Research Council, as a good native reclamation plant.

It is grown for seed (1.4-2 million seeds per kilogram), that is part of mixtures for grassland restoration after pipeline, oil well, or gravel pit use. It is hardy, with a 93% germination rate.

Pikas are alpine mammals related to rabbits that need to store lots of food for winter. They have been observed gathering alpine avens (Geum species) that is toxic to them as a food.

However, it appears to prevent the bacterial breakdown in the hay piles constructed by pikas, which layer the plants instinctively. The avens is safe for them to eat several months later, after decomposition, and in the meantime has helped preserve their food source through the winter.

MEDICINAL

CONSTITUENTS- *G. rivale* roots- tannins, including pyrogallol-type, alkaloids (0.03% dried), organic acids, glycosides, triterpenes, geoside, flavonoids , 8 phenolic acids and vitamin C (0.9 g/ kg).
aerial parts- tiliroside, cecropiacic acid, niga-ichgoside, gallic acid, ellagic acid, sterols, sucrose, 1-O-protocatechuoyl glucose, and 1-0-methyl-6-0-caffeoyl-beta-D-glucopyranose.
G. urbanum- roots- vicianose, gein. Vicianosidase is an enzyme that splits gein to eugenol and vicianose. Various phenolic glucosides including resorcinol, quinol, pyrogallol, phloroglucinol and catechol; as well as gallic, caffeic and chlorogenic acids are present as well. Up to 30% tannins.
G. aleppicum- whole plant- flavones, fatty acids, eugenol, gein, geoside.
Endophytes- stem- *Rhizobium gei* sp. nov; *Pseudoxanthomonas gei* sp. nov.
Root- *Sphingomonas gei* sp. nov; *Asticcacaulis endophyticus* sp. nov.

The various native avens roots are one of our better remedies for dysentery and chronic diarrhea.

It is a good remedy for bloody or odorous vaginal discharge, using the cooled decocted tea as a douche. For hemorrhoids, a retention enema works wonders.

As well, it will help to stop uterine hemorrhages, excessive menstruation and middle of the month bleeding like Cranesbill.

Avens is a good tea for irritation and inflammation of the stomach lining, and even ulcerative colitis, using either the dried leaf or stronger root tea.

Tiliroside, from aerial parts, reduce inflammation, via down regulation of iNOS and COX-2. Jin X et al, *Exp Ther Med* 2016 12(1):499-505.

Ellagitannins in the root decoction help formation of urolithin A, B and C by human gut microbiota.

Studies conducted by McCutcheon et al, at the University of British Columbia, found that *G. macrophyllum* root is a great fungal inhibitor (9 of 9), and showed activity against 9 of 11 bacteria tested, especially *E. coli. J Ethnopharm* 1994 44 and 1992 37.

Acetone extracts showed activity against gram-positive bacteria.

Large-leaved Avens fresh root tincture helps reduce fevers, in the manner of quinine. Use one half to one teaspoon in warm water every hour until improved. This same tincture can help improve and regulate liver and gall bladder function. It combines well with angelica root and silverweed root as a stomach tonic.

Dig the root as early in spring as possible. This is not always possible, unless identified the previous summer.

The leaves and stems showed activity against *Staphylococcus aureus*.

They found the plant active significantly reduces both protease and elastase activity.

Combine the dried root with dried bistort root for irritable bowel syndrome, as a warm infusion, or capsule product.

Purple or Water Avens (*G. rivale*) was studied for platelet activating factor (PAF) by Tunon et al, *J Ethnopharm* 1995 48(2). This herb and its cousin *G. urbanum* were found to be the most potent plants investigated *in vitro*.

All the avens are of similar composition and usage medicinally. Both *G. montanum and rivale* contain elastase-inhibiting activity, suggestive of benefit in skin health, collagen and cosmetics.

G. rivale leaves and roots show activity against gram negative and positive bacteria, as well as fungi. Parizzi et al, *Phytotherapy Res* 2000 14:7 This activity is probably due to its triterpene and/or flavonoid content.

Tiliroside may modulate the effects of antibiotics on MRSA (methicillin-resistant *Staphylococcus aureus*). Kuok CF et al, *Exp Biol Med* (Maywood) 2017 January 1.

The herb contains niga-ichgoside, a triterpenoid glycoside. Work by Kim YH et al, *Biol Pharm Bull* 2011 34(6): 906-11 found this compound attenuates cisplatin induced cytotoxicity by reducing oxidative stress in renal epithelial LLC-PK cells.

Water avens was written up extensively, by Dr. Cook. "Its action on the duodenum and mesenteries fits it for a class of cases to which few articles are applicable; and I am decidedly of the opinion that it will be found useful in *tabes mesenterica*, and in those forms of scrofulous looseness of the bowels which are dependent upon defective assimilation, and which often pass roughly as chronic diarrhea. This distinction between tonics to the digestive and to the assimilative apparatus, is one that has not heretofore been made; but it is one of importance, and those which act on the assimilative organs are so few as to deserve especial notice."

Water extracts of the root of *G. urbanum* have been found effective against *Staphylococcus aureus*. A water extract (20%) was injected into the bloodstream of cat and reduced blood pressure. Please don't do this to your own pet cat!

An ethanol extract was found to inhibit alpha-Synuclein fibrillation, and to partly disintegrate preformed fibrils. Lewy bodies and Lewy neurites primarily consist of this substance and are the major pathological hallmark of Parkinson's disease. Lobbens ES et al, *Biochim Biophys Acta* 2016 1864(9):1160-9.

Phloroglucinol has been found more effective than magnesium sulfate (Epsom salts) for treatment of patients with pregnancy-induced hypertension. Ai L et al, *Pak J Pharm Sci* 2016 29(4 Suppl.):1375-8.

It may be useful in treatment of retinal macular disease. Cia D et al, *J Cell Mol Med* 2016 20(9):1651-3.

The compound increases efficacy of sildenafil in diabetes-induced sexual dysfunction, and on its own reduced formation of advanced glycation end products. Goswami SK et al, *Sex Med* 2016 4(2):e104-12.

Wood Avens root infusions and decoctions have long been used for bleeding gums, gingivitis and periodontosis. Gemin A, a root constituent, shows modulating effect on the neutrophils function in reduction of bleeding of gums, via several pathways. Granica S et al, *J Ethnopharm* 2016 188:1-12.

The herb extract inhibits alpha-synuclein fibrillation, related to amyloid plaquing associated with dementia and Alzheimer's disease. Lobbens ES et al, *Biochim Biophys Acta- Proteins Proteom* 2016 1864: 1160-9.

Matthew Wood, in the *Earthwise Herbal:New World* (2009) writes. "The leaves and flowers of the beautiful little prairie avens are used by Native American people for inflammation and torsion of the ovary (Paul Red Elk, Yako Tahnahgah)….The root in decoction was used by other Native people for washing sore and inflamed eyes, sore throats, sore nipples from nursing, coughs, saddle sores, children's cankers, chapped lips, chicken pox, diarrhea, loss of flesh, (convalescence), externally to stop bleeding, and on stiff, sore muscles and joints."

HOMEOPATHY

Water Avens (*G. rivale*) is for severe jerking pains from deep in the abdomen to the end of the urethra. It is for affections of the bladder with pains in the penis. Like electric shocks and always occurring twice in succession.

The symptoms are made worse by eating, with imperfect digestion and assimilation. Excessive and depraved secretions, and relaxed mucous membranes are other symptoms.

DOSE- Tincture- 5 drops as needed. Based on self-experimentation by Hering.

ESSENTIAL OIL

Purple Avens (*G. rivale*) root contains essential oils, comprised mainly of cis-myrtanal (over 53%); and lesser amounts of pinene derivatives such as myrtanals, myrtenal, myrtanols and myrtenol.

Yield is about 0.04%, of reddish-brown oil with aromatic odor, and burning, bitter taste. The aerial parts are 34% 1-octen-3-ol.

G. urbanum is almost identical with eugenol content of root oil 69%. The aerial parts contain large amounts of aliphatic compounds with (Z)-3-hexenol at 38.4%.

FLOWER ESSENCES

Old Man's Whiskers flower essence deals with hair/aging/virility issues in men or for females who have issues relating to these aspects in their partners.   **ROCKY MTN**

Herb Bennet (*G. urbanum*) essence teaches the lessons of humility and modesty, especially useful for the profound extrovert.   **MIRIANA**

Avens (*G. triflorum*) is for precocious development of intellectual capacities with lagging emotional development; easily distracted or bored due to lack of heart attention and imagination; tendency to hyperactivity or attention deficit disorder.
                                                                      FLOWER ESSENCE SOCIETY

SPIRITUAL PROPERTIES

The star shape of the avens flower is reminiscent of the snowflake, which is a symbol of the Imbolc sabbat. Each snowflake is pure and absolutely unique. Similarly, the concept of creating from a pure space is at the center of Imbolc, which honors the generation of new ideas.   **JAMIE WOOD**

RECIPES

ROOT DECOCTION- Macerate one tsp of the dried root in one pint of boiled water. Drink between meals. For more serious conditions such as dysentery use up to a tablespoon; up to two tablespoons in more serious conditions.

For food poisoning and to help remove heavy metals, use small amounts more frequently.

The root can be boiled in milk, for those with a more sensitive system. The leaf is a more gentle and can be substituted when needed.

TINCTURE-5-15 drops. The spring root is the most fragrant, but the tincture can also be made in fall after the flowers have died back. Use a 1:4 ratio of dry root at 40%.

A tincture of the above ground leaves can be used; but is both weaker and less pleasant in flavor. Use a 40% alcohol to ensure minerals, tannins and essential oils are equally soluble.

Combine two parts avens root, with one part angelica root and silverweed root in brandy for a digestive tonic and convalescent pick me up. Take 25 ml in water before meals as an apertif, or one hour after for gas and poor digestion.

Also take 10 drops of tincture three times daily for halitosis or bad breath.

AVENS ALE- Boil one gallon water, remove from heat and add three pounds of malt extract, two pounds sugar and stir. Add three more gallons water and when 70 degrees Fahrenheit, pour into fermenter in which a muslin bag with two ounces dried or four ounces fresh avens root is placed. Add yeast and ferment for ten days. Siphon into bottles, add 1/2 teaspoon sugar, cap and store for two weeks. Drink.   **BUHNER**

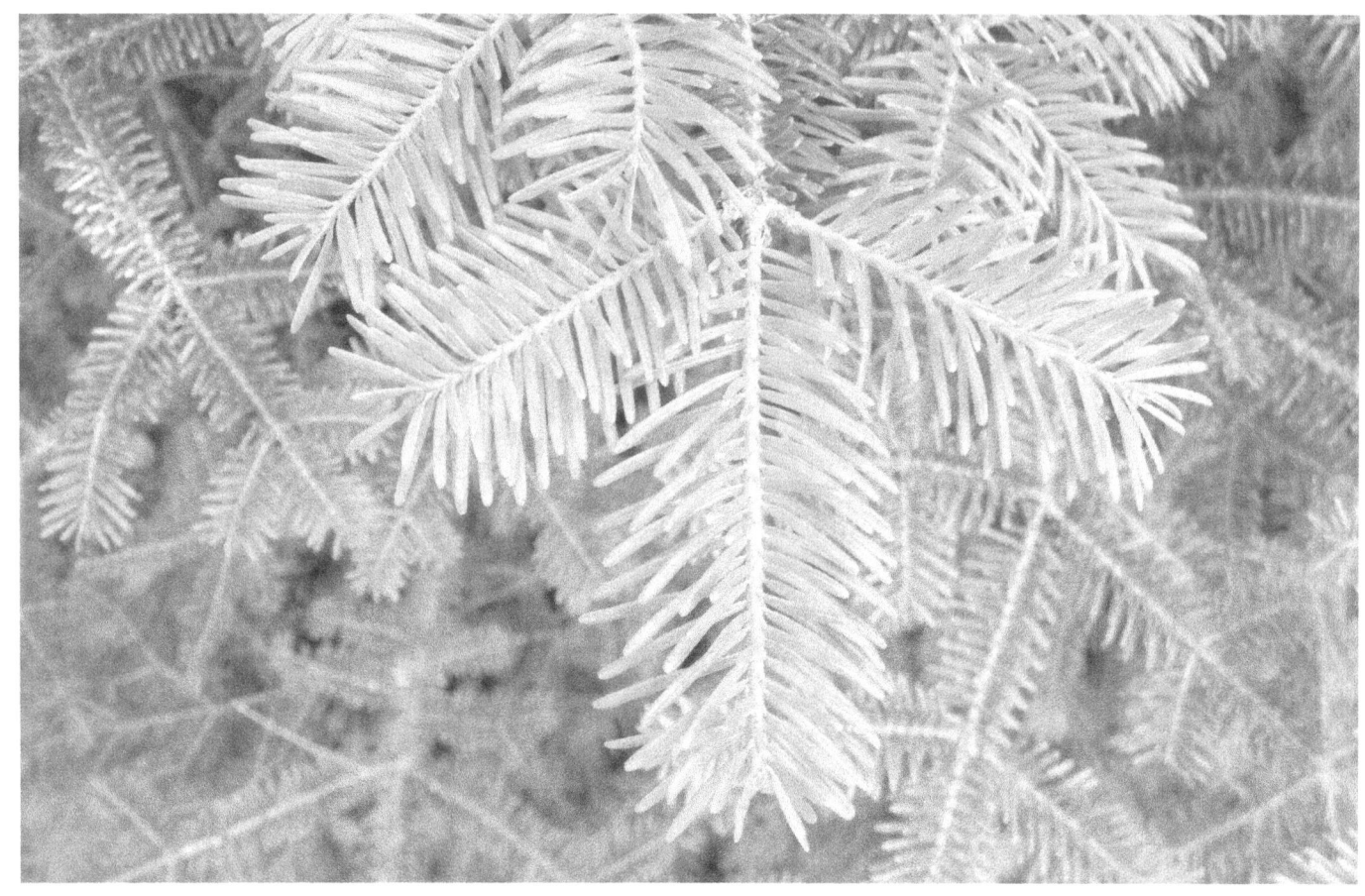

BALSAM FIR FLAT NEEDLES

BALSAM FIR
(Abies balsamea [L.] P. Mill)
SUB ALPINE FIR
(A. lasiocarpa [Hook.] Nutt.)
ROCKY MOUNTAIN ALPINE FIR
(A. lasiocarpa var. lasiocarpa [Hook.] Nutt.)
DOUGLAS FIR
(Pseudotsuga menziesii [Mirb.] Franco)
PARTS USED- bark resin, needles, roots.

Where the birds make their nests: as for the stork, the fir trees are her house.   **PSALMS 104:17**

Give me of your balm, O Fir-tree!
Of your balsam and your resin,
So to close the seams together
That the water may not enter,
That the river may not wet me!   **LONGFELLOW**

It is the time of year
When aspens shed their leaves
And decorate the fledgling firs
With golden tears.   **SID MARTY**

50

Abies is derived from the Latin **ABIRE** meaning "to rise" or "arising"; or **ALBEO** meaning "to go away" or "to depart", both in reference to the height some species attain. According to Dr. Daniel Pénoël the genus Abies means, "living for a long time", or "great longevity". Abies was the brother of the Irish king Ciladan.

Fir is derived from the Old Scandinavian **FYRI**, the Old English **FURH**, and the Danish **FYR**, meaning "fire", or firewood. The French name for fir is sapin, from the Latin sapientia meaning "wisdom".

Lasiocarpa is from the Greek **LASI**, meaning hairy or shaggy; and **CARPOS**, fruit, in reference to the rough textured cones.

Balsamea is from the Hebrew **BASHAM**, and the Arabic **BALASHAN**. The Romans made it **BALSAMUM** and then to the various English derivatives, balm, balmy, embalm. To preserve a dead body, "in balm", came from the Old French **EMBASMER**.

Balsam meant any fragrant oil or perfume, or resinous ointment that preserved, healed, or soothed. Balsam Fir is not considered a true Balsam, by some botanists/biochemists as it does not contain benzoic or cinnamic acid or their esters.

Likewise, Douglas Fir is not related to the true firs, and thus Pseudo, meaning false, and Tsuga meaning hemlock. The species was first noted and recorded by Menzies, the Scottish naturalist-physician and common name in commemoration of fellow Scotsman David Douglas. Menzies clipped off a twig in 1795, and upon his return to England, named it *Pinus taxifolia*. It was later given the binomial in his honor, but the tree is not a false hemlock, nor a fir, nor even a spruce. It is a member of pine family, but included here for my convenience.

There are two varieties, the so-called blue native to Rocky Mountains and interior, named *P. menziesii* var. *glauca*; and the coastal variety or green on the coast, *M. menziesii* var. *menziesii*.

The fir is A (ailm) in the Druidic tree alphabet, because it was a Yule tree, and represented the rebirth of the Sun. In German mythology, the God of the Forest, Vogesus dwelled in a fir tree. The tree signifies fortitude.

The Greeks used to have, in mythology, a fir tree, or Moon Goddess named Elate or Pitys. Hellenic writers later demoted her to a mere nymph in the usual transformation of every ancient Goddess into a tree to prevent some God from taking advantage of the human form. Pan's satyrs wore fir twigs in her honor.

In Poland, a female spirit, Dziwitza, roams the fir forests. Boruta, another wood spirit, is said to inhabit the Fir tree.

Fir symbolizes elevation and immortality, and birth date of January 15th; the cone represents order and December 27th.

Hildegard de Bingen mentions that "spirits of the air hate, and avoid more than in other areas, any place where there is fir tree wood. Magic thrives less and is less prevalent there than in other places."

One of my favorite childhood memories is from Nova Scotia. It is fall, late 1950s, and my grandfather and I are walking through the woods. Every once in a while, he will pause and mark a balsam fir, that will be harvested in November and shipped by rail to Florida as a Christmas Tree. Balsam Fir is the provincial tree of New Brunswick.

Balsam Fir is believed to be the original Christmas tree.

In the Hartz Mountains of Germany, young girls danced around the fir to prevent the escape of an imp who was concealed in the branches. Until he gave them presents, he was not allowed to leave, and may be the origin of Kris Kringle.

My relatives in Newfoundland call the tree Snotty Var, because of its sticky resin.

Balsam and Sub Alpine Fir often form hybrids in Alberta where their ranges overlap, and are used in a similar manner.

The Woods Cree call it **NAPAKAHSIHT**, or flat branch. I have also seen the tree called Gum Wood, or **PIKKOWAHTIK**. The pitch was used for irregular menses.

The Cree used the clear, fragrant resin from the bark blisters to treat cut, burns, and all manner of skin afflictions. It was combined with sturgeon oil as an ointment to treat tuberculosis; or taken internally for other respiratory conditions like colds, bronchitis and asthma. The bark is decocted for kidney and respiratory problems, usually in combination with roots or bark of other plants.

The Bush Cree call it a medicine tree, or infection fighter, **NAPAKÂSÎTA**. In the New Cree dictionary it is known as **SONI OKIHCIKAMEHK KOHPIKIT SIHTA**.

The resin was chewed to relieve heart and chest pains, including by the Chipewyan who call it **TS'U REKI**.

Sophie Thomas, a Sai'Kuz healer uses the pitch or sap of **TS'OOTSUN** for lung problems and tuberculosis.

The Cree sprinkled powdered needles on burns, cuts and blisters. Even the root was used, small pieces held in the mouth for relieving sores.

The Blackfoot know Alpine Fir as Sweet Pine and Holy Incense. The needle tea is used for chest colds, tuberculosis, and fevers. The bark is used for diarrhea in horses, and the needles used as a foot deodorant in moccasins. The cones are crushed into a powder and combined with fat and marrow for aiding digestion and served at social gatherings.

The Cheyenne used the fresh fir needles as incense, and burned them on coals while lightning and thunderstorms occurred to protect them; to chase away evil spirits; or revive the spirits of those with sickness and near death.

The needles were pounded into powder and combined with deer fat as a pleasant smelling hair tonic. Similar ointments were used for cuts, wounds, skin infections and ulcers, as well as bleeding gums.

The dry needle powder was used to treat open, running sores, baby powder, body scent and as a perfume and insect repellant for clothing and bedding.

Fir needles yellowed by the fungus *Melampsorella elatina* were burned as incense for ceremonial purpose. The smoke has an unusual, but delightful, scent.

The young shoots or dried bark were decocted and mixed with root of *Aralia nudicaulis* for leg ulcers, sores and cuts.

Alpine Fir resin is used as a poultice for sore backs, or to the stomach for internal bleeding.

The Blackfoot would collect the mounds of cone fragments left by squirrels and grind them to a fine powder. This was mixed with fat and marrow when melted and allowed to cool. This was given as a type of candy at social gatherings, as both a delicacy and aid to digestion.

The Gitksan of British Columbia used Alpine Fir, or **HOO'OXS**, bark blisters or the young cones. Picked in August, they were sliced and mashed as a purgative and diuretic in treating tuberculosis and gonorrhea.

Further east, the Iroquois combined a few drops of balsam fir resin in milk for colds, and mixed the gum resin with beaver kidneys to treat an unspecified cancer.

The Ojibwa mixed the resin with bear fat as an ointment for treating wounds, cuts and burns; or as a hair treatment. The Forest Potawatomi used the blister resin for colds and infusions of the bark for consumption (TB). They call it Peaked Top or **KEKI'NTEBA**.

The Mi'kmaq used fir cones to treat colic, and boiled the inner bark to wash sores and swellings.

The root was boiled for heart conditions.

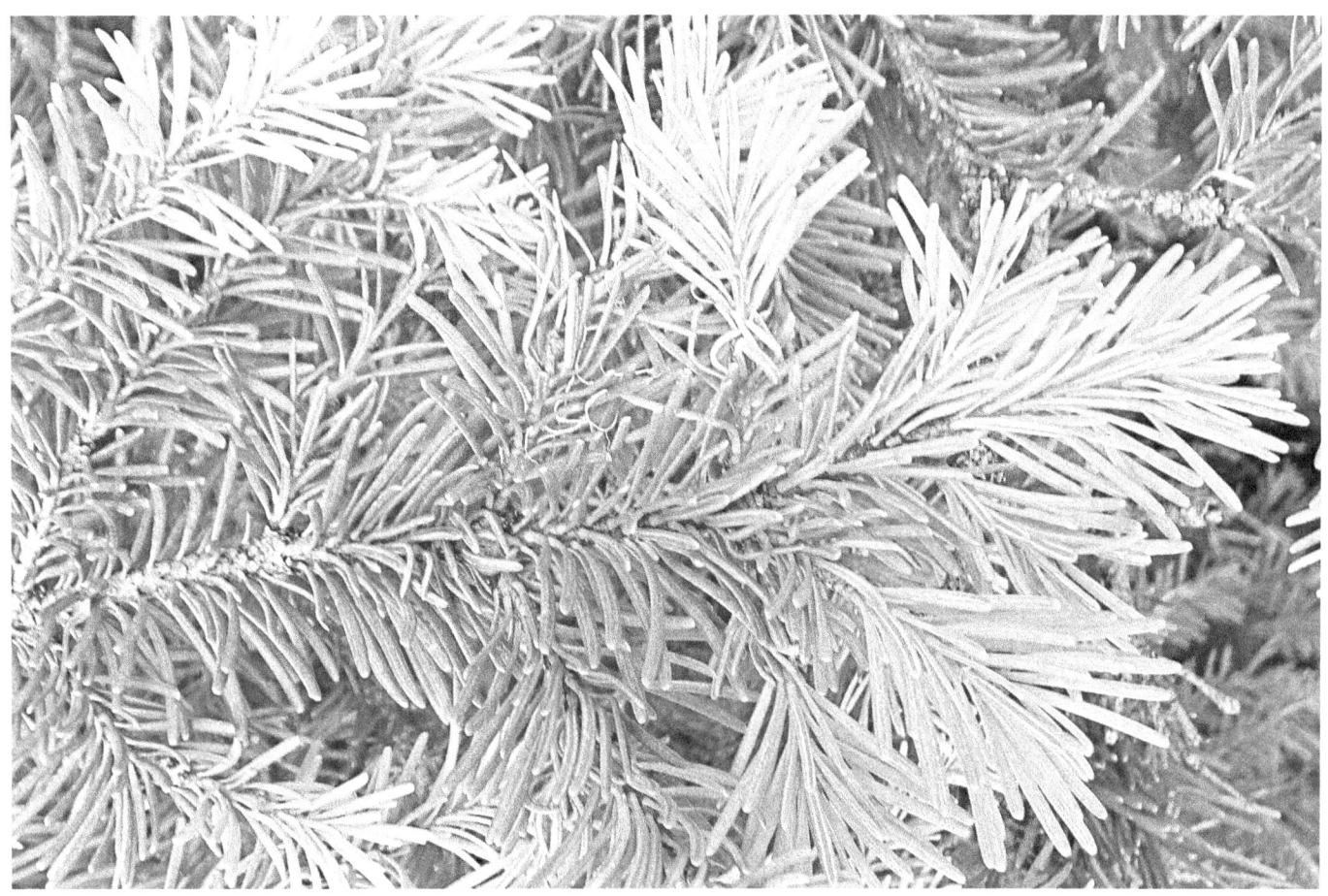

ALPINE FIR NEEDLES

The resin has been used in the past as a varnish to protect watercolour paintings. This clear resin is used, by wasps and bees, to waterproof their hives and provide anti-bacterial and anti-fungal protection.

Balsam Fir has a unique anti-feeding deterrent in the form of a juvenile hormone, jubavione. An insect feeding on Balsam Fir has no reproductive future, and hence it offspring will never graze on balsam firs.

This was discovered quite by accident when a researcher was traveling in the United States with one thousand larvae in his luggage. The larvae fed quite happily on newspaper, until ingesting the New York Times prevented pupation and they literally exploded. Further investigation revealed the pulp was from Balsam Fir, which contains jubavione in toxic levels.

Young firs protect themselves from rabbits, deer and moose by producing lasiocarpenone, a liver toxin.

Balsam fir is not as hard, heavy, or strong as spruce, and takes twice as long to dry as a construction material.

It is prized for pulp and paper, as its long fibres are useful in cardboard, newspaper and other paper products. Balsam fir branches, stripped of their needles act as a weather barometer, stand straight out for fair weather and point down for impeding rain.

Although similar in appearance, Sub Alpine and Rocky Mountain Alpine Fir are now considered distinctive, though formerly grouped together. The main difference, besides some chemical make-up is that the former is red under the bark, and the latter more tan colored.

Douglas fir (*Pseudotsuga menziesii var. glauca*) grows in the interior of British Columbia, and east to Calgary. They were more prevalent at one time, with one specimen from the Porcupine Hills near Nanton growing to

98 feet all, with a 70 inch diameter and living to 381 years old. Along the Bow River at the west end of Calgary are some specimens 350 to 400 years old.

They are larger on the west coast, with one tree felled in 1895 measuring 415 feet tall.

One other Douglas fir found on rocky cliffs near Jasper, has been determined to be over 700 years old.

Like all trees, Douglas fir root releases compounds that initiate mycelia spore germination.

These mycorrhiza form a symbiotic relationship with the tree, helping increase the uptake of nitrogen and phosphorus by some 7,000%, and produce polysaccharides that boost the tree's immune system, and daughter trees in same area.

Douglas Fir may be in symbiosis with as many as forty different species of fungi and spread hundreds of acres underground.

The tree forms a rare type of tri-saccharide sugar, 75-83% melezitose, but only in certain years.

In the hottest days of summer with warm nights, and on north facing slopes with adequate soil moisture, this wild sugar will begin to exude from the needles and congeal. It is honeydew, created by aphids that utilize sucrase enzymes.

The cones look like mice feet and tails are sticking out, and this was incorporated into a legend that involved the little rodents seeking shelter in the cones during a storm.

The Cowlitz placed the cones close to fire to appeal to the spirit for sunshine. The Skagit burned the cones to help direct the wind. The Swinomish decocted the needles as a general tonic tea. Other indigenous groups decocted the branches and drank the tea in the sweathouse for purification.

The bark is known as **ITHARIIP**, by the Karuk. They dried the new, needle tips of branches for gargle infusions, to treat tonsillitis and sore throats. The small branchlets are used as warp for forming fine baskets.

The Salish of southern Vancouver Island used the bark for respiratory ailments. Turner NJ & Hebda RJ, *J Ethnopharm* 1990 29(1): 59-72. It is known as **JSÁY (ch'sey')** to the Wsanec people of the Saanich pensinsula.

When available, it can be a nice addition to Fir Ale.

The tree symbolizes perseverance in the pursuit of knowledge, and a birth date of December 16th.

Douglas Fir releases a volatile oil from their needles in response to spruce budworm aggression. The firewood is prized, giving a hot, fast, smoke-less flame.

It was used traditionally to carve spoons, seal harpoon shafts, fire tongs, etc. The knots were moulded into curved hooks for halibut. The knots were steamed by placing them in a hollow kelp stem overnight, and then bending them to proper shape. After this, they were rubbed with animal fat to retain their desired shape.

The pitch was used to patch canoes and water containers, or a salve for wounds.

The trees regulate the amounts of individual and total terpene production based on the time of day, year, location and infestation, increasing terpenes by 500-600% between the middle of June and end of July, when budworms are most active.

Bornyl acetate increases from 0.25 mg/g to 1.0 mg/g fresh weight between June 18 and July 8th.

The trees vary the composition and production of terpenes every year, decreasing the ability of the insect to develop immunity to any one compound.

Collectively, the coniferous forests of the world release more than two trillion pounds of volatile terpenes into the atmosphere, with plants such as ragweed, yarrow and various artemisia contributing several trillion more. This falls with the rain, helping plants keep themselves and our ecosystems healthy.

Both Balsam and Alpine Fir seeds have a market for tree nurseries. Balsam Fir averages nearly 60,000 seeds per pound, while Alpine is closer to 35,000. If you think this is good, and are considering quitting your day job, realize that one cone of Balsam Fir contains about 134 seeds; or put another way, a yield of 37-46 ounces of seeds per bushel of cones.

In 1969, a patent was obtained in the former Czechoslovakia for the use of de-hydrojuvabione as an insecticide.

In 1985 a Japanese patent was granted for use the of polyprenyl compound from Abies leaves, as intermediates of mammalian dolichols.

Today, the yellow oleoresin from the bark blisters is still marketed as Canada Balsam, and used to seal microscope slides, and as a cement for clear glassware.

It should rightly be called true turpentine, because it is a combination of resin and essential oil, and does not contain any benzoic or cinnamic acid as mentioned above.

Two novel diterpenoid toxins have been found on an un-identified insect on the needles of balsam fir. They are 9alpha-hydroxy-1,8(14), 15-isopimaratrien-3-7,11-trione and 9alpha-hydroxy-1,8(14),15-isopimaratrien-3,11-dione.

Both of these toxins have been found to kill the spruce budworm cells and larvae.

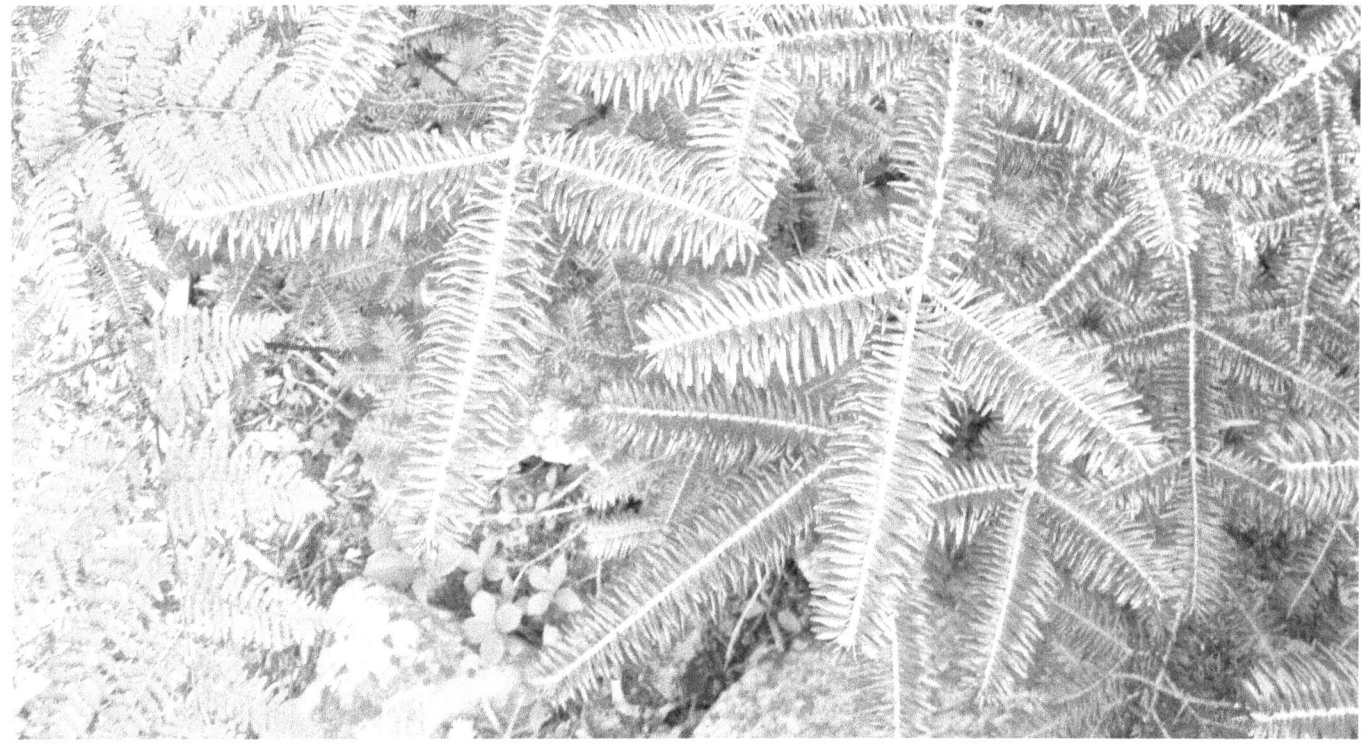

FIR NEEDLES

MEDICINAL

CONSTITUENTS *A. balsamea*- abienol, abietic acid, dehydroabietic acid, abietin (coniferin) abieslactone, camphene, limonene, pinene, alpha phellandrene and other monoterpenes, as well as sesquiterpenoids like dehydrojuvabione, and jubabione, Δ^3-carene, campesterol, beta sitosterol, triterpenoids, alpha and beta amyrin, allobetulin, betulin, and squalene.
Needles and shoots-fresh- 270 mg/100 g of reduced ascorbic acid.
A. lasiocarpa- sesquiterpenoids like 1'(Z) and 1'(E)-dehydrojuvabione; 2'dehydrojuvani-1'-ol, juvabiol, juvabione, lasiocarpenone, aromadendrin 3-galactoside
P. menziesii- bark- pseudotsuganol (flavonolignan), cinnamtannin A1(procyanidin oligomer)

Balsam resin was used traditionally in cough drops, and considered equal or superior to copaiba. It was official medicine in the U.S. *Pharmacopoeia* from 1820-1916. The gum resin from the bark bubbles can be boiled, and the steam inhaled to relieve sinus congestion, or added to a chest plaster in combination with other herbs.

The resin may be combined with canola oil (1:4), and used to relieve joint and muscle pain associated with arthritis, rheumatism and over-exertion.

This same oil combination is very useful for bacterial infections of the skin, and to soothe itching hemorrhoids, but should not be used on sensitive, granulating, or inflamed sores.

The bark was boiled and used as a poultice applied to boils, or taken as a decoction internally for infections, to purify the bowels and blood, and to treat everything from gout, to menstrual irregularity to coughs to worms. The mucilaginous, stimulating/relaxing tea can relieve soreness of the kidneys and urethra, as well as diarrhea.

Michaux said the resin caused inflammation and acute pain and if given "inconsiderately causes heat in the bladder". Dosage is important.

The tree can be tapped, and the sap boiled down to thin syrup for treating sore throats.

The inner bark was used as a tea for chest pains, gastro-intestinal inflammation, and difficult urinary infections.

The compound, abietic acid, may be of great value in treating allergies, due to its ability to inhibit lipoxygenase activity. Ulvsu et al, *Phytotherapy Research* 16:1.

The twig tea is considered a good laxative. The needles, containing pinenes, humulenes and beta caryophyllene, possess activity against *Staphylococcus aureus*. Pichette et al, *Phytotherapy Research* 20:5.

The inner bark was also dried, ground, and mixed with flour, or decocted with other herbs as a steam for delayed childbirth.

Use bark decoctions as a diaphoretic during flu.

The young buds contain picein, and have been used as a substitute for Balm of Gilead.

Fir needle infusions are useful for laxative effect.

Balsam fir alcohol and ether extracts shows activity against *Staphylococcus aureus*.

Abies and *Picea* species contain Δ^3-carene, a monoterpene also known as isodiprene. It is an oxytocin receptor agonist that is anti-inflammatory and induces uterine contraction.

Balsam fir inhibits, *in vitro*, CYP3A4 liver enzyme system suggesting it extends the half life of other herbs and drugs. This suggests, in theory, attention with certain prescription medications. Tam et al, *Can J Physio Pharmacol* 2011 89:1 13-23.

The compounds abietic acid, dehydroabietic acid and squalene, derived from the tree, help regulate liver cell glucose balance and may have application for the treatment of type 2 diabetes and insulin resistance. Nachar A et al, *Phytochemistry* 2015 117:373-9.

Abietic acid is a liver protectant and induces apoptosis in human cervical cancer (HeLa) cell lines. Ramnath MG et al, *Pharmacognosy Research* 2016 8(3):206-8.

It also improved the efficacy of Taxol on human melanoma cancer cells, suggesting an adjuvant in this deadly disease. Hsieh YS et al, *Am J Chin Med* 2015 43(8):1697-714.

It attenuates allergic airway inflammation in a mouse model of asthma, possibly by inhibition of NF-kappaB activation. Gao Y et al, *Int Immunopharmacol* 2016 38:261-6.

Early work suggests it may be useful in Chagas disease, demonstrating *in vivo* activity against *Trypanosoma cruzi*, and low toxicity. Olmo F et al, *Eur J Med Chem* 2015 89:683-90.

Dehydroabietic acid (DHAA) appears to be most effective. This compound is present in many pine and fir species. It is believed to be an anti-aging compound that mediates the direct activation of SIRT1, acting as a preventive against the aging process. Kim J et al, *Mol Cell Endocrinol* 2015 412:216-25.

DHAA reduces excitability in dorsal root ganglion neurons, suggesting benefit in the treatment of hyper-excitability disease. A number of conditions quickly come to mind, including ADD, ADHD, epilepsy, etc. Ottosson NE et al, *Sci Rep* 2015 5:13278.

DHAA is a positive GABA A receptor modulator, suggesting benefit in calming nervous conditions. Rueda DC et al, *Fitoterapia* 2014 99:28-34.

The compound induces gastric cancer cell death via oncosis and apoptosis. Luo D et al, *Biomed Res Int* 2016:2581061. Recent work has found abietic and dehydroabietic acids naturally occurring in cyanobacteria.

DHAA shows activity against drug resistant strains of *Staphylococcus epidermis*. Leandro LF et al, *J Med Microbiol* 2014 63 (pt12):1649-53.

Abieslactone induces cell cycle arrest and apoptosis in human hepatic carcinoma. Wang GW et al, *PLoS One* 2014 9(12):e115151.

Abies and *Larix* species contain coniferin or abietin, which upon digestion yields the active anti-PTH aglycone. Coniferyl alcohol inhibits PTH induced bone resorption and is anti-fungal. Angelica species, comfrey, beets, asparagus and larch all contain coniferin.

Cis-abienol (labdane diterpene) inhibits ornithine decarboxylase induction by 12-tetradecanoylphorbol 13-acetate.

Alpine fir needles contain aromadendrin 3-galactoside, also found in buckwheat seed.

Work by Ritch-Krc et al, found pure pitch of sub-alpine fir strongly active against *E. coli, Staphylococcus aureus, Pseudomonas aeruginosa, C. albicans* and *Aspergillus fumigatus*. J Ethnopharm 1996 52 151-156.

Douglas Fir (*Pseudotsuga menziesii*) bark contains various catechin derivatives that inhibit heart cAMP protein kinases. Polya GM and Foo LY, *Phytochemistry* 1994 35(6):1399-405.

Douglas fir bark contains pseudotsuganol with proven anti-hepatoxic properties. It is a plant growth regulator. Another bark constituent is cinnamtannin A1, which inhibits protein kinases.

Cinnamtannin B1 inhibits splenocyte proliferation, suggestive of immunosuppressive activity. It use or benefit in humans has yet to be determined. Chen L et al, *Evid Based Complement Alternat Med* 2014:365258.

Work by Towers et al at UBC, found fir tree extracts active against all 7 bacterial species tested. The Grand Fir, common in the province, showed similar results.

The bark contains 28-43% total extractives of various uses.

HOMEOPATHY

Balsam Fir is for delusion of being obstructed, from moving forward; or delusion of being persecuted, criticized or attacked.

There is anger at perceived rudeness of others. Issues of time, dreams and delusions of trees, upset over trees cut down, conflicts and mother issues.

Left side more affected, sensation of pressure presenting as gas, bubbles or lumps. Sensation as if top of brain will lift off from pressure, heavy and unable to hold it up.

Cold extremities, yet desire to go outside to get fresh air. Better standing, aversion to sitting, craving for meat and sweets.

DOSE- 30c potency. Proving by Christopher Sowton with ten provers in Canada in 2006.

Douglas Fir is for anxiety when alone, or delusions of being alone in the world, being despised, criticized or insulted. Hard feeling accepted, and isolated from people, anti-social, desire for company but aggravated by it.

Critical of small things, fear of opinion of others. Dreams of killing, being pursued, fights.

Increased appetite, tendency to overeat and then bulimia, sleepless with restless legs. Alcoholism.

Douglas Fir (*P. menziesii var. menziesii*) was proved by Steve Olsen, with sixteen provers at 30c in 1995. Krista Heron adds two cases in 1999.

ESSENTIAL OIL

Balsam fir yields about 1.0-1.4% of an essential oil, upon distillation of the young branches and leaves.

Material from a 15 year-old tree yields about 70% more oil than one over a hundred years old. Yield is highest in January to March, and again in September; and lowest from April to August.

Western Balsam Fir oil is 40% beta pinene, 12% alpha pinene, 12% bornyl acetate, 15% limonene, with minor components of camphene, and beta phellandrene. It has a specific gravity of 0.8800-0.8890, and a saponification number of 30.5 on average.

Balsam Fir oil is expectorant, analgesic, antiseptic, stimulating and toning. It helps relieve depression, and is uplifting in spirit.

Balsam Fir Oil was evaluated against several solid tumor cell lines and found active against all, with alpha humulene likely responsible for the cytotoxicity of the oil. Legault et al, *Planta Medica* 2003 69.

Alpha pinene, beta carophyllene and alpha humulene all show activity against *Staphylococcus aureus*. Pichette et al, *Phyto Res* 2006 20:5.

Fir needle oil is used in pet care deodorizing shampoos, such as 8 in 1 Perfect Coat Select Shampoo.

Alpine fir needle essential oil is from 23-51% beta phellandrene, 3-28% limonene, 5-20% beta pinene, and 5-21% bornyl acetate.

An absolute of the Balsam Fir is made by treating the needles and twigs with benzene to produce a concrete. This is washed with 95% alcohol to produce an absolute with balsamic, fruity and coumaric notes. This is dark green, and syrupy, very true to nature; like a freshly fallen tree, or Christmas tree.

The Oleoresin (see below) can be steam distilled, and yields from 15-25% of an essential oil. It is nearly colorless, and resembles templin oil, produced from silver fir cones.

It is composed mainly of alpha and beta pinene (21-44%), beta phellandrene (20%), camphene (4-11%), carene (7-35%) and limonene (3-20%), esters (bornyl acetate (9-23%), juvabione and alcohols. It has a specific gravity of 0.8605-0.8614.

The oil is used in certain ointments and creams as an antiseptic and treatment for hemorrhoids.

In France, the oil is used as a stimulant, and for its anti-spasmodic and anti-arthritic applications. It is antiseptic and anti-parasitic against ascaris worms. In sinusitis and rhinitis, it fights *Staphylococcus* bacteria. Recent work found the oleoresin active against *S. aureus* and MRSA (methicillin-resistant *Staphylococcus aureus*). Coté H et al, *Journal of Ethnopharmacology* 2016 194:684-89.

Abibalsamins, isolated from the oleoresin, show moderate cytotoxicity against A549 lung carcinoma cells. Lavoie S et al, *J Nat Prod* 2015 78(12):2896-907.

It was used, at one time, in dentistry as an ingredient in root canal sealers.

The oleoresin is a component of Collodion, a material substance for adhesive plasters in surgery for coating wounds and burns.

It is used as a fixative or fragrance in soaps, detergents, cosmetics and perfumes with maximum levels of 0.15% in soaps, and 0.2% in perfume. One example is Suave Shampoo with Balsam and Protein.

There is even some minor use in food and alcohol products.

Douglas Fir needles yield a pleasant essential oil composed of beta pinene, at twice the content of alpha pinene. In smaller amounts are limonene, 3-carene, p-cymene, myrcene, camphene (up to 30%), bornyl acetate (up to 35%) and gamma terpinene.

The oil has a somewhat citrusy-pineapple note that is very pleasant variation on the coniferous theme.

Bennet distilled needle oil and found it 31.5% geraniol, disguised by the presence of bornyl acetate. I'm not sure, but the presence of this percentage of geraniol does surprise me somewhat.

The essential oil is used for all manner of respiratory problem, including bronchitis, urinary tract infections and stomach cramps.

It helps support a healthy nervous system and has both an elevating and stabilizing effect on the mind and emotions.

It shows good fungicide activity, higher than commercial bifonazole. Activity against *Phomopsis helianthi* was noted by Vele Tesevic et al, *Serb Chem Society* 2009 74 10.

Studies have shown the wood essential oil to be active against *Actinomyces bovis*. Johnston et al, *Phyto Res* 2001 15:7.

WAX

Douglas Fir bark wax has a melting point of 59-63 degrees Celsius. It is harder than beeswax, and with chemical treatment can be make superior to carnauba wax.

The light, green brown wax could be used for polishes, internal lubricant for molded plastics, concrete additives, slow release fertilizer, carbon papers, as a fruit coating, or in cosmetics.

The specific gravity is 1.020, with an iodine value of 28-62, acid value of 58-80 and saponification value of 112-200, a very wide range indeed.

After removal of wax, the granulated bark fiber could be used as a plywood glue extender, or reinforcing fiber in plastics.

OLEORESIN

A liquid oleoresin can be collected from the bark vesicles of both balsam and alpine fir.

The blisters are punctured and drained from mid July to mid-August, and collected in glass or metal containers.

It is a pale yellow, to yellowish green transparent mass with a pleasant turpentine-citrus odor. It is used in Cologne and verbena compounds up to 10%, as well as a fixative in soap perfumes.

When exposed to air, it forms and dries a transparent varnish, but very slowly.

Due to its ability to dry to a brittle, clear glass-like residue, the oleoresin freed from the volatile oil above, and dissolved in xylene, is used for cement in lenses and prepared microscopic slides. At the turn of the 20th century, Quebecers were collecting twenty tons a year, but by the 1960s it was only fetching three dollars a pound. Optical lenses became cheaper and plastics replaced balsam oleoresin as cement.

It is used in some Balsam hair grooming products for its ability to stiffen hair and give it body.

HYDROSOL

The water left over from distillation of Balsam Fir can be used medicinally. To me, the smell is musky and cat urine-like, similar to the needles.

To others, it is woody and green. The pH is 3.8 to 4.0.

Suzanne Catty recommends adding one quarter to one half cup 2-3 times weekly in your bath, or foot soaks. She personally finds it of great help in combating SAD (seasonal affective disorder).

It is a general tonic, with mild diuretic effect, that supports the immune system and possesses mucolytic activity.

It may be used as the base of cough syrups, or as a compress for rheumatic, arthritic and joint pain, or soothing foot soak.

Mentally, the hydrosol is excellent as an addition to baths for "winter blues", and is "energetically expansive, and it promotes honesty of emotions", according to Catty.

FLOWER ESSENCES

Douglas Fir essence is for relatedness and finding one's place. It brings spontaneous energy and freedom to be oneself.   **GREEN MAN**

Arizona Fir (*A. lasiocarpa var. compacta*) essence helps us celebrate life and existence as spiritual based beings.
BAILEY

SPIRITUAL PROPERTIES

The Shasta Indians had another interesting use for the (Douglas) Fir. At their funeral ceremonies they danced about the body of their deceased tribes fellow with staves of Fir clasped firmly in their hands and Fir branches attached to their bodies. Why Fir staves and Fir branches? What did this tree have to offer that others didn't?

Was it the source of a kind of good luck charm? Or did it comprise a sort of preventative medicine? Or did it play both these roles simultaneously?   **WESTRICH**

Douglas fir's special teaching is how to enjoy your uniqueness and build your self-confidence, without being stuck in the trap of excessive ego, or pride. When you belittle yourself, doubt your abilities, or feel insignificant, Douglas fir helps you to stand tall and affirm your attributes or talents.

On the other hand, if your ego gets out of hand, Douglas fir teaches you about humility. It activates a quality of self-reliance and a quiet pride that looks inside for self-definition rather than to others, so that you can go about your business with poise and self esteem.   **CHASE & PAWLIK**

PERSONALITY TRAITS

Douglas Fir occurs as two distinct varieties: coastal and inland.

The coastal tree thrives in mild, moist conditions, where it can grow to 250 feet tall and six feet in diameter and live more than 500 years.

The inland variety, on the other hand, is hardened to a tougher existence, ready to withstand dry, cold interior conditions. There it grows more slowly and is much smaller than its coastal cousin.

Two very different lifestyles, and it would seem the coastal variety has the much better deal. But its existence is not without challenge. All that moisture creates a favourable environment for root rot disease, a great destroyer of this coastal king.

People are quick to compare their lifestyles with that of another. And often we feel ourselves falling short of another whose comfy existence seems replete with life's perks. But where you are today may have little to do with where you'll be tomorrow. And comparing your lifestyle to that of another is futile because you do no know that person's full situation. While your struggles may be more visible, another's may be hidden but equally hard.

G. MOHAMMED

Douglas fir oil is one of the primary oils to consider whenever anxiety disorder and primal fear is fueled by a sense of powerlessness- when one is open and exposed to life's buffeting winds and invasive factors and unable to find shelter from the storm sufficient to allow full flowering of the soul's creativity. Accordingly, the Douglas fir type is stalked by a recurring feeling of inferiority relative to his environment, society, etc…The Douglas fir type typically has a weakness in the chest, especially involving the rhythmicity of the heart/lung interaction. Thus, he tends to experience his feelings of anxiety and fear in his chest—a sense of profound uneasiness sometimes accompanied by rapid heart rate, palpitations and/or shallow, rapid breathing…In cases where male nurturing/protective influence has been historically deficient or lacking, Douglas fir is worthy of consideration, especially when anxiety and fear is reported as being experienced in the chest.

BERKOWSKY

At the most basic level, the Pseudotsuga-person seems to have lost the ability to create intimacy, or be nourished by intimacy. As the emotions are very alive, the starvation of love creates a pain that develops into feelings of loneliness, mixed with anger.

The person will express this as a deep sense of isolation and separation, of not belonging to anything or anyone.

It seems that Pseudotsuga will work only in cases where the people feel a fundamental separation from family, as if they do not belong and are rejected. This feeling starves them spiritually. They become angry and critical. They search for a 'fill-up' thus the bulimia.

STEVE OLSEN

Global aerosols are released from the modified leaves of balsam fir…the vast volume of pinene and its daughter compounds released into the global airway acts as an air cleanser and deodorant on a massive scale. The flush of this health-giving air affects all mammals, among which man is just one beneficiary.

BERESFORD-KROEGER

What has been explained from the botanical point of view also has a bearing on the significance of the symbolic nature of the Christmas tree. In putting lights on these trees we continue where nature left off. What else can the lights mean but making the tree radiant as if it were in bloom?… 'A tree can only become a flowering flame, man a speaking flame, an animal a moving flame,' says Novalis clairvoyantly in his Fragments…Symbolically speaking, we redeem the fir from its rigid, wood-bound state when we put lights on its hardened twigs. The tree itself is a symbol of mankind becoming entangled in the meshes of the material world and longingly awaiting redemption. Man's hopes speak from the Christmas tree.

GROHMANN

When you light up the tree on Christmas eve, making sure it is a fir and not a pine or spruce or hemlock, for we use all sorts of evergreens in our celebration, you may learn your fate, if you have courage to look at your shadow on the wall.

If the shadow appears without a head, it signifies that you are to die within the coming year. If you will cut off a branch and lay it across the foot of your bed, it will keep away nightmares. A stick of fir, not quite burned through, tends off lightning, and a bunch hung at the barn door keeps out evil spirits that want to steal the grain.

SKINNER

ASTROLOGY

Conifers are completely dominated by Saturn and the forces that inhibit growth processes, contract substance and harden form…The very needle shape only allows the smallest possible contact with the environment. Saturn governs the conifers and many of them reach sexual maturity only after the planet has performed on full cycle [twenty eight years]. Saturn's long rhythm also grants them long life. With their confined, hard shapes they can venture deeper into the winter, into the mountains and into the north than any other tree or shrub…Conifers have such an intimate part in the exchange of these mighty forces that their shape displays an even geometry that is reminiscent of the molecular structure of crystals or the physical patterns of starlight. These "green snowflakes' are much closer to the mineral world than their deciduous relatives.

HAGENEDER

MYTHS AND LEGENDS

The Saanich Story of How Douglas-Fir Got Pitch.

Pitch was a man who used to go fishing before the sun rose and retire to the shade before it became strong. One day he was late and had just reached the beach when he melted. Other people rushed to share him. Fir arrived first and secured most of the pitch, which he poured over his head and body. Balsam [grand fir] obtained only a little and by the time Arbutus arrived there was none left. Arbutus said, "I shall have to peel my skin every year and have a good wash to keep me clean." But just then ***XALS*** appeared and said, "You shall all be trees, and Fir shall be your boss. So now the arbutus sheds its bark every year, and fir has more pitch than any other tree.
NANCY TURNER 2005

A native American myth holds that each of the three-pointed bracts (on cones) represents the tail and back legs of a mouse that hid within the cone's scales, because the Douglas fir tree was kind enough to provide sanctuary for the creatures during forest fires. This myth also reflects the intermingling of the themes of protection and nurturing and the oil's resultant specificity for the feelings of vulnerability. **B. BERKOWSKY**

RECIPES

FIR ALE- Use the fresh spring tips and prepare, as for spruce beer. If you are fortunate enough to procure Douglas fir sugar, simply reduce sugar content from other sources in recipe.

BALSAM FIR SYRUP- Simmer 250 grams of balsam fir shoots in double the water, using a stainless steel pot, for twenty minutes. Remove from heat and let sit for further hour. Strain, and add one cup of honey. Return to low heat for 10 minutes; cool and bottle. Store in fridge. Excellent syrup for lung and intestinal congestion. Use one Tbsp as required. Shelf life of three months may be tripled using white sugar.

BARK DECOCTION- One cup chopped bark per quart of water. Simmer for 15 minutes, cool and strain. Drink warm in sauna or hot bath to stimulate sweating.

NEEDLE INFUSION- Three cups of needles to one quart of hot water. Steep for one half hour. Drink a cup morning and evening with meals for no more than three days.

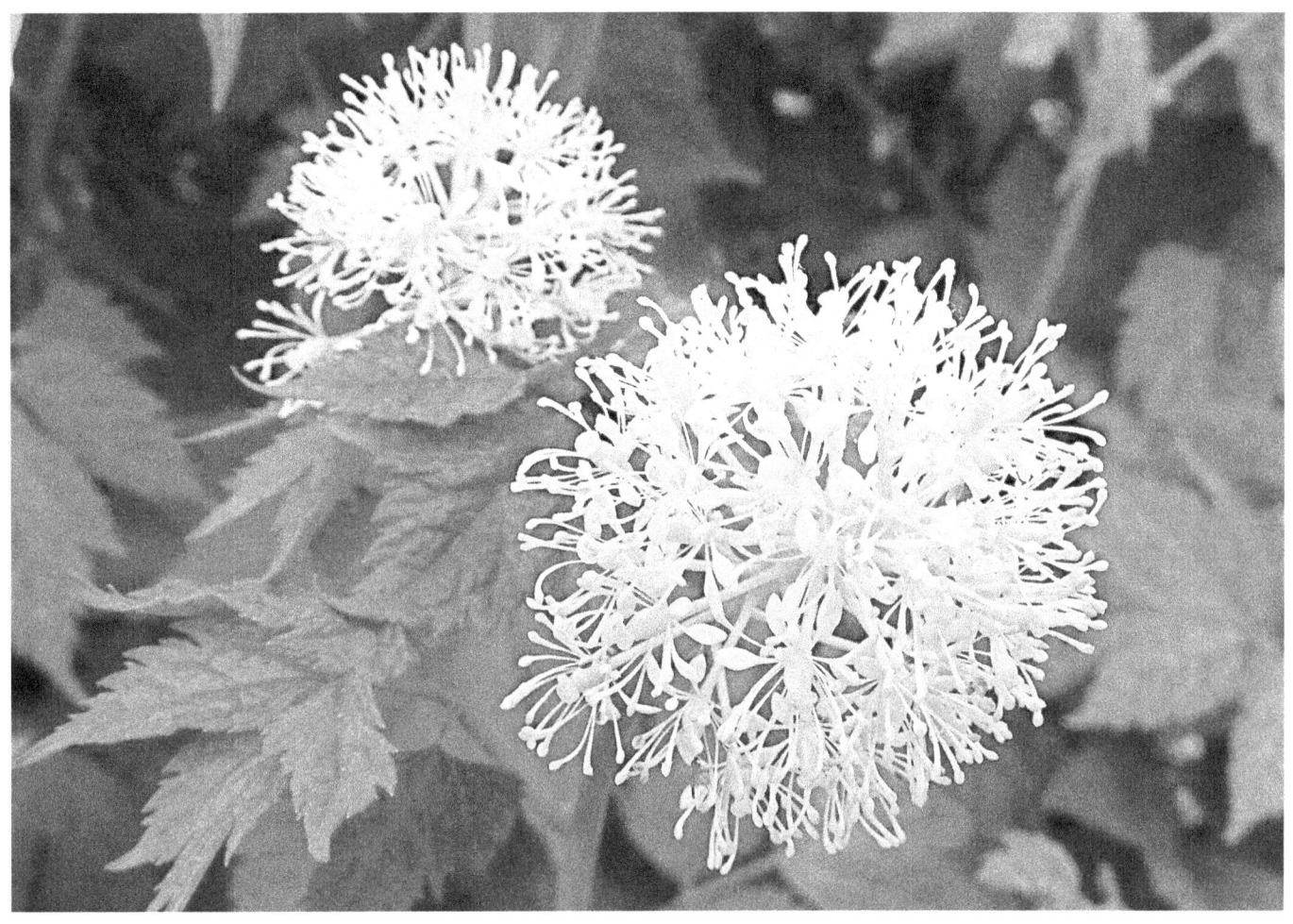

BANEBERRY FLOWERS

WHITE BANEBERRY
(Actaea rubra forma neglecta)
RED BANEBERRY
(A. rubra [Ait.] Willd.*)*
(A. rubra [Aiton] Willd. *ssp. arguta* [Nutt.] Hulten*)*
(A. arguta Nutt.*)*
EASTERN WHITE COHOSH
(A. pachypoda)
PART USED- root, flowers

World's use is cold, world's love is vain

World's cruelty is bitter bane; but is not the fruit of pain.   **ELIZABETH BROWNING**

Peter hopped over to smell of them. Then he made a wry face. They didn't smell good. No sir, he didn't like the smell of them.

Mrs. Grouse chuckled. "Those flowers are much like the berries they will turn into later-good to look at only," she said.

"Aren't the berries good to eat?" demanded Peter. Mrs. Grouse shook her head in a very decided way. "They are poisonous," she said. "I advise you never to try one of them".   **THORNTON W. BURGESS**

Baneberry comes from the Anglo-Saxon **BANA**, meaning murderous, or Teutonic **BANON** meaning, "that which causes death, or destroys life." The genus comes from the Greek word for elder, **AKTAIA**, due to the resemblance of the leaf shape. It may also derive from Actaeon, the mythological hunter turned into a stag by Diana, after he viewed her undressed. The stag was attacked and killed by wild dogs to complete the story.

Pachypoda means thick-footed, or thick-stalked. Podocarpa means, carpels with a foot or stipitate base; or simply put "with stalked-fruit."

The shiny white or red waxy berries are considered poisonous by many authors.

Although there has been no loss of life reported in the United States or Canada, European children have reportedly died after eating black baneberry (*A. spicata*) fruit. This is highly unlikely.

I have nibbled on both white and red berries, which are quite bitter, with no ill effect. A professor Muenscher wrote of *A. rubra*: "Eating six berries was sufficient to produce increased pulse, dizziness, burning in the stomach and colicky pains." I doubt he tried them himself.

Known as Herb Christopher, Toad berry or Troll Grape, the black baneberry was considered a bewitching or conjuring herb.

There is considerable confusion regarding the red and white berry plants taxonomically. *Actaea rubra* and *A. rubra f. neglecta* are the red and white berry forms found in western North America, up to the far north. The berries contain at least ten seeds.

White baneberry or cohosh (*A. pachypoda*) has white berries on red stems, and from 3-9 seeds.

Another species, *A. podocarpa*, is found in Appalachian hills and appears at first glance to resemble a short Black Cohosh (*A. racemosa*).

In 1903, Alice Bacon of Vermont experimented with the white berry (*A. pachypoda*?). She took increasing doses over a period of several days. The last batch caused "intense hallucinogenic displays with various blue shapes followed by confusion, incoherency, and dizziness. Other symptoms she reported were parched throat, difficult swallowing, an intense burning in the stomach with gaseous belches". She recovered after a few hours.

Black Bears have been observed eating the berries, with no apparent ill effect.

Natives of Alberta used the plant for rheumatism, but more as external applications to the affected areas than internally. The leaves were chewed and applied to bring boils to a head. Newborn babies were bathed in warm water, and the mouth, nostrils and eyes were washed with a root infusion, according to Al Burger.

The Blackfoot used baneberry root decoction for coughs and colds, or to treat their sick horses. The red form is called **SIXA-WA-KASIM**, and the white berry **SIXAS**. Like the Chipewyan, only the root of the white-berried plant was considered useful for medicine.

The Blackfeet of Montana call both red and white baneberry, "Black Roots", and decocted the root for coughs and colds.

The Saskatchewan Woods Cree call it **MASKOMINANATIK**. They used infusions of a small piece of the root to slow down excessive menstrual flow. A decoction of spruce needles and baneberry root was used as a purgative, and for various stomach complaints including constipation.

The Chippewa used **WAPKADAK**, white baneberry root, for convulsions in both adults and children; and for excessive menstrual flow.

The roots were rolled in basswood leaves and baked; and when black, an infusion was prepared. The Iroquois gave a root infusion to dogs that would not hunt anymore, and sprinkled on the head of young men to give them "right sense".

According to Smith, the Meskwaki name translates as sweet or squawroot, the latter name also used for Blue Cohosh, and in the same manner as a genito-urinary remedy.

Red Baneberry, known as **WI'COSIDJI'BIK**, or drawing root, was used for reproductive problems in men.

One ethnobotanist wrote the plant was used as a substitute for digitalis. "It is said to revive and rally a patient when he is at the point of death" (Sanders 2003:108).

The northern Chipewyan considered the red fruit poisonous and call it **JIE SLINI,** or "Bad Berry". Other members of this group consider the red berry to be the male and the white berry the female plant, much preferring the root of the latter.

The Thompson of British Columbia considered the white form particularly effective, and used the root for rheumatism, arthritis, and syphilis. Many elders say that you feel rough and sick the next day, but the following you are much better.

The Gitksan call the plant **SGANMAA'YA SMEX**, meaning "black bear berry plant."

The Quinault chewed the leaves and spit them onto a boil to bring it to a head. They call it **PA'MASIM**, meaning cold. The Quileute used the leaves in a similar manner, and called the plant **KOLOQWIXI** meaning, "open the place".

The Okanagan decocted the root for rheumatism and emaciation.

The Cheyenne used decoctions of the root to increase a mother's milk supply, often combining it with lungwort (*Mertensia*).

The dried roots were scalded in hot water in which fat had been boiled to leave them covered with a thin film of grease. This preserved the root's strength.

The Cheyenne believed that children that took "Sweet Medicine" would grow up to be of good mentality, strong and patient. An alternate name was **MOTSE?EOTSE** meaning, "about raising children." The cultural hero and prophet, Sweet Medicine or Sweet Root Standing, named the plant after himself. He lived with the Cheyenne for 445 years, and upon death transformed his sacred powers into the plant.

The root was used in decoction to destroy lice, fleas, and mites externally, and taken internally for blood and improving appetite.

It was combined with *Psoralea* species, *Koeleria cristata* and yellow root medicine for sores.

The root is sweet and later, somewhat acrid/bitter with a bit of a licorice taste. Fresh slices of the mature root are slightly pink.

The dried root is made into a strong tea in the southwestern United States. A bit is drunk and the rest is used as a wash for acute arthritis and swollen joints. Traditionally, wild tobacco powder was moistened with this tea as a poultice, held in place with cheesecloth. The ripe seeds were combined with pine pitch and placed as a plaster in front and behind the ear to treat facial neuralgia. The seeds, when roasted and powdered, were added to a soft-boiled egg for diarrhea, vomiting and tenesmus.

Headaches due to eyestrain, may respond to weak root decoctions of red or white baneberry. It is worth noting that hens and ducks will die from eating the berries; but herbivores appear to eat them without difficulty. A number of birds enjoy them with no problem. The flowers yield no nectar, but are rich in pollen.

Salicylic acid appears to increase levels of actein in rhizomes, suggesting cool willow or aspen bark decoctions may be useful supplement, for your neighborhood patch.

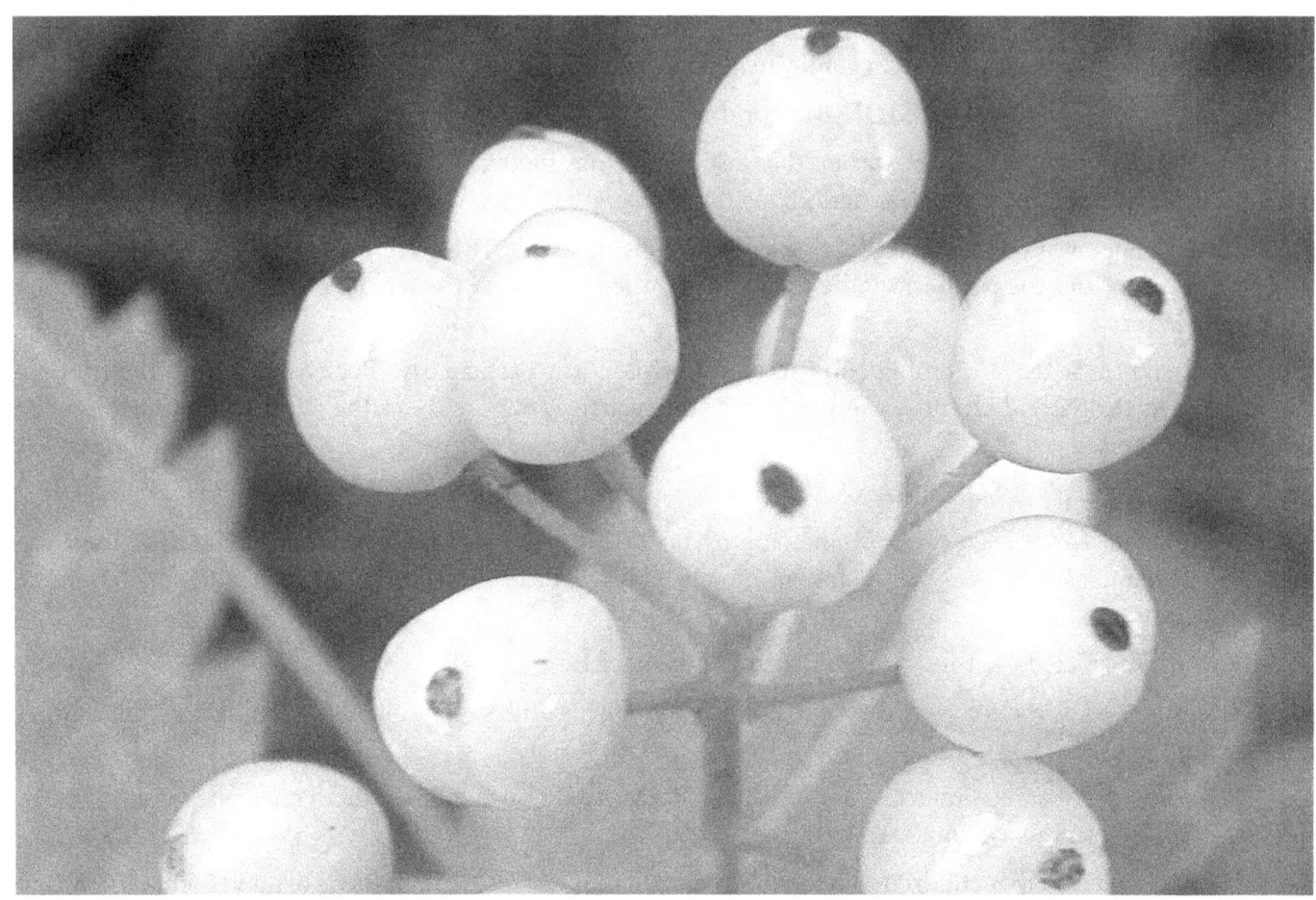

BANEBERRY- WHITE BERRIES

MEDICINAL

CONSTITUENTS- two resins present in the root resemble those in black cohosh, a close cousin. The root of *A. rubra* contains 11 xylosides of 12, 9, 19-cyclolanostane type triterpenoids including rubraside A, and a beta sitosterol glucoside, as well as 13 beta-acetyloxycimigenol. Also contains cimicifugic acids A and B. Polyphenols (2.92% dry weight).
The seeds and fruit contain trans-aconitic acid, actein, nonadecane, caffeic and chlorogenic acids, triterpene glycosides and proto-anemonoid type compounds.
A. pachypoda- root- polyphenols (0.36% dry weight), including fukonolic acid and cimicifugic acid A, as well as 12, 9,19 cyclolanostane type triterpenoids including 7,8-dihydroactaeaepoxide 3-O-beta-d-xylopyranoside, 12-deacetoxyactaeaepoxide 3-O-beta-d-xylopyranoside, and 12 beta-acetoxycimigenol.
A. podocarpa- root- podocarpasides A-J, polyphenols (1.71% dry weight), especially cimicifugic acids A and E.
A. spicata- root- corytuberine, magnoflorine, actein, trans-aconitic acid.

Eclectic herbalists suggested Baneberry be used in depleted nervous systems associated with reproductive problems. These include headache, insomnia, melancholy and convulsions.

Combine six parts valerian root with one part fresh root tincture for sleep issues associated with muscle aches and pains.

The white cohosh fresh root is very active and will produce, in excess, violent vomiting. It acts upon the female reproductive organs specifically, including ovarian neuralgia or tenderness. It is useful as a preparation for birthing and Dr. Fulton recommended it for birthing after-pains.

White cohosh root tincture is an emmenagogue, and combines well one part with four parts wild licorice root for PMS. Kuts-Cheraux, in *Naturae medicina and naturopathic dispensatory* (1953) mentions the root as a gentle nerve tonic, useful in anorexia nervosa. This makes sense, as the berry and root have shown ability to suppress activity of the vagus nerve.

The use of red baneberry root tincture was suggested by Professor Scudder, to treat dysentery, diarrhea and colic. It was used where there was desire to urinate, but without success.

Michael Moore suggested the rhizome is similar to black cohosh, and is useful for its anti-inflammatory, antispasmodic and sedative effects. "Use Baneberry tincture (10-15 drops to 4X a day) for any rheumatoid-like dull ache in the uterus, joints and muscle insertions. Think *cold*. If covering up with a shawl or getting warm helps the condition, use some Baneberry…Baneberry may also help a dull orbital headache, and like black cohosh, it is supremely useful for crampy, late menses with vague pains in extremities. Also like its relative, it seems to fool the brain into thinking there is some used estrogen floating around, slows down the hypothalamic demand for more hormone, and for three or four hours at a time can often back off hot flashes and/or dark, morbid rushes during a tiresome menopausal glitch."

It is a peripheral vasodilator and should not be used during pregnancy.

The fresh root tincture combines well with trillium root or licorice root for menopausal hot flashes.

Marija Helt writes about her personal experience with single drops of tincture in *Herbaria Monthly* April 14, 2017. "My limited experience so far in playing with Banebarry root…

One drop of root tincture was enough to feel its sedating effect, and I immediately noticed a sense of my heart center, similarly to taking Clematis. Perhaps not surprising, given Baneberry's know effects on the heart.

On the reproductive side of things, Black Cohosh has a definite effect on my cycle: It messes up and gives me sore boobs. Lo and behold, one drop of Baneberry root tincture three times a day for less than a month was enough to mess up my cycle and give me sore boobs. To be more specific, it's really the menses that shift, becoming quite a bit more drawn out. So it's perhaps not *my* herb, but it may be a good one for those clients in my practice that respond well to Black Cohosh."

Cimifugic acids A & B show cytotoxic activity against cancer cell lines. Yim SH et al, *Arch Pharm Res* 2012 35(9): 1559-65.

Cimifugic acid exhibits stronger hyaluronidase inhibition than rosmarinic acid. Iwanaga A et al, *J Nat Prod* 2010 73(4):573-8.

Hyaluronidase inhibition reduces the degradation of hyaluronic acid, reducing inflammation, angiogenesis, etc. This explains, in part, the traditional use of the root for snakebites, particularly from rattlesnakes.

They also inhibit activity of elastase, associated with breakdown of elastin, associated with cardiovascular and skin health. Löser B et al, *Planta Medica* 2000 66(8):751-3.

Fukinolic acid and cimifugic acids A and B prevent collagen degradation by collagenase or collagenolytic enzymes, for wound healing and reduction of inflammation. Kusano A et al, *Biol Pharm Bull* 2001 24(10):1998-201. This may explain, in part, its use for improved joint function, and reduction of cartilage wear and tear.

Actein may arrests angiogenesis, associated with breast cancer growth. Yu GG et al, *Sci Rep* Oct 12;6:35263. It alters the activity of the ER 1P3 receptor, induces calcium release and modulates NFkappaB and MEK pathways. Einbond LS et al, *Fitoterapia* 2013 91:28-38.

Actein exerts a synergistic effect on growth inhibition of breast cancer cells when combined with doxorubicin or 5-flourouracil. It enhanced induction of apoptosis by paclitaxel and two other drugs, in digitoxin, and inhibits Na+-K+-ATPase. Einbond et al, *Planta Medica* 2006 72 (13); Einbond et al, *Phytomed* 2008 15:6-7; Einbond et al, *Biochem Biophys Res Commun* 2008 375:4.

It displays suppressive effect on breast cancer and early liver cancer. Xi R et al, *Biomed Pharmacother* 2017 88:242-51.

Actein shows anti-HIV activity. Sakurai et al, *Bioorg Med Chem Lett* 2004 14(5):1329-32.

Actein arrests human leukemia HL-60 cell lines and possesses low toxicity. Wu D et al, *Molecules* 2016 21(8). It also inhibits glioma cell growth via a mitochondria-mediated pathway. Yuan LQ et al, *Cancer Biomark* 2017 doi:10.3233. And may be useful in gastric cancer. Yang ZC & Ma J, *Biochem Biophys Res Commun* 2016 November 30.

Actein is lipophilic, suggesting the need for alcohol extractions.

The compound inhibits cell proliferation and migration in human osteosarcoma (bone cancer), by inducing cell apoptosis (programmed death). Chen Z et al, *Med Sci Monit* 2016 22:1609-16. Work by Einbond LS et al, *Fundam Clin Pharmacol* 2009 23(3):311-21 on rats, found actein activated a statin-like response to cholesterol and inhibition of human HepG2 liver cancer cells.

The powdered root is a good counter-irritant in the manner of a mustard plaster. The powder is mixed with hot water, applied to affected area, and covered with heated towels. Use with caution to avoid blistering.

Methanol extracts of the whole plant of Red Baneberry are effective against *Bacillus subtilis, E. coli,* and *Cladosporium cucumerinum.* Water decoctions showed action against only *B. subtilis.* Bergeron et al, *Int J Pharmacognosy* 1996 34(4).

One compound in *A. rubra* root showed moderate anti-complement activity in work by Zulfigar et al, *Planta Med* 2006 72:14.

Actaea spicata is a European species. It contains trans-aconitic acid; found to inhibit cancer cell lines. Nikonow et al, *Pharm Zentralh* 1964 103:8 601.

HOMEOPATHY

Red Baneberry (*A. spicata*) is quite useful in homeopathic preparation as a rheumatic remedy.

Specifically it is for the small joints, where there is a tearing or tingling pain. This pain is made much worse from touch or motion.

Often, there is pain in the wrist, ankles, or swelling of joints from the least movement. Accompanying this, there may be a lame feeling in the arms, and a slight feeling of paralysis in the hands.

Asthma that is exaggerated by cold, or weakness after eating may also indicate this remedy. A pulsating pain in either kidney, or vascular spasms, are also indications for using actaea.

It is an ancillary remedy in stomach carcinoma.

DOSE- Third potency is best. The mother tincture is made from the root, gathered in May before flowering.

This is sometimes given to women, in the manner of black cohosh, as a preparative for efficient delivery in the last month. First proving by Petroz in France in 1834.

ESSENTIAL OIL

Although the author is not aware of attempts to make essential oils from members of the Actaea, an interesting study was conducted in Sweden in 1987.

Floral fragrances of *A. spicata, A. rubra* and others were studied by gas chromatography. Fifteen closely related monoterpenes were discovered.

These are, in descending concentration, mycrene (44.7%), benzyl alcohol (12.6%), nerol (11.4), and smaller amounts of geranyl acetate, geraniol, ocimene, limonene, farnesene, and neryl acetate.

The related Cimifuga simplex essential oil is composed of 27..57% m-acetanisole, 6.84% (E)-cinnamaldehyde, 5.58% paeonol, 5.07% caproic acid, and 3% atractylone.

FLOWER ESSENCE

White and red baneberry flower essences combine to heal and reveal the soul qualities of guilt.

Religious experiences often lead individuals to believe in the concept of original sin, resulting in feelings of guilt.

This flower essence is useful for those who continue to sabotage their happiness through inappropriate response to loving and caring for others. There is a death wish that is only obvious through the choices made in day-to-day life; but not necessarily expressed verbally. **PRAIRIE DEVA**

Baneberry flower essence helps us interface with the fairy kingdom and initiate plant-spirit journeys; for attuning deeply with the plant kingdom; helps calm hyperactivity and excitable states.
DELTA GARDENS FLOWER ESSENCE**S**

White Baneberry (*A. pachypoda*) flower essence is for blood health, especially helpful information to the white blood cells as they defend the body against infectious disease and foreign bodies.
GREEN HOPE FARM

SPIRITUAL PROPERTIES

Red Baneberry was called Sweet Medicine by the Cheyenne. The Cultural Hero and Prophet, Sweet Medicine or Sweet Root Standing, named this plant for himself, stating that it would help bring up children.

Sweet Medicine reputedly lived 445 years with the Cheyenne. Upon his death, he transformed his sacred powers into this plant. To this day, Cheyennes keep this root in the Sacred Arrow, Sacred Hat, and Sun Dance bundles, thus benefiting from Sweet Medicine's sacred powers. With the Sacred Arrows, he said to the Cheyennes: "Don't forget me. This is my body I am giving you. Always think of me."

In a holy ceremony, the priest (?) bites a tiny fragment of the root and spits it upon his hands and those of other priests, thus throwing Sweet Medicine's power at them and blessing their hands for sacred tasks. As the priest does this, the others avert their eyes, because the sacred root would blind them if they saw it.

PERSONALITY TRAITS

Consider the lesser-known Western cohosh or Red baneberry (*Actaea arguta*) an equivalent to Black Cohosh. Morphologically and therapeutically the two plants appear nearly identical. Although there is no particular study to confirm the two plant's correspondence, empirical observation, confirms this. American herbalists familiar with under-utilized native plants have been using Western cohosh as an equivalent to Black cohosh for a number of years. It rivals the latter's potency and therapeutic sphere.
CHARLES W. KANE

RECIPES

TINCTURE- A dry root tincture is made one part root to five parts 40% alcohol; the preferred fresh root at 1:3 at 80% alcohol. 1-20 drops daily. The fresh root tincture can be a mucous membrane irritant in large amounts. It is somewhat acrid, but sweet at the same time. Use 3-6 drops in water as an emmenagogue. Combine one part with four parts wild licorice root for PMS or hot flashes- 20 drops up to six times daily.

DECOCTION- 1-2 fluid ounces, up to four times daily from the dry root. One heaping tablespoon of dried root to one point of water simmered for 20 minutes.

Do not use with pregnancy or chronic hypotension. Large doses may cause frontal headaches.

LINIMENT- Take two ounces of ground root to 70% rubbing alcohol. Add twenty drops of birch oil. Shake well. Use externally.

CAUTION- If you suspect the berries have been eaten, symptoms will appear within a few hours to days. Excruciating pain and inflammation followed by blisters or open sores in the mouth, lips, tongue and throat. Larger amounts can cause vomiting with bright red blood, severe diarrhea and cramping, excessive blood tinged urine, hallucinations, and even grand mal seizures. Induce vomiting, followed by milk or egg white as demulcent. The hospital will want to check renal function and electrolyte levels.

BEARGRASS
(***Xerophyllum tenax*** [Pursh] Nutt.)
(***Helionas tenax*** Pursh.)

Xerophyllum is from the Latin Xeros meaning dry (as in Xerox- dry paper copying) and phyllon meaning leaf. Bears will eat the fleshy leaves in spring and hence the common name.

The roots were eaten by various groups of natives for food, either roasted or boiled, but not very pleasant. The decoction was used as a hair tonic and to soothe pain of inflammation. Further evaporated, the residue, rich in saponins, was used as soap.

The long, thin leaves were used to weave cloth or baskets.

The herbaceous, perennial is rare and endangered. If you visit Waterton National Park in early summer, you would be surprised to hear of its endangerment, but that is probably the only place on the Canadian prairies that it will be found in any numbers.

The flowers are large, white and star-shaped, and only bloom every five to seven years. When they do, the hillsides are covered with their scent and beauty. It is a magnificent vista.

The plant reproduces mainly by extension of shallow rhizomes that then form new plants that take up to five years to mature and flower. Squirrels chew the flower stalks and eat them. Grizzly bears have been found to use the grass leaves as nesting material for winter dens.

In some unprotected areas of the United States, the leaves are wild-crafted and sold to the floral trade.

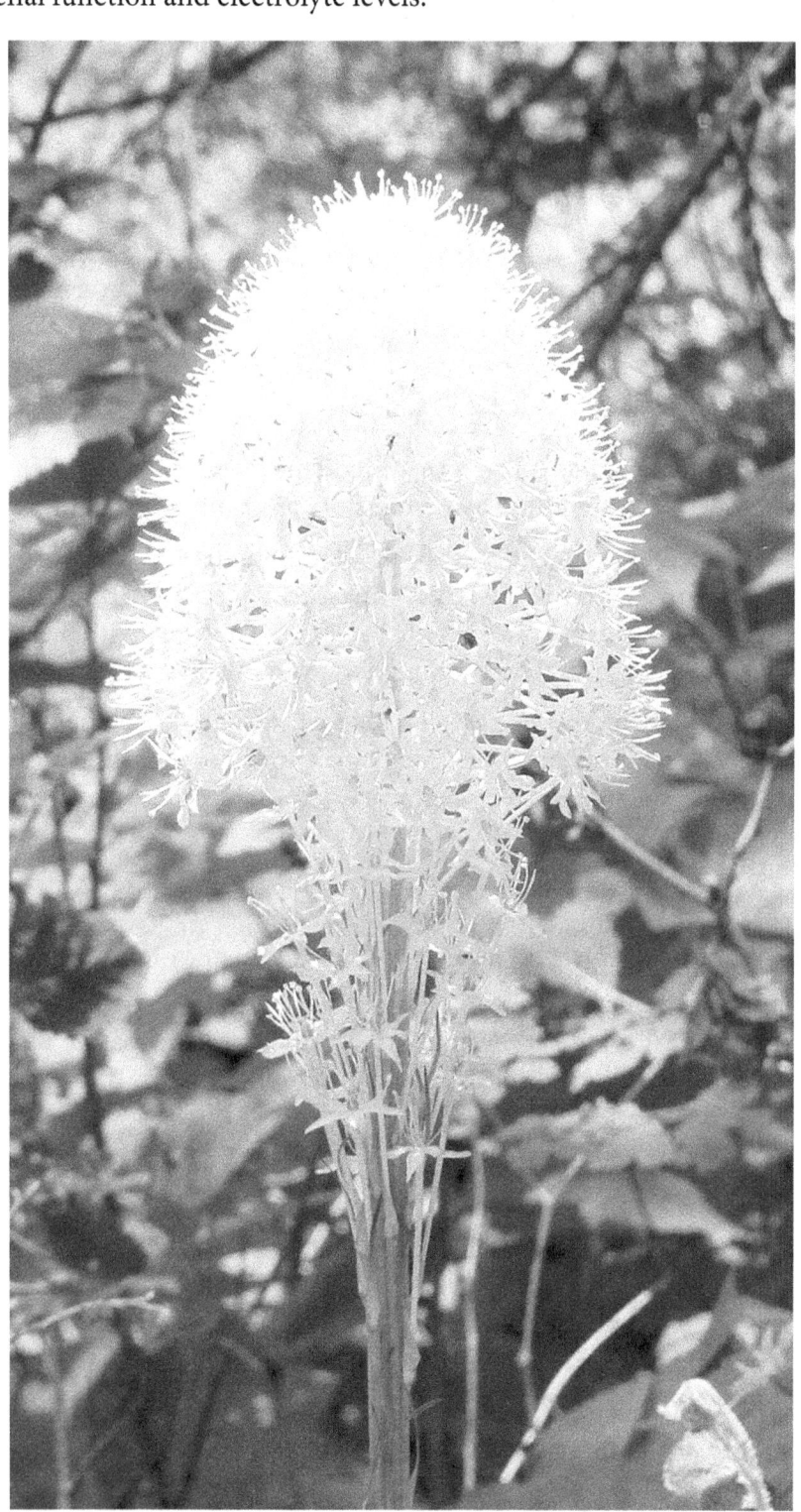

BEARGRASS IN BLOOM

The leaves were traditionally harvested in spring, soaked in water to make them pliable and woven into hats and capes.

The Thompson tribe know it as both Squaw Grass, and Bear Grass, **S/PE?EC PE& S/YIQ-M.**

The root and leaf were both used by various Western tribes to treat liver and gallbladder problems.

Pregnant Wintun women chewed Beargrass in order to ensure the birth of a strong baby boy. This may have some basis in fact, as research has shown that during a very early state of fetal development, a flood of testosterone or its absence, may dictate sexual dominance.

Beargrass contains plant steroids known as ecdysones that influence hormonal production, mainly 20-hydroxyecdysone.

The roots or rhizomes are astringent and help contract blood vessels. The chewed roots are applied as poultice to open, bleeding wounds. The washed root was rubbed into a lather and used to bathe sore eyes.

HOMEOPATHY

Xerophyllum is useful for those with a dull or confused mind. They forget names, or write the last letter first, as well as misspell common words, like dyslexia.

The head is full and stuffed up, with sinus and forehead pain. The eyes are painful and smarting, as if sandy. Vision related to close work is impaired and unable to focus.

The face is bloated in morning, with puffy eyes.

Stomach is full and heavy, with vomiting around 2 p.m.

There is lots of gas and flatulence, and yet small hard, lumpy stools with much straining and bearing down rectal pain.

Urine is difficult to retain, with dribbling during walking, and frequent night-time urination.

The female suffers a bearing down sensation with inflamed vulva, itching, and increased sexual desire. This is tempered with ovarian and uterine pains, as well as leucorrhea.

The back feels hot deep down to the spine with muscular weakness of the knees, and much trembling and stiffness in limbs.

The skin may be the major indication, with erythema, vesication and intense burning, stinging and itching. The skin is rough and cracked, and feels like leather.

Dermatitis around knees, or swelling of the inguinal glands and behind knees are other indications of its use.

The various indications are made worse by cold water, and in the afternoon and evening. Symptoms are better in morning, from moving affected areas and by application of hot water.

DOSE- Sixth potency and higher. Compare with poison ivy and grindelia as some symptoms are close. The mother tincture is made from the whole fresh plant in flower. Proving by Arndt with ten students of the Hahnemann College of the Pacific in San Francisco with 1x, 3x, 6x, and 12x potencies in 1903.

A summary of proving is found in Plants volume 3, page 587 by Vermeulen and Johnston.

FLOWER ESSENCES

Beargrass flower essence is especially useful for children or adults suffering dyslexia.   **PRAIRIE DEVA**

Beargrass fosters our knowing that no outside influence can overpower our deeply held intentions. It keeps us steadily centered in our hearts.   **DESERT ALCHEMY**

WHITE BEARD TONGUE
(*Penstemon albidus* Nutt.)
SMOOTH BLUE BEARD TONGUE
WAX LEAF PENSTEMON
(*P. nitidus* Dougl. ex Benth.)
YELLOW BEARD TONGUE
(*P. confertus* Dougl. ex Lindl.)
SHARP LEAF BEARD TONGUE
(*P. acuminatus* Dougl. ex Lindl.)
SHELL LEAF BEARD TONGUE
LARGE FLOWERED PENSTEMON
(*P. grandiflorus* Nutt.)
WHITE BEARDTONGUE
TALUS SLOPE PENSTEMON
(*P. digitalis* Nutt. ex Sims)
SLENDER BLUE BEARD TONGUE

PIN CUSHION BEARD TONGUE
(*P. procerus* Douglas ex Graham)
FUZZY-TONGUED PENSTEMON
CRESTED PENSTEMON
(*P. eriantherus* Pursh.)
LILAC FLOWERED BEARD TONGUE
SLENDER BEARD TONGUE
(*P. gracilis* Nutt.)
SHRUBBY PENSTEMON
SHRUBBY BEARD TONGUE
BUSH PENSTEMON
(*P. fruticosus* [Pursh] Greene)
ALBERTA BEARD TONGUE
(*P. albertinus* Greene)
PARTS USED- whole plant, seeds

These are rather dull looking and unrefined penstemons. The pride of the family, however, has passed away into the rich house of penstemons, and must therefore be looked for as *P. barbatus*.   **REGINALD FARRER**

The prairies we have passing through in Manitoba were then called the weedy prairies on account of the number of tall flowering plants that grew upon them. Before us, while we stayed at Rat Creek, extended a flat plain, twelve miles wide without a house, and one unbroken mass of tall flowering plants; **PENSTEMON**, sunflowers, goldenrods, asters. In the next 150 miles we passed through a beautiful country and to us Easterners it looked as if it were a perfect garden.   **JOHN MACOUN**

Penstemon means five stamens, from the Latin **PENTE**, for five; and **STEMON**, for stamen or thread. It may also originate from the Greek **PEN**, for missing and **STEMON** for thread, referring to the stamens within the tubular blossoms. The original name was Pentstemon, which makes more sense.

Procerus means tall and slender. Confertus is Latin for crowded; alluding to the dense flower head. Nitidus is from the Latin meaning shiny, smooth or clear. Eriantherus means woolly anthers.

Beard Tongue is named for the fact that of the 5 stamens in the flower, one is sterile and bearded, like a hairy lower lip that protrudes from the flower.

Beard Tongues are a large group of hardy perennials on the prairies.

Shell Leaf Beard Tongue and White Beard Tongue are frequent additions to urban gardens, due to its much larger flower. Shrubby Penstemon is a small rare bush, or shrub, the rest are herbaceous in nature. Slender Beard Tongue extends up into the Peace Country, while White Beard Tongue is found in the southeast corner of Alberta.

The Thompson tribe used Yellow Beard Tongue (*P. confertus*) root decoctions as a purgative. The stems and leaves were roasted and powdered for sprinkling on sores, cuts and wounds. The outer stem and root bark was decocted as a stomach remedy.

Some Okanagan tribes boiled the flowers and rubbed them on arrows as an indelible blue dye.

Shrubby Penstemon (*P. fruticosus*) is found on the dry, rocky slopes of the mountains. It was used by the Shuswap for urinary and bladder complaints; and by others as a wash for arthritis, rheumatism, eyes, or sore, itching scalp.

A small piece of the fresh root was used directly on toothaches.

The leaves and flowers were often added to layer cooking pits, to flavor wild onions, and balsamroot.

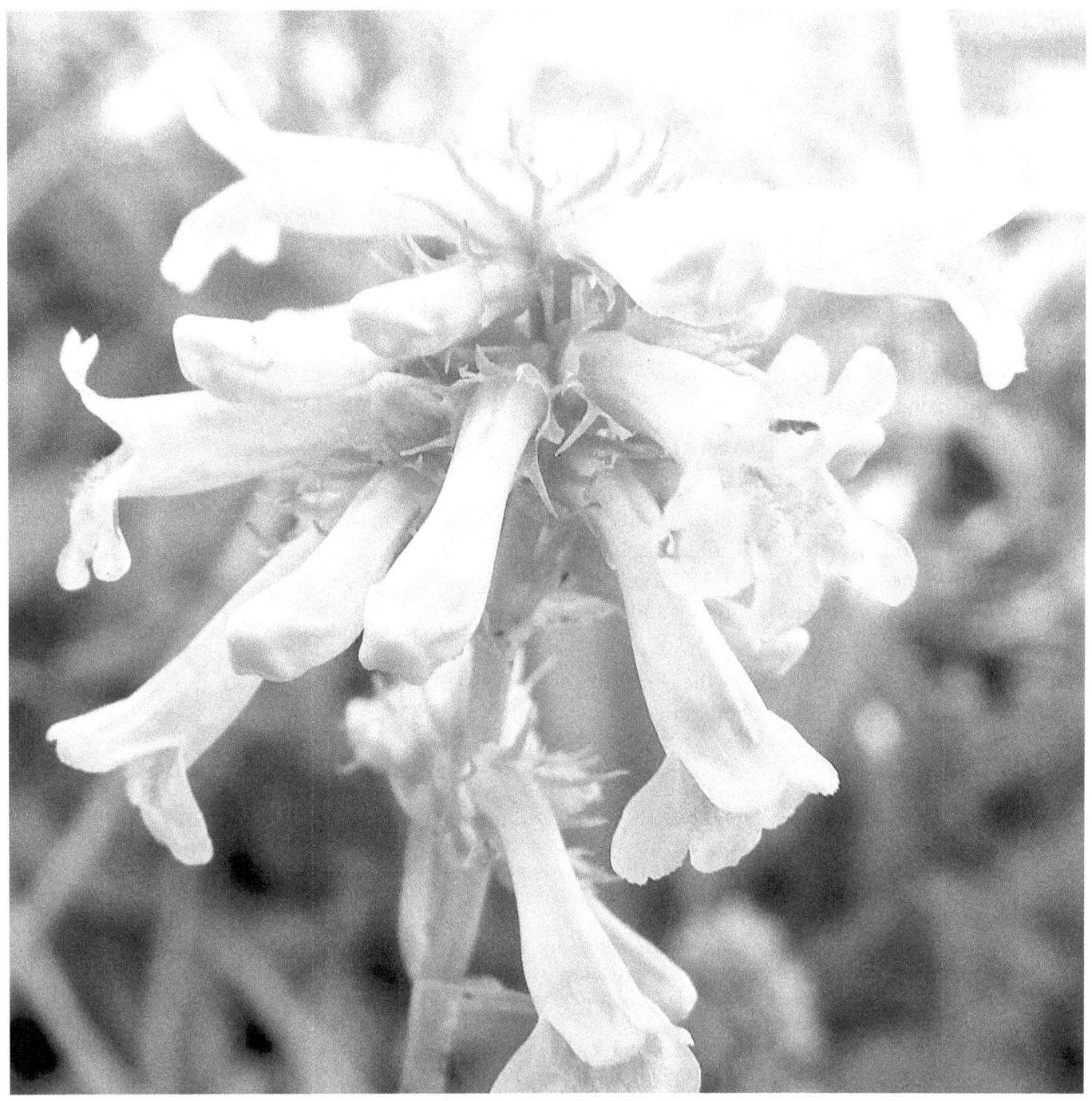

YELLOW BEARD TONGUE (*P. confertus*)

The Okanagan used the leaves as padding in moccasins. The Stl'atl'imx rubbed the leafy branches on Nodding onions to "get the whiskers off" and give them a better flavor. Various other tribes, including the Secwepemc used the branches for flavoring in pit cooking.

Shell Leaf Beard Tongue (*P. grandiflorus*) root was decocted by the Dakota for chest pain (heart?). Several tribes, including the Kiowa and Pawnee called it Wild Foxglove. This makes sense, when you realize the plant contains digitoxin-like compounds.

The Kiowa decocted the roots for stomach trouble, while the Pawnee made a leaf decoction for chills and fevers.

The Navaho combined Indian Paintbrush and Penstemon blossoms as an infusion for treating the pain of centipede bites.

The Blackfoot of Montana drank warm infusions of *P. acuminatus* to help stop vomiting, stomachache and cramps. It is called Tastes Like Fire, or **AT-SI-PL-KOA** due to its flavor.

It is a beautiful plant that appears sliver white from a distance. The stems are pink, with shades of yellow-green, the bracts are reddish green, the flowers are azure blue while the tube remains pink.

Slender Beardtongue (*P. gracilis*) root was known as snake's medicine, or **ZUZE'CA TAPEJU'TA**, by the Lakota, who used it traditionally to treat various reptile bites.

The related *P. barbatus* is rubbed on rabbit sticks by Zuni throwers to ensure success.

The related *P. gentianoides* has been used traditionally for inflammation and migraines. Work by Dominguez et al, *J Ag Food Chem* 2005 53 found methanol extracts with significant anti-oxidant activity.

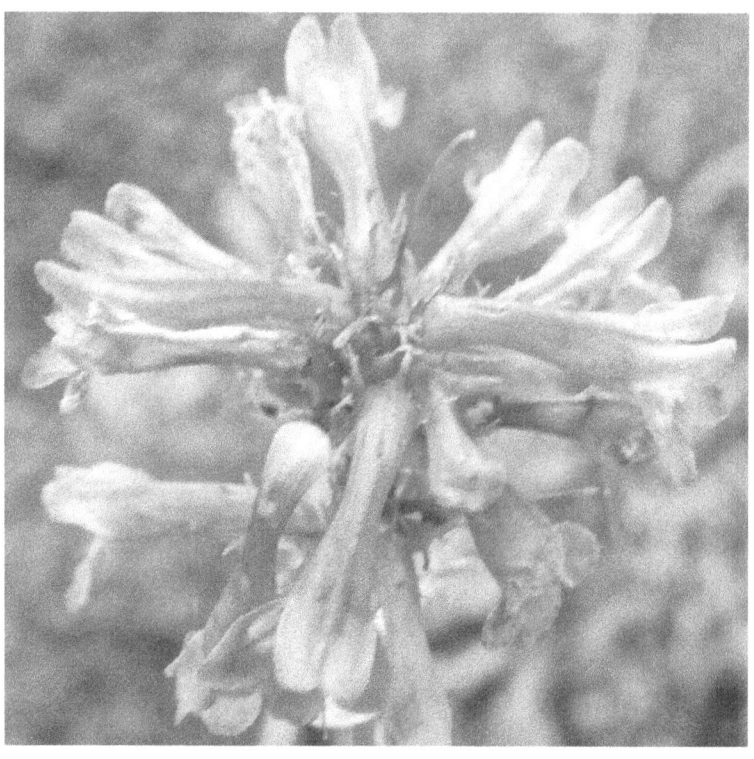

PENSTEMON PROCERUS

White Beardtongue was introduced by the University of Nebraska in 1983, as "Husker Red", due to its red foliage. It was named the 1996 Perennial Plant of the Year.

MEDICINAL

CONSTITUENTS - *P. albidus*- whole plant- various acetyl digitoxin-like substances, catalpol-like derivatives.
P. nitidus- leaves-various cardenolides and cardiac glycosides including digoxin, 10-hydroxycornin, verbascoside (1.7% dry wt), 10-hydroxy-epihastotoside, echinacoside (0.2% dry wt), and 10-griselinosidic acid; iridoid glucosides including cornin (verbenalin), hastatoside, beta-dihydrohasatoside, and 10-hydroxycornin.
root- lanatoside C
P. confertus- confertoside, dihydro-serruloside, 7-hydroxyebuloside, 8-epi-hydropenstemide, penstemide and 2-o-(8'-hydroxy-2,6-dimethyl-2E,6E-octadienoyl) di-hydropenstemide. The iridoid glycosides are of the valeriana type.
P. grandiflorus- leaf and flower-desacetyl lanatoside-C, acetyl digitoxin-like glycosides, gitoxin
root- lanatoside B-like glycoside, as well as above.
P. procerus- leaves- penproside A and B- phenylpropanoid glucosides; two iridoid glucosides euphroside and plant-arenaloside.
P. eriantherus- iso-scrophularioside (iridoid glucoside); 10-cinnamoylaucubin.
P. fruticosus- leaves-two C9 iridoids, aucubin and eurostoside, six iridoid glucosides, and two C10 iridoids, mussaenoside and 2'-cinnamoylmussaenoside; three phenylpropanoid glucosides, two acetophenone derivatives, and cis and trans forms of 10-O-p-methoxycinnamoylaucubin.
Various other cardinolides and cardiac glycosides appear in thin layer chromatography, but have not been positively correlated with known substances.
P. venustus- root- taxisterone, 20-hydroxyecdysone, makisterone A and C, and venustone, three iridoids and three phenylpropanoids.
P. linarioides- leucosceptoside A, aceteoside, poliumoside (glycosides); plantarenaloside (iridoid)
P. digitalis- stansioside (iridoid glycoside), orobanchoside, martynoside, diginpenstroside.
P. barbatus- leaf- echinacoside (5%), verbascoside (11%).

All Penstemon species have some medicinal benefit.

P. venustus, which grows wild in Montana and Idaho, contains ecdysteroids, as in the Silene genus. These compounds are hormonal growth factors, used for muscle building in athletes, and worthy of further study.

Penstemon venustus and *P. fruticosus* contain a number of compounds active against six gram positive and gram negative bacteria, as well as three human pathogenic fungi. Zajdel SM et al, *Nat Prod Res* 2013 27(24): 2263-71.

Shell Leaf Beard Tongue (*P. grandiflorus*) roots and stems have been water extracted, and show activity against gram-positive bacteria.

The fresh plants make useful poultices for bites, bruises, etc.

On a practical level, all Penstemon can be gathered fresh and wilted; combined with an equal volume of olive or canola oil and sun infused for at least a week or two.

This can be strained and heated enough to add the right amount of beeswax to make a salve. In cold climates, use a crockpot for 3-4 hours with low heat and lid removed.

This is an excellent remedy for irritations of the skin, anus, and lips.

Penstemide exhibits potential anti-tumour activity against P-388 lymphocytic leukemia cells. The compound exhibits anti-inflammatory activity similar to indomethacin. Dominquez M et al, *Pharm Biol* 2011 49(2):118-24.

Plantarenaloside shows cytotoxicity against THP-1 leukemia cell lines. Rana A et al, *Nat Prod Res* 2014 28(8):593-6. It also shows neurite differentiation or neurotrophic activity for PC-12 cells. Yu ZW et al, *Zhongguo Zhong Yao Za Zhi* 2005 30(17):1335-8.

Echinacoside, also present in Echinacea species, has a neuroprotective effect on regulating the stress active signals in mice models of Parkinson's disease. Zhang J et al, *Neurochem Res* 2016 December 15. The compound inhibits glutamate release in cerebrocortical nerve synaptosomes, and suppression of protein kinase C activity. Lu CW et al, *Int J Mol Sci* 2016 17(7).

Eurostoside exhibits significant activity against hepatitis C virus. Zhang H et al, *J Nat Prod* 2009 72(12):2158-62.

Mussaenoside possesses anti-inflammatory activity through NFkappaB in-activation. Lee DS et al, *Arch Pharm Res* 2014 37(7):947-54. It prevents the elevation of E-selectin, thus reducing pro-inflammatory response. Vogl S et al, *Evid Based Complement Alternat Medicine* 2013:2013:395316.

Verbascoside (found also in mullein) and 4"-0-acetylverbascoside are present in *P. centranthifolius*. Ye et al, *Phytother Res* 24:5 found the two compounds inhibit bacterial biofilm of *E. coli*.

Aceteoside (verbascoside) shows inhibitory activity against protein kinase C alpha, indicating possible anti-tumour activity. The IC value is 9.3.

Verbascoside inhibits xanthine oxidase, associated with uric acid and gout. Wan Y et al, *Int J Biol Macromol* 2016 93(PtA):609-14.

Verbascoside and martynoside exhibit strong inhibition of acetylcholinesterase and butyrylcholinesterase. The breakdown of these compounds is believed related to formation of senile plaque, dementia and Alzheimer's disease. Cespedes CL et al, *Food Chem Toxicol* 2013 62:919-26.

These two compounds also prevent red blood cells from free radical damage (sport- induced anemia) in a mice study. Zhu M et al, *Int J Sports Med* 2010 31(8):537-41. They reduce skeletal muscle fatigue, especially verbascoside. Liao F et al, *Phytother Res* 1999 13(7):621-3.

Martynoside is a potent anti-estrogenic in MCF-7 breast cancer cells, and induces nodule mineralization in osteoblasts. It also showed anti-proliferative effect on endometrial cells, suggesting it may be an important natural selective estrogen receptor modulator. Verbascoside (acetoside) is also anti-estrogenic to breast cancer cells and osteoblasts. Papoutsi Z et al, *J Steroid Biochem Mol Biol* 2006 98(1):63-71.

Both compounds inhibit ACE, angiotensin-converting enzyme, contributing to possible treatment for hypertension.

Catalpol, also found in Mullein, *Plantago lanceolata*, and various species of Veronica, is present in many species of Penstemon.

Catalpol stimulates production of adreno-cortical hormones that increase the production of sex hormones. It also ameliorates diabetic induced atherosclerosis, probably due to inhibition of oxidative stress inflammation and anti-fibrosis. Liu JY et al, *Am J Transl Res* 2016 8(10):4278-88.

Growth factor receptor-bound protein 10 (Grb10) negatively regulates insulin-like growth factor 1 receptor, a pathway critical for cell growth, apoptosis and implicated in kidney disease. It may play a role in diabetic nephropathy. Work by Yang S et al, *PLoS One* 11(3)::e0151857 found catalpol significantly abrogated elevated Grb10 in diabetic kidneys.

Catalpol, in diabetic mice, showed benefit against lipid and glucose disorders including insulin resistance. Bao Q et al, *Korean J Physiol Pharmacol* 2016 20(2):153-60.

Catalpol inhibits the formation of senile plaques in the brain, suggesting its benefit in Alzheimer's disease. Huang JZ et al, *Mol Med Rep* 2016 13(1):491-6.

Peri-menopausal and menopausal women can benefit from Penstemon species tinctures at one to two teaspoons per day.

Cornin exerts a protective effect against myocardial ischemia. Xu Y et al, *Braz J Med Biol Res* 2016 49(2):e5039. It has been shown, in vitro, to induce angiogenesis in human brain microvascular endothelial (HBMEC) cell lines via programmed P13K/Akt/eNOS/VEGF signaling. Kang Z et al, *Food Chem Toxicol* 2013 58:340-6.

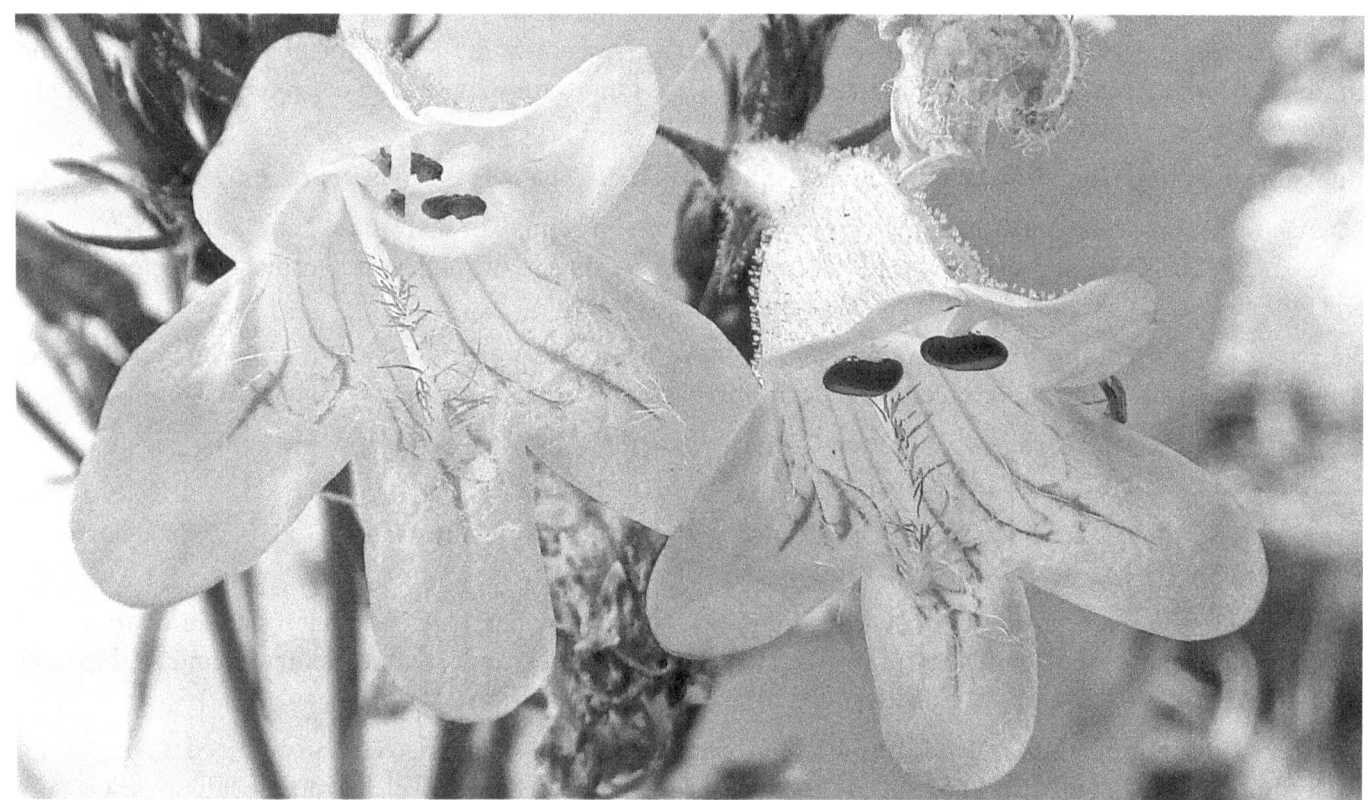

PENSTEMON DIGITALIS

ESSENTIAL OILS

The floral scent of *P. digitalis* and its nectar is strictly (S)-(+)-linalool.

SEED OIL

The seeds of White Beard Tongue contain up to 20% oil containing 58% oleic acid, 7.6% of a conjugated octadecaienoic acid, and 34% of non-conjugated octadecadienoic acids.

HYDROSOL

Hydrosols of various Penstemon species ccan be useful for application to mosquito bites, tick bites, as well as cracked skin, itching and eczema.

One dropper in water twice daily can be useful as a menopause or peri-menopausal tonic.

FLOWER ESSENCES

No flower essences have been researched from local Penstemons. Both Mountain Pride (*P. newberryi*) and Penstemon (*P. davidsonii*) have been well researched by the Flower Essence Society, but these are warm climate cousins.

Rhonda Pallasdowney has examined the properties of Palmer's Penstemon, and Scarlet Penstemon in *The Complete Book of Flower Essences*.

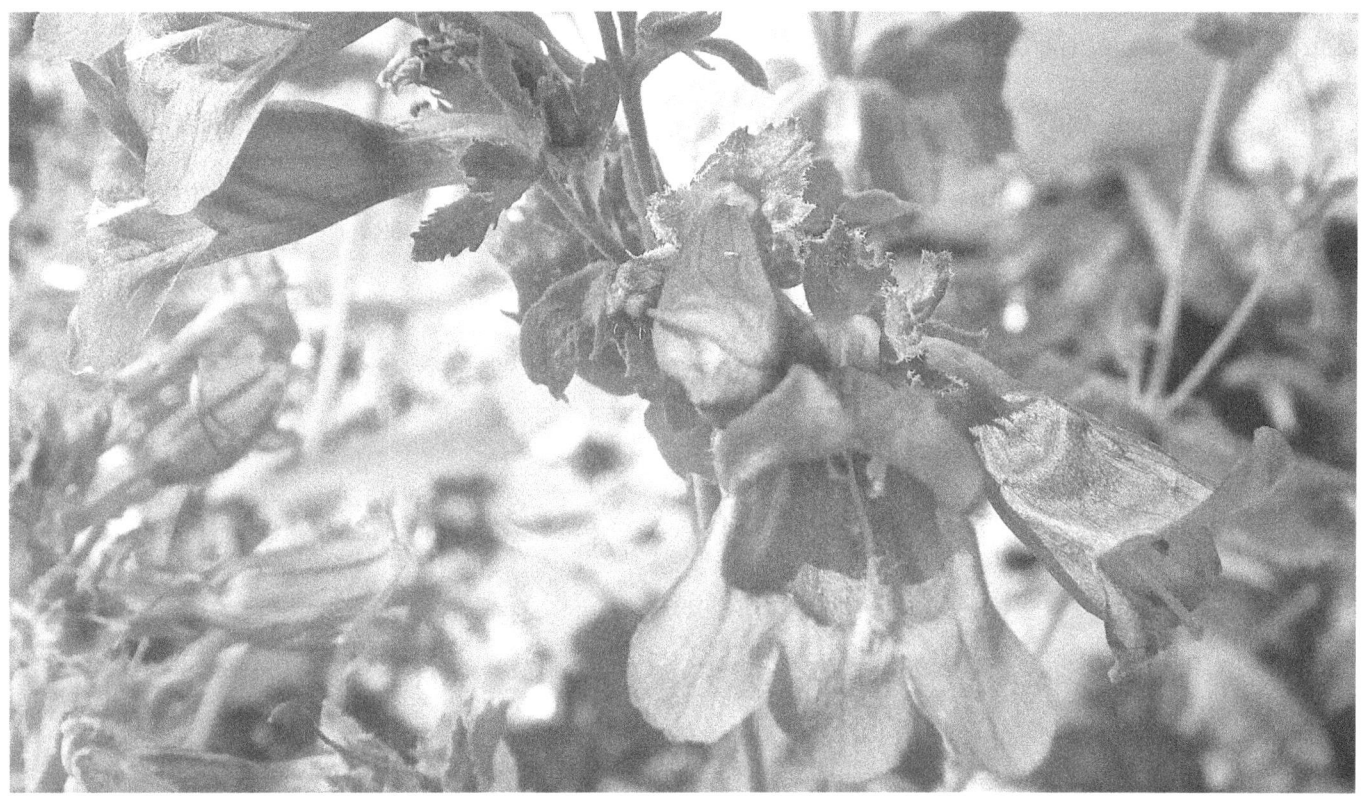

PENSTEMON SERRULATUS

SPIRITUAL PROPERTIES

After their Christianization, the Cahuilla Indians prized the Hummingbird's Kiss (Penstemon spp.) mainly as an ornamental plant, which they displayed at funerals and other church functions. Records are silent on the subject of its prior use as a medicine but it's probable, nonetheless, that the medicinal properties of this plant were well known to these and other desert Indians as well as to the settlers who learned their ways.

Today a concoction made from this herb is used as a soothing application for the skin. Mashed and blended, it's sometimes mixed with other ingredients such as olive oil and used as a lotion for the treatment of rashes, cold sores, chapped hands, and other epidermal irritations. **WESTRICH**

The spirit of the Penstemon flower is full of vital, fluid, pulsating life force. Listen to the message of the Penstemon and make an intention to bring more physical activity into your daily life. **ECLARE**

DOCTRINE OF SIGNATURES

The blue coating on the leaves corresponds to the throat chakra, and the mouth, throat, esophagus and thyroid. The throat area relates to creativity, associated with the right hemisphere of the brain.

The pink colour of the flower relates to the heart centre, which stimulates compassion and positive self-expression. These chakras together are a signature of speaking or expressing ourselves from the depth of our hearts rather than through our heads and emotions.

The bud of the flower has a line through the centre that separates the upper and lower petals, resembling a tight jaw line. I have used this essence for myself and others in treating TMJ. The flower itself, in full bloom, resembles an open wound. The fuzzy yellow head looks like a soft tongue.   **PALLASDOWNEY**

The tongue is a forceful aggressive-defensive symbol because it is the only organ of the body that can be so startlingly displayed. The extended tongue in Maori art and Hakas (war dances) expresses challenge and defiance (as does everyday tongue-poking), and it is also a common sexual symbol in primitive art, such as fertility "pole figures" from Borneo. The protective god Bes in Egypt appears with a protruding tongue, which is believed to ward off evil. There is a strong symbolic link between tongues and flames—both are red, active, consuming, and creative-destructive – thus the Indian fire god Agni is shown with seven tongues. The tongue can also symbolize language, eloquence or wisdom; in Egyptian funerary art, extended tongues allowed the dead to speak to the gods. Some animal effigies with protruding tongues invoke rain.   **JACK TRESSIDER**

RECIPES

TINCTURE- 1:3 at 50% for fresh flowering plants. 1-2 tsp. as needed.

NODDING BEGGAR TICKS
NODDING BUR MARIGOLD
BUR MARIGOLD
TICKSEED
(*Bidens cernua* L.)
SPANISH NEEDLES
(*B. bipinnata* L.)
BURR MARIGOLD
TRIFID BURR MARIGOLD
WATER MARIGOLD
WATER AGRIMONY
THREE-LOBE BEGGAR TICKS
SWAMP BEGGAR TICKS
(*B. tripartita* L.)
PURPLE STEM BEGGAR TICKS
(*B. connata* Muhl. ex Willd)
TALL BEGGAR TICKS
COMMON BEGGAR TICKS
(*B. frondosa* L.)
TALL BEGGAR TICKS
WESTERN STICKTIGHT
(*B. vulgata* Greene)
HAIRY BEGGAR TICKS
BLACK JACK
(*B. pilosa* L.)
PARTS USED- seed, roots, and whole flower in bloom.

He wrapped himself in quotations—as a beggar would enfold himself
In the purple of Emperors.   **RUDYARD KIPLING**

Bidens is from the Latin, meaning "double-toothed", in reference to their barbed prongs so difficult to remove from clothing. Cernua may be from the Latin **CERNUUS** meaning nodding or drooping. **PINNATUS** means feathery, while bipinnate means twice pinnate or leaves arranged on either side of stem, opposite each other. Frondosa means lush or abundant in growth. Vulgata is variation of vulgare, meaning common. Connation is the developmental fusion of petals forming a tubular corolla. Tripartita means composed of three parts. Pilosa means hairy.

Bidens species are used for healing around the world. *Bidens pilosa* is the most well known and studied, but a few other species are native or have found their way north. Those are the ones I use for medicine. Some are annuals and others perennial.

Spanish Needles, *Bidens pilosa* and Purple Stem Beggar Ticks are introduced species found in Ontario and Quebec and south. Tall, Nodding and Swamp Beggar Ticks are all native to my region of northern prairies. Tall Beggar Ticks (*B. frondosa*) is common, yet introduced.

The Cherokee chewed the leaves of Spanish needles for sore throat. Infusions were prepared to rid the body of parasites. In Curacao, plant decoctions are taken as a female aphrodisiac and emmenagogue.

Tall beggarticks (*B. frondosa*) young leaves and stems are cooked and eaten, as a vegetable, in Japan.

Both Tall beggar ticks and Spanish needles were prescribed in the United States as emmenagogues, and for the treatment of laryngeal and chest complaints.

Tall beggar ticks leaves have been used traditionally as an infusion for croup; the heated leaves placeed over the chest and neck as a poultice. A hot infusion of the seeds is more useful in whooping cough.

The seeds of the latter in tincture have been used in amenorrhea, dysmenorrhea and other uterine difficulties. Infusions of the root are helpful in severe coughs.

In Russia and Brazil, a heated poultice or fomentation of Nodding beggar ticks is used for throat and chest complaints, including laryngitis, croup and bronchitis.

Palpitations of the heart, and nervous insomnia in children are helped.

In Ghana, the fresh leaf juice is squeezed into the eyes and ears for reducing inflammation. Indigenous healers use the plant for prostate tumors.

In South Africa, the young shoots are chewed to relieve rheumatism.

Burr marigold is introduced and somewhat rare on the prairies. It has been used in China for eczema, heart ailments, and chronic dysentery. It was known as Water Agrimony in old herbals, and used for bladder ailments, gravel and stones, and an excellent remedy for ruptured blood vessels.

Culpepper wrote: "It is called in some countries Water Hemp, Bastard Hemp, and Bastard Agrimony; Eupatorium and Hepatorium, because it strengthens the liver, modifies the hardness of the spleen, and strengthens the lungs exceedingly... country people give it to their cattle when they are troubled with the cough or broken winded". Culpepper noted burr marigold or beggarticks were prescribed for "the fever- the gravel or stone of both kidney and bladder [and as a] styptic in bleedings."

Dr. King recommended infusions of the plant for heart palpitations.

Externally, the herb is used in Russia for treating alopecia, or lack of melanin in skin.

When the dried herb is burnt, the flowers give a cedar odor that acts as an insecticide and incense. The plant is a cadmium accumulator, suggesting phytoremediation potential.

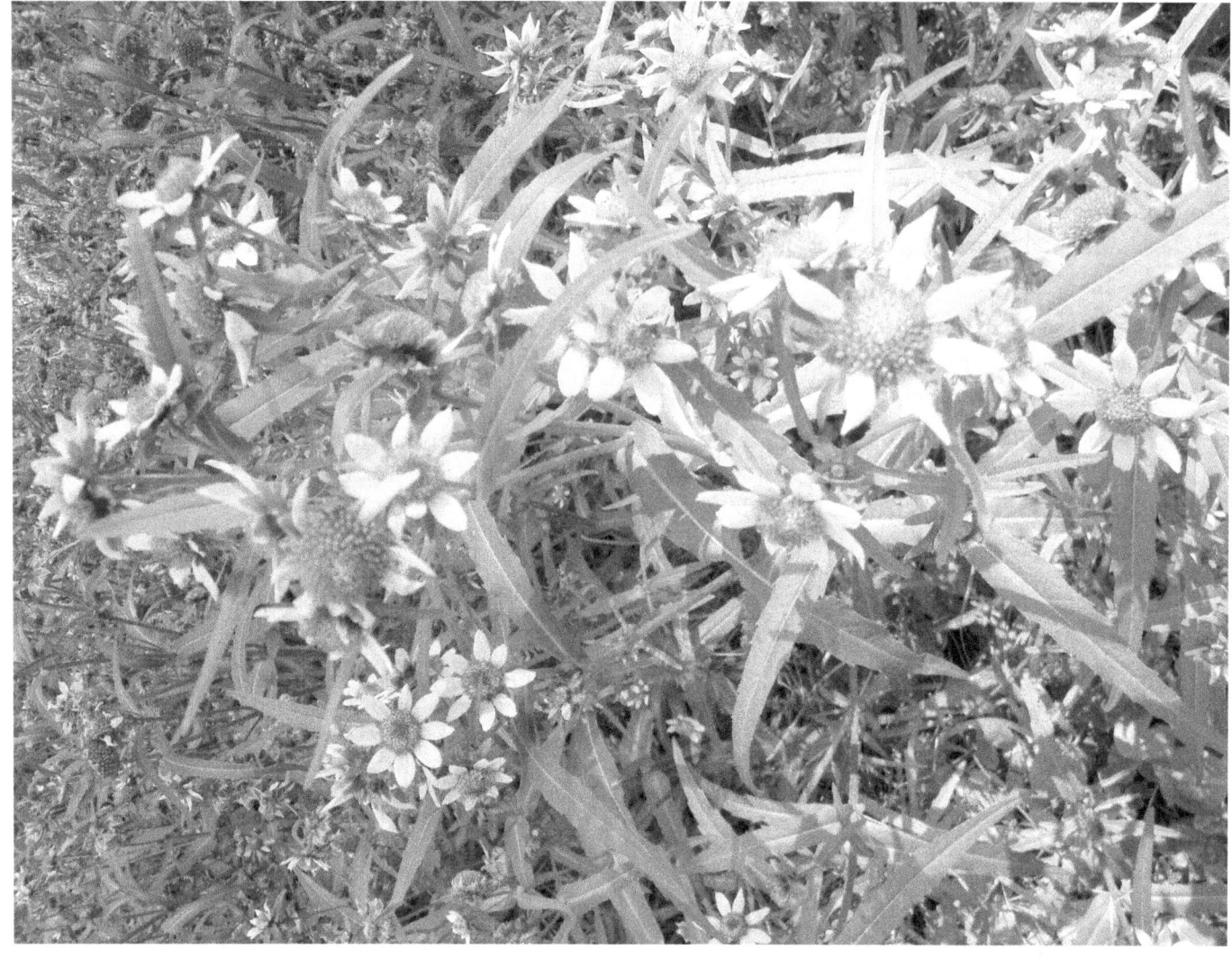

NODDING BEGGARTICKS

In China, *Bidens bipinnata* is often substituted for *B. pilosa*, going by the name ***HSIEN-FENG-TSAO***. Both herbs are used to remove toxins, clear heat, eliminate stagnancy, and fight skin infections.

It is used in flu-like conditions, swollen and sore throats, bowel and hemorrhoid inflammation, and epilepsy in children.

Hairy Beggar Ticks is eaten as a potherb and used as a tea substitute, in that country.

It is considered anti-bacterial and used for bug bites, diarrhea and unhealthy granulations. It is sometimes called Black Jack, or **KUEI CHEN GAO**.

Although introduced to North America, it is found in Ontario and Quebec, down the eastern seaboard and from Florida across the south to California.

In Brazil, the herb is considered a liver protectant, and used to treat malaria in the Amazon Basin. Garrafadas is the maceration product of the plant in alcohol, with alcohol soluble acetylene and flavonoids involved.

In the summer of 2000, while photographing plants around Alberta, Randy, Mors and I found three Bidens species, *B. cernua, B. frondosa and B. tripartita,* all growing together on the banks of the South Saskatchewan River, a rare event indeed.

Nodding Bur Marigold is often found on land that is covered with water in winter, and dries up in summer.

MEDICINAL

CONSTITUENTS - *B. cernua*–cernuol, cerbiden, chalcone glycosides, oils, gallic and oxalic acids, rutin-7-glucosides, iso-okanin-7-glucoside, cernuole, sulfuretin, maritimetin, quercitrin, and some as yet unnamed phenolic astringents. Flavonoid content in the leaves is a high 2.31%. Also contains phenyl heptatriyne- a potent anti-fungal.

B. frondosa- 56 constituents including chlorogenic acid, sulfuretin, marein, coreopsin, maritimetin, okanin, butein, luteolin, and a glycoside of 1,12,12-trihydrocytri-deca-4,6,8,10-tetrayn-2-ene. The seed oil is 34% of dry weight.

Five new acylated glucosides of chalcone (namely okanin 4-O-(6"-O-acetyl-2"-O-caffeoyl-beta-D-glucopyranoside), okanin 4-O-(2"-O-caffeoyl-6"-O-p-coumaroyl-beta-D-glucopyranoside), 4-O-methylokanin 4'-O-(6"-O-p-coumaroyl-beta-D-glucopyranoside), 4-O-methylokanin 4'-O-(6"-O-acetyl-beta-D-glucopyranoside) and 4-O-methylokanin 4'-O-(6'-O-acetyl-2"-O-caffeoyl-beta-D-glucopyranoside)) have been isolated from the fresh leaves. An aurone, 3',4', 6, 7-tetrahydroxyaurone is also present.

B. tripartita- aerial parts- 3 polyacetylenes, 2 thiophene derivatives, tridecane derivatives including trideca-1,12-dien-3,5,7,9-tetrain; linoleic acid, engenol, acetylene, xanthophylls, ocimene, 2'-hydroxy-4,4'-dimethoxy-chalcone, chlorogenic acid, luteolin, cynaroside, flavomarein, butin, buteine, scopoletin, umbelliferone, sterols, a flavonoid-isocoreopsin; and traces of an unstable cosmene. Also rich in iron, phosphorus and other minerals, volatile oils, tannins, and water-soluble polysaccharides. A flavonoid glycoside isolated from the herbage was identified as 7-O- beta -D-glucopyranoside (R-2) isoocanin ((R-2) flavanomarein). Flowers- the flowers contain only about half the flavonoid content of leaf, but exert twice the anti-oxidant activity. seeds- lysine (4.8-5.4%), fatty oils.

B. bipinnata- 24 compounds including alkaloids, tannins, saponins, flavonoids, including flavanomarein, cyanroside and luteolin; three phenylpropanoid glucosides, sterols, quercitin, maritimetin, esculetin, numerous glucopyranosides, bidenosides, isookanin. Butein is a yellow pigment present in the flowers of many *Bidens* species.

B. pilosa- phenyl-1, 3, 5-heptatriyne, phenylheptatriyne, friedelin, friedelan-3 beta-ol, phytosterin B, beta amyrin, esculetin, lupeol.

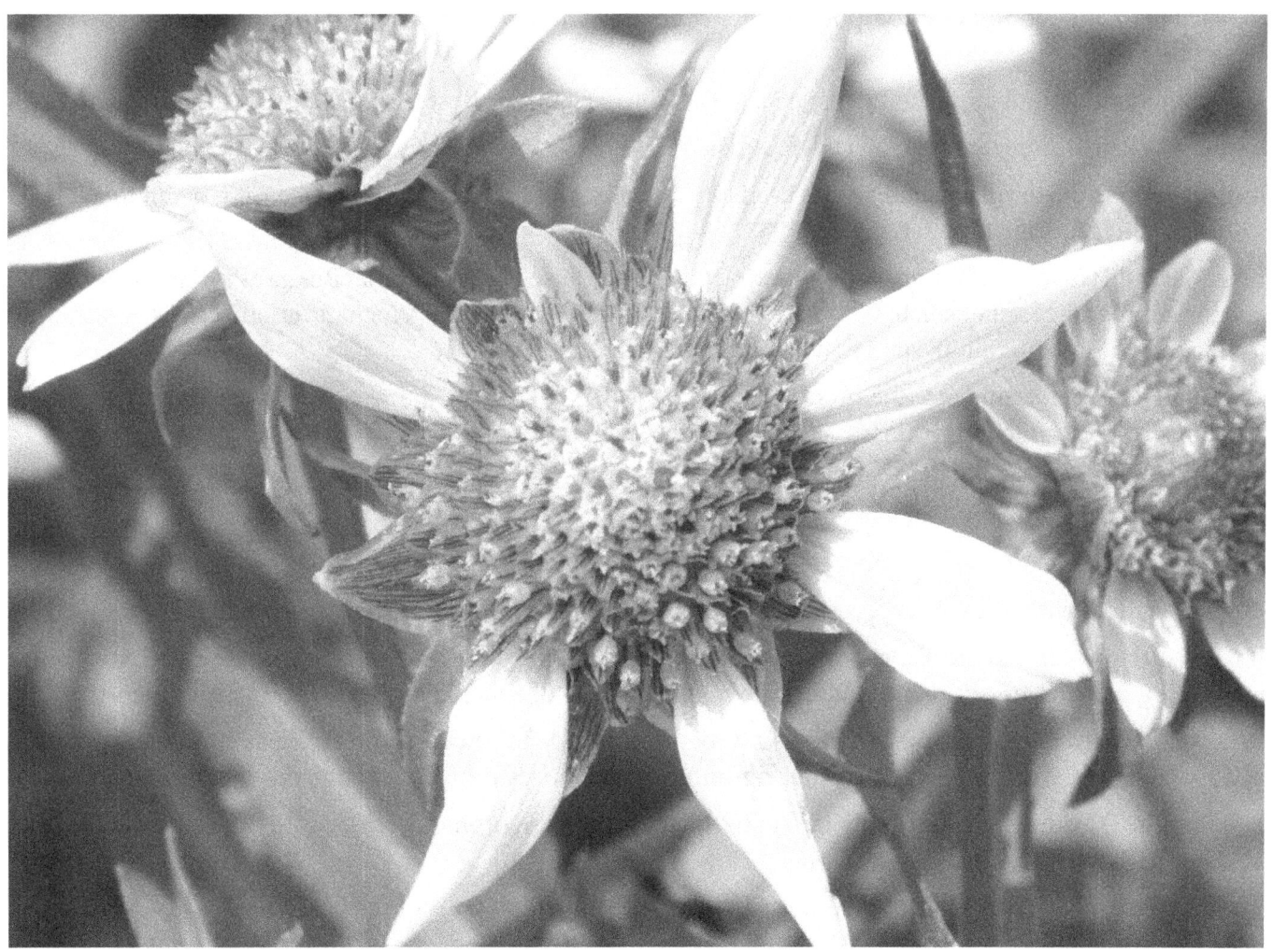

NODDING BEGGARTICKS

Nodding Beggartick seeds have been used historically for menstrual difficulties, including amenorrhea and painful periods. They combine well with Lady's Mantle to treat menorrhagia.

Infusions of the root have proven useful in severe coughs, including whooping cough. Acute bronchitis, asthma, hay fever and other respiratory infections also respond to the root or whole plant.

The whole plant as an infusion or tincture is useful for relieving irritation, inflammation, pain and bleeding of the urinary mucus membrane.

For benign prostatic hypertrophy (BPH), Bidens reduces the irritability and inflammation in the manner of nettle root.

Retention enemas reduce rectal irritation and help tone and shrink connective tissue in the area.

Matthew Wood says that "as a pungent aromatic it thins and warms the fluids, as a bitter it moves stagnant fluids and phlegm, and as an astringent it tones relaxed and swollen tissue".

Investigations of the plant using alcohol extracts reveal activity against Gram positive bacteria. Cernuol, isolated from aerial parts of *Bidens cernua* (collected from Ukraine) exhibited activity against *Microsporum canis* and seven *Trichophyton spp.* (MIC values of 10-20 mcg/ml), *Epidermophyton floccosum* (10 mcg/ml), *Candida albicans* (50 mcg/ml), *C. krusei* (100 mcg/ml) and seven Gram positive bacteria (5-10 mcg/ml). *Fitoterapia* 1998 67 9:1.

Hladun NP et al, *Mikrobiol Z* 2002 64(6):57-61 found cerbiden possesses anti-fungal activity against *Candida* species, sensitive and resistant to nystatin, amphotericin B, and clotrimazole.

Rybalchenko et al, found one compound, phenyl heptatriyne, active against 125 strains of yeast and fungi. *Fitoterapia* 2010 81(5):336-8.

This compound, found in many Bidens species, is highly effective against *Escherichia coli* (*E. coli*).

Earlier work by Bishop and MacDonald, found activity against *Staphylococcus aureus*.

In the Ukraine, the dry powdered herb is used as a water extract for treating skin rashes. It is given to adults as a diuretic and sudorific for internal use.

Burr Marigold (*B. tripartita*) leaf and shoot extracts have been used medicinally in Russia as a diuretic, sudorific, and for improving metabolism. In Germany, the aerial parts are used in gout, hematuria, and colitis. It combines well with Beth Root (Trillium spp.) and Sea Holly for blood in the urine.

Although it does not influence the production of uric acid like Devil's Club, this herb helps remove excessive amounts in gouty afflictions by increasing the kidney's excretion.

The herb has potent anti-diabetic activity and should be examined more carefully. Orhan N et al, *Iran J Basic Med Sci* 2016 19(10): 1114-24.

Washes of the plant are useful against staph infection, and can be used as an eyewash, or sitz bath.

It has been used with limited success for conditions of alopecia, applied externally as a wash.

It will help stop blood in the urine, or stool, as well as from gastric ulcers and lung. It combines well with other herbs like Cranesbill, or Agrimony in ulcerative colitis, and with Shepherd's Purse in cases of heavy menstruation.

When used for treating digestive conditions, it is best combined with a carminative such as coriander, or ginger. The herb combines well with calamus root, agrimony and comfrey for bleeding mucous membranes.

It is used in TCM for tracheal cough, laryngitis, pharyngitis and chronic dysentery. It is known as **LONG BA CAO** or Wolf's Grasp Weed.

The herb infusion or decoction has been used successfully in palpitations of the heart.

Studies from Russia seem to indicate that the wild isolated plants have significantly greater medicinal value than those grown in plot settings.

The herb contains compounds that mimic acyl-homoserine lactone and operate as a quorum sensing agonist. Tolmacheva AA et al, *Acta Pharm* 2014 64(2):173-86.

Both leaf and flower contain natural antioxidants that may have application for medicine or food. Wohiak et al, *Acta Pol Pharm* 2007 64:5.

Water extracts of the aerial parts possess significant anti-inflammatory, and analgesic properties. Pozharitskaya et al, *Phytomed* 2010 17(6):463-8.

Extracts show anti-thrombin and anti-cancer activity. Goun EA et al, *J Ethnopharm* 2002 81 337-342. The herb shows activity against both gram positive and negative bacteria. Tomczykawa et al, *Folia Histochemica et Cytobiologica* 2008 46:3.

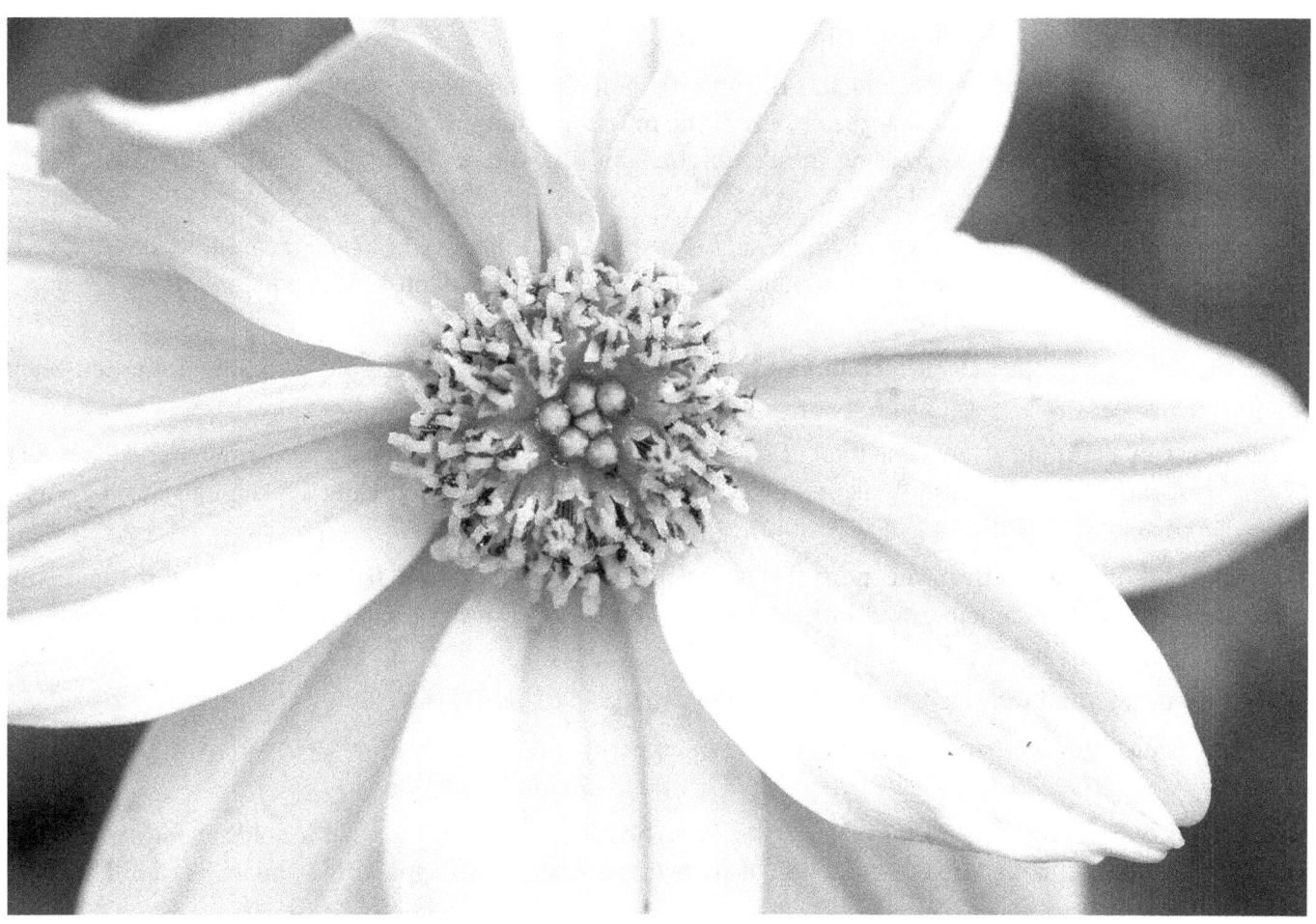

TALL BEGGAR TICKS FLOWER- CLOSE UP

Tall Beggar Ticks (*B. frondosa*) was screened, for broad anti-bacterial activity in Korea, by Kim et al 1993; with very positive results against both gram negative and positive bacteria. Earlier work by Bishop and MacDonald, in the former *Canadian Journal of Botany* 29 found acetone and ether extracts effective against *Staphylococcus aureus*.

Because it contains five acetylated glucosides, the work of Brandao et al, *Journal of Ethnopharmacology* 1997 57(2) may be relevant. They found Bidens species with 6-14 acetylenes were very active against parasites, and protozoa, whereas plants with three or less were inactive.

Work by Christensen and Lam, *Phytochemistry* 1991 20 11-49 found ethanol extracts of *B. frondosa* show 91% inhibition of malarial parasites at 50 micrograms per ml. Burr Marigold was 87% at same concentration and *B. bipinnata* 71% against *Plasmodium falciparum*.

Known in Japan as **SENDANGUSA**, the stem and leaves are used for treating colds, fevers and dysentery.

Maritimetin has been found to inhibit iodothionine deiodinase; the same as aureusidin in snapdragon, and bracteatin in straw flower.

Sulfuretin is found in this herb and nodding beggar ticks. Research has shown it to promote osteoblast differentiation and facilitate *in vivo* bone regeneration. Auh QS et al, *Oncotarget* 2016 7(48):78320-30.

It appears to promote apoptosis and cell cycle arrest in human cancer cell lines. Poudel S et al, *Biochem Biophys Res Commun* 2013 431(3):572-8.

An aurone derivative in herb has been found to possess anti-oxidative activity.

Recent work by Le J et al, *Molecules* 2015 20(10):18496-510 identified new compounds with anti-inflammatory activity, bringing total of identified fractions to fifty six.

Spanish Needles is a very effective mucous membrane tonic. Michael Moore wrote the herb has, "the ability to tighten, shrink and tonify the structural cells of the mucus membranes thereby preventing congestion and edema, while simultaneously increasing circulation, metabolism, and healing energy of the functional cells of those tissues."

This has been shown recently in work by Bo et al, *J Pharm Pharmacology* 2012 64:4. Flavonoids from this herb may be useful in improving micro-vascular inflammation, by reducing cytokine production, in *Henoch-Schonlein purpura* patients.

This condition is most prevalent in children, with 50% of cases under six years old, and 90% under ten years of age.

Recent work by Fei WJ et al looked at total flavones from Hairy Beggar Ticks (below) and how they can protect against vascular damage in this population by inhibiting NFkappaB, and reducing TNFalpha and NO levels. *Zhongguo Zhong Xi Yi Jie He Za Zhi* 2016 36(2).

It can be used for urinary tract infections (UTIs), helping clear up irritation, pain and congestion after acute infection is resolved. It combines well with cranberry or blueberry leaves, or uva ursi, depending upon the pH of urine.

It will help tighten and tone bladder tissue thus preventing recurring UTIs.

Spanish Needles (*B. bipinnata*) has shown benefit on experimental arthritis in rats, in work conducted by Liu et al in 1964.

Recent work by Shen AZ et al, *BMC Complement Altern Med* 2015 15(1):437 found flavonoids in herb ameliorate adjuvant-induced arthritis through induction of synovial apoptosis. This appears to validate its traditional use in arthritic conditions.

The plant is used in Traditional Chinese Medicine, and known as **NIEN SHEN TSAO** or **KUEI CHIN TSAO**. I have also seen it as **GUI ZHEN CAO**, 鬼針草 , and **GWAI JAM CHOU**.

Nien Shen Tsao or Nian Shen Cao (stick to the body weed) is confusing, as this teralso refers to *Desmodium sambuense* and *D. caudatum*.

The herb is used for its neutral properties and bitter flavor, in wind dampness, dispersing stagnant blood and invigorating it.

Rheumatoid arthritis, sprain, diarrhea, hepatitis, acute nephritis, as well as sore stomach and throats, all fit the picture pattern for use. It may be useful addition for irritable bowel syndrome.

The leaves are diaphoretic and emetic, and were used traditionally for relieving croup.

Dr. Craig, an early Eclectic physician, used the leaves as a fomentation to stop bleeding. He also used a wash for hemorrhoids, nosebleed, or bleeding gums. A neti pot of infused herb may help chronic or acute sinusitis.

The seeds are a diffusive stimulant and relaxant, promoting expectoration, soothing and sustaining to the nervous system, with some degree of benefit in light cases of painful or deficient menstruation.

The seed tea is generally taken as a warm infusion.

The root is a toning expectorant in cases of chronic cough.

Water extracts of the leaves and stems reveal activity against both yeast and gram positive bacteria. The flowers and stems inhibit *Staphylococcus aureus*. In parts of Ecuador, it is used for its tranquilizing effect.

Spanish Needles is used medicinally in Hawaii. **HO'OKO'OLAU** leaves are made into a tea that is taken in the morning for reviving failing appetite. Regular usage is said to prevent stroke. The compound isookanin is a potent inhibitor of alpha amylase with IC_{50} of 0.447 mg/ml.

Work by Wang et al, discovered five compounds in the herb that show inhibition of two leukemia cell lines HL-60 and V397, with an IC_{50} of less than 60 mcg/ml. *Zhong Yao Chi* 1997 20:5.

Isoquercitin, derived from this herb, was found to inhibit the progression of human liver cancer, *in vivo* and *in vitro*. Huang G et al, *Oncol Rep* 2014 31(5):2377-84.

Other work found anti-tumor activity against human hepatic carcinoma and human cervical carcinoma (HeLa) cell lines. Yang QH et al, *Afr J Trad Complement Altern Med* 2013 10(3):543-9.

Work by Zhong et al, *J Pharm Pharmacol* 59:7 confirms anti-oxidant and significant anti-hepatoxic activity.

Herbal extracts inhibit the growth of mouse cervical carcinoma U14. Zhu LH et al, *Afr J Tradit Complement Altern Med* 2013 10(4):66-9. Human application is unknown.

Butein is found in the flower petals and has been found to inhibit NADH oxidase and the activity of auccinoxidase.

Hairy Beggar Ticks (*B. pilosa*) is widely used in Traditional Chinese Medicine. It is known as **BAI ZI REN** (Cantonese) or **BAAK JI YAN** (Mandarin). In Taiwan, it is referred to as **HSIEN FENG TSAO**. It is also referred to as **SAN YE GUIZ HEN CAO**, meaning three leaf bidens.

It has been used for moving pathogens to the surface of body, clearing heat, removing toxins and eliminating stagnancy. It has been traditionally used for influenza, sore throat, intestinal conditions, including hemorrhoids, as well as dysentery and jaundice. It has been used traditionally, for over forty diseases around the world.

The compound phytosterin B has been found to lower blood pressure.

Since this book is focused on northern plants, I will share just a few of the recent studies.

Ethanol extracts inhibit prostaglandin synthesis. Jäger AK et al, *J Ethnopharm* 1996 52(2):95-100. This suggests benefit in headache and inflammatory conditions.

Hot infusions show activity against herpes simplex virus 1. Chiang LC, *Am J Chin Med* 2003 32(3):355-62. The polyacetylenes in this herb are one of the few natural substances reported to inhibit cytomegalovirus, a herpes virus that causes problems in immune compromised individuals.

An oral feeding of the herb to mice suppressed tumor metastasis and myeloid-derived suppressor cells. By communicating with bone marrow cells, this herb should be investigated further for adjunct treatment of metastatic cancers. Wei WC et al, *Sci Rep* 2016 6:36663.

Work by Chang JS, *Am J Chin Med* 2001 29(2):303-12 found hot water extracts inhibit five leukemia cancer cell lines.

The herb may be useful for androgen deficient dry eyes, based on work by Zhang C et al, *Cell Physiol Biochem* 2016 39(1):266-77. A cooled, strained infusion in an eyecup would be worth a trial for improving tear quantity, maintaining tear film stability and inhibiting inflammation of the lacrimal gland.

Isoquercitrin from this herb inhibits bladder cancer progression by regulating the P13K/Akt and PKC signaling pathways. Chen F et al, *Oncol Rep* 2016 36(1):165-72.

It may be useful adjunct in colorectal cancer, based on work of Wu J et al, *Journal of Nat Med* 2013 67(1):17-26.

The herb and isolated compound suppress adipogenesis and lipid content in adipocytes and mice via down regulation of Egr2, C/EBPs and PPARgamma pathways, suggesting benefit in obesity. Liang YC et al *Sci Rep* 2016 6:24285.

The plant has potential for use in treating diabetes. Work by Yang WC, *Evid Based Complement Altern Med* 2014:698617 looked at the pharmacology and phytochemistry in great detail.

The related *B. alba* contains a protein that appears active against colorectal cancer cell lines. Ong PL et al, *Food Chem Tox* 2008 46:5. The content of phenylheptatriyne of *B. alba* var. *radiata* leaves growing in Florida, is highest in October. Cantonwine EG, Downum KR, *J Chem Ecol* 2001 27(2):313-26.

ESSENTIAL OIL

Nodding Beggar Ticks produces an essential oil with a very important compound called cernuole. It's chemical nature is 3-methoxy-4- (1,5-dimethylhex-4-enyl)-6-methylphenol. At dilutions of 5-20 milligrams per litre, cernuole was found active against both gram postive bacteria and dermal fungi. It is considered one the most anti-microbial active sesquiterpene compounds known.

Bur marigold (*B. tripartita*) has been CO_2 extracted; yielding 0.6% of dry weight. The extract contained 1.34% essential oils, 26% nonsaponifiable substances, and 0.087% tocopherols. The lipid fraction included sterols, phosphatides, cabohydrates, wax (21%), and glycerides (52.5%).

The flower heads have been steam distilled and contain over 16% p-cymene, as well as lesser amounts of beta caryophyllene, and humulene epoxide. The fresh herb contain contains 38% allocimene, 30% (Z)-beta ocimene, and 8.5% alpha phellandrene, as well as eugenol and cosmene.

Work by Kaskoniene V & Maruska A, *Acta Chim Slov* 2015 62(1):1-7 found beta ocimene (40-46%) the main volatile, with alpha pinene, p-cymene, and beta-elemene also present in significant amounts. The essential oil exhibits anti-fungal activity.

The roots have been steam distilled and found to be strongly anti-fungal. The oil contains 15% alpha pinene, 9.3% beta-bisabolene, 6% p-cymene, 5.7% hexanal, 4.6% linalool, 3.4% p-cymene-9-ol, 2.6% beta-elemene, 2.2% 2-pentylfuran, and 2.1% silphiperfol-6-ene.

Common Beggar Tick yields an essential oil that shows activity against a number of microbes including *S. aureus, Listeria monocytogenes, Bacillus subtilis, Pseudomonas aeruginosa, Salmonella enteritidis,* and *Enterobacter aerogenes*. Rahman et al, *Int J Food Sci Tech* 2011 46:6 1238-44.

Spanish needles (*B. bipinnata*) was steam-distilled with a yield of 0.15% from the aerial parts.

The oil consists of 17.6% thymol; 16.8% beta caryophyllene, 14% gamma-cadinene; 12% gamma elemene; 10.5% alpha humulene; and smaller amounts of delta cadinene, delta elemene, methylthymol, alpha and beta pinene, alpha cubebene.

Hairy Beggar Ticks has been found to increase PGE_2 secretion in human gingival fibroblast studies. Studies in Northern Cameroon suggest the leaf essential oil may be useful for as natural pesticide for stored food.

The leaf and stem oils are rich in sesquiterpenes with the leaf oil rich in caryophyllene oxide (37%), beta caryophyllene (10.5%) and humulene oxide (6%) and the stem rich in hexahydrofarnesyl acetone (13.4%), delta cadinene (12%) and caryophyllene oxide (11%).

SEED OIL

Common Beggar ticks (*B. frondosa*) seeds contain 34% oil.

Work in Bulgaria, looking for genetic pools to improve sunflower seed yield, led to the analysis of 14 different plots of *B. tripartita* and their seed oils.

Linoleic acid, oleic acid and the amino acid lysine were in the range of 64.0-73.8, 18.3-23.4 and 4.83-5.45%, respectively.

FLOWER ESSENCES

Beggar's Tick (*B. alba*) helps us to end kowtowing to other's plans for use and carries us away to follow our own destiny. This essence is also supportive for clearing and cleansing of the kidneys, urinary tract and prostate.
GREEN HOPE FARM

Bidens essence is useful in helping households to interact harmoniously. It will allow you to claim your own space in a healthy way. It impacts psychological boundary issues related to family.
CHARISSA'S CAULDRON

RECIPES

INFUSION- Two to four ounces prepared at 1:20 ratio. Up to four times daily.

TINCTURE- 20-40 drops up to four times daily in acute cases; less in chronic. Dry plant tincture is 1:5 at 45% alcohol; fresh plant 1:3 at 60%.

CAUTION- Extremely nasty necrosis and severe skin burns have been reported by Terzioglu et al, *Internet J Alt Med* 3:2 from external application of *B. tripartita*.

BERGENIA
ELEPHANT EARS
SIBERIAN TEA
LEATHER BERGENIA
HEART LEAVED BERGENIA
(*Bergenia crassifolia* [L.] Fritsch)
(*B. cordifolia* [Haw] Sternb.)- no longer accepted.
MILE'S BERGENIA
HIMALAYAN BERGENIA
(*B. milesii* Baker)
(*B. stracheyi* [Hook.f & Thomson] Engl)
FRINGED BERGENIA
HAIRY LEAF BERGENIA
WINTER BEGONIA
(*B. ciliata* [Haw.] Sternb.)
(*B. ligulata* [Wall.] Engl.)
PARTS USED- leaves, flowers, roots

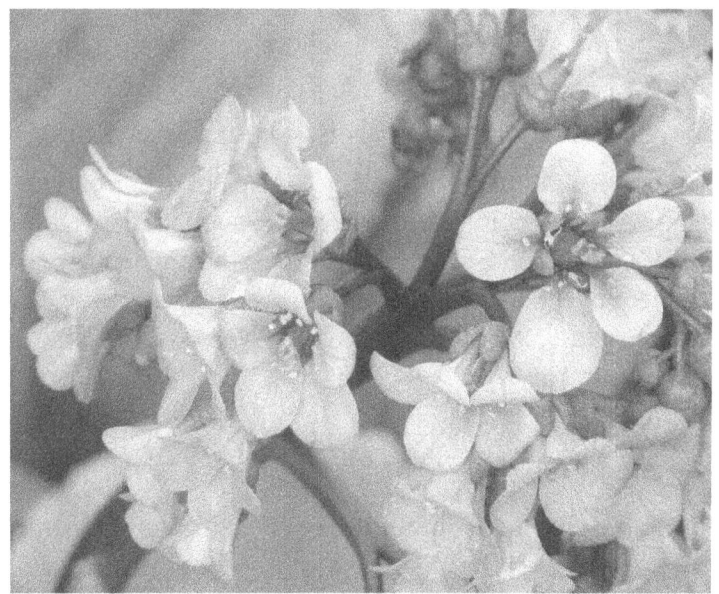
BERGENIA FLOWERS

God is not troubled by one who is conservative or liberal, and He certainly never inclines His ear toward a donkey or an elephant.
MAX LUCADO

Bergenia is named after Karl August von Bergen, an 18th century Botany professor from Frankfurt. He wrote several texts on medical botany, including *Flora of Frankfurt* in 1750.

Cordifolia means "heart-shaped"; and crassifolia "thick leaved". Saxifraga is Latin meaning "growing in rocky crevices". Ciliata means hairy or fringed.

A common nickname, Pigsqueak, came about when it was discovered that a swine-like noise could be obtained by stroking the large leaves between index finger and thumb.

Another common name, Leather leaf was linked to the plants earlier use in tanning and dying leather.

Bergenia has always been one of my favorite garden perennials. The large green leaves turn a reddish golden in fall and because they are evergreen they persist through the winter snows. It is widely grown in gardens throughout my hometown of Edmonton.

The plant is native to Siberia, and produces beautiful rose to purple flowers in May. It thrives on all types of soil, low maintenance, but grows larger when it has damp feet. It is known as **BADAN** in Russia.

It has been widely used in that country for colds, gastritis, enterocolitis, headache, diarrhea and fever. The rhizomes are decocted and the water used for periodontal disease, gingivitis, stomatitis and bleeding gums.

The leaves are dried and used as a beverage, usually in form of tea. The young leaves are green, second year are brown and third year turn black. The latter are preferred and known as Chagirsky tea, due to the reduced content of tannins.

The rhizomes are official in Russia. Infusions are recommended for excessive menstruation, bleeding after miscarriage or abortion, and cervical erosion treatment.

It is suggested to strengthen capillary walls, local vasodilation, decreased blood pressure, and heart health.

It appears to meet the historical definition of an adaptogen. That is, an adaptogen must produce a non-specific response. For example, increase the power of resistance against stressors; have a normalizing effect regardless of the nature of pathology; and be non-toxic and innocuous and not influence normal body functions.

The fresh, green leaves are poulticed in Tibet and applied to sunburn and UV damage.

In TCM (traditional Chinese medicine), the thick leaf, known as **HOU YE YAN BAI CAI**, is used to supplement vacuity and staunch bleeding, relieve coughs and asthma, and alleviate dizziness and hemoptysis.

The roots and rhizomes are official medicine in Mongolia, and used for typhoid, lung fever and inflammation, as well as stomach, intestinal disorders, and diarrhea.

The root of *B. ligulata*, a closely related plant that grows in the Himalayas up to 7000 feet, is used as an antidote to opium. It is combined with honey and applied to the gums of teething children. The root or rhizome is used for kidney stones, combined with diuretic and antiseptic herbs. One of its names **SHILABHED** means, "dissolving or piercing stones", in reference to its effect on kidney stones, or rocky terrain where the plants grow. Water/alcohol extracts inhibit calcium oxalate and calcium phosphate aggregation and formation. Lipschitz WL et al, *Pharmacol Exp Ther* 1943 79-97.

The rhizome is cool and bitter.

In India, the flowers are boiled and pickled.

Two other species from the region, *B. ciliata,* and *B. stracheyi* are hardy to the prairies, but may not keep their evergreen leaves through the winter. In several books, *B. ciliata* and *B. ligulata* are considered synonyms for the same species.

The former is found in the temperate Himalayan valleys between 800-3000 metres.

Bergenia stracheyi is native to Afghanistan and Uttarakhand, and found on alpine slopes between 3300-4500 meters. Traditionally, a fine powder of roots is made into a paste with pine resin and applied to ripen boils.

Leaf yields of *B. crassifolia* vary between 1.1 and 2.5 kilograms per square metre, and the rhizome yield between 1.5 and 3.3 kilograms.

Mile's Bergenia is supposed to be hardy to zone 7 and higher. It grows in Edmonton, which is zone 3, in sheltered spots. *B. ciliata/C. ligulata* is hardy to zone 5 and is also found in local gardens.

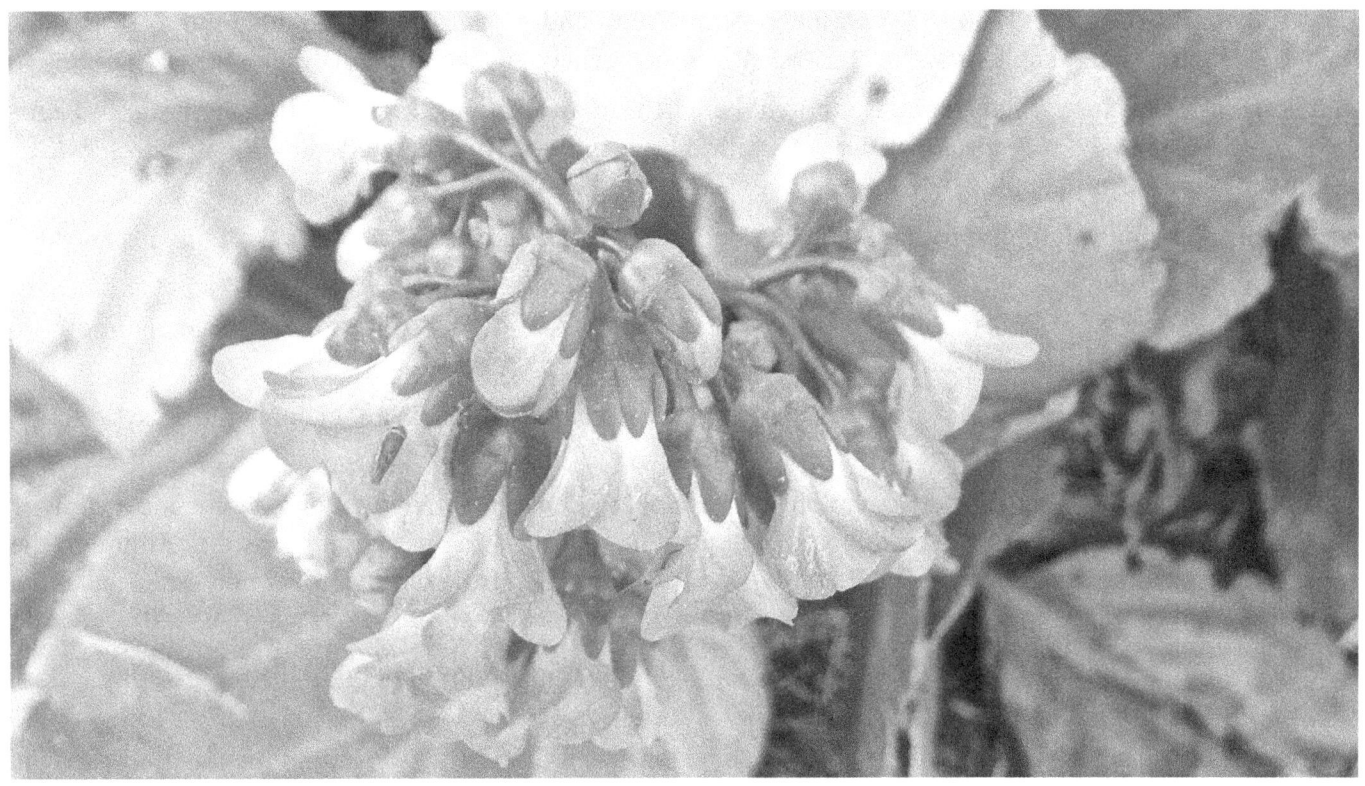

BERGENIA CRASSIFOLIA FLOWER AND LEAF

MEDICINAL

CONSTITUENTS- *B. crassifolia* root- bergenin (6-10%), (+)-catechin-3-O-gallate, proanthocyanidins, tannins, quercitin, arbutin (1.8-2.3%) bergenan (polysaccharide).
The green leaves contain 5.1% bergenin, 55% ellagitannins, 29% gallic acid, 11% flavonoids, bergenan, bergapten, norathyriol, norbergenin, trihydroxycoumarin, caffeoyl quinic acid, acetyl salicylic acid, the glucoside rhododenrin (betuliside) and 10.6% arbutin (older leaves up to 22%)
Gallic acid is primary compound in black leaves.
A complete phytochemistry of over 100 constituents is found in work by Shikov et al, *Phytomedicine* 2014 21:1534-42.
B. ciliata roots- beta sitosterol, bergenin, gallolylated leukoantho-cyanidin-4-(2-0-galloyl) glucoside, gallic acid, metarbin, glucose, mucilage, tannins, beta sitosterol, flavonoids.
leaves- berginin (3.1%), quercitin, kaempferol,their 3-rhamnosides,quercetrin, and afzelin; arbutin derivatives and beta sitosterol , paashanolactone
B. ligulata rhizomes- bergenin, afzelechin, paashaanolactone, arbutin, catechin, gallic acid, albumin (7.75%), glucose (5.5%), mucilage.
B. stracheyi- (+) catechin-3-gallate, beta sitosterol and bergenin.
B. hissarica root- five anthraquione derivatives including aloe-emodin, its 8-0-beta-glucoside, physcion, chrysophanein and emodin 1-0-beta-D-glucopyranoside.
Leaf- aloe-emodin, physicon, aloe emodin 8-O-beta glucoside, chrysophanein, and 1-O-beta-D-glucopyranosyloxy-6,8-dihydroxy-3-methylanthraquinone.

The various species all exhibit similar profiles and can be used interchangeably. Some species have more identified compounds, with bergenin, common to all.

A dry extract of the over-wintered black leaves increased the working capacity of white rats by 30%, and showed both anti-stress and immune stimulating properties in mice.

Work by Popov et al, *Phytother Res* 19:12 identified bergenan, a polysaccharide as possessing immune stimulating and phagocytic activity *in vivo*.

Bergenin, an iso-coumarin lactone, is obtained from the root and used in Russia, Tibet and parts of Eastern Asia to treat chronic bronchitis, gastroenteritis, and various gynecological inflammations.

Bergenin has been closely studied and is reported beneficial as an anti-hepatotoxic, anti-arrhythmic and anti-ulcer agent. Lim et al, *Pharmacology* 2001 63:2 found bergenin restores depleted glutathione stores in liver helping remove harmful toxins.

Bergenin, taken orally, inhibits product of pro-inflammatory Th1 cytokines. Nazir N et al, *J Ethnopharm* 2007 112:401-5.

It inhibits COX-2 but not COX-1, which is somewhat surprising considering content of salicylates. Numomura RC et al, *J Brazil Chem Soc* 2009 20:1060-4.

Like the epigallocatechin gallates of green tea, bergenin has been found useful in augmenting the lipolytic action of agents acting on the adrenergic system.

While studies have shown no direct stimulation or measurable adrenergic activity, it markedly enhances lipolysis induced by norepinephrine and even opposes the lipogenic (or fat building) action of insulin. Although the exact action is unknown, it is believed to involve increased norepinephrine binding to fat cells. This makes it a useful addition to weight loss formulas where it is desired to avoid CNS stimulation.

Bergenin exhibits significant anti-anxiety activity, comparable to diazepam, in animal studies. Singh J et al, *J Ethnopharmacology* 2017 195:182-7.

In a study comparing bergenin and dexamethasone on chronic bronchitis, it was found they both worked via similar, but slightly different, effect on BCAA metabolism. Ren X et al, *Mol Biosyst* 2016 12(6):1938-47.

Bergenin ameliorates acute lung injury by inhibiting NFkappaB activation. Yang, SQ et al, *Journal of Ethnopharmacology* 2017 200: 147-255.

Bergenin reduces renal inflammation and block TGF-beta1-Smads pathway, in ameliorating diabetic nephropathy in rats. Yang J et al, *Immunopharmacol Immunotoxicol* 2016 38(2):145-52.

Bergenin is regenerative of pancreatic beta cells. Kumar et al, *Fitoterapia* 2012 83(2):395-401.

Ethanol/water extracts of the rhizome inhibit human pancreatic lipase activity, and exhibit anti-oxidant properties as well. Ivanov et al, *Fitoterapia* 2010 Oct 3.

A 70% alcohol tincture of the rhizomes inhibits ACE 1, or angiotensin 1-converting enzyme. Ivanov et al, *Khimija Rastititel'nogo Syr'ja* 2011 2:165-72.

It is often called Siberian Tea *(B. crassifolia)*, and used in veterinary medicine for various digestive and gastrointestinal disorders in calves.

Leaf infusions of *B. crassifolia* have been shown to inhibit gram positive and negative bacteria and mycobacterium. Leaf washes have been used for skin leishmaniosis.

Ethanol extracts of both root and aerial parts show activity against *Candida albicans*.

Kokoska et al, *Journal of Ethnopharm* 2002 82:51-3, found it one of the most anti-microbial of 16 Siberian plants tested, with activity against *Bacillus cereus, Candida albicans, E. coli, S. aureus* and especially *Pseudomonas aeruginosa* at very low concentration.

A Russian study by Fedoseeva et al reported on the anti-microbial activity of the dry leaf extract. The MIC for various bacteria was 0.1 g/ml, whereas a decoction of uva ursi at the same concentration only affected 78% of gram negative and 56% of gram positive bacteria.

Water-soluble extracts of the root show activity of mitochondrial ATP dependent potassium channels. Mironova et al, *Bull Exp Biol Med* 2008 46:2.

According to Dr. King, the celebrated Eclectic physician, bergenin is a valued nerve tonic, "its action being intermediate between quinine and salicin".

The arbutin content of aerial and below ground parts is increased in Leather Bergenia, when the total removal of aerial parts is done in early May, without damaging the growing tip. Querctin and kaempferol content remains much the same.

Berganan is a pectin polysacchride, found in both leaves and root, containing about 80% D-galacturonic acid. It appears to possess immunostimulating activity. Popov SV et al, *Phytother Res* 2005 19(12):1052-6.

Arbutin levels are much higher than those in Uva ursi leaves. The best extraction method for arbutin is to use alkalized water and ultrasound treatment. It has a disinfecting activity similar to Uva ursi or bearberry leaves. It also inhibits tyrosinase and is useful in skin-whitening cosmetics, by inhibiting production of melanin.

Arbutin, of course, inhibits bladder cancer, protects sperm from cryodamage, and is highly antioxidant. Bladder cancer is rapidly increasing in North America.

Ethanol extract of the rhizome are cytotoxic to human lymphoblastoid Raji cells, and slightly more efficient that green leaf tinctures.

The leaf extracts reduce both systolic and diastolic blood pressure. Makarova & Makarov 2010. *Molecular Biology of Flavonoids: Manual for Doctors*. Lema Pub. St-Petersburg, pages 272-290.

Pedunculagin was found cytotoxic against human chronic myelogenous leukemia (K562), human promyelocytic leukemia (HL-60), mouse lymphoid neoplasm (P388), mouse lymphocytic leukemia (L1210) and sarcoma 180 cells lines.

Infusions of the fermented leaf show increased glucose utilization and decreased lactate levels in mice. Shikov et al, *Journal Funct Foods* 2010 2:71-6.

The same author found both black and fermented leaf decreased appetite and energy supplementation by up to 40% in fat induced obese rats. *Phytomed* 2012 19:1250-5.

Another study found black leaves increased treadmill running time in rats, similar to Siberian ginseng (*Eleutherococcus senticosus*), a long proven, efficient adaptogen.

Galloyl glucosides, from leaf, inhibit hepatitis C virus, in vitro. Zuo GY et al, *Antiviral Chem Chemother* 2005 16(6):393-8.

The green leaves are cerebral protective, in rat studies of experimental hypoxia. The protection is believed associated with normalization of succinate-dependent energy production and rapid metabolic cluster reactions. Khazanov VA & Shmirnova NB. *Bull Exp Biol Med* 2000 1:63-65.

Related plants from the Himalayas such as *Bergenia ligulata* are used medicinally. The root is diuretic, demulcent and astringent; and used for kidney stones, tuberculosis and liver complaints.

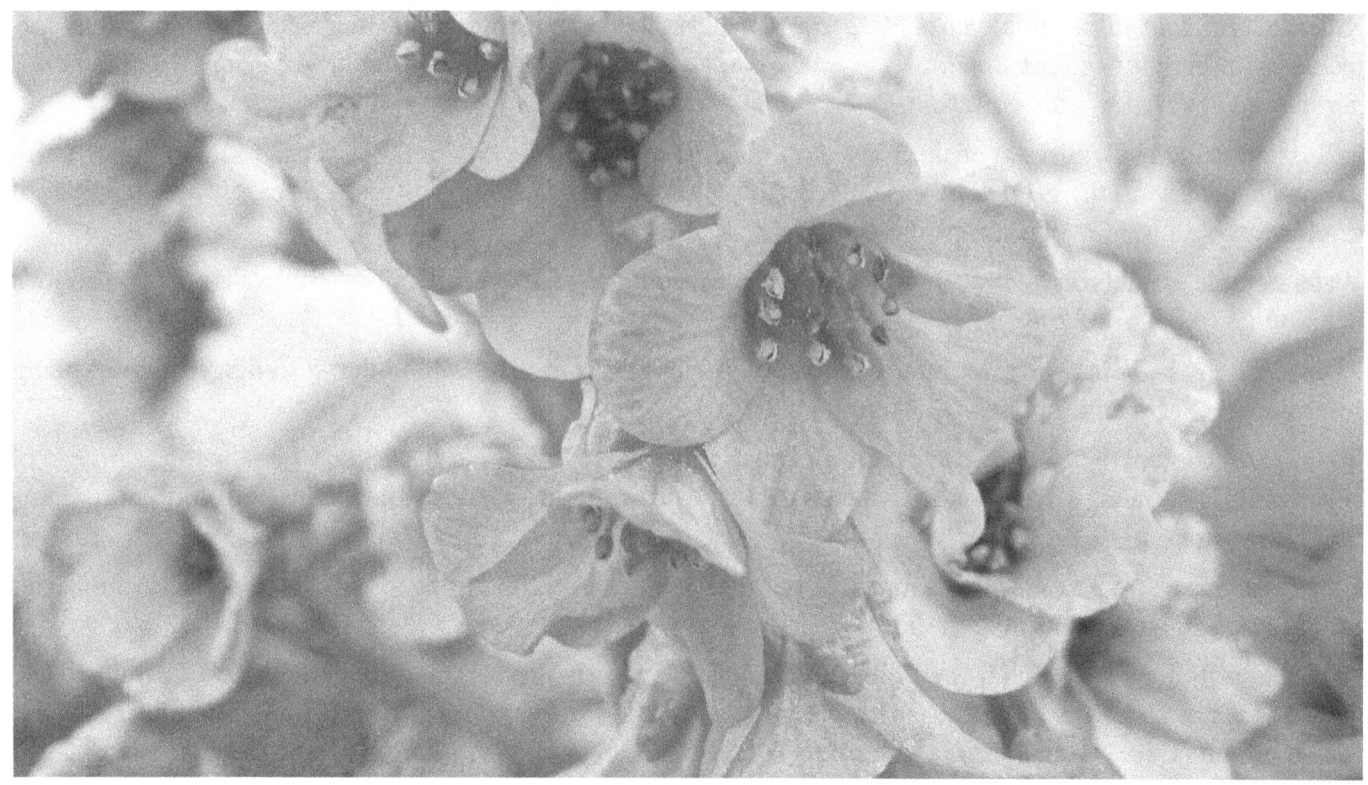

FLOWERS OF BERGENIA CRASSIFOLIA

Juice or powder of the whole plant is given to treat urinary complaints, while a juice of the tannin rich root is taken for hemorrhoids, asthma, as well as urinary trouble. The dose is about six teaspoons three times daily. The squeezed root is boiled and the filtered water taken for gout, and indigestion.

Pastes of the root are applied to backache. The root powder, about three teaspoons, is taken with warm water as an anthelmintic.

It is also anti-inflammatory. *Phytochemistry* 1998 47:5.

Rajbandani et al, *Journal of Ethnopharmacology* 2001 3:74; and *Pharmazie* 2003 58(4) showed significant anti-influenza activity from *B. ligulata*.

Fifty percent inhibition at only 10 mcg per ml was exhibited. Partial protease inhibition activity was also indicated.

Alcohol extractions of the root of *B. ligulata* have shown anti-cancer activity in rats; but insignificant anti-lithic activity dissolving stones in male rats.

The latter study, by Garimella et al, *Phytother Res* 2001 15:4 reported weak stone dissolving activity. Despite the rodent study, the root is used extensively in India for kidney stones.

Bashir et al, *J Ethnopharm* 122:1 found the herb inhibited calcium oxalate crystal aggregation.

Work by Joshi et al, Urol Res 2005 Mar 25, showed water extracts of this herb and Puncture Vine (*Tribulus terrestris*) inhibit the growth of calcium phosphate stone formation. More research is needed.

The compound (+)-afzelechin, derived from rhizomes, is an alpha glucosidase inhibitor. Saijyo et al, *J Oleo Sci* 2008 57:8.

Root extracts of *B. ciliata* induce hypotension in dog studies, and significant diuretic effect in rats.

Work by Sinha et al, *J Pharm Pharmacol* 2001 53:2 found methanol extracts *of B. ciliata* rhizome to possess anti-inflammatory potential. The extracts were approximately 75% as powerful as the phenylbutazone used as a standard.

The same group found anti-tussive activity. *Phytomedicine* 2001 8:4. And to complete publication requirements for the year, the anti-bacterial activity was tested, and reported by the same author in *Fitoterapia* 72:5.

Water alcohol extracts show activity against herpes and influenza viruses, as well as moderate protease inhibition. Rajbhanddari et al *Evid Based Compl Altern Med* 2007 Oct 25; *Journal Ethnopharm* 2001 74 251-55.

Recent work by Kakub et al, *Phytotherapy Res* 21:12 suggests the rhizome may be of use in gastric ulcers.

Rhizome tinctures show activity against breast, liver and prostate human cancer cell lines. Rajkumer et al. *J Pharm Res* 2011 4:2.

The herbal drug **PASHANBHED** consists of the dried rhizomes of *B. ligulata*, *B. ciliata*, and *B. stracheyi*. The rhizomes have no significant anatomical differences.

The name Pashanbhed is contraversial as it has been assigned to various herbs, including *B. ligulata*, *Kalanchoe pinnata*, *Coleus aromaticus* and *Rotula aquatica*.

They are considered a tonic for use in fever, diarrhea and pulmonary affections.

The leaves of *B. ligulata* are hemostatic.

An 80% tincture of the rhizome inhibits alpha glucosidase, suggesting benefit in treating blood sugar conditions. (+)-afzelechin is considered the primary inhibitor.

Berginin, isolated from rhizomes of *B. stracheyi*, show anti-arthritic activity, in part, by balancing Th1/Th2 cytokines. Bergenin and norbergenin inhibit the production of pro-inflammatory Th1 cytokines (IL-2, IFNgamma, TNFalpha), while potentiating anti-inflammatory Th2 cytokines (IL-4 and IL-5).

The roots of *S. hissarica* are used in Uzbekistan as astringents, with hemostatic and anti-phlogistic activity. They are mainly used in gastrointestinal and gynecological conditions.

Aloe emodin is an anthraquinone component of *Bergenia* spp. roots and rhizomes. It is laxative, boosts the immune system, and possesses anti-inflammatory and anti-microbial activity.

Dar Lesa is a low calorie, non-alcoholic carbonated beverage made with Bergenia leaves, *Polygonum* ssp. and the tops of yarrow. This drink was developed at the Kemerovo Technological Institute of the Food Industry for patients with diabetes mellitus.

Work by Majurnikova et al, *Voprosy-Pitaniya* 2000 69:1-2 evaluated the Russian beverage at two clinic in involving 25 patients, who were given one glass every day for two months.

Results showed a marked improvement in their condition, with the beverage being recommended for inclusion in the diet of diabetes mellitus patients.

The related *B. himalacia* shows stimulation of insulin release from INS-1 cells at 20 mcg/mL. Hussain et al, *Phytother Res* 2004 18:1.

Bergenin is found, as well, in Large Flowering Astilbe (*A. macroflora*), and exhibits the same anti-inflammatory property.

ESSENTIAL OILS

The green leaves *of B. crassifolia* contain 0.05% essential oil, consisting of 3-methyl-2-buten-1-ol (26.5%), hexadecanoic acid (16%), dodecanoic acid (10%), linalool (5.63%), octadecadienoic acid (4.1%) and minor volatiles.

In another study both green and fermented leaves were distilled and yielded 0.012% and 0.010% respectively. The oil of fermented leaves consists mainly of alpha-bisabolol oxide B, and increased levels of alpha terpineol, geraniol, linalool and nerolidol by 1.7 to 2.9 fold.

Essential oil from roots of *B. ligulata* contains 97 compounds, including (+)-(6S)-parasorbic acid (47%), isovalaric acid (6.25%), (Z)-asarone (3.5%) and terpinen-4-ol (3%). The rhizomes contain only berginin and beta-sitosterol.

The root oil is a natural insecticide.

The rhizome of *B. stracheyi* yields 0.13% essential oil, consisting of 3-methyl-2-buten-1-ol (52.7%), beta-eudesmol (7.44%), damascenone (3.2%), caryophyllene (2.75%) and phytol (2.57%).

FLOWER ESSENCES

Pig Squeak (*B.cordifolia*) flower essence is for situations of betrayal, and helping one trust one's own experience. It is for when one finds oneself unwillingly embroiled in other's emotional issues, and the feeling of confusion, bewilderment and betrayal that can be engendered. It helps enable one to trust one's own inner experience and guidance, so that one can be uncompromising in one's own actions, and immune to the false opinion of others. **CHRISTCHURCH** FLOWER ESSENCE**S**

Bergenia essence assists us to perceive the inaudible frequencies of the living earth, a bandwidth of sounds heard primarily through our listening hearts. Bergenia gently re-directs us away from passing bright ideas by focusing any scattered or tangential thinking. It also balances water disparities (edema/dehydration) in the body. **RAVEN ESSENCES**

Bergenia (*B. crassifolia*) flower essence is useful for those who have endured or suffered early trauma. It helps to "toughen" the etheric shield around those who have been exploited, victimized, or abused in psychological or physiological manner.

It may also be useful, combined with fleabane essence, for individuals that feel "weathered" or "weary" of life's demands, helping restore a sense of relaxation and harmony to everyday demands. **PRAIRIE DEVA**

RECIPES

DECOCTION- rhizome- One to two tablespoons three times daily of 1:20 decoction.

TINCTURE- dry rhizome- 1:4 at 40% alcohol and 10% glycerin.

Fresh leaf tinctures, either green, brown or black are prepared at same ratio.

Research on *B. ciliata* rhizomes found 50% alcohol tincture gives highest yield after 21 days.

BIRD'S FOOT TREFOIL
(***Lotus corniculatus*** L.)
PARTS USED- flowering tops

Lotus is from the Greek **LOTOS**, of several legumes. Corniculatus means, "with small horns", and refers to the small seedpods.

The Lotus-eaters of mythology ate fruit from a shrub that inspired happy indolence. Bird's foot refers to the slender seedpods appearance, while trefoil alludes to a similarity with red clover, also known as trefoil.

Dioscorides called it Coronopus and wrote it, "is a little herb, somewhat long, spreading upon the ground, have leaves indented; and this is also eaten as a pot herb, being sod; having a thin root, binding, which being eaten is good for coleiaci(ileocecal valve)."

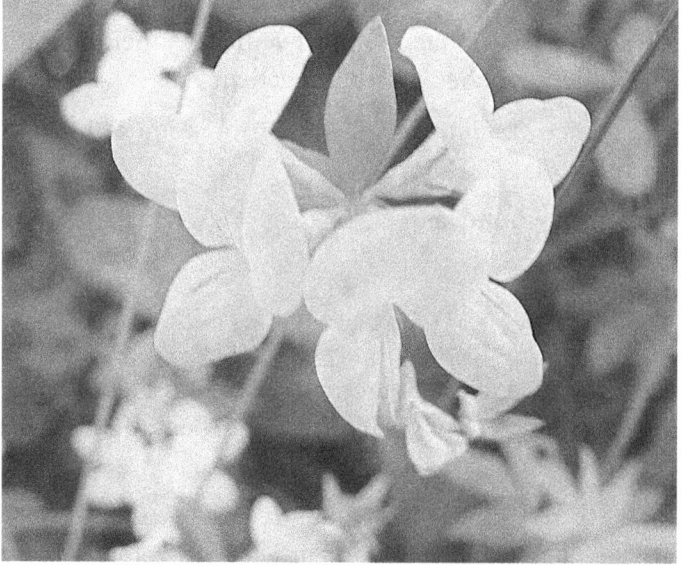

BIRD'S FOOT TREFOIL IN FLOWER

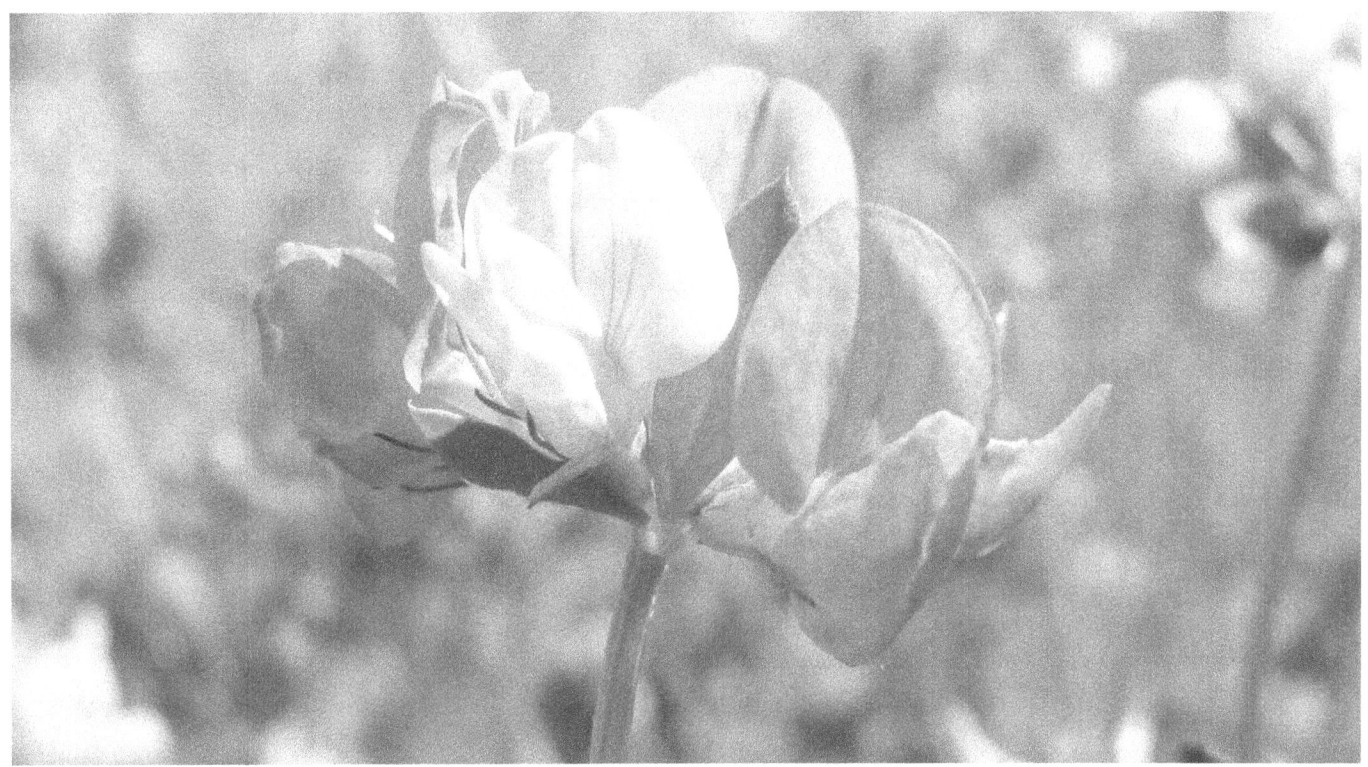

BIRD'S FOOT TREFOIL CLOSE UP OF FLOWERS

In Ireland, it was known as No Blame by school children, who believed its possession would save them from punishment. It has come to symbolize revenge, and birth date of December 23rd.

Bird's foot trefoil is grown as pasture herbage, and one of the few fodder plants to contain condensed tannin (CT). It has a high nutritive value despite moderate protein content. CT binds plant proteins in the rumen, reducing their solubility and degradation by rumen bacteria. CT improves the flow of plant protein to the intestine and increases availability of essential amino acids by 60% compared to other forage. These condensed tannins are up to 3% dry weight of pro-anthocyanidins.

The feeding value of this plant has equaled or surpassed alfalfa and other good legume hays when fed to dairy cattle and sheep.

Additionally, milk from cows fed trefoil hay contains more carotene, vitamin A, and tocopherols than milk from clover or timothy fed cows.

In sheep, the condensed tannins help increase lactation, promote wool growth, and encourage weight gain.

Field trials conducted by Banuelos et al, *Lotus Newsletter* 1992 23 in the San Joaquin Valley, indicate that bird's foot trefoil is an excellent plant to remove excessive boron and selenium from the soil.

Recent work by McCutcheon and Schnoor (Eds.*) Phytoremediation: Transformation and Control of Contaminants* Wiley-Interscience 2003 found the plant hyper-accumulates TPH and PAHs from soil, suggesting bioremediation possibilities.

Bird's foot trefoil is more tolerant than other legumes to drought, water-logged, saline, acidic, and calcareous soils, and is excellent for planting on highway right of ways.

Leaves and flowering tops were once the source of blue and yellow dyes respectively, for woolens and cottons. An excellent honey is said collected from the plant blossoms.

In Kenya, the herb is used traditionally for sore eyes, coughs and is anti-spasmodic.

One bonus of a patch of bird's foot trefoil is the control of internal parasites in livestock.

Reported by Niezen et al, *International Journal of Parasitology* Aug-Sept 1996 is a three-year study of bird's foot trefoil as an anthelmintic. More information can be obtained from the author at <u>Niezenj@agresearch.cri.nz</u> .

Another study by Marley et al, at the U of Wales looked at lambs feeding on pastures rich in chicory and birds foot trefoil. They found fewer heleminth parasites than the control pasture of ryegrass and white clover. *Vet Par* 2003 112. Min & Hart *J Animal Science* 2003 81 102-9 found similar results.

It is interesting to note that when it is grown in warmer climates, it generates cyanide to prevent herbivore devastation. Like white clover, the further north and harsher the climate, the less need for the plant to display cyanogenic properties, and thus less toxicity to animals and humans.

MEDICINAL

CONSTITUENTS- It contains flavonoids that comprise up to 1.9% of the dry plant weight; while the condensed tannin content is 1.1-3.9% of dry weight. Epi-catechin (67%), epigallo-catechin (30%), and minor amounts of catechin and epi-afzelechin (flavan-3-ol) units are linked together with C4/C8 interflavanoid bonds. Also contains phyto-alexins like sativin and vestitol, as well as quercitrin.
The first two can be further developed in hairy root culture by adding glutathione to the water.
The seeds contain trypsin inhibitors, like crown vetch and saponins. The latter has been broken down to yield rhamnose, xylose, glucose, galactose, glucuronic acid, and soyasapogenols B, C and E.
flowers- gossypetin 8 rhamnoside.

The French herbalist, Henri Leclerc first discovered, and reported the medicinal properties of this herb. He recommended an eyewash of sweet clover to treat an attack of pink eye in a woman suffering from insomnia and heart palpitations.

By mistake, the distraught patient made a tea of bird's foot trefoil, drank it, and discovered her nervous troubles disappeared within the week!

Recent research indicates this plant contains constituents similar in nature to those in passionflower.

Further study is required, but it appears that the sedative, anti-anxiety, anti-spasmodic and tranquilizing properties may be similar. The plant is considered by some to have exhilarating properties; and may be useful in cases of neuro-vegetative dystonia, anguish and depression. It supports parasympathetic nervous system balance.

The plant is a central nervous system sedative, useful for treating tachycardia, anxiety, depression and insomnia.

It is sympatholytic and musculo-trophic, with a neurotropic, anti-spasmodic nature.

Research by Achola et al, *International Journal of Pharmacognosy* 1995 33:3 found methanol extracts of the aerial parts show both intestinal and cardio-relaxant activity in laboratory studies. A fall of diastolic blood pressure, with a lesser fall of systolic pressure was observed in lab animals. Infusion is made 1:32 and taken cool 30 ml at a time.

Externally, the plant can be made into a poultice to reduce skin inflammation.

The flowers of some cultivars contain traces of prussic acid, creating mild toxicity in the flowering stage, but are innocuous when dried as silage or hay.

The gossypetin 8 rhamnoside, from the yellow pigment of the flowers, is anti-bacterial against *Pseudomonas mattophilia*. Quercitrin, common to many plants, inhibits lens aldose reductase, suggestive of maintaining good eye health.

Hexane and ethyl acetate extracts show activity against *Bacillus subtilis, Enterococcus faecalis* and *Acinetobacter calcoaceticus*. Dalmarco et al, *Int J Green Pharmacy* 2010 4:2.

A lectin from the seeds showed a strong anti-proliferative activity towards human leukemic (THP-1) cancer cells, followed by lung cancer (HOP62) cells and HCT116. Studies confirmed the lectin induced apoptosis, and inhibited cell migration. Rafiq S et al, *Phytomedicine* 2013 21(1): 30-8.

Epiafzelelechin may be useful for osteo-protection. Wong KC et al, *J Chromatogr B Analyt Technol Biomed Life* 2014 967:162-7. Epiafzelelechin increased the area of mineralized bone nodules, and along with epicatechin promotes osteoblast proliferation, as well as protected myoblast cell apoptosis against hydrogen peroxide. Zeng X et al, *Phytomedicine* 2014 21(3): 217-24.

It also acts as COX inhibitor, with about one-third the anti-inflammatory activity of indomethacin. Min KR et al, *Planta Medica* 1999 65(5):460-2.

FLOWER ESSENCE

Bird's Foot Trefoil flower essence is helpful for instilling greater self-esteem. **MIRIANA**

SPIRITUAL PROPERTIES

Of all the plants in this area, the little trefoil is the least understood in herbal terms. Its action is not at the physical but at the aetheric level.

It is able, when taken internally as a tea made from the root and leaves (steep in near boiling water two minutes), to open the aetheric body to energy inputs from higher levels, and to bring the energies of the aetheric, and the thus the physical, into better balance. It is recommended for all cases of exhaustion, chronic tiredness, lack of 'spunk' or energy, apathy, and listlessness, and also nervousness and edginess.

In the case of this plant, the most useful factors for combating tiredness are not in the flower. What is in the flower is a wonderful capacity to overcome a tendency toward drunkenness and other forms of self-obliteration, for it can improve the self-image to the point where such blotting out of reality is no longer needed.

The flower is used by making a tea and this should be drunk whenever the individual feels the urge to take alcohol or drugs. The plant can be transplanted indoors, and 'tricked' into maintaining at least some blooms for most periods of the year. **HILARION**

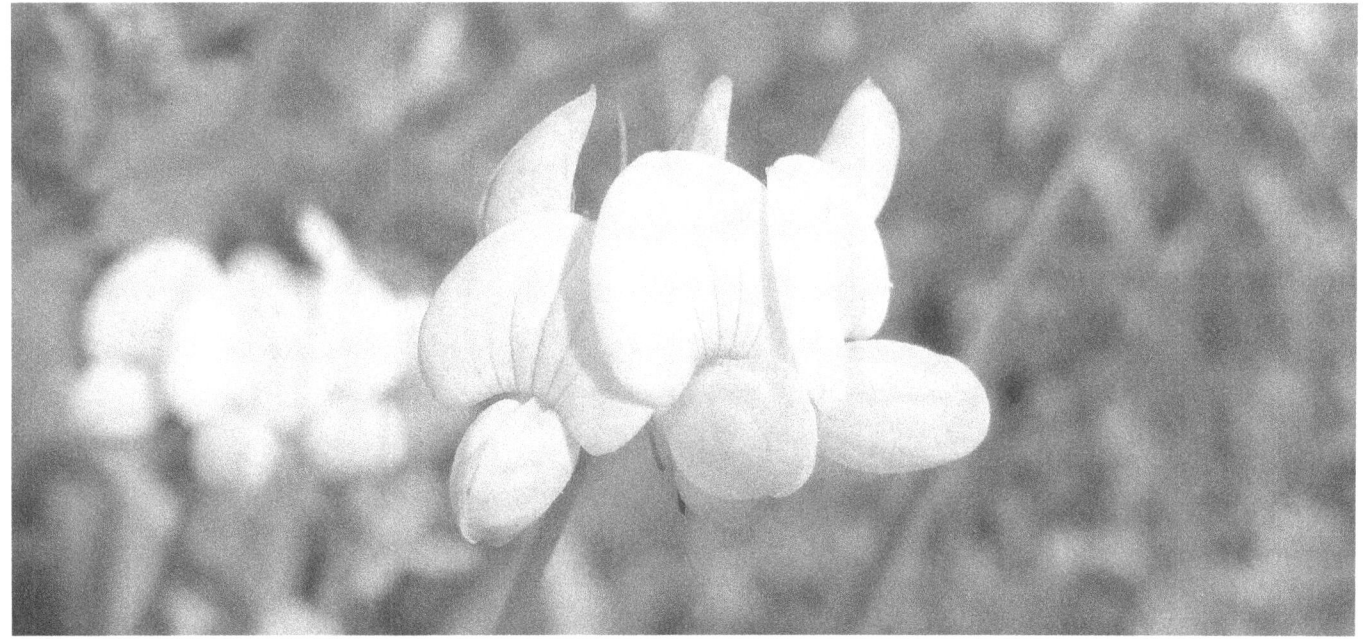

LOTUS CORNICULATUS

PERSONALITY TRAITS

Trefoil is one of our earliest symbols of trinitarian divinity; going back to 2500 BC.

The symbol was sacred to many Indo-Europeans, including the Celtic Irish who had a God of the Trefoil, **TREFUILNGID TRE-EOCHAIR.**

His spirit produced three special trees, and was called the Triple Bearer of the Triple Key.

This symbol was assimilated in the legend of St. Patrick, as a shamrock for the Christian trinity.   **WALKER**

RECIPES

INFUSION- one part dried leaf and flowers to 20 parts water. Steep for 10 minutes and drink one half cup or more at body temperature one hour before bedtime.

TINCTURE- 20-40 drops as needed. Prepare fresh at 1:4 and 60% alcohol.

WESTERN BISTORT
AMERICAN BISTORT
MOUNTAIN MEADOW BISTORT
PINK PLUMES
(*Polygonum bistortoides* Pursh.)
(*Bistorta bistortoides* [Pursh.] Small)
ALPINE BISTORT
(*P. viviparum*)
(*B. vivipara* [L.] Delarbre)
WATER SMARTWEED
SWAMP SMARTWEED
WATER KNOTWEED
(*Persicaria amphibia* [L.] Delarbre)
SMARTWEED
MARSH PEPPER SMARTWEED
ARSESMART
(*P. hydropiper* [L.] Opiz)
LADY'S THUMB
MANY KNEES
RED LEG
(*P. maculosa* Gray.)
KNOTGRASS
COMMON KNOTWEED
PROSTATE KNOTWEED
PIGWEED
DOORWEED
(*Polygonum aviculare* L.)
PALE SMARTWEED
PALE PERSICARIA
(*Persicaria lapathifolia* [L.] S.F. Gray)
RUSSIAN KNOTGRASS
DEVIL'S SHOESTRING
STRIATE KNOTWEED
(*Polygonum erectum* L.)

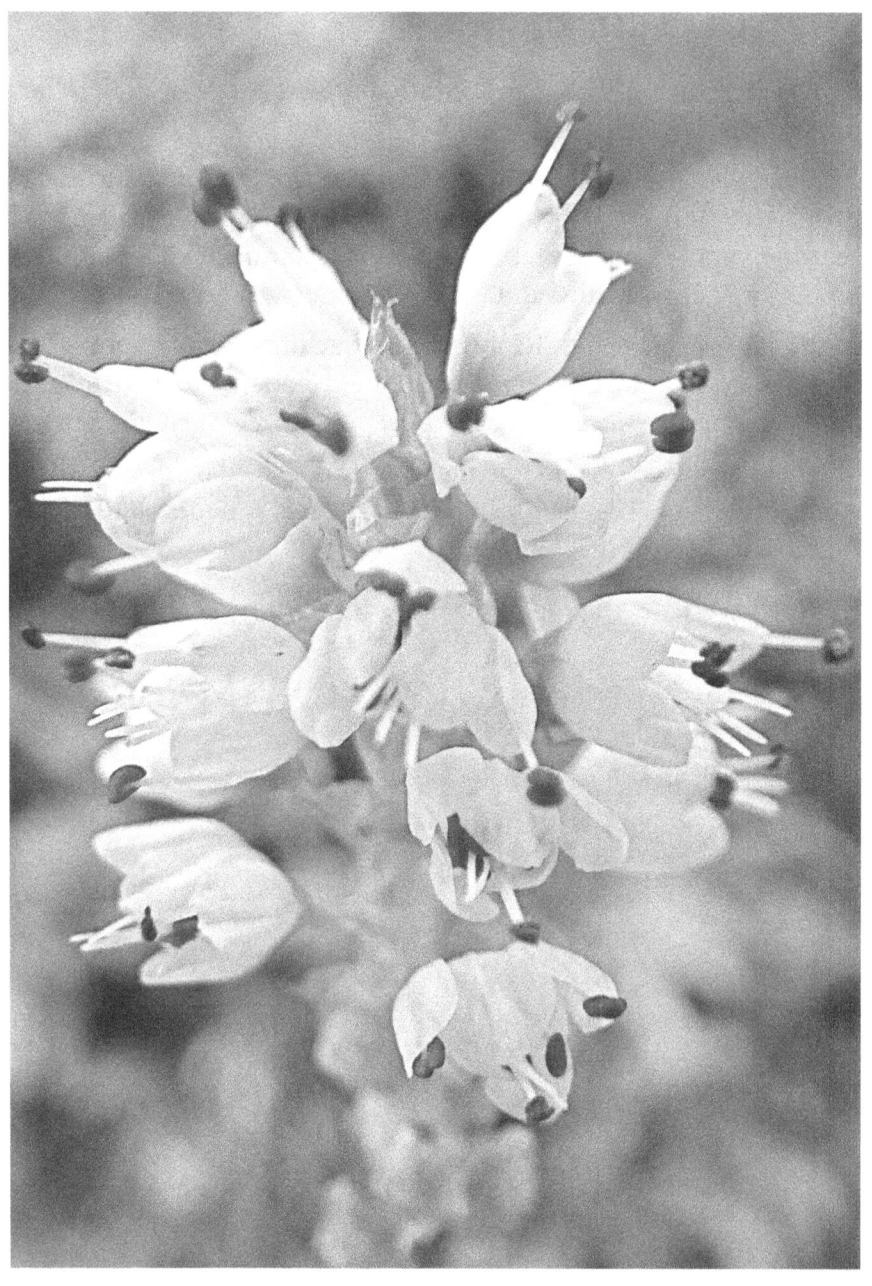

ALPINE BISTORT FLOWERS

98

BUSHY KNOTWEED
TALL KNOTWEED
(*P. ramosissimum* Michx.)
DOTTED SMARTWEED
(*Persicaria punctata* [Elliot] Small)
PARTS USED- Seeds, roots, leaves and flowers

Knotgrass carpets every dooryard and fringes every walk, and softens every path that know of the feet of children.
J. BURROUGHS

Get you gone, you dwarf,
You minimus, of hindering knot-grass made.
SHAKESPEARE

Polygonum literally translates as "many joints or knees" in reference to the numerous angular stems. *GONU* means knee, as in genuflexion; **POLY**, for many. It may also mean "many offspring", from the Greek **GONOS** meaning, seed or semen; as in gonad; in reference to the prolific seed formations.

Smartweed is derived from the Old English **SMOERTEN**, to bite, while Knotweed probably refers to the flower clusters that appear like tiny knots.

Viviparum means "live birth".

Bistort is derived from the Latin **BIS** for twice, and **TORTA** meaning, twisted. Aviculare means, "small birds". *Lapathifolium* is derived from **LAPATHI**, meaning sorrel or dock-like, also referring to the leaves. *Persicaria* comes from the Latin **PERSICUM**, meaning "a peach", in reference to leaf shape. *Muhlenbergii* is named in honor of the Reverend Heinrich Muhlenberg, a noted naturalist. *Coccineum* means scarlet, due to the crimson-striped stems.

Lady's Thumb may derive from the leaves bearing a design that someone thought was the thumbprint of the Virgin Mary. The Christian faith has used this many times throughout history, in attempts to usurp ancient traditions and faiths.

This group of plants has undergone some taxonomic changes in last while, with many *Polygonums* now placed in *Persicaria* genus.

All are members of the buckwheat family and contain seeds that are nutty and flavorful. They may be collected and used like sesame or poppy seeds in recipes. In Nepal, the seeds of **KHALTI** are pickled for later use.

They also are used for birdseed and to fatten poultry.

Bistort may have white or pink tinged flowers leading some taxonomists to name Pink Plumes as *B. bistorta* and Western Bistort as *B. bistortoides*. They are the same plant, with great variation in height due to geographic elevation. The herb is circumpolar.

Bistort rhizomes are tasty, and almond- like, and were used by the Blackfoot for soups and stews. It is called **EK-SIK-A-PATO-SPI** meaning, "look back"; perhaps due to the twisted nature of the root. It is somewhat flat on two sides, pleated, and folded on itself. The black peel is bitter at the top, but the white flesh inside is mild, crisp and starchy.

The northern Slave name is Arctic Ground Squirrel Potato, **TSELI YANESHI;** or Hoary Marmot Potato, **DEDIE YANESHI.**

The Dena'ina of Alaska name is **TL'ANALYI** meaning, "that which lays in a crescent shape." They chewed the root after eating fish eggs to clean their teeth.

The Cheyenne call it "tasteless potato", but nevertheless gathered, peeled and dried the root for food. The tubers are roasted for food by Inuit of Yukon and Alaska.

The Russians called it "Serpentine", because of the root shape. In times of famine, it was a valued food that due to the rich content of tannins, also shrunk the intestines, and reduced the amount of food needed to relieve hunger.

In England, a traditional pudding, *Easter Ledges*, is made from dried bistort, to aid conception and prevent abortion.

Herb Pudding or Yarby Pudding, made from the boiled leaves in broth with barley and chives, is served on Easter Day.

Yorkshire and Cumbria Dock Pudding is made with bistort, nettles, onions and oatmeal, and after simmering, strained and allowed to cool. It was then sliced and fried with bacon. Yum!

Around the villages of Hebden Bridge and Mytholmroyd in the Calder Valley of Yorkshire, is held an annual world championship dock pudding contest.

An Anglo Saxon text from the 10th century records:

"If a woman drink, while fasting, the juice of this plant three times a day with wine for the space of eleven days after her last menses, and the man do the same before he lies with her, she shall conceive and the child shall be male."

In Shakespeare's day, the plant juice was used for nasal polyps, and rubbed on horse's teeth to prevent decay.

The dried root was used for incontinence, headache, diphtheria and diarrhea.

Henry's *Medical Herbal* (1814) lists it as "the strongest vegetable astringent known."

Bistort, along with Rowan, is associated with the 10th Norse Rune, Nyd Not.

Bistort grows along the mountain chains down to the Southwestern United States, where it is known as *Yerba del Pescado*, or Herb of Fish.

Thinly sliced root help keep dill pickles firm when added at processing time.

Alpine Bistort root is probably our most important high mountain survival food, followed by woolly lousewort. The small nut-like roots vary from mildly bitter to sweet and taste like hazelnuts. Where found, it is plentiful and would give good nutrition to those who know. The small bulblets can also be picked off and eaten, especially in fall when they turn purple and ripe. They are nutty, but astringent. Water is recommended when eating.

The Alpine bistort has sterile flowers at top of the stem. Below the flowers are tiny bulblets, or baby plants that grow while attached. When they fall off they root themselves.

The Inuktitut word **SAPANGARALANNGUAT** means "imitation small beads", as the un-ripe bulblets were strung for jewelry. The rhizome is known as **UQPIGAIT**, a prized edible.

Historically, in both China and North America, various bistorts have been used for treating jaundice and cholera.

Patients were wrapped in sheet soaked with hot decoctions of the plant at the first symptom.

In the doctrine of signatures, the significance of the plant's flexible joints cannot be overlooked for treating swollen joints. Nor can the use of the spotted leaves for pimples and acne.

The Cree call Water Smartweed **KAMITHWACOAHTIK** and used the powdered root to cure blisters in the mouth. The Chippewa used the same plant for unspecified stomach pain. Tanners in Russia and the western United States made use of the astringent roots for tanning animal hides.

The Ojibwa dried the flowers and add it to their hunting smoking mixture, to attract deer.

The Meskwaki used the root combined with leaves of wild tobacco as an antidote for peyote overdose. The name translates as "white or water potato." Various native tribes would prepare the herb without heat, believing the active principle is destroyed from high temperatures.

The Blackfoot call it Bitter root, or **AIKSIKKIKSI**. The root is chewed for sore throats and after a short time a numbing occurs. This property can be used for early stages of colds, ear and headaches, and as a powder for ceremonial singers.

Two distinct varieties of Water Smartweed have been recognized. Long root Smartweed is found along shorelines and has bright crimson-pink flower over 4 cm long, and hairy stems. Water Smartweed (*P. amphibia*) is more aquatic, pink, small flowered, floating leaves and smooth stems.

Lady's Thumb leaf was used, after its introduction from Europe, by the Cherokee to relieve poison ivy. Numerous tribes made use of the fresh leaves to wash sores and skin infections. Gargling the leaf tea cured throat and mouth sores.

The powdered leaves were also given to children to kill pinworms. The long, lance shaped leaves are distinguished by a purple triangular blotch in the middle of some of them.

The Ojibwa used a flower and leaf decoction for treating stomach pain; while others used it for heart, stomach and kidney stone problems.

The Karuk used it for back pain, with the plant signature of vertebrae fitting together, hence common name joint weed.

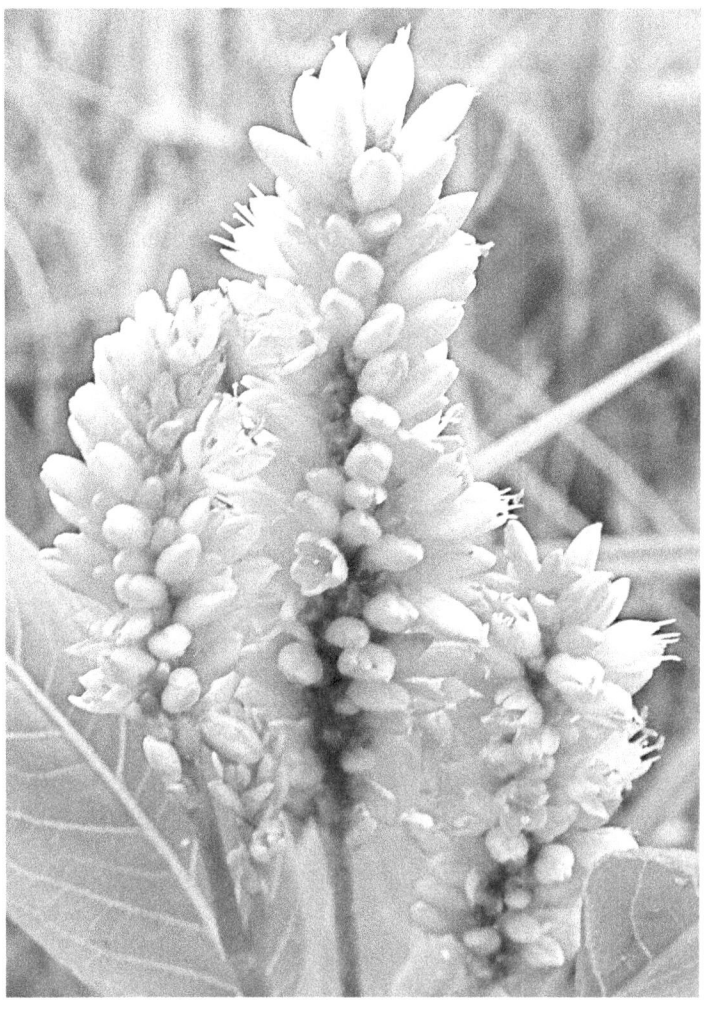

LONG ROOT SMARTWEED

During the Middles Ages, it was believed that Lady's Thumb had the extraordinary ability to change the seat of disease from one part of the body to another.

In Gaelic, the plant is known as *Lus Chrann Censaidh*, or herb of the cruxifixion, as it was supposedly spotted, with His blood.

In Brazil, the leaves and stems are used to treat hemorrhoids and diarrhea; while in Ecuador, the herb is infused as an insecticide.

Smartweed was used as a rubefacient by the infamous alchemist Paracelsus, and by the also famous 16th century Italian botanist Mattiolus, who used the fresh juice on open wounds of animals to repel flies and heal the skin. He suggested placing smartweed on fresh meat to protect it from insects. From ancient Greece comes the belief that a handful of the herb placed under the saddle of a horse will allow the animal to travel for some time before feed or water.

Smartweed (*P. hydropiper*), according to Thomas Green, "cures those little ulcers in the mouth commonly called the thrush".

The leaf was used for toothache or as a counterirritant like mustard plaster on affected areas.

The leaves and young shoots have been traditionally dried and ground up for a pepper substitute. This should be done in moderation due to some toxic compounds.

The seeds, however, are non-toxic and numerous. They can be sprouted.

101

In Japan, the seedlings are used to garnish white-fleshed raw fish- known as **TADE,** and the red-purplish color is, of course, highly desired. The sprouts, known as **MEJISO** or **BENITADE** are served with sashimi in higher end restaurants. The expressed juice is used as a dip sauce for raw river fish.

Polygodial improves the flavor of mints such as chewing gum, as well as beverages for a cooling sensation.

In parts of India, the plant is used to poison fish. Polygodial is a biodegradable insecticide used for treating aphids, wheat galls (*Anguina tritici*) and other insects.

In one study, application of 25 grams per hectare raised winter barley yields from 3.83 to 5.22 tonnes per hectare.

According to M. K. Hard, in a 1848 publication, an extract of Smartweed and Tansy in equal parts, thickened with equal parts of Black Cohosh and Cayenne, were formed into pills and taken three times daily as an emmenagogue.

In Traditional Chinese Medicine, Smartweed (*P. hydropiper*) is called **LA LIAO**, and is used to remove dampness and food stagnancy associated with indigestion. The whole plant is used in decoction for dysentery, enteritis, heat stroke and rheumatic arthralgia.

The poet and scientist Chang Hua noted in 290 AD, "where the smartweed grows abundantly, there must be plenty of haematite (ferric oxide) below."

In Mexico, infusions are used as a diuretic, and put into baths for those suffering rheumatism.

Big Root Lady's Thumb (*P. amphibia*) root decoctions were given to women of the Fox tribe, when the birth of the baby injured the womb. The Ojibwa infused **AGONGO' SIMINUN** for stomach pain.

Pale Smartweed (*P. lapathifolia*) is an annual common near sloughs on the prairie. Greenish white to pale pink flowers are produced; resembling a lizard's tail. The seeds are a flattened brown, and average about 800-1500 per plant.

The presence of seeds at several Danish excavation sites indicates that pale smartweed seeds were gathered and stored for food in the Iron Age.

The jointed stems were eaten in Ireland for a condition known as **BRIOS BRONN**, very similar to **BRIOSE BRUN,** a name for cattle lameness caused by phosphorus deficiency.

The Potawatomi tribe infused the whole plant to cure fevers. John Lame Deer, a Lakota healer, noted, "for a stomach ache we use **TAKU-SASALA**- the smartweed. It's good for cramps and the runs."

In Nepal, *P. lapathifolia var. lanata* produces a soft white mass, a froth-like soap, applied to burns, as well as used for bathing and washing clothes.

The ripe seeds, which are circular and biconcave, can be stripped and ground into flour. The mild tasting leaves are edible raw or steamed.

Knotgrass (*P. aviculare*) has been used as food since prehistoric times (Renfrew 1973), and for flour during the Middle Ages in Poland. In 1950, two peat diggers in Tollund Fen in Denmark, found a perfectly preserved 2000 year-old corpse. His stomach contained a high amount of knotgrass seed.

A related plant yields a blue dye resembling indigo, and is used for this purpose in Japan (*P. tinctorium*).

Knotgrass and its fibrous roots were used as a quinine substitute in both northern and middle Africa.

Both Pliny and Dioscorides named it **SANQUINARIA,** for its ability to stop bleeding.

Knotgrass was known in Europe as the "hindering knotweed" from the belief that it would hinder the growth of children. The seeds were said to be emetic and cathartic.

The herb was known as *prosperpinaca* and *unfortraedde*, meaning "un-trodden to pieces" in the Old English Herbarium written over 1000 years ago. It was recommended the herb be simmered slowly in wine for vomiting blood, and the fresh juice for pain in the sides, earache and softened with butter for a woman's sore nipples.

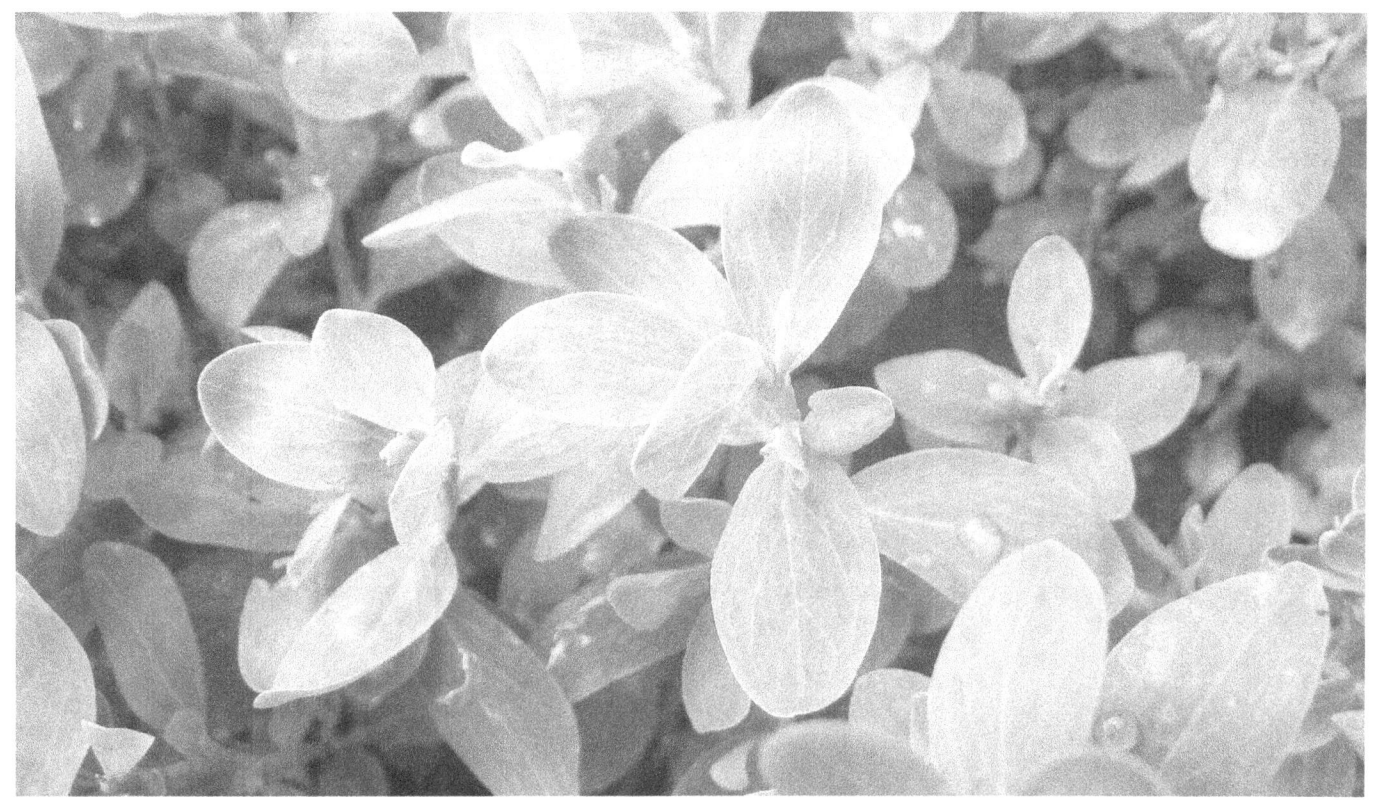

KNOTGRASS

The 17th century Scottish herbalist, Salmon, believed knotweed "effective against bleeding and kidney leakage… makes the nerves and tendons more flexible… (and) cures gout if taken correctly morning and night."

The Iroquois used the introduced Knotweed (*P. aviculare ssp. depressum*) as a decoction mixed in the feed given to heifers to restore their milk. They also infused the plant with Silverweed for treating loose stools in babies.

Various tribes used the root for children's diarrhea, painful urination, the leaf as a warm infusion for stomachache. The Cherokee even rubbed the plant on their children's thumbs to prevent sucking.

The Karuk used either fresh or dried plant as tea for back pain, according to elder Josephine Peters.

Bushy Knotweed, a lime green plant that habitats wet flatlands was used by the Navaho-Ramah. They infused the whole plant and drank it warm for stomach aches.

Knotgrass (*P. aviculare*) has been used in traditional Chinese Medicine as a diuretic for over 2,000 years, and known as **PIEN HSU**, or sometimes **PAI HUO LA**, meaning White Peppery Knotgrass; and even **PAI LA LIU**, meaning White Peppery Willow.

In Tibet, the herb is called bri-ta-sa-dzin.

In Argentina, the plant is called **SANGUINARIA**, and used traditionally as a depurative in rheumatism and syphilis; as well as an astringent, diuretic and in cases of menstruation.

In Peru, the green herb is combined with *Malva parviflora* as part of a green chili sauce that I really enjoyed with barbequed chicken, while living there many years ago.

The packaged herb is known as Weidemannscher, or Homeriana tea.

The seeds can be hand stripped and ground into flour.

Recent studies from China indicate roots of *P. officinale* produce hypoglycemic effect in diabetic mice by decreasing the hepatic liver glucose output.

Other Polygonums, such as *P. orientale* contain beta sitosterol glucosides active against cancers of the stomach, intestine and liver, and *P. perfoliatum* that contains cardiac glucosides active against cancers of the esophagus, gastrointestinal tract and prostate.

The related *R. obtusifolius* is used as a cold infusion by the Kofans of Brazil for "pains around the heart".

The leaf of *P. punctata* is used in parts of Ecuador as a skin rub to remove light or dark spots. It is also known as **ERVA DE BICHO, CATAIA** and **PIMENTO DO BREJO** in Brazil. There it is used to treat hemorrhoids and rheumatism, and an abortifacient, diuretic and emmenagogue.

Ethanol extracts suggest benefit as anti-histamine, anti-inflammatory, antipyretic and hypotensive.

Native to Saskatchewan and Manitoba (I have not found it in Alberta), it was used as a whole plant decoction for stomach pain, as well as gastrointestinal problems, pain and swelling in legs and joints and "loss of senses during menses".

All of the Smartweeds and Wild Buckwheat help rebuild soil, even better than cultivated Buckwheat. Sow the seed, available from seed mills, and plow under at the start of flowering.

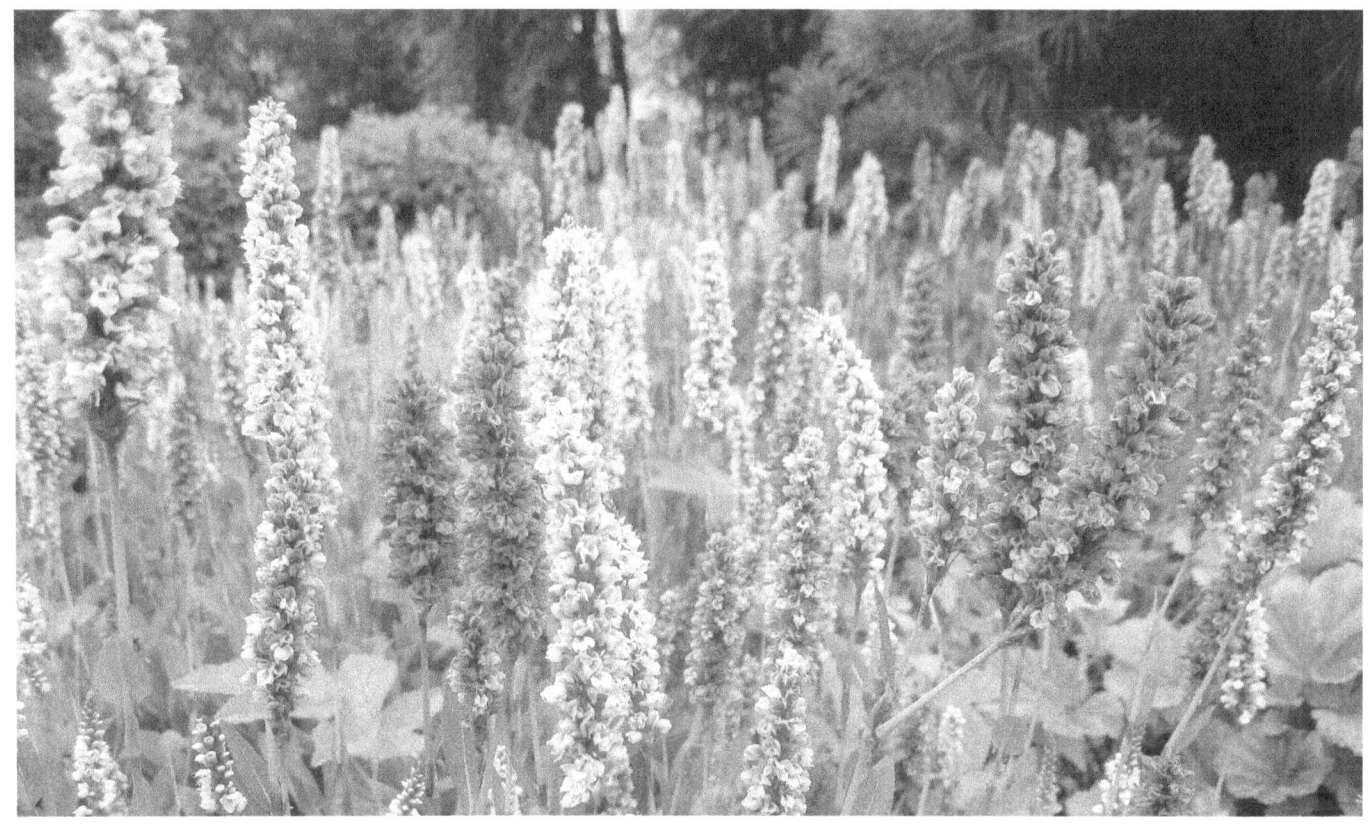

BISTORT

MEDICINAL

BISTORT
(*B. bistortoides*)

CONSTITUENTS- rhizome- 15-36% tannins, bistortaside A, mainly catechins; gallic, ellagic, caffeic, silicic and polygonic acid, phenolic compounds, quercitol, phlobaphene (a red-brown pigment), starch, phlotoglucinol, methylanthraquione, 5-glutinen-3-one, friedelin, 3beta-friedelinol, friedelanol, various flavonoid glycosides, a trace of emodin, kaempferol, avicularin, procatechuic acid, and quercimeritrin; 24(E)-ethylidencycloartanone, 24(E)-ethylidenecycloarten-3alpha-ol, 24-methyl-enecycloartanone, beta sitosterol, gamma-sitosterol, and beta-sisosterone.

Due to lack of polygodial in leaf and flower, the plant has been moved, taxonomically, to *Bistorta* genus.

Infusions of fresh leaves in cold water are useful in coughs, colds and gravel. Hot tea will alleviate suppressed menstruation both by drinking and applying hot fomentations to the lower back.

At body temperature, the same tea makes a useful douche for feminine itching, pain, and whitish discharge.

A study in 1994, confirmed the anti-inflammatory activity of bistort in both acute and chronic edema. It makes an excellent decoction gargle for inflammations of the mouth and throat; as well as inflammatory bowel complaints like dysentery, and chronic, but not acute, diarrhea.

John Christopher mentions it removes mucoid coating from the intestine that allows new mucus with increased immune properties to take its place.

Michael Moore writes, "the high altitude packer who awakes in the morning with a distended or relaxed uvula (usually a mouth breather) will find that chewing on a fresh or dried Bistort root will shrink it and get rid of that half-swallowed, slippery choking sensation."

Work by Duwiejua et al, *Planta Medica* 1999 65(4):371-4 isolated the two main active anti-inflammatory compounds as friedelanol, and 5-glutinen-3-one.

Follow up by Ahn-Jungsu et al, *Korean Journal of Pharmacognosy* 1999 found the anti-inflammatory constituents exhibit greater activity than aspirin.

In the previous year, the same author, in same journal published a paper regarding the ability of bistort to inhibit the activity of 3alpha hydroxysteroid dehydrogenase involved in the metabolism of dihydrotestosterone that creates benign prostatic hypertrophy.

There is ongoing research into the potential use of bistort as an anti-viral that helps to induce interferon-like activity. Smolarz et al, *Acta Pol Pharm* 1999 56:6.

Bistort tincture shows cytotoxicity against the rarely studied liver carcinoma cell line (HCCLM3). Intisar A et al, *Afr J Tradit Complement Altern Med* 2012 10(1):53-9.

Bistort has been used traditionally for tuberculosis, bronchitis with abundant secretions, intermittent fevers, prostate congestion, urethritis, and enuresis, or bed wetting.

Several species including *B. bistortoides, P. hydropiper, P. lapathifolia* and *B. vivipara* exhibit high inhibition of xanthine oxidase, suggesting benefit in uric acid and rheumatic gout conditions. Orban-Gyapai et al, *Phytother Res* 2015 29(13):459-65.

Bistort root is used in Chinese medicine, known as **TZU SHEN** in Mandarin, for severe infections involving toxicosis with boils, abscesses, sore throats, etc. It is sometimes called **TAO KEN TS'AO**, Inverted Root Grass, **CAO HE CHE**, meaning Snakeweed, or **QUAN SHEN**, Fist Root.

Its warm, astringent properties can be put to good use in external wounds and hemorrhage.

It is an important medicine in cervical lymphadenopathy and various other swellings.

Combine bistort, cranesbill, and fireweed as a salve for bleeding hemorrhoids.

Drink the infused tea internally and apply the salve after each bowel movement.

Combine with comfrey root as a drawing poultice for abscesses, injured tendons and broken fingers.

The root is also dried and finely powdered; and used as a styptic on cuts. The powder combines well with clay for treating sore bruises, strains and sprains.

Put the dried root powder into #00 capsules and use 2-3 capsules 3-4 times daily for ulcerative colitis, irritable bowel syndrome (IBS), and other intestinal as well as excessive menstrual bleeding. For IBS, combine with equal parts of wild ginger root.

Recent studies have found the roots suppress degranulation of mucosal mast cells, suggesting a source of benefit in food allergies, ulcerative colitis, etc. Zaidi SF et al, Pak *J Pharm Sci* 2014 27(4 Suppl):1041-8.

Bistort combines well with calamus or gentian root for intermittent fevers. The powdered leaves have been used successfully, killing pinworms in children.

The fresh root is decocted and is good for treating irritations of the vagina in the form of a warm, well-strained douche.

Bistort is considered in TCM to be very useful in tumors and the early stages of cancer. Mice studies indicate activity against sarcoma 180 cell lines.

Friedelin shows activity against *Mycobacterium tuberculosis*. Chinsembu KC, *Acta Trop* 2016 153:46-56. Other research suggests it may be a useful anti-ulcer agent. Antonisamy P et al, *Eur J Pharmacol* 2015 750:167-75.

The compound 3beta-friedelanol is more active against human coronavirus than actinomycin D. Chang FR et al, *Nat Prod Commun* 21 7(11):1415-7.

Veterinarians recommend the wounds or sores on horses be washed with decoctions; and that flies avoid them and do not molest them, even in the heat of summer. Font Quer, P. *Plantas Medicinales* 1962.

WATER SMARTWEED
(*P. amphibium*)

CONSTITUENTS- tannins (dried stems 17%, root 21%), leucoanthocyanins, caffeic and chlorogenic acids, saponins, hyperoside, kaempferol, quercitin, avicularin, flavonoids, saponins, luteolin-7-O-glucoside, quercimeritrin, quercitin-3-O-beta-glucuronide, quercitin-3-O-alpha-rhamnosyl- (1—> 2)-beta-glucuronide.

Water Smartweed is very effective in the treatment of atonic hemorrhage that follows abortion or miscarriage. It is somewhat less effective in uterine conditions of chronic standing like endometriosis. On the long term however, it has definite effect in persistent low volume bleeding that sometimes accompanies peri-menopuase.

Infusions in cold water make an excellent gargle for sore mouths and spongy gums, again due to tannins.

Fresh crushed leaves make a reliable mustard plaster substitute.

Chronic skin ulcers and staph infection respond to water smartweed and pineapple weed infusion washes.

Fomentations relieve flatulence and colic.

The various flavonoids in Water Smartweed inhibit thrombocyte aggregation, through an effect on cyclo-oxygenase.

Millspaugh, in *American Medicinal Plants*, suggests *P. amphibium* resembles sarsaparilla in its qualities, and has been substituted for it. Not sure about that.

Sardari et al, *Pharm Bio* 1998 36:3 found anti-fungal activity against *Candida albicans*.

The flower extracts show activity against *Staphylococcus aureus* and *C. albicans*. Borchardt et al, *J Med Plants Res* 2008 2:5.

Smolarz et al, *Phytother Res* 17:7 found the plant stimulates human lymphocyte proliferation, a measure of immune response.

Other work by Smolarz et al, *Phytochem Anal* 2008 19(6):506-13 found it active against leukemia cancer cell lines, especially its two glucuronides.

Avicularin is present in Bistort, Knotweed and Water Smartweed. Studies have shown it is a sucrase enzyme inhibitor, suggesting benefit in reducing postprandial glucose and insulin peaks. Abedlhady MI et al, *Pharmacogn Mag* 2016 12(Suppl 3):292-6.

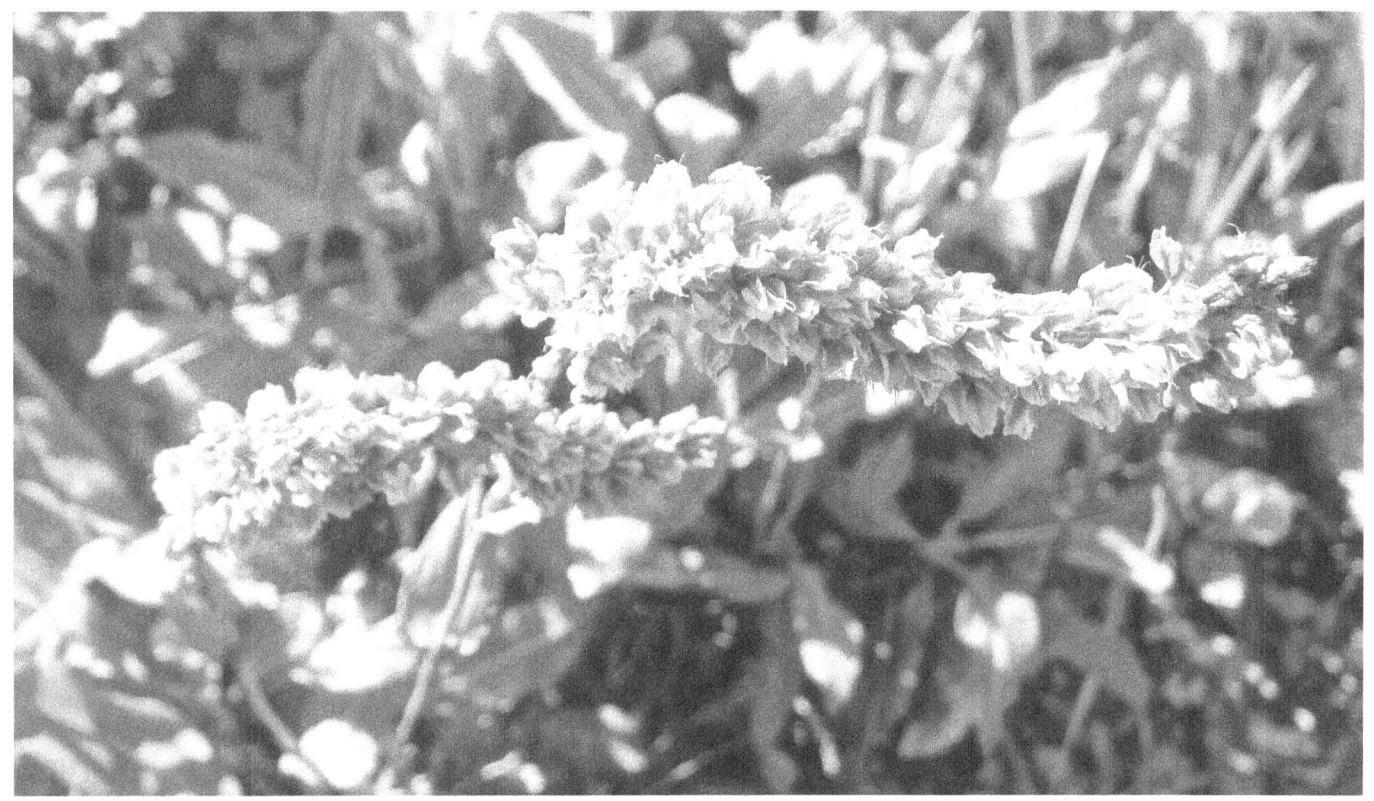

KNOTWEED FLOWER- GOING TO SEED

SMARTWEED
(*P. hydropiper*)

CONSTITUENTS- leaf and flower- drimane sesquiterpenes (11-ethoxy-cinnamolide) polygodial (tadeonal), polygonolide (isocoumarin), persicarin, isotadeonal, warburganal, valdiviolide, (6S, 9S)-roseoside, and fuegi; various flavanol aglycones with antioxidants like quercitin 3-sulphate, kaempferol, isorhamnetin 3,7-disulphate, tama-rixetin-3-glucoside-7-sulphate, and rhamnazin; hydropiperosides A-B, vanicosides A, B and E; 7,4'-dimethlyquercitin, 3'-methylquercitin, quercimeritrin, galloyl quercitrin, quercitin, isoquercitrin, hydropiperside, flaccidine.
whole plant- persicarin, rhamnazin, isotadaeonal, quercimeritrin, tadeonal, dendocarbin L, (+)winterin, (+)fuegin, changweikangic acid, futronolide, 7-ketoisodrimenin, 3beta-angeloyloxy-7-epifutronolide, polygonumate, vanicosides B, F and E, 5,6-dehydrokawain, aniba-dimer-A, (+)-ketopinoresinol, isalpinin, cardamonin, pinosylvin, 2-desoxy-4-epi-pulchellin.
Seed- polygonic acid, polygonal, isodrimeniol, isopolygodial, confertifolin, tannins, flavonoids.
At full bloom the aerial parts contain the maximum polysaccharide content (10% of dry weight); composed of nearly half galacturonic acid and half rhamnose with five other minor monsaccharides.
The fresh flowers contain about 6.2 mg/g of polygodial. Several members of the Persicaria genus contain this compound, but in much lower amounts.
root- hydropiperoside, polygonolide (an isocoumarin)

Smartweed contains stimulating, diuretic, antiseptic, diaphoretic and emmenagogue properties.

Dr. Eberle, one of the early Eclectic physicians, found teaspoon doses of the tincture, given 4-5 times daily, most effective in treating amenorrhea.

He noted that it caused an increase in the heat of the body, with bearing down pain and sense of fullness in the pelvic region.

It will definitely re-establish absent periods in young women, or menstruation delayed by shock or cold.

A cold water infusion has been used for treating gravel, colds and coughs.

Hot infusions are good for a bad cold, taken daytime and before bed.

Studies conducted by Kubo et al, at the University of California, Berkley in 1993, showed that polygodial and warburganal extracts from Smartweed, when combined with low concentrations of anethole from, increased 32 fold, the activity against *Candida albicans*. A 64-fold increase was noted by combining polygodial and sorbic acid found in unripe mountain ash berries. Anethole is, of course, a major component of sweet cicely root, fennel and anise seed. Perillaldehyde is also synergistic with polygodial, and found in perilla leaf.

On its own, the herb shows activity against *C. albicans* 50%, a similar potency to miconazole. Lin et al, *J Ethnopharm* 2012 July 31.

Tommy Bass, noted Appalachian herbalist, suggested long ago that the herb was an accelerator for other herbs. He was right!

Polygodial activity against fungi is strongly increased in acidic conditions. Work by Lee et al, *Planta Medica* 1999 65:3 confirms its powerful anti-fungal activity against growing and non-growing *Candida albicans*. Significantly, this antifungal activity was not diminished in the presence of ergosterol. It is found useful in creams for treating athlete's foot. Confertifolin, derived from the leaves, shows activity against a number of pathogenic fungi in work by Duraipandiyan et al, *Pharm Biol* 2010 48:2.

Polygodial also exhibits synergistic anti-fungal effect when combined with EDTA, a food preservative. Kubo et al, J Ag Food Chem 2005,53. Work by the same author found this compound active against *Bacillus subtilis* and *Salmonella choleraesuis*. *Phytother Res* 19:12.

Polygodial possesses the antifungal activity of maesanin and improves antibiotic effect of actinomcyin D and rifampicin by helping cell transport.

Polygodial shows activity against chronic myeloid and acute B lymphoblastic leukemia cell lines. Fratoni E et al, *Naunyn Schmiedebergs Arch Pharmacol* 2016 389(7):791-7.

Derivations of polygodial may be useful against apoptosis-resistant cancer cells. Dasari R et al, *Eur J Med Chem* 2015 103:226-37.

Polygodial triggers glucocorticoid-like effects on pancreatic B cells, in a similar but milder way than adverse effects of dexamethasone. Barrosa KH et al, *Chem Biol Interact* 2016 258:245-56.

Similar to 6-gingerol, piperine and capsaicin, the compound polygodial inhbits TRP channels associated with trigeminal sensations of numbness and tingling. Beltran LR et al, *Front Pharmacol* 2013 4:141.

Early studies by Nickell (1960) reveal smartweed inhibits both gram positive and negative bacteria.

Rhamnazin inhibits proliferation and induces apoptosis of human Jurkat leukemia cells, in vitro. Philchenkov AA et al, *Ukr Biochem J* 2015 87(6):122-8.

The compound inhibits angiogenesis and proliferation of breast cancer cells MDA-MB-231, in vivo and in vitro. Yu Y et al, *Biochem Biophys Res Commun* 2015 458(4):923-9.

Dr. Thomas Ogier, *Charleston Med J* 1846:1, found Smartweed tincture useful in treating an obstinate case of amenorrhea. One teaspoon three times daily in water led to a yellowish discharge on day six which continued until day ten when her menses came. Dosage was reduced and menses lasted six days.

Smartweed has been studied in Russia since 1912, when Piorovsky, a pharmacist, noticed folk herbalists using the plant to stop uterine and hemorrhoid bleeding. It has been a part of official herbal medicine ever since; and a commercially prepared liquid extract for stopping uterine bleeding is available by doctor's prescription.

This includes atonic postpartum bleeding, abortive bleeding and menopausal bleeding.

It has been used traditionally in delayed menstruation, or for amenorrhea in teenage girls to help promote healthy menstrual flow when periods are absent for several months.

When Smartweed and Plantain are combined, infused and cooled, the tea can be taken three times daily for female complaints and menopausal transition.

Experiments in England, showed the herb suppresses the production of sperm and of gonadotropins and estrogens when given to mice.

Root extracts were found by Indian researchers to have embryotoxic and anti-implantation effects on rats. The root powder is used extensively for preventing pregnancy in parts of the world. Work by Hazarika et al, *Contraception* 2006 74:5 appears to confirm its activity.

The powdered leaves can be used on athlete's foot, or if not available the dilute tincture as a wash.

Compresses of the fresh juice can be applied to open wounds and to help draw infection and pus; while fresh plant poultices can be applied to the back of the head to treat headaches.

Studies conducted in Japan indicate *P. hydropiper* leaves contain sulfated flavonoids with potent inhibition against lens aldose reductase and related enzymes. This inhibition may be effective in preventing cataract formation in diabetes. *J Nat Products* 1994 59:4.

The leaves also possess significant anti-oxidative properties, due to the flavonoid compounds, with galloyl quercitrin the most powerful identified to date. Tamarixetin-3-glucoside-7-sulphate also possesses strong anti-oxidant activity.

A boiled extract of the plant exhibited greater anti-oxidant activity than all other plants tested. Chan et al, *Chin Med* 2008 3:1.

The herb is strongly anti-inflammatory and may be useful in relieving gastritis, via suppression of Src/Syk/NFkappaB and IRAK/AP-1/CREB pathways. Yang et al, *J Ethnopharm* 2012 139:2 616-25.

Work by Kim et al, Int J Cosm Sci 2007 29:6 found the whole plant exhibits anti-elastase activity and inhibits MMP-1 m KNA expression in human fibroblast cells.

The most active flavonoid is isorhamnetin 3,7-disulfate. Further studies show it exhibited non-competitive inhibition against glyceraldehyde and NADPH.

Drimane-type sesquiterpenes have been studied for their ability to inhibit chymotrysin as well as acetyl and butrylcholinesterase enzymes. Sultana et al, *Planta Medica* 2011 77:16 1848-51. Futronolide appears most active. Recent work by Miyazaki Y, *Biosci Microbiota Food Health* 2016 35(2):69-75 confirmed the herb exhibits anti-acetylcholinesterase activity and immune stimulating effect. He suggests the herb is a functional food candidate for prevention of dementia.

Extracts have shown the ability to help stop bleeding and to lower blood pressure. Dobelis et al 1986.

Dr. John Christopher, an early teacher, says the herb "produces a sensation of heat in the stomach, increases the force of the heart, raises arterial tension, promotes surface warmth and the secretions of the bronchial, renal and uterine areas."

In Germany, various Smartweed preparations are used for treating bleeding of the womb, menstrual bleeding, and bleeding hemorrhoids and diarrhea. The plant is an active vaso-constrictor. Persicarin possesses anti-thrombotic activity.

This makes it valuable in normalizing excess or deficient urinary flow associated with bleeding and hemorrhages. Persicarin may be useful for severe vascular inflammatory diseases, such as sepsis or septic shock. Kim TH et al, *J Cell Physiol* 2013 228(4):696-703.

It also shows significant neuroprotective activity in glutamate injured cortical cells. Ma CJ et al, *Phytother Research* 2010 24(6):913-8. The compound, also known as isorhamnetin 3-sulfate, is found in dill seed and weed.

Millspaugh says that the fresh leaves, bruised with Mayweed (*Anthemis cotula*) and a few drops of turpentine oil, make a speedy vesicant that is highly esteemed.

It also is used for diuretic and rheumatic complaints. It helps to break up arthritic nodes in the joints.

In parts of Europe, it was used to remove kidney stones, similar to the use of hydrangea or gravel root.

Dr. William Salmon in the Great English Herbal of 1710 writes that it is a "specifik known by manifold and huge experience to be a peculiar plant against gravel and stone, whether in reins or bladder".

Ethyl acetate extracts of the whole plant show significant antinociceptive, or pain relief activity. Work by Rahman et al, *Fitoterapia* 73:7-8 identified pain-relieving properties.

Polygonolide is also a possible fertility regulator, with anti-inflammatory potential.

Warburganal is a sesquiterpene dialdehyde in smartweed with cytotoxic, insect anti-feedant, and antibiotic activity. It is a potent anti-fungal.

Combined with polygodial, it is useful for control of aphids, albeit with a half-life of three weeks. Warburganal is patented as a virus genome in-activator.

The various sulphated flavonoids have been studied in Japan by Yagi et al, for anti-oxidant properties. More research is needed on this important herb. A recent study by Kuroiwa et al, *Food Chem Tox* 44:8 found an increase in mast cell production associated with its use.

Traditional Chinese Medicine uses the seed of Smartweed, for its warm, pungent properties.

It is called **LIAO SHIH**, or **LA LIAN** and helps warm the stomach and spleen, clears vision, resists wind cold, causes water Ch'i to descend, and dispels pathogenic bacteria from the superficial muscles.

Polygonic acid, present in both the herb and seed is easily destroyed by heat or drying.

The dry seed is decocted or ground into a powder for treating tumors, scrofula, scalp lesions, stagnant undigested food, palpable masses in the stomach, edema and toxic lesions.

The seeds contain cardamonin, a compound that represses proliferation, invasion and causes apoptosis of prostate cancer cells. Zhang J et al, *Apoptosis* 2017 22(1):158-68.

It exhibits novel anti-allodynic and anti-hyperalgesic effects throught the activation of the opioid system, both centrally and peripherally. Sambasevam Y et al, *Eur J Pharmacol* 2017 796:32-8. This is worthy of further investigation, considering the considerable harm associated with opioid drugs.

It also appears to protect against ulcerative colitis, due to reduced inflammation. Ali AA et al, *Pharmacol Rep* 201 69(2):268-75.

The seeds will germinate more easily if the testa is removed, a potassium nitrate wash (0.2%) is used and varying day/night temperatures are introduced.

KNOTGRASS
(P. aviculare)

CONSTITUENTS- caffeic, chlorogenic, vanillic, sinapic, salicylic, ferulic, gallic and ellagic acids, caffeic acid, rutin, avicularin (0.2% dry tops), uglanin (kaempferol-3-0-arabinoside), hyperoside, umbelliferone, scopoletin, juglanin, astragalin, betmidin, vitamin E, 4-hydroxyphenacetic and protocatechuic acids, anthraquinone, b-coumaric acid, quercitrin, quercitrin hydrate, quercitin-3-galactoside, avicularin, aviculin (a lignan glycoside), (-)-loliolide, vitexin, isovitexin, rhamnazine bisulphate, 6-methoxy-plumbagin, sitosterol, oleanolic acid, 5,6,7,4'-tetramethoxyflavanone and essential oils.
Knotgrass is a rich source of minerals.
A Russian study found (mg/kg) for boron 13, sodium 980, magnesium 2230, aluminum 354, silicon 677, phosphorus 400, potassium 3441, calcium 1472, manganese 7, iron 70, copper 2506, zinc 588, strontium 13, molybdenum 4, barium 25, and lanthanum 14. Trace amounts of vanadium, cobalt, nickel gallium, zirconium, silver, tin, and cerium were also detected. *Voprosy Pitaniya* 1994 1-2.
Polysaccharide content is maximal during the full bloom; the principle components being galacturonic acid and arabinose.
Flavonoids during flowering range from 0.65-2.3% in aerial parts, and from 0.47 to 4.4% in leaves; and during vegetative growth from 0.88 to 3.65% dry weight.

Knotgrass is a good cooling and moistening diuretic, with slight astringent properties that relieve diarrhea, and kill pinworms. Urinary infections, vaginal ulcers and trichomoniasis are likewise treated, using a warm douche in the latter cases.

Its silicic acid content helps strengthen the connective tissue of the lungs; and help make it one of the most effective remedies for affections of the bronchial tubes and lungs. Its soothing and healing effects relieve coughs, loosen phlegm, and reduce irritation and tickling of the throat.

Dr. Valnet suggests it relieves the thirst in diabetics and controls blood sugar levels. It has been shown to increase resistance to tuberculosis, and reduce hyperacidity.

Knotgrass tincture reduces varicose veins of recent origin quite effectively. Various ointments containing Knotgrass are now used to treat roseola, and flabby or dry skin.

This could be related to the ability of (-)-loliolide to rescue senescence in human dermal fibroblasts, suggesting use in ameliorating tissue aging or age-associated disease. Yang HH et al, *Arch Pharm Res* 2015 38(5):876-84. Earlier work by same team found quercitin-3-O-beta-D-glucuronide inhibited cellular senescence.

In Uruguay, Knotgrass is used for hypertension and used to reduce the viscosity of blood.

It has been found in pharmacological studies to be an active ACE inhibitor.

Extracts show anti-thrombin and anti-cancer activity. Goun EA et al, *J Ethnopharm* 2002 81 337-342.

Cancer of the stomach, breast or kidneys may respond to knotgrass ingestion.

Its high mineral content makes it useful in osteoporosis formulas, combining well with horsetail for both bone building and with purslane for fibromyalgia.

Recent studies indicate it is an acetylcholinesterase inhibitor, suggestive of benefit in Alzheimer's disease.

Studies in Poland in 1984 showed that knotgrass is an interferon inducer in mice. Reatival is an herbal product from Yugoslavia with proven oxygen radical scavenging activity, according to Stajner et al, *Fitoterapia* 1997 68:3.

The formula consists of Knotgrass, peppermint, wormwood, sage, black elderberry, and others.

Knotgrass is used in Korea traditional medicine as an anti-pyretic, anti-parasite, to treat obesity, hypertension, and a diuretic. Water extracts possess hepato-protective properties.

A tincture may protect against the development of atherosclerosis, based on work with mice. Park SH et al, *J Ethnopharm* 2014 151(3):1109-15.

Work the previous year found a tincture give to high fat diet induced obese mice, suppressed lipogenesis in adipose tissue, inhibited fat accumulation and increased antioxidant activity. Sung YY et al, *Evid Based Complement Altern Med* 2013:626397.

It is used as a tea, and known commercially as Weidemannscher tea and Homeriana tea. It was used toward the end of the 19th century in Germany and Austria for asthma and bronchitis.

Today, the herb tea is still recommended for laryngitis, sore throats, and bronchial congestion and inflammation. It has shown benefit in treating gingivitis. Begné MG et al, *J Ethnopharm* 2001 74 45-51.

In China, Knotgrass is known as **BIAN XU** (Mandarin), or **BIN CHOK** (Cantonese). A tea is considered a good remedy for painful, burning, scanty dribbling urination, in cases of urethritis, lithiasis and chyluria. It combines well with Umbrella Polypore (*P. umbellatus*) mushroom, Water Plantain rhizome and Dianthus for urinary problems, with Plantain seed and Amur Bark for jaundice and damp heat depression, and with Gas Plant (*Dictamus spp*) and Amur Bark for eczema.

It is used in combinations for weeping eczema and is effective against dysentery and parotitis. The herb is an anti- ascaridiasis agent, and in cases of bloody, vaginal discharge taken both internally and as a douche.

One study involved 108 patients with bacillary dysentery treated with a paste of knotgrass, internally, with 104 recovering within 5 days. *J Chin Herb Med* 1972 2:24.

It also shows inhibition against *Staphylococcus aureus, Pseudomonas pyocyanea, Bacillus typhosus* and various skin fungi.

The herb, and its active compounds of quercitrin hydrate, caffeic acid and rutin induce cutaneous wound healing in work by Seo SH et al, *Phytother Res* 2016 30(5):848-54.

The leaf and stem exhibit activity against both gram negative and positive bacteria, and various fungi except *Candida albicans.*

Work by Salama et al, *Saudi J Bio Sci* 17(1):57-63 found the constituent panicudine active against *Bacillus subtilis, Salmonella paratyphi, S. typhi* and *Staphylococcus aureus.* Leaf extracts showed better activity.

Water extracts have been shown to have an inhibitory effect on prostaglandin biosynthesis and platelet activating factor (PAF) induced exocytosis.

An alcohol extract induced cytotoxicity in MCF-7 human breast cancer cell line, due to up regulation of P53, down regulation of Bcl-2 proteins, and induced apoptosis. Habibi RM et al, *Daru* 2011 19(5):326-31.

The plant is useful both internally for a wide variety of parasitic and fungal infections including tapeworm, hookworm, pinworm, roundworm; and externally for skin disorders like tinea, scabies, weeping eczemas, general skin itching and vaginal trichomonas.

Externally, a decoction is made and used as a wash, douche or compress. When available the fresh juice or thawed ice cube juice is best.

For damp heat associated with genital itching, or pruritis the herb is combined with *Kochia* seed.

As a tincture it is used internally for restoring and resolving a variety of kidney and bladder problems, such as cystitis, urethritis, nephritis, and other acute urinary tract infections; and is similar in action to horsetail for toning connective tissue. A good combination to unblock painful urination is Knotweed and Chinese Pink (*Dianthus chinensis*). Both have a downward draining action and resolve damp heat.

Anthraquinones isolated from Knotweed also bind Calcium and reduce the production of urinary stones. It combines well with Creeping Jenny (*Lysimachia species*) for painful, stony urinary dribbling.

A study by Nan-JiXing et al, found *P. aviculare* extracts reduced fibrotic liver formation considerably after bile duct ligation. This could prove invaluable to the millions of individuals who suffer after gall bladder removal. The full report is available in *Biological and Pharmaceutical Bulletin* 2000 23:2.

The compound juglanin reduced inflammatory response involved in hepatic injury in fructose fed rats. Considering the human connection between high fructose corn syrup ingestion and fatty liver, this should be looked at more closely. Zhou GY et al, *Biomed Pharmacother* 2016 81:318-28.

Juglanin is found in black walnut husks in much larger amounts.

It removes mild catarrh of the respiratory tract; as well as oral and pharyngeal inflammations as a gargle. One study looked at the effectiveness of *P. aviculare* on gingivitis in 60 male dental students. The herb extract was gargled twice daily for two week, with significant decrease in gingivitis. Gonzalez et al, *J Ethnopharm* 2001 74:1.

It was traditionally used as a perspiration inhibitor in cases of tuberculosis.

It acts as an astringent in diarrhea, enteritis and hemorrhoids; as well as staunching bleeding in postpartum hemorrhage, uterine bleeding or blood in sputum. For this is combines well with Shepherd's Purse.

Knotgrass has been shown to have anti-fibrotic activity induced by bile duct ligation. Nan et al, *Bio Pharm Bull* 2000 23:2. All liver enzymes showed reductions of 40% compared to control group.

It appears to reduce the kidney toxicity associated with acetaminophen. Sohn SH et al, *Environ Toxicol Pharmacol* 2009 27(2):225-30.

Note the content of astragalin, found in Astragalus species.

Be careful in urinary difficulties associated with abdominal weakness. Knotgrass is contraindicated in cold, deficient conditions, and pregnancy.

LADY'S THUMB
(P. maculosa)

CONSTITUENTS- a sesquiterpene, isotadeonal, tannins (25-30% of root), pyrogallic tannins coumarins, isoquercitin, hyperosides. From the seeds is derived 5,7-dihydroxychromone.

The leaves contain a high amino acid count; suggesting they make suitable forage.

Lady's thumb is mildly astringent, mucilaginous and diuretic; and a useful skin wash in chronic eczema and arthritis. It is warming and drying in nature.

Water extracts of both the flowers and leaves reveal activity against gram positive and mycobacterium.

Matthew Wood contributes a great deal to the use of this plant in The Earthwise Herbal.

"Indications for lady's thumb have been worked out by my friend Lise Wolff. She says that it is indicated when there is a dark spot in the center of the tongue or a dark line down the central crease. This usually corresponds to depression of the digestive powers or stagnant blood involving the spine. The characteristic stomach emotions are present.

The person worries, is a worrier, and the stomach is "all tied in knots". Food allergies are common. The membranes are dry and digestion is poor. There may be a history of unresolved mononucleosis…vaginal dryness. It is a remedy for infertility because it eliminates stagnate blood from the uterus and increases secretion. Stagnant blood in the lower spine and pelvis. Cancer when there is a black spot in the middle of the tongue.

A friend of mine had cancer of the colon, removed by surgery. She had a big black spot in the middle of the tongue. I gave her tincture of lady's thumb and the spot disappeared. She did many other things as well. Neither the spot nor the cancer has returned. That was five years ago."

The fresh plant juice is caustic, so caution is advised.

Work in Argentina confirms the traditional use of the plant for fungal infections. Derita M & Zacchino S, *Nat Prod Commun* 2011 6(7):931-3.

PALE PERSICARIA
(P. lapathifolium)

CONSTITUENTS- dihydrochalcone, lapathosides A-D, hydropiperoside, vanicoside B, lapithinol, lapthone, angelafolone, valafolone, melafolone, various 6'-methoxy chalcones, as well as kaempferol/quercitin glucosides, and galactosides (interesting flavonoids).

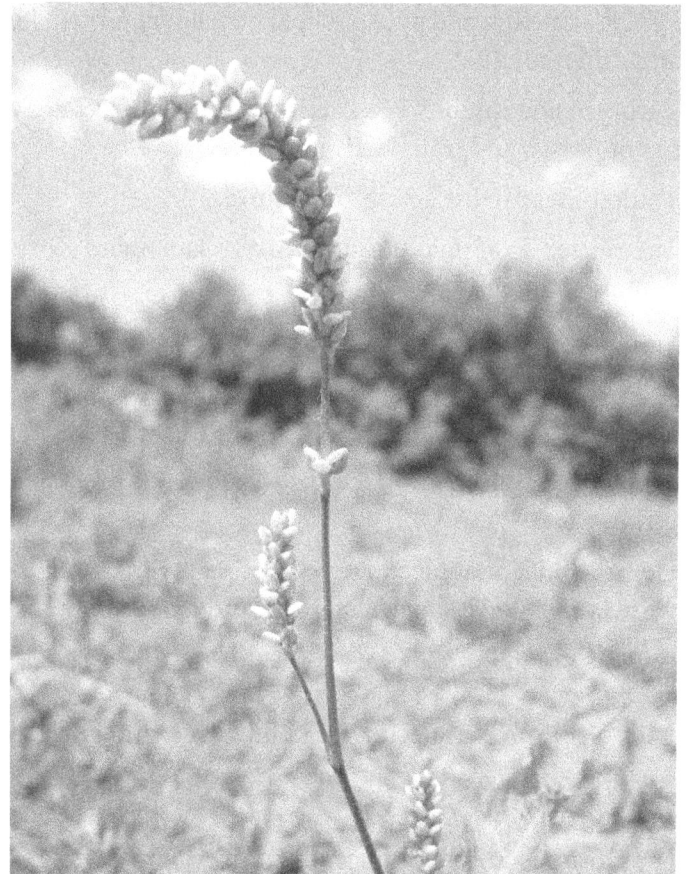

PALE PERSICARIA

Ethanol and water extracts of the flowers, leaves, root and stems show activity against both gram positive and myco-bacterium.

Work by Takashaki et al, *Cancer Lett* 2001 173(2):133-8 identified vanicoside B and lapathoside A as significant inhibitors on Epstein Barr virus early antigen activity, suggesting a cytotoxic activity. Skin tumors were inhibited by vanicoside B.

Vanicoside A & B show inhibition of beta-glucosidase, suggestive of use in diabetic conditions.

The herb inhibits xanthine oxidase, suggestive of use in gout and issues with uric acid.

The herb contains pinostrobin that at 1 mcg/M shows 88% inhibition of human leukemic cancer cells. Smolarz et al, *Z Naturforsch* 2006 61:7-8.

The plant is a hyper-accumulator of manganese, suggestive of phyto-remediation.

RUSSIAN KNOTGRASS
(P. erectum)

Infusions of Russian Knotgrass are useful in children's diarrhea, as the astringency of the leaves soothe this summer complaint.

A little summary is in order thanks to the work of Matthew Wood. *P. aviculare* is mucilaginous and cooling, *P. bistortoides* is warming and intensely astringent, *P. hydropiper* is warming and stimulating, and *P. persicaria* is warming and mucilaginous.

The related *P. pensylvanicum*, from the US eastern seaboard, was screened for PKC inhibition, and as an ethanol extract is active with an IC_{50} of 38 ug/ml.

PKC is a calcium and phospholipid dependent protein kinase involved in signal transduction and cell proliferation and differentiation.

Verbascoside inhibits PKC activity and demonstrates anti-neoplastic activity. It appears that PKC plays a role in apoptosis, and trans-activation of HIV.

Vanicosides are the active compounds.

The related *P. perfoliatum* is native to Japan and Korea but introduced into the eastern USA in the 1940s. It contains vanicosides.

HOMEOPATHY

P. amphibium (P. amphibia)

Smartweed is used for bleeding, whether it is excessive bleeding at menstruation, or lack of bleeding in young girls.

Hemorrhoids that bleed are relieved with Smartweed. In the female the hips feel drawn together. Menopausal women may have superficial sores and ulcers on their lower extremities.

P. persicaria (P. maculosa)

Lady's Thumb is a specific for kidney colic and gravel. Externally, it is used for gangrene.

P. aviculare

Knotgrass is an introduced weed in Alberta. It's greatest use is in the treatment of tuberculosis and other intermittent fevers. It is useful in arteriosclerosis and abnormal redness of the skin due to irritation and dilation of capillaries. Use tincture doses.

P. lapathifolium (P. lapathifolia)

Pale Smartweed (Lapathum) is used in cases of leucorrhea with constriction and expulsive effort through the womb and pain in the kidneys.

DOSE- For all the above, tincture doses.

P. hydropiper

Burnett, who prescribed *P. hydropiper* under its name Persicaria urens, regarded it as a splenic, and as useful in old cases of syphilis. As a splenic he found it often required in cases of gout; and in gouty eczema with much irritation he used it with much benefit in the 6th, 12th and 30th.   **CLARKE**

Polygonum punctatum (Persicaria punctata) is for great depression, followed by excessive irritability. It is for a gloomy view of life and dislike of change and excessive dread of death. There are dreams of have a severe headache, and waking with one.

The left side is more affected. Great thirst and appetite for cold water but produces nausea. Moderate exercise brings on profuse sweating and trembling.

Swollen glands, pains like a 'tremulous electrical movement'.

Feeling of strangulation in neck of bladder, tongue as if swollen, lots of tearing and burning pains.

DOSE- Self experiment by Joslin on chewing the leaf in 1854 and taking a tincture of leaf in 1856. Proving by Payne and one other male with tincture in 1858. Self experiment by Cameron with tincture in 1865. Clinical symptoms arranged by homeopath Bayard in 1885.

Polygonum sagittatum is used as a diuretic and has been used successfully for renal colic and relieving pain caused by sand and gravel.

Symptoms reported by Boger include itching of hard palate, making one wish to scratch, especially right side of palate. Dryness and slight roughness of throat. Lancinating pains along the spine, and a burning downward on inner side of right foot and in front of ankle.

ESSENTIAL OIL

Steam distillation of lady's thumb (*P. persicaria*) yields 0.053% of a volatile oil consisting of fatty acids, with acetic and butyric acids isolated in the form of their silver salts. The rest of the oil contains a camphorous-like substance named persicariol.

Smartweed (*P. hydropiper*) essential oil contains 1,4 cineole, alpha and beta pinene, borneol, bornyl acetate, camphor, carvone, cinnamic acid methyl ether, cinnamic alcohol, fenchone, p-cymol, phellandrene, poligonone, terpineol and confertifolin.

The latter, steam distilled from the leaf, shows activity against *Enterococcus faecalis* as well as various fungi. Duraipandiyan et al, *Pharm Bio* 2010 48:2 187-90.

Essential oil from leaves and flowers inhibit acetylcholinesterase and butyrylcholinesterase, suggestive of use in the treatment of Alzheimer's disease. Ayaz M et al, *Lipids Health Dis* 2015 14:141.

The oil contains confertifolin, which may be useful as part of superior natural mosquito repellants or to kill larvae in water sources.

Confertifolin shows activity against *Enterococcus faecalis* and a variety of fungi.

An essential oil can be obtained from Knotgrass (*P. aviculare*). It appears in several early Arabian perfume recipes, under the name Red Robin.

Bistort expresses different essential oils at various phases of development. Fresh aerial parts yield from 0.004-0.01%. During vegetative stage the predominant oil is 3 methylbut-3-en-1-ol, during flowering linalool, and during fruiting dodecanoic acid and its methyl esters. The oil shows minor anti-microbial activity.

HYDROSOLS

A water may also be distilled from Smartweed (*P. hydropiper*) that, if drunk often, will cure jaundice completely, drive out all the scummy matter and gravel retained in the kidneys, and cleanse and sweeten sharp scorbutic blood as well. Externally, this water is very useful for all manner of old, proud, stinking wounds and fistulous sores if they are rinsed with it or irrigated with it while it is warm. **SAUER**

The distilled water, drank to the quantity of a pint or more in a day, has been found serviceable in the gravel and stone. It is a diuretic of considerable efficacy, and has frequently been administered with success in the jaundice, and the beginning of dropsies.   **THOMAS GREEN**

Arsesmart when distilled "has been found better for gravelly complaints than a great variety of drugs taken… to little purpose."   **BORLASE**

Distilled (Bistort) water stops bloody flux and diarrhea, and withstands poison and contagion. If you drink one ounce or more of this water, it even has the power to stop bleeding, and will promote the healing of old, corrupt, stinking, spreading sores if they are bathed with it frequently. In this same manner, (Bistort) water can even be used for cancers of the back and the nose.   **SAUER**

Bistort root water is used to heal deep wounds, staunch bleeding, coughs, evil humors of the breast, pissing with pain, as a wash for frozen feet, stings, nose polyps, congealed blood and wounds. For the latter, combine 16 parts bistort, two parts chervil and two parts hemp water.   **BRUNSCHWIG**

Knotgrass distilled water…is accounted one of the most sovereign remedies to cool all manner of inflammations, breaking out through heat, hot swellings and impostumes, gangrene and fistulous cankers, or foul filthy ulcers, being applied or put into them; but especially for all sorts of ulcers and sores happening in the privy parts of men and women.   **CULPEPPER**

Brunschwig recommended knotgrass water, distilled from the herb and roots for stopping diarrhea, ague with heat, pain in wounds, increasing urine flow, worms in children, inflamed eyes, lukewarm for earaches, and black blains.

He suggested Lady's Thumb hydrosol for hemorrhoids.

PLANT OIL

Water Smartweed (*P. amphibia*) is composed of 36mg/100 grams dry weight of lipids. This breaks down to 33% neutral, 41% glucolipids, and 24% phospholipids.

The latter, in turn is nearly 47% phosphotidyl choline and only 1.7% phosphotidyl serine.

FLOWER ESSENCES

Bistort is very grounding. It relieves disorientation and helps increase emotional resiliency. It is a general strengthener.   **PEGASUS**

Bistort is for trust in surrendering control. Patterns of fear within that create the need to always control others and self are helped. It is for lack of trust, great inner turmoil and resistance in allowing life to unfold.   **CANADIAN**

Bistort is for those with tendency to self-destruct during times of personal change. There is an overly emotional response to the change process. These people loose their direction and tend to forget it is part of what they have worked toward. Those working to free themselves from past attitudes and emotions would benefit.   **BAILEY**

Knotgrass (*P. aviculare*) is used mainly as an essence for stomach problems and also for the joints, remember it when you need to flexible and bend in certain situations.   **OLIVE**

Knotweed flower essence is for those feeling grumpy and out of sorts.   **ROCKY MOUNTAIN**

Smartweed essence is for those who believe that since they were hurt before they will be hurt again. These people hide away and withdraw from perceived dangers of being with others.   **DESERT ALCHEMY**

Bistort operates with the higher mental body – specifically: new ideas, new structures, new concepts. It helps the ability to change one's mind comfortably and creatively without any sense of doubt or loss or anxiety.
HIGH SIERRA

Knotweed essence is for issues of insecurity, especially relevant to puberty and teenage years.   **MIRIANA**

Bistort flower essence is helpful for unfinished conflicts, and acts as a soul patch for those who cannot forgive the past.   **MIRIANA**

SPIRITUAL PROPERTIES

Knotweed is for vital aspiration and union with the divine.   **MOTHER**

Bistort helps one apply lessons of working to spiritual awareness. Making use of what has been learned, it encourages spiritual integration. Concepts of religious doctrine are merged; so that the person may more easily find what is true and important.

Because of alignment with higher truth, there is greater discernment of whether another person is saying the truth. This is not from a place of judgment, but an ability to know whether the statements are in harmony.

It is wise to use bistort in certain forms of agriculture, such as growing herbs in a greenhouse. Mists made from this plant will protect plants rare, or difficult to grow.   **GURUDAS**

Knotweed has the ability to dissolve a number of blockages in your path. This can often be the simple things such as little annoyances or difficulties. A strengthening of positive affirmations may also develop. Those who work with affirmations and yet struggle to truly feel or know them, are greatly aided by this herb. This dissolving effect may also remove negative thought forms, though here it is not so much in the etheric or emotional body as in the mental body.

This is similar on the spiritual level, in that if one dissolves and empties there can be a filling effect, a way one is strengthened with the positive nature that one receives, as negative thought forms dissipate and positive ones replace them.

It is like wishful thinking. This is a way in which intuition is displaced with these positive thought forms. The action of this herb in tea form, or in a very dilute concentration of the juice, even prepared homeopathically at 2X or 3X potency, has a balancing and self governing effect in which these affirmations are taken in balance.

Petrochemical and heavy metal miasms are eased.   **GURUDAS**

Write down all your cares and concerns on a piece of paper. Place some Knotweed in an envelope with the letter and put it on your altar. Leave it there for a week and then burn the envelope. Allow the Knotweed to absorb all the emotional pain expressed in your letter and allow the fire to transform it.   **S. GREGG**

PERSONALITY TRAITS

BISTORT (Yerba del Pescado)

Fish have become symbols of the most sacred significance and mystical import during the progress and interpretation of Christianity. The fish was even a symbol of Christ in primitive and medieval Christian art. The origin is to be found in the initial letters of His names and titles in Greek, which together spell the word for fish. It was said to be represented in the oval-shaped figure pointed at both ends, and formed by the intersection of two circles, also known as the *Visica piscis*, which is common in ecclesiastical seals, and as an aureole in paintings surrounding figures of the Trinity.

CURTIN

The family name, Polygonaceae, is derived from poly-gonum, meaning 'many knees', based on the swollen joint-like stem nodes. This encapsulates the theme. A joint is a break in a stable structure to provide flexibility. The knee, however, is unique in that while being flexible it must also provide stability. It must master two opposites, suddenly and unaccountably changing between flexible and stable, depending on the needs of the body at any moment. Tasked with achieving diametric opposites, a knee's function is to provide flexible stability and stable flexibility, an almost impossible feat of biologic engineering.

Capricious, changeable, unpredictable, contrary and given to whims is hardly surprising when trying to please two opposing duties or desires.

VERMEULEN

RECIPES

DECOCTION-One tablespoon of root, to one pint of water. Simmer fifteen minutes. Take one tablespoon several times daily.

INFUSION- Cold infusions are made by covering the plant with water, and sitting overnight. If need be the water is slowly warmed before drinking. Up to four ounces three times daily. NOTE- the constituents of all the aerial parts of plants are quite heat sensitive.

TINCTURE- 10-15 drops 3x daily. Smartweed tincture is made 1:5 at 45% alcohol. Fresh plant is best, but dried works as well. Use 30-60 drops as needed. Fresh seeds of smartweed require immediate crushing and high level alcohol to retain polygodial content. Avoid during pregnancy.

POWDER- 1-5 "OO" capsules of dried powder several times daily.

Caution- Knotgrass (*P. aviculare*) has shown some indication as a human abortifacient. Do not use in pregnancy.

BLACK-EYED SUSAN
GLORIOSA DAISY
BROWN-EYED SUSAN
(*Rudbeckia hirta* L.)
(*R. hirta var. pulcherrima* Farw.)
TALL CONEFLOWER
GREEN-HEADED CONEFLOWER
CUTLEAF CONEFLOWER
THIMBLEWEED
(*R. laciniata* L.)
(*R. ampla* A. Nels.)
(*R. laciniata var. ampla* [A. Nels.] Cronq.)
PARTS USED- flower, leaves, and root

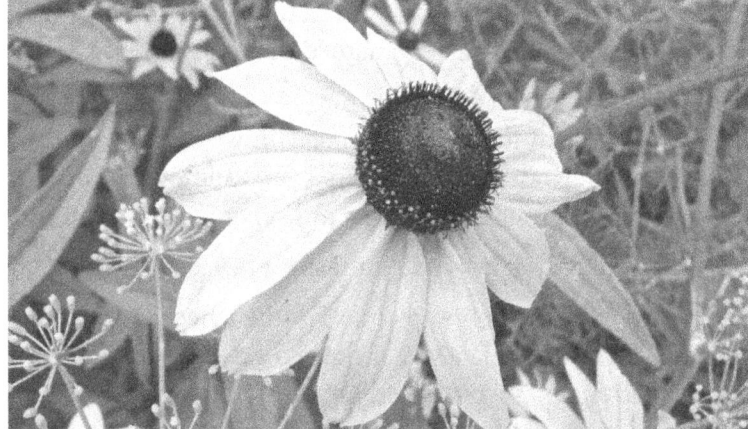

BLACK EYED SUSAN

Merry, laughing black-eyed Susans
grow along the dusty way.

M. WAIT

All in the dawn the fleet was moor'd,
The streamers waving in the wind,
When Black-eyed Susan came on board,
Oh where shall I my true love find?
Tell me, ye jovial sailors, tell me true,
If my sweet William, if my sweet William
Sails among your crew?

JOHN GAY

Rudbeckia is named after the famous Swedish botanist/scientist Olaf Rudbeck whose son, of the junior name, was a friend and patron of Linnaeus. The Elder Rudbeck founded the Uppsala Botanic Garden, while his son was a professor at Uppsala University. They produced a volume of the known plants of the early 1800s, complete with thousands of woodcuts, destroyed by fire in 1702. Carl von Linne, later Linnaeus, came there to study medicine in the 1720s, and moved into the son's house and earned money tutoring four of the professor's 24 children. The elder Olaf wrote a book Atlantikan, that claimed Sweden as the locale of Plato's Atlantis, but he was also a fine scientist that helped identify the lymphatic system.

It is interesting to note that before Linnaeus created his system of classification this plant, like many others, was given a long, multi-worded Latin phrase name or polynominal.

Rudbeckia hirta, for example, was known as *Chrysanthemum Marilandicum, caule & Foliis hirsutis Hieracii, flore magno, pluribus petalis radiato, disco granti protuberanate*; a real mouthful to say the least.

Hirta is from the Latin meaning rough or hairy, referring to the stem. Lanciniata means lance-leafed.

The common name came from a popular English ballad written around 1720, by John Gay. His musical, The Beggar's Opera, was performed, in England, more than any other play of the 18th century.

Black-eyed Susan is common throughout the prairies, and children cannot resist picking bouquets of the yellow-petal and chocolate brown-centered flowers.

It is a short-lived perennial, biennial, or even an annual. Actually the yellow petals are sterile florets. The actual flower is the small cluster in the middle.

It is said that the flower migrated east, as the buffalo began disappearing. True, but actually, the plant moved east when the forests of eastern America were cleared, and later, when introduced for erosion control by state governments.

Both the Cherokee and Iroquois used root infusions for pinworms in children, for which purpose it combines well with pineapple weed. Infusions were also used externally to bath ulcerous sores, and soothing sore eyes.

The plant leaf infusion was used traditionally for increasing urination and a mild stimulating effect on the heart.

The root tea was also used as a wash to heal sores, and swellings; including saddle sores of horses. In New Mexico, the root has been used traditionally to alleviate menstrual cramps and referred back pain.

The Potawatomi know it as Black Eyeballs, or **MEMAKATE'NÎNGWEÛK**.

Hot infusions were taken to cure colds and flu. The fresh juice from the root was dropped into the ear for earaches. The roots were decocted for use as a heart medicine in an unspecified manner.

Tall Coneflower is more hairless, with deeply cut leaves, growing on the plains from Montana through to Manitoba, and south. Both species are hardy to -40° C.

The Chippewa steeped the root of Tall Coneflower with Arrowhead for indigestion, while the flowers were dried and used as a moistened poultice with goldenrod and Anise Hyssop for burns. They call it **GIZUSWEBIGWAIS** meaning, "it is scattering", or Yellow Flower, **WEZAWAB-GONIK**.

The Cherokee ate the steamed leaves of Souchon as it is known, as a spring tonic, and to give them strength. It is zesty, to say the least.

It was also called **AHWI AKATA**, meaning Deer Eye. The root decoction was used for weak or inflamed eyes, snakebite, and swellings.

Eclectic physicians used it for kidney infections, difficult urination and related problems.

Black-eyed Susan is the official state flower of Maryland. Lord Baltimore's colours were gold and black, as are the Orioles of baseball, and the bird itself.

It was voted the 11th showiest wildflower in a 1940s poll of naturalists and botanists.

In 1999, *Rudbeckia fulgida* "Goldsturm" was named perennial plant of the year, and is fully hardy to zone 3.

Black-eyed Susan is a prolific seed producer, but they are extremely small, counting nearly 3.75 million per kilogram.

MEDICINAL

CONSTITUENTS- *R. hirta*-eupaline and eupatoline (flavonoids), 3, 4', 5-trihydro-3',6,7- trimethoxy-flavone, ambrosanolides, coumarin, thiopheneacetylenes, sodium salicylate, thiarubrine A, various trimethyoxy-flavones, patulitrin, patuletin-7-glucoside, salicylic acid, chlorogenic acid and quercetagetin.
Flowers- three phenolics acids, two phenolic acid esters, four flavonol glycosides and a trimethylated flavonol, rudbeckolide.
roots- di-thiacyclohexadienes and thiophenes.
R. laciniata root- rudbeckianone, rudbeckolide, nor-sesquiterpene, bisabolen-1,4-endo-peroxide, 1 beta-hydroxy-8-epi-ivangustin, alantolactone (1%), 5-6-dihydro-4-5-dehydro-alantolactone, isoalantolactone, bisabolene-1-4-endoperoxide, alpha curcumene, 5-hydroxy-alpha-curcumene, eremophila-1(10)-11(13)-dien-12-8-beta-olide, 8-alpha-(H)-seco-eudesmanolide, lasidiol angelate (crispane), alpha beta and gamma selinene, beta humulene, trideca-12-ene-2-4-6-8-10-pentayne,
plant- squalene, methyl ether coumarin, beta amyrin, germacrene D, rudbeckianone, 13-oxo-1-2-3-4-didehydro-cacalol, phytol.
seeds and pericarp- 38% protein

Black-eyed Susan benefits the immune system in a manner similar to Echinacea. It is interesting to note that the term Rudbeckia was at one time associated with Echinacea species, but not since the 1840s. In laboratory studies, the extracts stimulated phagocytic activity of macrophages, showing anti-bacterial properties. Spleen weight also increased in laboratory animals.

A 1994 study by Bukovsky et al in the former Czechoslovakia found alcohol extracts of flavonoids possess immune modulating effect.

More recent studies in Germany have shown root extracts of Black eyed Susan to have higher immuno-stimulating effect than either *Echinacea angustifolia* or *E. gloriosa*.

Thiarubrines from the root show strong anti-bacterial and anti-fungal activity. An interesting study at the University of British Columbia in 1989 showed that the antibiotic effect was only effective when activated with UV-A light. This leads to interesting possibilities of study.

Generally, Black-eyed Susan is a stimulating diuretic, with mild cardiac stimulation as a side effect. It increases the volume of urine, but does not increase the amount of solids removed.

A recent study of the phenolic metabolites in flowers, gives scientific credence to the use of the herb for inflammation. Michael BR et al, *Nat Prod Res* 2014 28(12):909-13.

Quercetagetin is both anti-bacterial and an inhibitor of RNA/DNA polymerase and reverse transcriptases of RLV and HIV.

The compound exhibits strong anti-oxidant, anti-diabetic and anti-lipimic activity. Wang W et al, *J Food Sci Technol* 2016 53(6):2614-24.

It shows anti-viral activity against the Chikungunya virus, that causes extreme arthritis in some individuals. Lani R et al, *Antiviral Res* 2016 133:50-61.

Chlorogenic acid in *R. hirta* is anti-viral and has a similar structure to Tamiflu and Relenza, well-known neuraminidase inhibitor drugs. Jaiswal et al, *Phytochem Analysis* 2011 22:5 432-441.

Patulitrin inhibits HeLa cancer cell lines. Kashif M et al, *Pharm Biol* 2015 53(5):672-81.

Rudbeckolide, present in both species, is a potent anti-oxidant.

The closely related Tall Coneflower (*R. laciniata*) is used in the American Southwest for delayed menstruation, where there are cramps and headaches. It is also used for vaginal discharge and dull, aching uterine inflammation, according to Michael Moore.

"Unlike Echinacea (and like Balsam Root, another Echinacea-like remedy), lance leafed Coneflower stimulates secretions, respiration, and the skin and kidneys, thereby helping to excrete the very waste products its immunostimulus helps create (unlike Echinacea)… The root of *R. laciniata* has a history of use for painful menstruation in New Mexico, and in fact it has been recommended by *parteras* when Immortal is unavailable and birthing contractions have slowed or stopped prematurely.

I can't vouch pro or con for this, but I can for its value in stimulating dry, suppressed menses at the end of the month with inadequate progesterone magnitude and duration."

It is also used for chronic urethritis, and as a bladder tonic. The compound lasidol angelate was formerly found in parsley and called crispane.

The root can be combined with other herbs to relieve indigestion.

Tall Coneflower contains alantolactone, also found in Elecampane species. Work by Ding Y et al, *J Hematol Oncol* 2016 9(1):93 found this compound selectively targets leukemia stem cells and may be useful in acute myeloid leukemia.

Previous work by this researcher found alantolactone induces apoptosis in colorectal cancer cells. Jiang Y et al, *Oncol Lett* 2016 11(6):4203-7 found this compound induces apoptosis in human cervical cancer cells.

The compound is active against herpes simplex virus, lung squamous cancer cells, breast cancer cells; and is known for its vermifuge activity for whipworms, pin worms, etc.

Alpha curcumene induces apoptosis of SiHa ovarian cancer cell lines. Shin Y et al, *Toxicol Res* 2013 29(4):257-61. It also is cytotoxic to both K562 human chronic myelogenous leukemia and LNCaP human prostate carcinoma cell lines. Nishikawa K et al, *Biosci Biotechnol Biochem* 2008 72(9):2463-6.

Dr. King, an Eclectic physician of the 1800s wrote "Thimbleweed is a valuable diuretic, tonic and balsamic. Useful in many diseases of the urinary organs and highly recommended in strangury, Bright's disease, and wasting or atrophy of the kidneys".

Both plants exhibit activity against gram positive bacteria in the leaves. Work by Bishop and MacDonald, *Can J Botany* 29 found alcohol extracts active against *Staphylococcus aureus*.

CAUTION- Do not use during pregnancy.

SEED OIL

The seed oil of Black eyed Susan yields 20% and is composed of 4% conjugated and 67% non-conjugated linoleic acids. It also contains 11% of a saturated fatty acid.

Tall coneflower seeds contain 26% oil composed of 60% non-conjugated linoleic acid, 4% saturated acid, and 26% octadeconoic acid.

ESSENTIAL OIL

An essential oil has been extracted from the closely related Tall Coneflower (*R. laciniata*) that grows in the open woods of Manitoba and south.

It is rich in alpha pinene, limonene, beta-phellandrene, and bornyl acetate.

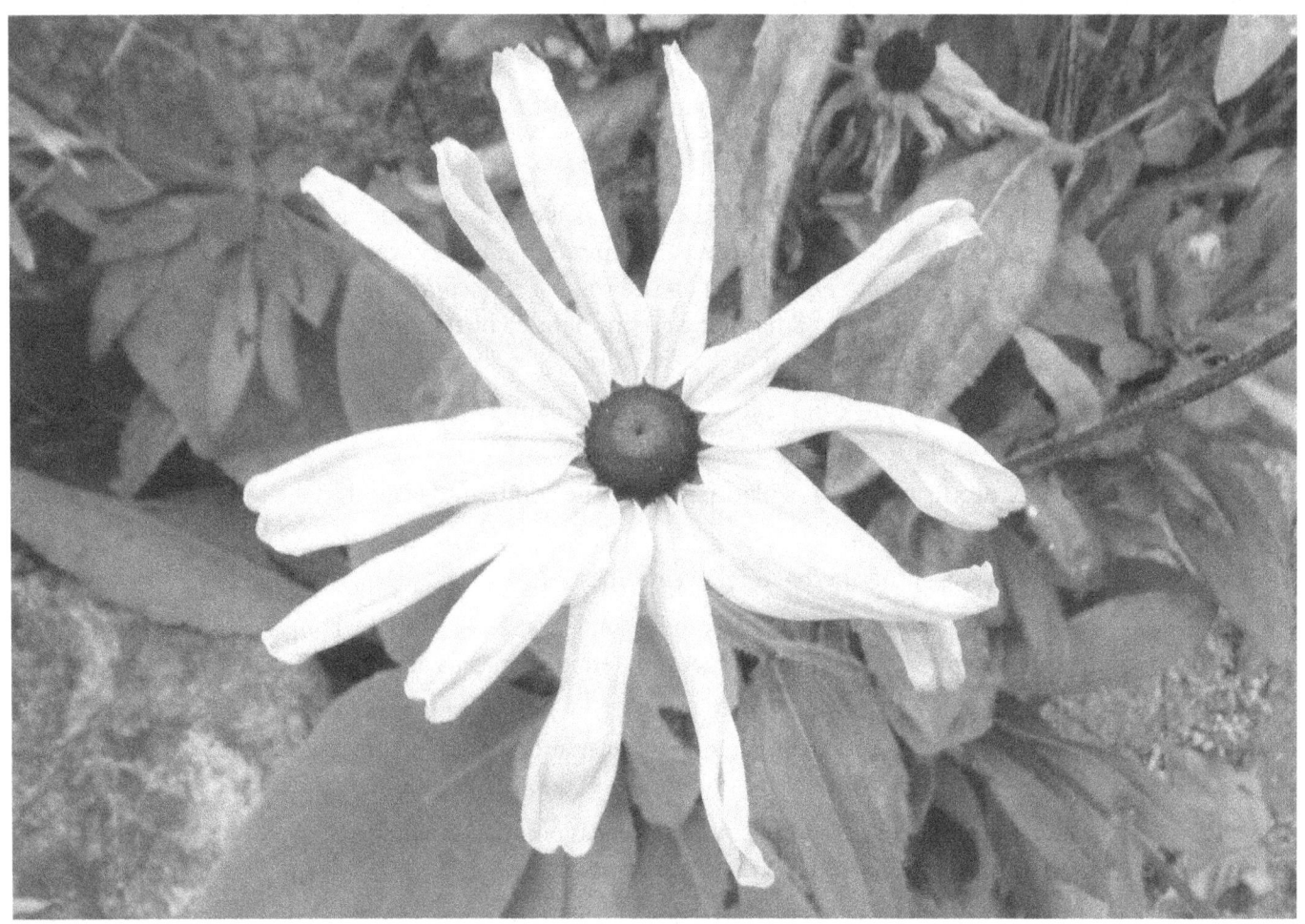

BLACK EYED SUSAN

FLOWER ESSENCES

Black-eyed Susan flower essence alleviates low self-esteem. It helps generate a sunny disposition, self-sufficiency, and emotional stability. It has a calming effect on one undergoing shock, or when used with meditation. **PEGASUS**

Black-eyed Susan is for avoidance or repression of traumatic or painful aspects of the personality. It helps awaken and gives penetrating insight into deep emotions whenever resistance comes up in self therapy, counseling or dream work. **FLOWER ESSENCE SOCIETY**

Black-eyed Susan flower essence improves vision, opens the heart, more openness to Leo energy, and seeing the God in everyone. **JADE MOUNTAIN**

Black-eyed Susan flower essence may be helpful for those who misuse their personal power, feel stuck in "hairy" situations, or tend to over-analyze situations or let emotions cloud their judgment. **LIVING FLOWER**

Black-eyed Susan could be considered the keeper of the realm of childhood magic. It's the place where love never dies, where your secret friends live, where the best aspect of your early childhood imagination takes shape and root.
HIGH SIERRA

Black Eyed Susan essence is for restless and impatient people. Their excessive demands create constant emotional setbacks.
MIRIANA

SPIRITUAL PROPERTIES

Black-eyed Susan is for first turning of the vital towards the Divine light. The vital prepares itself to be transformed.
THE MOTHER

Black-eyed Susan, perhaps the most spiritual of all the species of wildflowers, is inhabited generally by a spiritual substance drawn, not from the aura of the plant, but from the planet Venus. That planet is surrounded, continually, by the vibrations of Christ-Love, and therefore, it will be understood that the tiny entity in each of these plants also partakes of the same purity and love.

By drinking once daily, a tea made by pouring near-boiling water over the petals of one flower, the heart chakra can be opened up immeasurably, and man can learn to love with the same universality that all the higher beings can project.

A dab of oil can be placed on the heart chakra for a short period. Start with a few minutes, and slowly lengthen to 15 minutes.
HILARION

Black-eyed Susan's unique wisdom vibration can help aggressively clear away what is no longer serving you on the emotional plane. What I mean by "aggressively" is that the dynamic isn't exactly gentle and gradual: it's more like an energetic purgative of nonphysical (i.e., emotional and spiritual) toxins, which can cause some upsets as our lives shift to meet our newly cleansed outlook and mental state…Black-eyed Susan can help us stay grounded, calm and energetically healthy, especially when we feel beset by harsh or challenging environments or situations…And if we've been feeling lopsided in either directions or unable to integrate our bright and shadowy aspects for any reason, black-eyed Susan can help.
TESS WHITEHURST

PERSONALITY TRAITS

The glorious prairie daisies are the essence of reliability but with such exuberant charm that we would grow them even if they were to fold after only one season. In fact, clumps go on for years…some gardeners are snotty about yellow. I used to be one of them…As a fine art student I arbitrarily decided to give yellow a miss for a whole year until I was told, rather pointedly, that yellow was the colour of spirituality.
C. KLEIN

DOCTRINE OF SIGNATURES

The dark core spreading out into light petals is symbolic of this plant's ability to bring release and of the shadow-self embracing the light. The dark core also represents the darkness of the earth and our connection with our root chakra; this is the energy center that connects us with the earth and helps us build a foundation for understanding who we are and what direction we will choose in our lives.

The yellow halo or crown is symbolic of our conscious awareness and our ability to embrace a light and higher power. The yellow petals also represent the solar plexus chakra, which gives us our ability to think and reason, to find our purpose in life, and to empower ourselves.

The coarse, hairy stem and leaves represent our rough, "hairy", potentially dangerous risks, losses and injuries.
PALLASDOWNEY

HERBAL POETICA

All in the dawn the fleet was moor'd,
The streamers waving to the wind,
When Black-eyed Susan came on board,
Oh where shall I my true love find?
Tell me, ye jovial sailors, tell me true,
If my sweet William, if my sweet William
Sails among your crew!

JOHN GAY

Merry, laughing black-eyed Susans
Grow along the dusty way,
Homely, wholesome, happy-hearted
little country maids are they.
Fairer sisters shrink and wither, 'neath the hot midsummer sun,
But these sturdy one will revel till the long, bright days are done.
Though they lack the roses sweetness
And the lily's tender grace,
We are thankful for the brightness of each honest, glowing face,
For in dry and barren places, where no daintier blooms would stay,
Merry, laughing black-eyed Susans cheer us on our weary way.

MINNIE C. WAIT

RECIPES

INFUSION- of the root or leaves- Use one tsp. to pint of hot water. Like mullein, the leaves contain irritating hairs that should be strained through a coffee filter or the like.

DOSE- One half cup when needed.

TINCTURE- 10-20 drops up to three times daily. The tincture is prepared from the fresh whole plant at 1:4 and 50% alcohol.

BLADDERWORT, GREATER
(*Utricularia vulgaris* L.*)
(**U. vulgaris ssp. macrorhiza** [Le Conte] R. T. Clausen)
FLAT-LEAVED BLADDERWORT
(*U. intermedia* Hayne)
SMALL BLADDERWORT
(*U. minor* L.)
HORNED BLADDERWORT
(*U. cornuta* Michx.)
PARTS USED- whole flowering plant

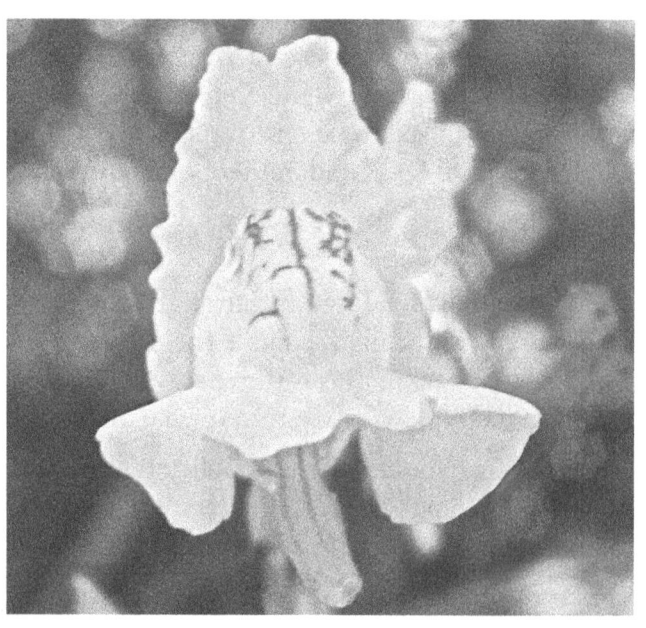

BLADDERWORT

Utricularia is from the Latin **UTRICULUS**, meaning "small or little bottle". Vulgaris means common; while macrorhiza means large rooted.

Bladderworts are perennial plants of the water or mud, in the case of U. cornuta. They are found in the tiniest of ditches, as well as ponds and sloughs.

The name Bladderwort is due to the collection of translucent bladders along the stem. These are windows of death to a variety of larvae, crustaceans, and fresh water shrimp. They are draw through a trap door into the pods, where they die a slow death, and are converted into a soupy juice of nitrogen for the plant. More than 50% of their prey are algae and pollen grains.

The plant does this by closing the pod door, and removing half the water from the bladder. This, of course, creates a strong negative pressure inside. When an insect touches the trigger hairs, the door springs open, and water rushes to fill the vacuum, carrying the meal along. It closes again, in 0.02 seconds. Then, the plant releases enzymes, and dinner is served! It is an ultra fast trapping device.

Resetting the trap takes 20-40 minutes in warm water and up to several hours in cold.

Bladderwort has some potential as a bio-control agent for mosquitoes, in areas where larvicide is neither feasible nor desirable. Ponds containing *U. minor* have significantly lower counts of mosquito larvae and eggs than those without. Angerilli and Beirne, *Can J Zoo* 1980 112.

The bladders are filled with water, until the plant is ready to bloom. Then, they fill with air, like miniature balloons, and carry the plant to the surface.

The bladders are green and translucent when empty, but turn dark purple to black when digesting organisms.

In times of drought, the bladders also serve as a reserve source of water. Microscopic water animals, called rotifers, perch themselves on the non-trigger bristles of Bladderwort traps, and rotate their cilia to capture even smaller prey.

It is possible that cellulase breaks down algae in the bladders as another source of food.

The Slave living near Great Slave Lake call the plant Water Berry, or **TUE DZHI**. They decocted the plant and used it to wash sore legs.

The Dena'ina of Alaska name is similar, **TANAGHA** which means, "water eye".

Thoreau was less enamored with the plant and called it "a dirty-conditioned flower, like a sluttish woman with a gaudy yellow bonnet". I believe he remained a bachelor all his life.

Small Bladderwort (*U. minor*) is dried and powdered for an inebriating drink in Ladakh, India. This region has a lot of regional specialties, this one is known as Lingeatzish. The dried, powdered leaves are roasted on a flat rock, and then mixed with water in a glass bottle and buried in the sand for two weeks. It is very inebriating and can cause death when taken in excess.

In areas of the world where rice is harvested, bladderwort is used as a poultice for wounds, due to its mild astringent effect.

The bright yellow, toadflax-like flowers last only one day, and after fertilization the developing pod is pulled down into the water for ripening and release of seed. The plant rarely sets seed, but reproduces by overwintering buds (turions) that release and drop into the mud to begin again the next spring.

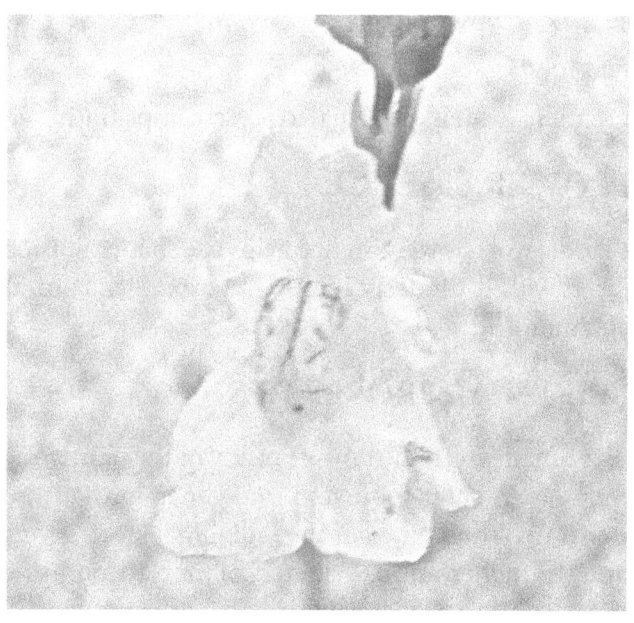

GREATER BLADDERWORT

MEDICINAL

CONSTITUENTS- *U. vulgaris*-organic salts, aucubin, catapol, tannins, essential oils; 2 novel iridoid esters (6-0-p-coumaroyl aucubin and 10-0-caffeoyl aucubin); glucolipids including monogalactosyyliacylglycerides, digal-actosyldiacylglycerides, cerebrosides, apigenin, luteolin, diosmetin, 6-hydroxyluteolin, carotenoids, and iridoid monoterpenes such as globularin, scutellarioside II, phenylpropane derivatives such as 1-p-cumaroyl glucosides; cyanidin (zyanidine), coumarin and flavonoids. *U. intermedia*- spermidine (alkaloid)

The most common fatty acids in the three glycolipids are palmitic, stearic and linoleic acids.

Diuretic, and vulnerary uses are noted for the plant.

The various flavones in *U. vulgaris* have both anti-inflammatory and anti-bacterial activity. It was used previously for urinary tract disorders with inflammation.

Externally, the plant is used for burns, and various skin inflammations, mouthwashes and cosmetic applications.

Active substances in the plant increase gall bladder secretions.

Cerbrosides are found in many plants, and especially in some medicinal mushrooms including Hericium species, Turkey Tail and others. Cerebroside E, from the fruiting body of Lion's Mane (H. erinaceus) reduced cisplatin induced kidney toxicity in LLC-PK1 cells and significant inhibition on angiogenesis in HUVECs. This suggests the beneficial effects in cancer treatment. Lee SR et al, *Bioorg Med Chem Lett* 2015 25(24):5712-5.

Hydrolysed catalpol and aucubin modulate STAT3 signaling pathway and enhance apoptosis in human myeloid leukaemia cells. Kim MB et al, *Phytother Res* 2015 29(3):434-43.

Diosmetin is a potent muscle relaxant and anti-spasmodic. Mendel M et al, *Eur J Pharmacol* 2016 791:640-6.

It reduced amyloid beta associated with Alzheimer's disease, in an oral mouse study. Sawmiller D et al, *J Neuroimmunol* 2016 299:98-106.

Diosmetin may be a key target of cell apoptosis in HepG2 human hepatoma cancer cells. Liu B et al, *Mol Med Rep* 2016 14(1):159-64.

It may alleviate chronic asthma and pulmonary fibrosis via unique pathways. Ge A et al, *Life Sci* 2016 153:1-8.

Luteolin inhibits human lung cancer A549 cell lines via arrest of cell proliferation at G_1 phase, and apoptosis. Zhan G et al, *J Food Sci* 2016 81(10):H2578-86. Luteolin is commonly found in a multitude of medicinal herbs and food.

Cyanidin exhibits potential to prevent cisplatin-induced nephrotoxicity. Gao S et al, *Cancer Lett* 2013 333(1): 36-46.

FLOWER ESSENCE

Bladderwort flower essence helps use shatter illusion through clear inner knowing; promotes discernment when faced with dishonesty in others; strengthens our ability to perceive the truth regardless of the confusion that surrounds it.   **ALASKA**

SPIRITUAL PROPERTIES

A tea made from the flowers of any of the numerous Bladderwort species can be very helpful in all cases of poor memory, mental confusion, and general exhaustion. The effect of the spiritual substances in the flowers is to unite all of the minds of the individual more strongly together: the lower mind (conscious and subconscious) and the higher mind. Instances of mental confusion and tiredness almost always arise from a poor connection between the various mental levels of the individual and this charming little plant offers a wonderful gift for all who suffer in this way. There may be some cases of "mental incompetence" or "retardation" that can also be aided by this plant. The tea is to be drunk once daily before retiring.

The key to determining the use of this flowers lies in the bladders, since these were meant to symbolize the brain.
HILARION

PERSONALITY TRAITS

In digestive activity, insect-eating plants can challenge any animal stomach. Not only the living muscle tissue of insects is digested, but raw, minced or roasted beef or veal. Even strong cheese, tough gristle, nitrogen rich plant seeds, pollen, fragments of bone and tooth enamel cannot resist their powers of digestion. On farinaceous, sweet and sour substances are not digested.
STREHLI

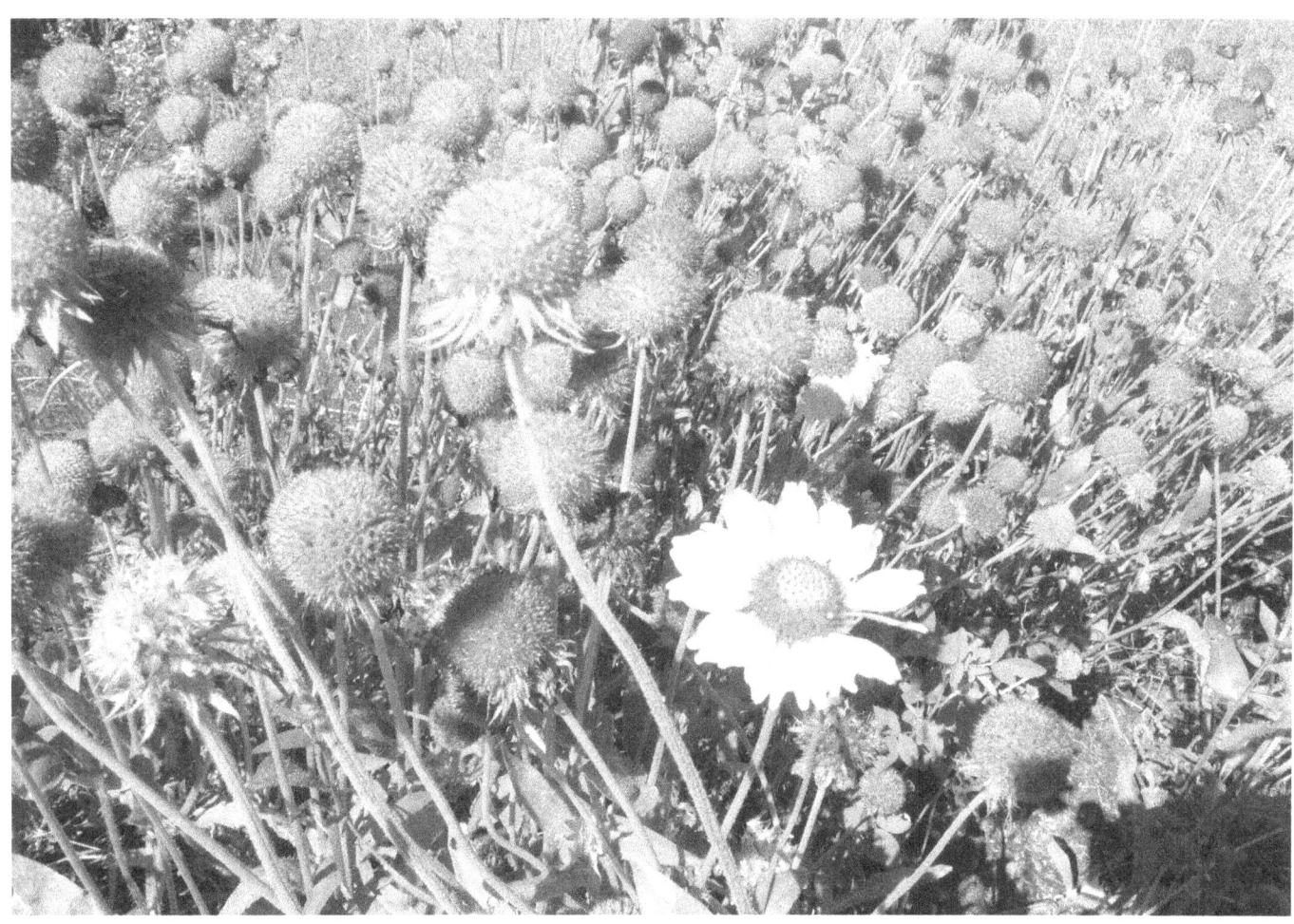

WILD BLANKET FLOWER (*G. aristata*)

GAILLARDIA
(***Gaillardia* X *grandiflora** Van Houtte)
COMMON GAILLARDIA
BLANKET FLOWER
GREAT BLANKET FLOWER
(**G. aristata** Pursh)
INDIAN BLANKET
ROSERING GAILLARDIA
FIREWHEEL
(**G. pulchella** Foug.)
PARTS USED- flower, leaves

I think sitting behind a keyboard can be a security blanket. **LIA ICES**

Gaillardia is named after M. Gaillard de Marentonneau, a French magistrate and patron of botany.

Aristata is from the Latin meaning "bristly or bearded"; referring to the numerous bristles on the seeds. Pulchella means pretty. Mason bee (*Schinia masoni)* is named for its discovery in 1896 by John Mason, a Denver-area butterfly collector.

G. aristata is the native perennial, while *G. pulchella* is a nursery annual, with daisy like flowers of red, orange and yellow. They do well in full sun, and poorer soil; and start well from seed; and root cuttings. *G.* x *grandiflora* is a garden hybrid.

Terry Willard writes, "to our ancestors, this plant represented the health, earthiness and wholesomeness of the common people".

Blanket Flower was used traditionally by the Thompson as a decoction for headaches, and general indisposition.

The Blackfoot used root infusions for stomach and bowel problems, and for sore eyes, or nose drops. Footbaths were also made from the flower heads. The root decoctions were also used to relieve saddle sores on their horses.

The chewed, powdered root is used for skin problems, and a tea from the plant was applied to sore nipples of nursing mothers.

Their close neighbors, the Stony drank the herb tea to relieve menstrual problems.

Root Woman, a great herbalist from Saskatchewan, says it is considered a good luck plant, used medicinally for sunstroke. The ripe seeds were cracked and warmed as incense.

The Blackfoot rubbed the flowers on rawhide bags to waterproof them. The roots were decocted for hair health and eyewash for horses.

The Secwepemc used the plant as part of a dandruff shampoo.

Various tribes of the British Columbia interior knew it as "little salmon eyes". The whole plant was lightly toasted, pounded with bear grease and applied to mumps.

The Okanagan drank a tea to cure kidney problems and bathed in it attempting to cure venereal disease.

Poultices were applied to the back and other affected areas for relieving pain, saddle sores on horses, and even falling hair.

Steedman, in her study of the Thompson tribe in 1930, said it was used for divination. "If a person is sick the whole plant is boiled for a considerable time, and if the decoction remains whitish or clear the person will die. If the decoction is reddish, or well-colored, the person will get well".

The Cheyenne used the flowers as a sunstroke medicine.

Today, it is both a nursery crop for back yard gardens, and a reclamation plant for oil well, gravel pits, and other sites of restoration, in both the open prairie, and openings in Aspen parkland.

It is said that Luther Burbank was walking a short distance from his train searching for plant and it pulled away without him. Eventually all was corrected and railway officials were apologetic. Burbank said. "It really doesn't matter, I've got my gaillardia."

It is grown as a seed crop, yielding 350,000-450,000 seeds per kilogram.

Most ornamental varieties are variation of *G. grandiflora*, a tetraploid without confirmed medicinal value. The plantlets may be useful in phyto-remediation. Work by Watharkar AD & Jadhav JP, *Ecotoxicol Environ Saf* 2014 103:1-8 found detoxification and decolorization of textile dye mixtures.

*Gaillarida aristata, Echinacea p*urpurea, Red Fescue (*Festuca arundinacea*) and alfalfa (*Medicago sativa*) may be useful for treatment and remediation of petroleum hydrocarbons. Liu R et al, *Environ Eng Sci* 2012 29(6): 494-501.

Recent taxonomic detective work by J. von Raison, from Dusseldorf, Germany suggests that Blanket Flower is more closely related to the Arnica genus than previously thought.

Blanket Flower has very few plant or insect pests. One moth, called the Mason Bee, is the sole host, and exactly matches the mottled red centers. It is only found on flowers, to my knowledge, growing around Boulder Colorado.

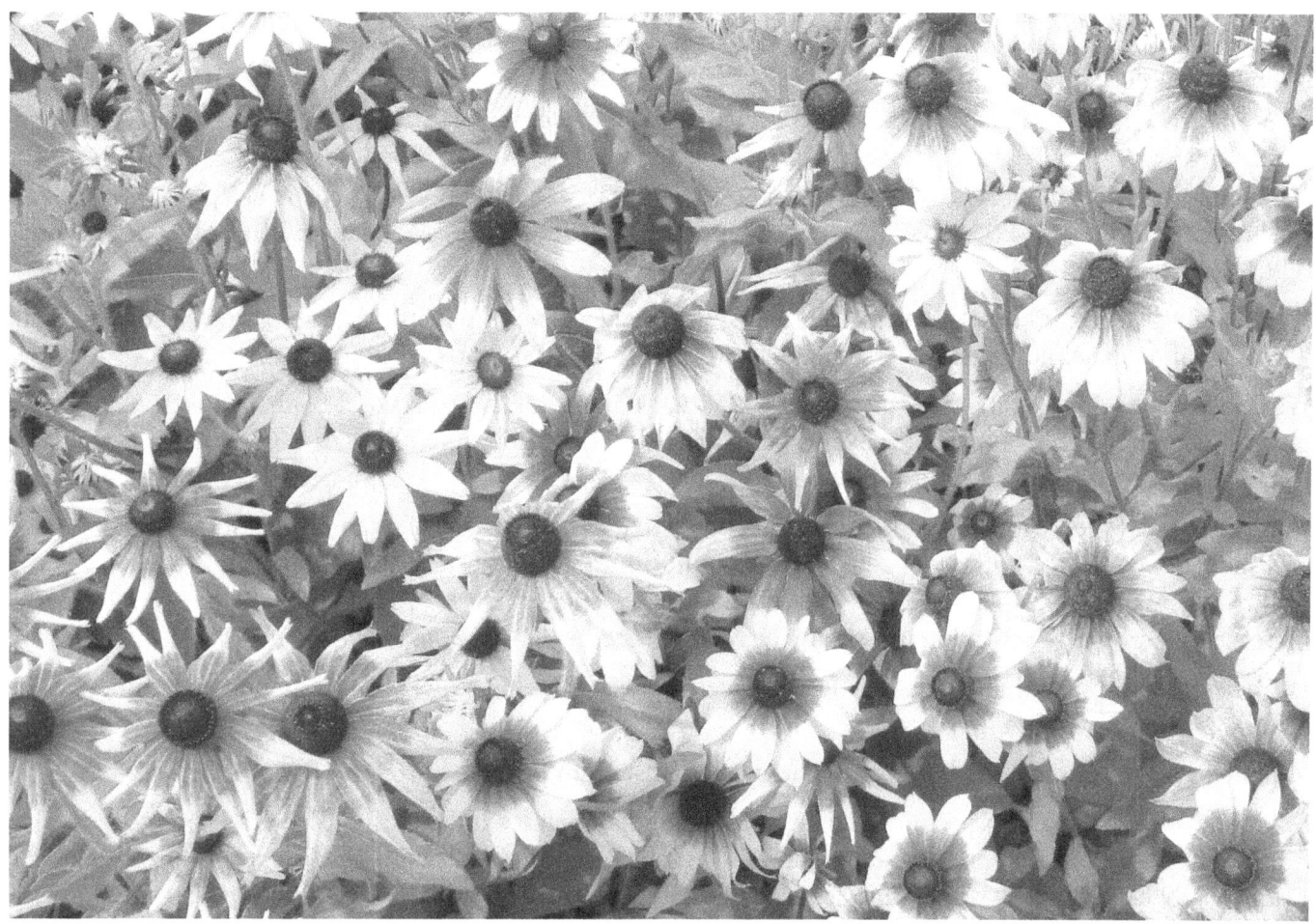

CULTIVATED, HYBRIDIZED BLANKET FLOWER

MEDICINAL

CONSTITUENTS- *G. aristata* flowers and leaves- pseudoguainolides, including 11 beta H-dihydro-4-epineopulchellin; apigenin, methoxyflavone, isoquercitrin, swertisin, 9-0-desacetylspathulin-2-0-(2-methyl-butanoate) and sesquiterpene lactones like gaigranin, gaigrandin, spatulin, pulchellin. Leaves contain 3-epi-isotelekin, neopulchellin, 6alpha-hydroxyneopulchellin, beta sitosterol-3-o-beta-D-glucoside, apigenin, quercitin, eupafolin, kaempferol-3-methoxy-7-o-alpha-L-rhamnoside, apigenin-7-O-beta-D-glucopyranoside, alpha amyrin and beta-sitosterol
Stems contain malonated anthocyanins.
The plant is very rich in carotenoids, yielding 1.34 grams per kilogram.
This includes over 36% of trans-monoepoxy-beta-carotene, nearly 30% cryptoxanthin isomers, 9.3% flavaxanthin, 9% zeaxanthin, 6.3% cis-monoepoxy-beta-carotene, 4% auro-xanthin, and 3.7% beta-carotene.
G. pulchella- swertisin, neopulchellidine, pulchellidine, and various sesquiterpenoids including gaillardin, isogaillardin, neogaillardin, pulchellin and pulchelloids.
G. megapotamica- helenalin & dehydroleucodine (sesquiterpene lactones)

Various studies have been conducted on Gaillardia all over the world, with promising results.

Polish studies by Gill et al in 1981, found that *G. artista* leaves and flowers contained anti-bacterial, anti-fungal and anti-cancer fractions. Follow up studies in 1995 by Adekenov in the Republic of Kazaskhstan, again found *Gaillardia arista* exhibited anti-neoplastic properties.

McCutcheon et al, *J Ethnopharm* 1992 37 found moderate activity against six of 11 bacterial strains, including MRSA.

Studies conducted by Inayama et al in Tokyo, seem to indicate that the non-sesquiterpenoid constituents, especially methyl caffeate, may be responsible for the anti-tumor activity. *Chem Pharm Bull* 1984 32(3):135-41.

Gaillardin has been identified as both cytotoxic and anti-tumor agent. It appears to inhibit proliferation of breast cancer cells via inducing mitochondrial apoptotic pathways, suggesting its value in cancer chemoprevention or treatment. Fallahian F et al, *Cell Biol Toxicol* 2015 31(6):295-305).

Gaillardin shows cytotoxicity and apoptosis on human breast cancer (MCF-7), hepatic (HepG-2), non-small cell lung carcinoma (A-549) and colon adenocarcinoma (HT-29) cell lines. Moghadam MH et al, *Z Naturforsch C* 2013 68(3-3):108-12.

It also shows strong inhibition of acetylcholinesterase, suggestive of use in treating or prevention of senile dementia and Alzheimer's disease. Hajimehdipoor H et al, *An Acad Bras Cienc* 2014 May 14.

Work by Salama MM et al, *Nat Prod Res* 2012 26(22):2057-62 identified several compounds in *G. aristata*, including neopulchelllin and 6alpha-hydroxyneopulchellin, that show activity against breast MCF7 and colon HCT116 cancer cell lines.

Pulchellin is a type 2 ribosome-inactivating protein that shows promise, as an adjuvant, in breast cancer treatment. Mice treated with pulchellin showed significant immune system activation with increased release of IFN-gamma and Th2 cytokines (IL-4 and IL-10); and decreased levels of IL-6 and TGF-beta levels. It also increased macrophage activation in work by de Matos DC et al, *BMC Complement Altern Med* 2012 12:107.

Extracts of the flower inhibit melanogenesis, suggesting usefulness in suppressing skin pigmentation. Kim M et al, *BMC Complement Altern Med* 2015 15:449.

Water extracts of *G. pulchella* leaves reveal activity against gram positive bacteria.

Swertisin, derived from this species, is anti-oxidant, anti-inflammatory and has been used for diabetic conditions. The compound appears to promote differentiation of pancreatic progenitors in beta islet cells in the pancreas. Dadheech N et al, *PLoS One* 2015 10(6):e0128244; *Evid Based Complement Altern Med* 2013:280392. Reversal of hyperglycemia was noted after transplant of newly generated islet-like cells in to diabetic-induced mice.

It shows strong anti-hyperglycemic action, in rat studies, due to stimulation on in vivo insulin secretion. Folador P et al, *Fitoterapia* 2010 81(8):1180-7.

Work by Oh HK et al, *J Psychopharmacol* 2016 Oct 11 suggests it may be useful in managing the symptoms of schizophrenia, including sensorimotor gating disruption and cognitive impairment. These behavioral outcomes, in a mice study, may be related to Akt-GSK-3beta signaling in the prefrontal cortex.

The compound may also be useful in memory impairment due to its adenosine A1 receptor antagonistic property, and perhaps useful in dementia and Alzheimer's disease. Lee HE et al, *Behav Brain Res* 2016 306:137-45.

The compound 3-epi-isotelekin shows significant inhibition of *Mycobacterium tuberculosis*. It is found in several Rudbeckia species and elecampane root (*Inula helenium*). Cantrell CL et al, *Planta Medica* 1999 65(4):351-5.

Sesquiterpene lactones from *G. megapotamica* and *Artemisa douglassiana* induce apoptosis (programmed cell death in *Trypanosoma cruzi*, implicated in Chagas disease. Jimenez V et al, *Phytomedicine* 2014 21(11):1411-8.

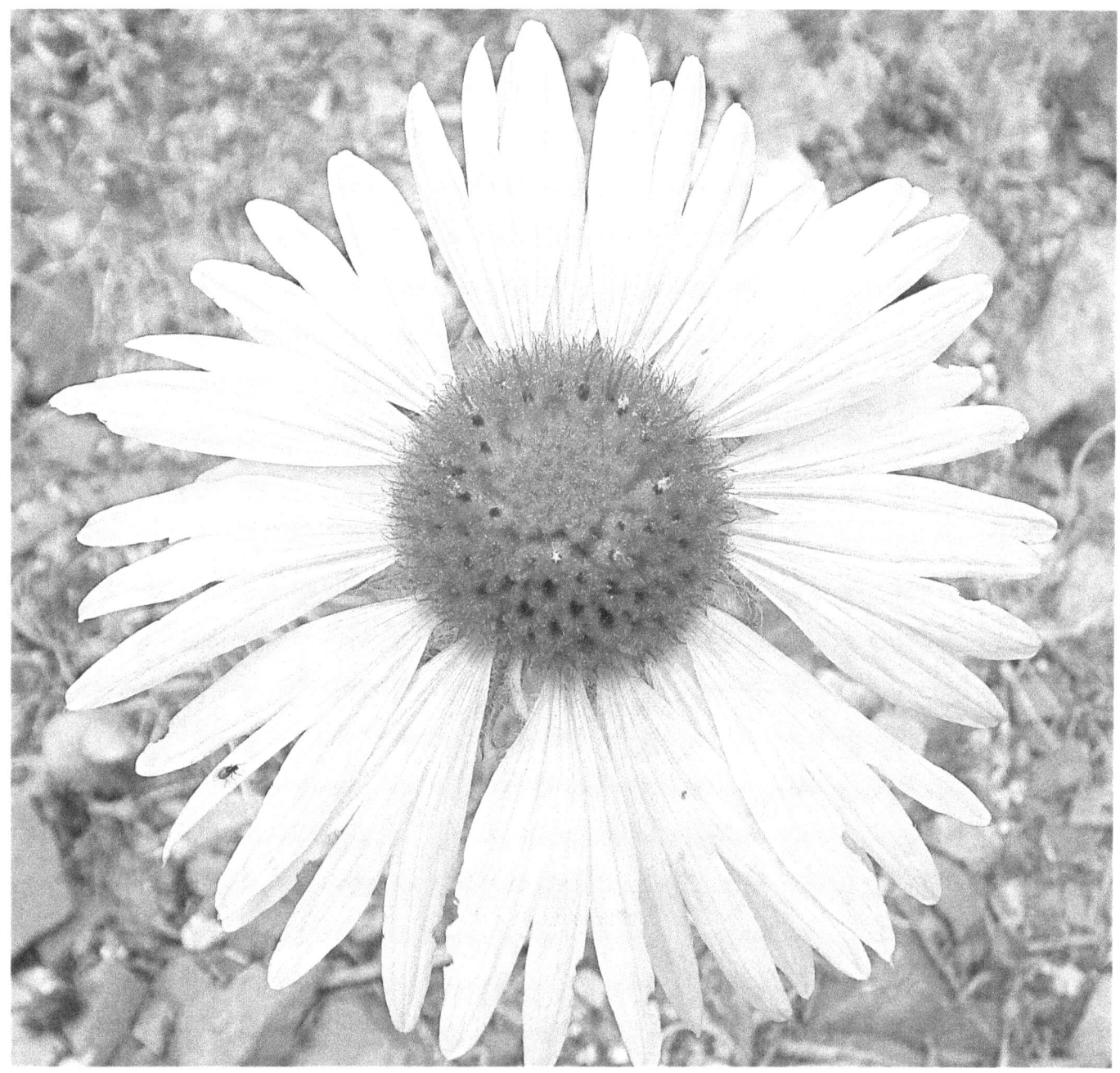

GAILLARIDA ARISTATA

ESSENTIAL OIL

An essential oil was obtained from *G. pulchella* flowers by hydrodistillation. Twenty-eight compounds were identified with n-hexadecanoic acid (27%), phytol (7.58%) and cyclopropane-octanoic acid, 2-[[2-[(2-ethylcyclopropyl) methyl]- methyl ester (6.73%).

The oil exhibits anti-oxidant activity. Yao XT et al, *J Oleo Sci* 2013 62(5):329-33.

SEED OIL

The seed oil of *G. aristata* contains up to 28%; and is composed of 68% linoleic, 1% linolenic, 16% oleic, and about 10% of saturated acids like palmitic and stearic.

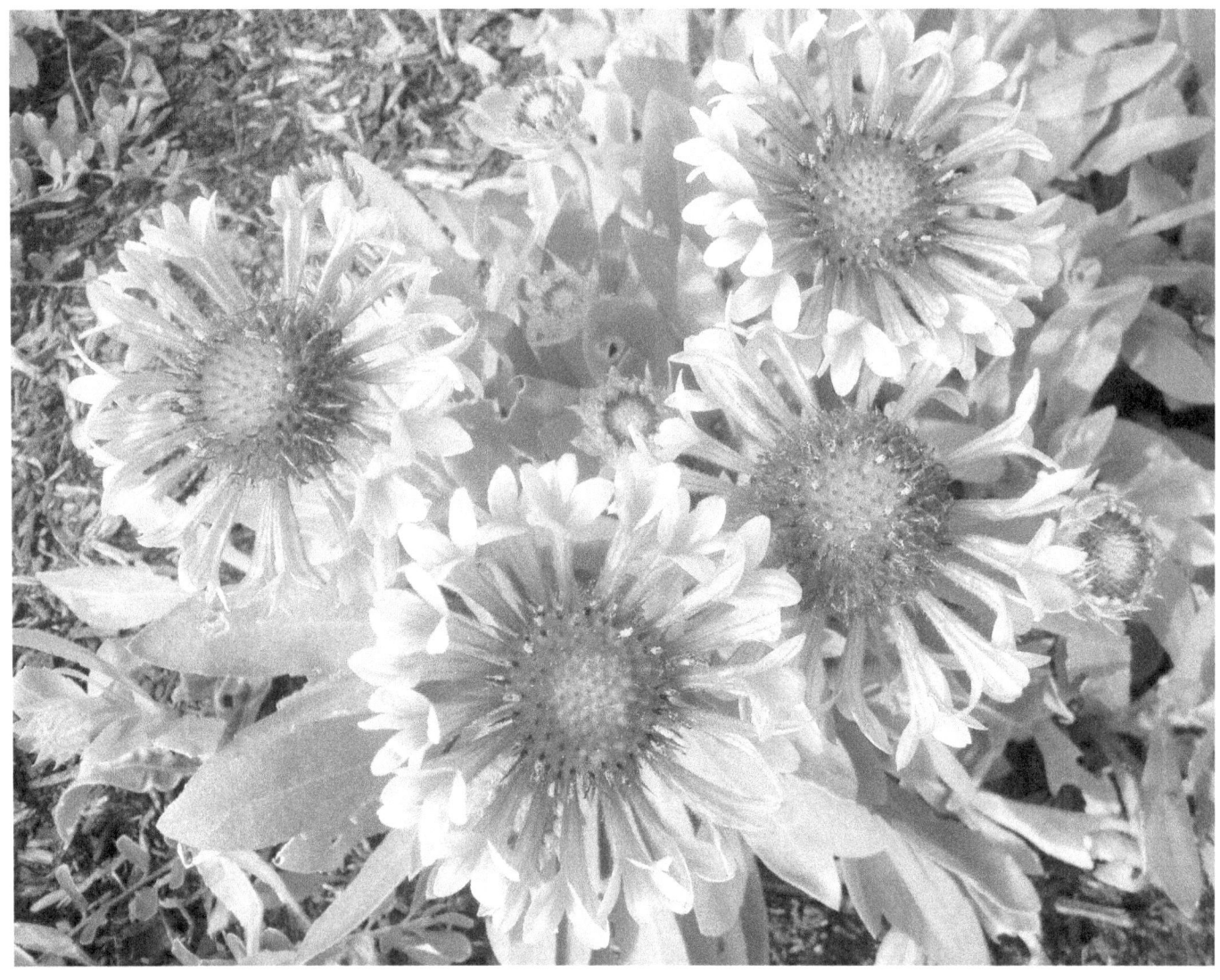

CULTIVATED HYBRID

FLOWER ESSENCES

Gaillardia flower essence enhances our determination to succeed against all obstacles, and use our " stubborn" nature to accomplish the Joy of Completion.

Macrophage activity, the dinosaurs of the immune system, may be enhanced to increase and engulf damaged or foreign cells. **PETITE FLEUR**

Blanket Flower (*G. pulchella*) flower essence is for those who feel inhibited or shut down, need an energy boost, experience depression, low vitality, and lack creativity, joy and love of life. **LIVING FLOWER**

Blanket Flower essence helps outdoors people feel less awkward in social settings, especially if dress is fairly formal. **ROCKY MTN**

Gaillardia essence provides a safe, secure blanket that enhances healing, and protects by sealing energetic leaks and tears. **WILD ROSE**

Gaillardia is good for increasing one's sensitivity to self and other and seeing the "big picture". Excellent for meditation, enhancing immune system, and helpful in cleansing and detoxing. **RAVENWORKS**

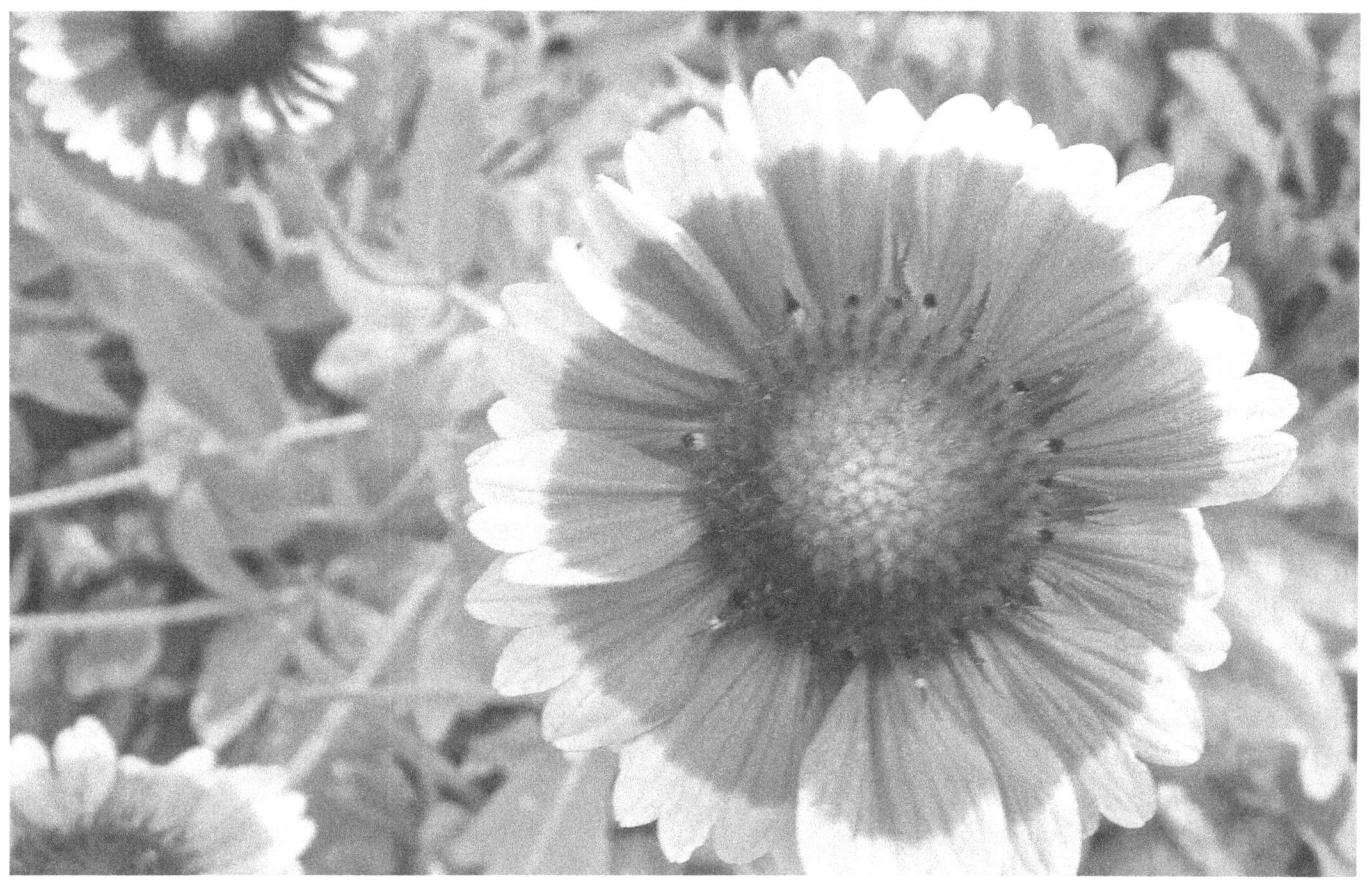

CULTIVATED HYBRID

DOCTRINE OF SIGNATURES

The bright yellow and reddish orange colors of the plant resemble the fiery, colorful elements of the sun, correlating with the solar plexus, spleen and root chakra. The fiery presence of the blanket flower represents a joyful, creative expression of life, with warmth and exuberance.

The flower is positive expression of feeling the warm fire glowing within to without, giving the signature of a strong, healthy vital life force.

The golden-yellow dome-shaped center represents the brightness within the core and the sun-like ability to embrace radiance, compassion and light.

Another signature is the warm sensation felt in the solar plexus, spleen and abdomen when drinking the flower essence.   **PALLASDOWNEY**

RECIPES

DECOCTION- One tsp of dried root to one pint of water. Simmer slowly for twenty minutes. Drink one-half cup as needed. For footbaths, you may double the dosage.

INFUSION- leaf and flower- Use 1:20 ratio of dried or fresh herb to water. Steep ten to twenty minutes. Hot infusions are mildly diaphoretic, cool infusions more diuretic.

TINCTURE- aerial parts in early flower stage. Make fresh tincture at 1:4 ratio and 40% alcohol. Twenty to forty drops up to four times daily as tolerated.

BLUE BUTTONS
FIELD SCABIOUS
CLODWEED
GYPSY ROSE
DEVIL'S BIT
(*Knautia arvensis* [L.] Coult.)
(*Scabiosa arvensis* L.)- no longer accepted
SWEET SCABIOUS
LADY'S PINCUSHION
GYPSY ROSE
MOURNING BRIDE
(*S. atropurpurea* L.)
PAPERMOON
STAR FLOWER
(*S. stellata*)- no longer accepted
(*Lomelosia stellata* [L.] Raf.)
DOVE SCABIOUS
SMALL SCABIOUS
LESSER FIELD SCABIOUS
DOVE PIN CUSHION
(*S. columbaria* L.)
PARTS USED- root, whole herb

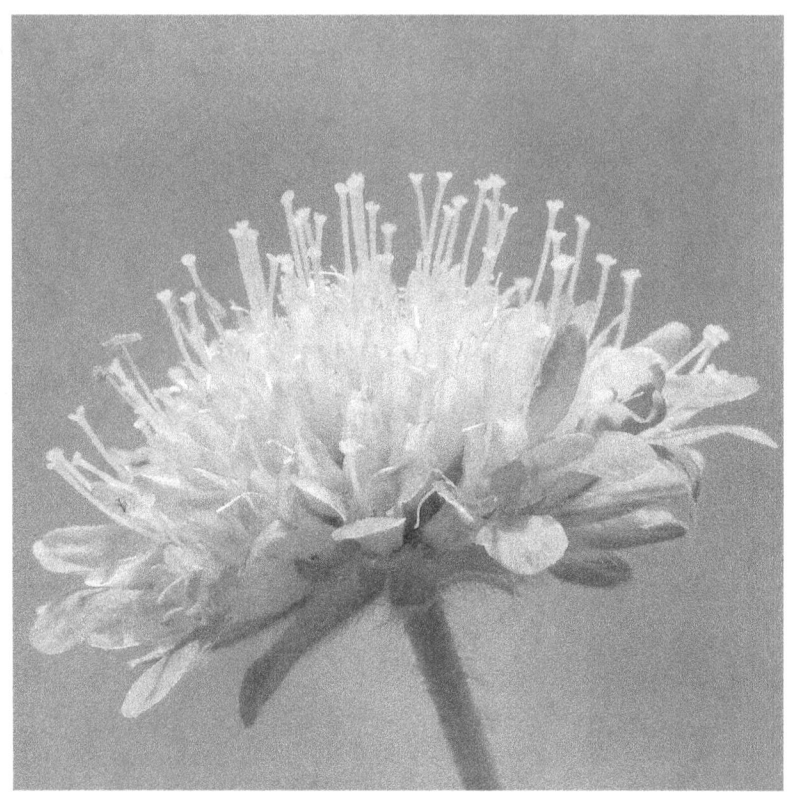

BLUE BUTTONS

America: It's like Britain, only with buttons.   **RINGO STARR**

We made the buttons on the screen look so good you'll want to lick them.   **STEVE JOBS**

Knautia is named after Dr. Christian Knaut, a Saxon botanist and physician of the 17th century. Arvensis means, of cultivated fields. Scabious is connected with scab, or scabies; or from the Latin **SCABERE** meaning, to scrape or scratch. Scabious also means rough, pertaining to the itchy hairs covering the stem and leaves.

Devil's Bit comes directly from the devil, who was jealous of the plants valuable medicinal efficacy, and bit off a piece of the root in an attempt to make it worthless. So they say!

The first year root looks like a carrot or radish, but gradually becomes woody, with the bottom decaying, and the top looking as if it had broken away.

Blue Buttons are a rough-looking, perennial, introduced from Europe. It is often overlooked as a weed and yet has large, attractive mauve-blue blossoms. It looks, at a distance, somewhat like Bachelor Buttons.

Culpepper says "the decoction of the roots taken for forty days together, or a dram of the powder of them taken at a time in whey, doth (as Mathiolus saith) wonderfully help those who are troubled with running or spreading scabs, tetters, ringworm, yea, though they proceed from the French poc ".

He also thought the plant "very effectual for coughs, shortness of breath, and other diseases of the lungs- a decoction of the herb, dry or green, made into wine and drunk for some time together, is good for pleurisy".

According to the signature of plants, the hair-covered stems indicated their use in allaying tickles and irritations of the throat.

Culpepper said that the fresh herb bruised and applied to carbuncles, would dissolve them in three hours. A decoction removed stitches and pains from the side.

The whole plant is considered cleansing and antiseptic, and used for treating skin conditions and female ailments.

The Gaelic name translates as blue lad. In Scotland the plant was used in ointments for skin problems including gangrene and dandruff.

The roots are fomented and applied to bruised, weak sinews and old sores on farm animals. Older herbals mention that the pale blue flowers turn bright green at the touch of a lighted match. I'll have to try!

Buellin, in his *Booke of Simples* 1562, wrote of the frog's fondness for Scabiosa, under the leaves of which they "shadow themselves from the heate of the daie, popping and plaiying under these leaves, which to them is a pleasant Tent or Pavillion".

Culpepper considered the Small Scabious or Lesser Field Scabious (*S. columbaria*) to be of similar use.

Sauer, in his *Compendius Herbal*, gives some insights into the medicinal uses of Lesser Scabious in 18th century Philadelphia.

The plant was used primarily for chest and lungs, removing phlegm and easing expectoration.

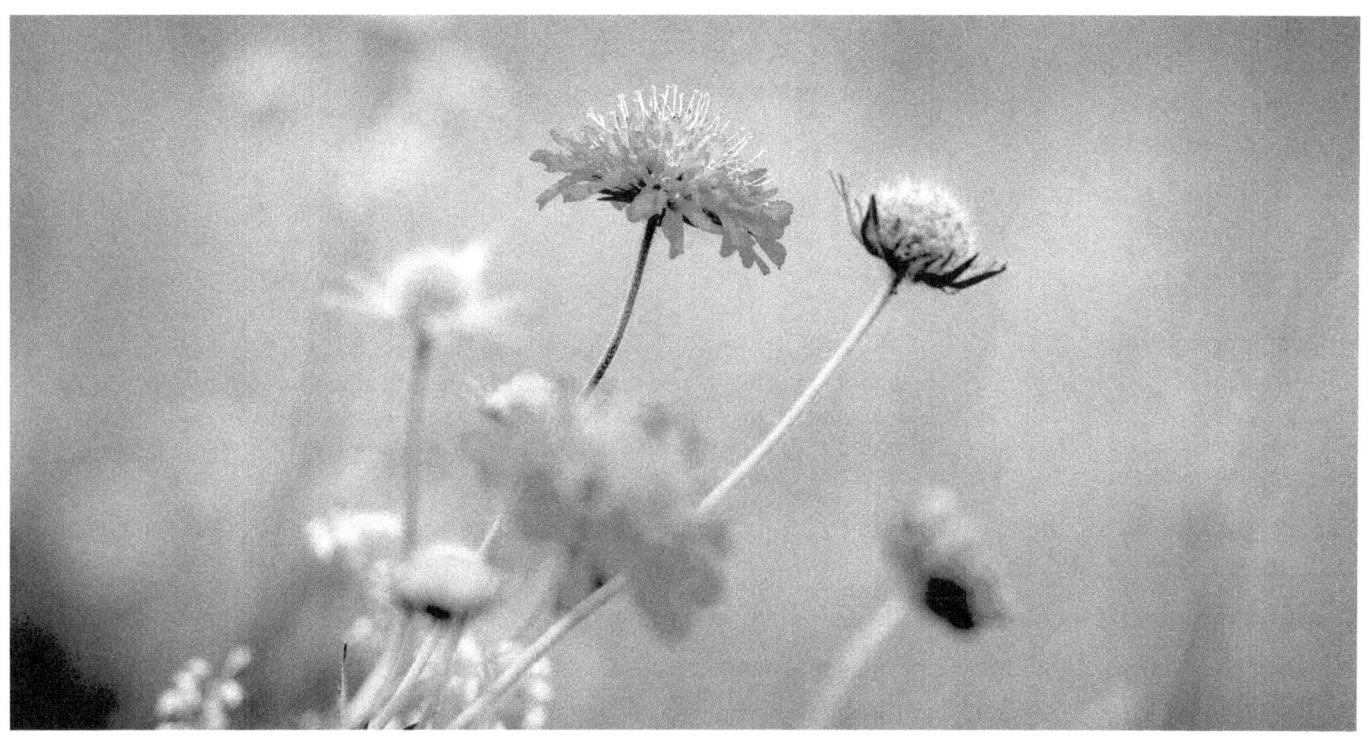

SMALL SCABIOUS

It was put into lye and then used to wash the head to get rid of mites in the hair.

For old fistulas, and weeping sores, both the root and leaf of Lesser Scabious are combined with Avens root, Celandine root, Speedwell, Agrimony and Sanicle.

Root decoctions were, according to Grieve, considered a cure for all sores and eruptions, the juice being made into an ointment for the same purpose.

Dr. Withering wrote, "a strong decoction of it, used in continuance, is an empirical secret for gonorrhea."

The plant contains a rich source of tannin and bitter compounds.

It has been used in homeopathy for chronic skin conditions and eczema, and was considered, in the pas,t to be one of the finest skin remedies available.

The introduced European plant was used by various Native tribes of Eastern Canada for treating leucorrhea, and general maladies of the head.

Lesser Scabiosa found its way to Africa. Fresh root infusions were used for colic, dyspepsia and heartburn. To treat venereal disease, the pulverized root was mixed with paraffin as an ointment.

The dried root has been powdered and is said to be like a pleasant smelling baby powder.

Devil's Bit (*S. pratensis*), with honey-scented flowers, has been used traditionally as a menstrual regulator.

Both Sweet Scabious and Papermoon are introduced annuals, available through nurseries for seasonal planting. The former has such a rich, honey scent that the cut flowers are almost overwhelming indoors. They prefer limed soil.

Dove Scabious is a hardy perennial that can be found in gardens and nurseries.

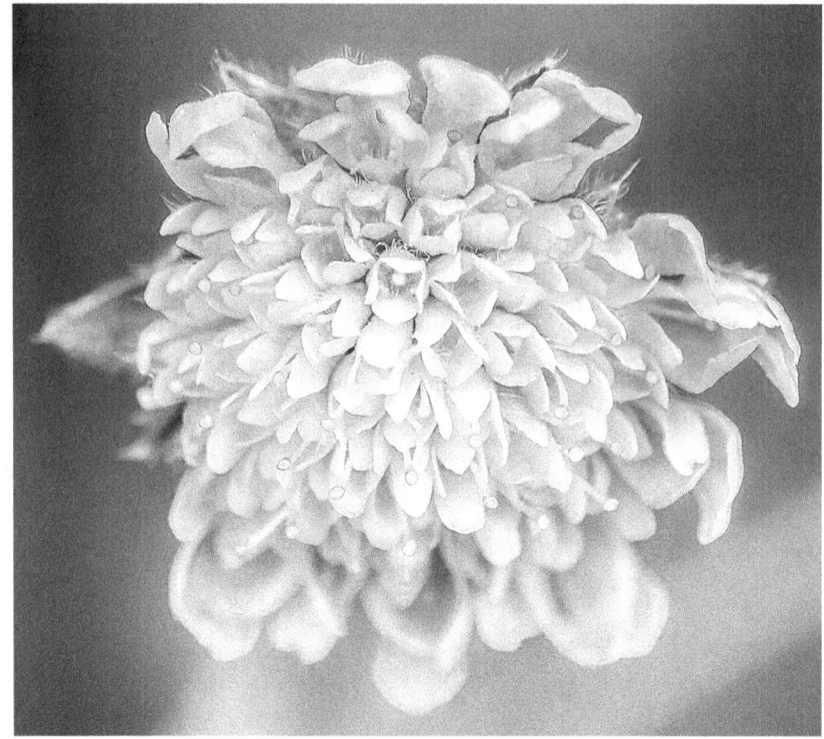

DOVE SCABIOUS

MEDICINAL

CONSTITUENTS- *K. arvensis*- aerial parts- various triterpene saponins including knautiosides A & B; iridoid monoterpenes including dipsacan; flavonoids such as leucanthoside, and luteoloside, tannins, triterpenes such as ursolic acid, polyphenols including caffeic acid and luteolin-7 glucoside, cryptochlorogenic acid, chlorogenic acid, 2-O-trans-caffeoylhydrocitric acid, isovitexin 7-beta-D-glucopyranoside, 7,4'-dihydroxy-5-methoxyflavone-6-C-beta-D-glucopyranoside, 3,5-O-dicaffeoylquinic acid, 4,5-O-dicaffeoylquinic acid.

Blue Buttons has an astringent, antiseptic and expectorant quality. In large amounts, it is purgative so be careful with dosage.

Blue Buttons is used for chronic skin diseases, such as eczema, fissure, itching anus, urticaria, scabies and favus.

It is used for cleansing and healing of ulcers, for contusions and inflammation.

Expectorant uses include coughs and throat complaints.

The plant decoctions ease bladder inflammation, cystitis and other urinary tract infections, when drunk at body temperature.

The leaf and flower infusions are mild enough for infants suffering through chicken pox, measles; helping to resolve the condition more easily and quickly.

Extracts of *K. arvensis* have been screened for anti-fungal activity by Kowalczyk et al, published in *Herba Polanica* 1999 45:2.

Activity against *Candida albicans, Rhodotorula rubra* and *Aspergillus fumigatus* is believed related to the polyphenolic compounds, especially flavonoids. Maybe. The seed oil contains capyrlic acid, a known anti-fungal. And chlorogenic acid, found in aerial parts, is a potent anti-fungal, inducing apoptosis. It appears to induce potassium efflux, leading to apoptotic volume decrease and G2/M cell cycle arrest in *C. albicans*. Yun J et al, *Biochim Biophys Acta* 2016 1861(3):585-92.

Small Scabiosa (*S. columbaria*) herb and root are used together. It has some similarity to Pleurisy root, but is probably less effective, and is not a relaxant expectorant in cases of asthma.

Peter Holmes suggests that the remedy is a cross between Pleurisy root and Plantain leaf in its main actions. I like the analogy.

It is effective for bronchial conditions with heat, pain, coughing and asthmatic wheezing as in Pleurisy root, but is also useful in various skin conditions addressed by Plantain.

These include dry skin eruptions, pruritis, eczema, scabies, boils, ringworm, skin blemishes, and carbuncles; as well as skin wounds and infections.

As a mouth gargle, the plant is useful in throat and gum infections.

The related *S. tschiliensis* contains triterpenoid saponins that exhibit strong inhibition of pancreatic lipase in vitro. Zheng et al, *J Nat Prod* 2004 67:4.

HOMEOPATHY

Blue Button types are indisposed to work, are sulky, morose and have no idea what to do.

There is heat and perspiration before going to sleep, burning pains in esophagus and stomach, worse on waking in morning.

It feels as if a spider web is inside the head, heat over the face, especially the forehead.

Throat is raw, worse from talking, which causes coughing.

Headache in morning, but on waking better from coffee.

DOSE- tincture to 3x. Proving by Stager with two females and three males in 1899-1900.

SEED OIL

The seeds of *K. arvensis* contain about 25% oil, of which some 33-40% is in the form of capric and caprylic acids. These acids are being increasingly sought after, for lubricants of high quality, and in the preparation of some valued dietary fats and supplements.

Caprylic acid is an aggressive anti-fungal and is often used for chronic yeast infections, including *Candida albicans*, both topically and internally in enteric coated capsules.

Most of these oils are of a tropical nature, so a locally grown source would be welcomed by the natural oleo-chemical industry.

HYDROSOL

The distilled water of Scabious is very good for coughs, sores in the chest, and pleurisy. It will purify the chest and lungs of all phlegm and pus, when taken often in four or five tablespoon doses. It cleanses the blood of all impurities, for which reason it is quite useful to those inclined toward leprosy or who are afflicted with the French Pox.

It will gently get rid of the purples and measles in children, provoke a mild sweat, and strengthen the heart against miasmas… Scabious water is a good healing remedy for wounds, injuries and open sores in the privates of man and woman if a small cloth is dipped in it and laid warm over the hurt.　　　　　　　　**SAUER**

Scabious water helps pleurises and pains, and pricking in the sides; Aposthumes, coughs, pestilences, and straitness of the breast.　　　　　　　　**CULPEPPER**

Scabious water is made from the flower and root, and is good for abscess of the breast, as well as causing larger breasts.　　　　　　　　**BRUNSCHWIG**

FLOWER ESSENCES

Field Scabious (*K. arvensis*) flower essence helps bring transformational wisdom. It quiets thinking and purifies unnecessary thoughts through the earth. It also brings a connection to higher serene spheres and lets this reflect in one's surroundings so the support and warmth of others can be received.   **BLOESEM**

Field Scabious flower essence helps when exploring and learning about other levels of existence.   **BRYNAHERB**

Field Scabious essence helps to assign and arrange our own thoughts, as well as cleanse our aura.   **MIRIANA**

ASTROLOGY

In other plants, the principles of formation leading to the development of sympetalous plants deeply penetrate plant growth. Not only do the petals of the individual flowers fuse, but the flowers of inflorescences also join together into one higher unit. In this way, the flower heads of the globe daisy, the teasel family and the composites develop. The far planets are even more pronouncedly manifest here. The flowering impulse takes hold of the plant with such intensity that the stems and leaves that usually stretch far up into the region of the flowers are stunted. In the teasel family, particularly in the scabious…the individual blossoms of one flower head are tightly crowded in a bowl-shaped "calyx" of simple leaves. There the blue or purple blossoms turn to all directions of the sky. In the flower heads of the scabious, the lowest blossoms with their tubes and petal-like edges become rather large.   **KRANICH**

RECIPES

COLD INFUSION- For chronic eczema- Take four teaspoonfuls of herb to 500 ml of water. Let sit for ten minutes, and drink throughout day.

STANDARD INFUSION- Take 30 grams of dry herb to one litre of hot water. Strain and cool. Take one cup three times daily.

The concentration of phenolic acids is higher after acidic hydrolysis.

BUCKBEAN
BOGBEAN
(***Menyanthes trifoliata***)
PARTS USED- leaves, rhizomes

I think of the bog as a feminine goddess—ridden ground, rather like the territory of Ireland itself.   **SEAMUS HEANEY**

Buckee, Buckee, biddy Bene
Is the way now fair and clean?
Is the goose y gone to nest?
And the fox y gone to rest?
Shall I come away?   **OLD NURSERY RHYME**

Menyanthes may be from the Greek "**MENANTHOS**" for moon or month flower; due to life of flowers or related to the menstrual cycle. Some texts suggest it was first named by Theophrastus, the Greek botanist. **MENYEIN**, means disclosing, and **ANTHOS**, flower, in allusion to the sequential opening of flowers.

Other authors believe Menyanthes is derived from the Greek **MINUTHO**, to diminish, for the short-lived flowers.

Buckbean is from the Dutch *"Boksboon"* or the French *"Bouc"* for Goat's Bean. Bogbean, by which it is commonly known, has similar foliage to broad beans. It originally was called "goat's bean" from the French **BOUC**.

It also should be noted that **SHARBOCK**, the German term for scurvy is considered a possible origin of the word.

It is abundant in western Canada, but easily passed by in mosquito-infested bogs and swamps it inhabits. The delicate whitish-pink flowers give off a very unpleasant odour when in bloom.

Alaska natives use the rhizomes as an emergency food supply; just as the Laplanders made bread from the powdered root. Flours from buckbean can be substituted for wheat and other grains that may cause nutritional allergies, where the plant is plentiful.

Early herbals list the leaf as a hop substitute in beer; one Swedish recipe from 1824 suggests one part buckbean for every eight parts hops. Today, the bitter principles are used in liqueurs.

The leaves are best collected in flower, but since they produce for three months, this is not really a problem. Root could be used as long as they are not over harvested.

Native tribes of this region made decoctions of the stem and root for stomach sickness; especially if there was spitting of blood. Other tribes drank the tea to put on weight lost during the flu.

The Kwakiutl of British Columbia decocted and drank the root water for stomach troubles. In Scotland, stomach ulcers were likewise treated.

For constipation, the root is boiled until the water is thick and dark. One teaspoon at a time is given.

Buckbean leaves make an effective facial steam for acne, or suitable rinse for oily hair.

The dried leaves are also a common smoking ingredient, blending well with mullein, clover, coltsfoot, bearberry and others.

Johannes Franckenius wrote in 1613, that bogbean decoctions remove all visceral obstructions, act as an emmenogogue and diuretic, kills intestinal worms, and was an efficacious remedy in scrofula.

Seed decoctions were used traditionally for rheumatism.

Cullen suggested using the root for obstinate skin affections of a cancerous nature; applied externally in the form of a poultice.

Boerhaave, it is said, cured his gout by drinking the plant juice in whey.

Studies from the former USSR indicate bogbean successfully removes mercaptan compounds from pulp and paper wastewaters.

Buckbean contains mitsugashiwa lactone, found to induce the catnip response in cats.

It was believed that drinking buckbean herbal tea every day makes you live longer. Who's to say?

MEDICINAL

CONSTITUENTS- numerous anthraquinones including emodin, aloe-emodin, chrysophanol, menyanthin, and secologanin, menthiafolin and dihydro-foliamenthin glycosides, sweroside, choline, tannins 3%, physcion, menthiafolin, franula-emodin, rhamnicoside, seco-iridoid and alaterin. Alkaloids like gentianin E, gentianadine, gentiatibetine and gentianlutine are present. Various phenolics such as ferulic and caffeic acids, p-hydroxybenzoic and protocahtechuic acids also present.
Fats such as palmitic acid, phytosterin and ceryl alcohol; flavonoids such as rutin, hyperoside, trifolin; pigment like carotin; enzymes such as invertin and emulsin; a terpenoid lactone loliolide, various triterpene glycosides such as lupeol, betulin, betulinic acid, and beta amyrenol; coumarins like scopoletin, scoparone and braylin; as well as mitsugashiwa lactone and deoxyloganin.
Root- betulinic acid 0.8%. betulin, loganin, foliamenthin, sucrose, loganetin, pentosans, pectin, meliatin, inulin, alpha spinasterol, alpha and beta lupeol were identified.

Buckbean is very useful in conditions where digestion and blood quality are involved. The herb is cooling, bitter, cleansing and detoxifying. Because its chief action is to clear old stagnation, it is somewhat similar to gentian root, in both a vagolytic and sympathomimetic manner.

In fact, when you look at the chemical composition, the herb could be a cross between rhubarb and gentian. Emodin and aloe-emodin are valued compounds for a variety of health conditions, including cancer prevention and treatment.

It is useful for pitta/kapha tendencies in Ayurvedic tradition, and for damp heat and liver Qi stagnation from TCM.

Recent Swedish studies confirmed that decoctions of buckbean showed inhibitions of inflammatory models *in vivo*, and *in vitro*. Huang et al, *Yao Hsueh Hsueh Pao* 1995 30.

This makes it useful in difficult conditions like fibromyalgia; combining well with Actaea rubra root.

Buckbean stimulates the sympathetic deficient and sedates excessive parasympathetic nervous systems. It is worth a trial in cases of anorexia, combining well with calamus root. It also works well for amenorrhea in women with vacuity of the blood or the spleen, and hence the older German name **MONATSBLUME**, or Moonflower.

Buckbean's bitter principles give it good action for spleen, liver and intestinal obstruction. Deoxyloganin, for example, possesses laxative properties.

As a bitter digestive stimulant, it promotes appetite, taken in cold water ten minutes before meals. This makes it useful for frontal headaches associated with eating fatty foods, and indigestion or constipation associated with biliousness and bloating.

The bitter index of Bogbean is 2.5-3 times less than Gentian at one part to 4-10 million. Caffeic and ferulic acid are bile stimulants.

Sweroside, assisted by loganin, appears to be one the constituents that give this plant strong hepatoprotective effect. Luo et al, *Chem Pharm Bull* (Tokyo) 2009 57:1.

Sweroside attenuates cholestatic liver injury by restoring bile synthesis, transport to normal levels and suppressing pro-inflammatory response. Yang QL et al, *Acta Pharmacol Sin* 2016 37(9): 2128-28.

It may also be useful for osteoporosis, by helping proliferation of osteoblasts. Sun H et al, *Fitoterapia* 2013 84:174-9.

As a diaphoretic, taken in hot water, it is used for treating intermittent fevers and acute viral infections. The German name **FIEBERKLEE** means Fever Clover, indicating a long usage for remittent or intermittent fevers.

The lymphatic glands begin to drain, and with its diuretic action, bogbean is suited for many chronic arthritic and rheumatic conditions, which find their origin in poor fat and protein digestion.

The fresh juice of the leaves is specific for gouty rheumatism.

Because it detoxifies pelvic lymphatic congestion, buckbean is often helpful in uterine disorders, migraines of liver origin, menstrual irregularities and hemorrhoids. Individuals with allergy or food sensitivities, associated with constipation and indigestion may benefit.

In some ways, it is similar to blue flag, in the treatment of biliary migraines, but less purgative in nature.

Studies out of Lithuania in 1989 suggest buckbean be further studied for possible anti-tumour activity. Water and alcohol extracts show the plant exhibiting activity against gram-positive bacteria, particularly *Staphylococcus aureus*.

Buckbean also relieves wheezing and asthmatic congestion by stimulating expectoration.

Skin problems that stem from stagnation, including dry flaky skin, eczema, and psoriasis respond to buckbean combined with goldthread, or Oregon grape root.

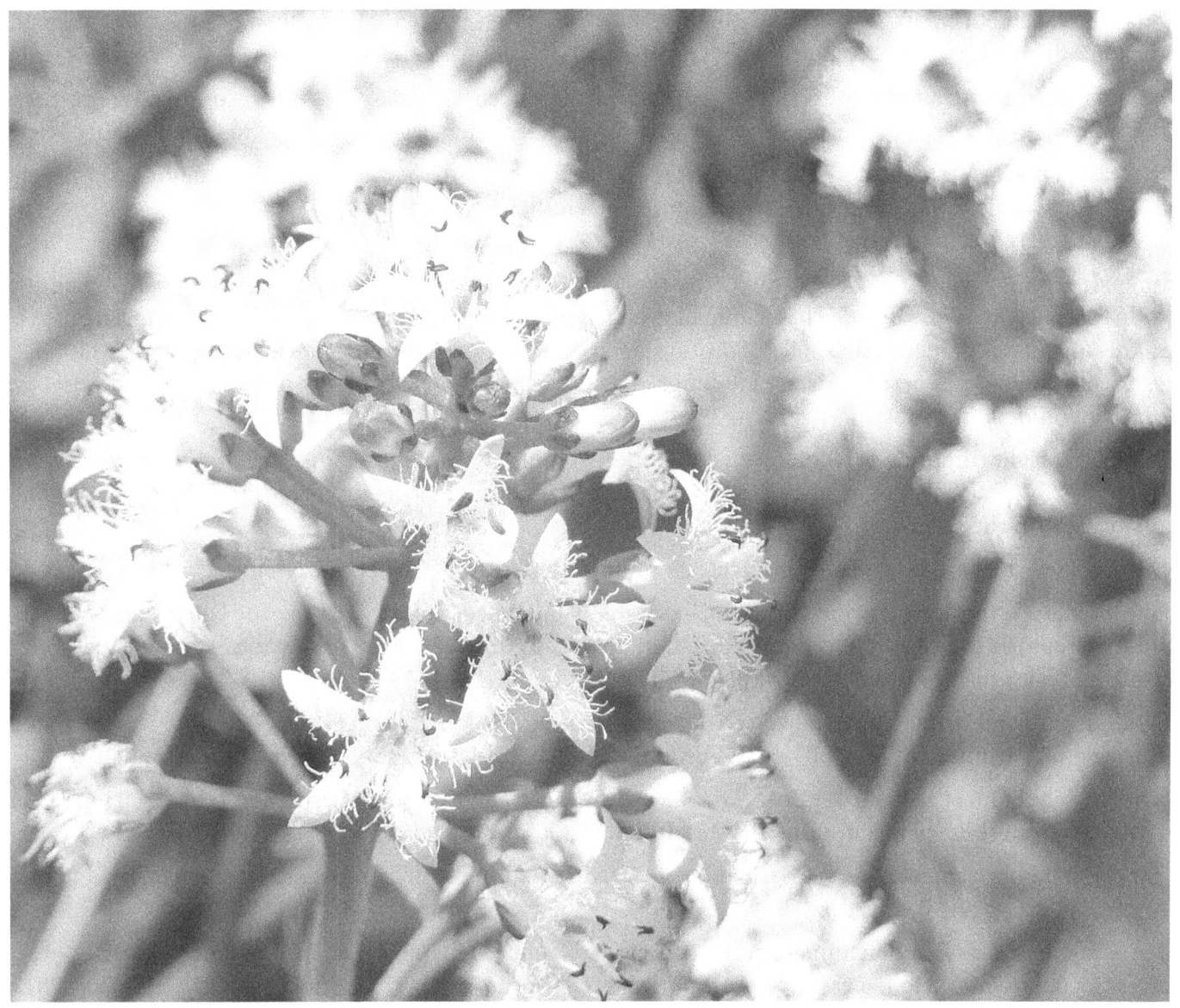

BOGBEAN IN FLOWER

Externally, a poultice of buckbean leaves can help soothe festering skin sores, herpes pain, and reduce glandular swelling. A shampoo patent on the market contains buckbean leaf extract for anti- bacterial properties, and dandruff control.

Buckbean combines well with baneberry root externally for achy joints, including osteoarthritis. Gentianine, a leaf alkaloid has been shown to have pain killing and tranquilizing effects in labs.

Gentianadine reduces blood pressure and decreases inflammation. Dr. Bastyr used buckbean leaf tincture, 15 drops three times daily, for hypertension.

Buckbean has been noted to demonstrate hemolytic activity and may increase risk of bleeding in those taking warfarin or similar blood thinners.

Remember, buckbean leaf is for chronic conditions and will severely irritate colitis, or acute diarrhea conditions. In the Highlands of Scotland, the herb is used for stomach pains, including ulcers, but caution is advised.

Aperient, tonic candies are marketed in Europe for infants that contain 0.25% menyanthins, derived from bog bean.

In Japan, the herb is known as either **SUISAIYO**, or **MEISAI**. In early herbals, the intake of the plant was said to induce drowsiness, a quality after which it is named.

Although its main traditional use is to strengthen the stomach, it is also used for insomnia, indigestion, intermittent fevers, headaches, earaches, amenorrhea, jaundice, edema, gout, scabies and ulcerated furuncles.

The leaf tea may help shingles. J. V. Cerney relates that a working man, "had an eruption of painful little blisters along his lower ribs on his right side. They followed in a line along his ribs and became agonizingly painful to the point where he couldn't do his job." He was completely cured using buckbean leaf tea.

Tunon H et al, *Phytomedicine* 1995 2(2):103-12 suggested bog bean root decoctions be used for glomerulonephritis (kidney tubule inflammation). Such inflammations often result during strep infections. The exact mechanism is unknown, but it is thought that platelet activating factors (PAF) and leukotrienes are involved. Ortiz et al, 1987. Or perhaps it works in part by elastase inhibition. The roots have been found to possess hemolytic properties, due to an unidentified substance.

Two out of eight compounds found in the roots show significant inhibition of prostaglandin synthesis, with 2-14 times the potency of aspirin. This makes the root an important analgesic agent; and explains in part the folkloric use in rheumatism.

The decocted rhizome shows benefit in acute glomerular nephritis. Bohlin et al, *J Ethnopharm* 1993 38 2-3.

Like birch bark, the herb contains betulinic acid, betulin and lupeol. Recent work on the latter, suggest it may induce apoptosis in head and neck cancers, and may re-sensitize cells that had previously progressed under cisplatin. Bhattacharyya S et al, *Cell Oncol* (Dordr) 2015 doi: 10.1007.

Betulinic acid and betulin have shown activity against melanoma cancer and HIV-1. Betulinic acid inhibited prostaglandin synthesis at IC50 of 101, and betulin at 119 microM, suggesting anti-inflammatory activity.

Work by Lindholm et al, looked at Bogbean for its anti-cancer activity against ten human cancer cell lines. The herb was one of seven with anti-tumour potential out of 100 plants studied. *Journal Biomol Screen* 2002 7:4.

Chrysophanol has been found cytotoxic to drug sensitive and multi-drug resistant T leukemia cancer cells. Ozenver N et al, *Planta Med* 2016 (S01):S1-S381.

The compound, also found in Rumex species and rhubarb, induces apoptosis, and shows synergistic effect with cisplatin and paclitaxel to increase apoptosis of JEG-3, choriocarcinoma cells. Lim W et al, *J Cell Physiol* 2017 232(2):331-9.

Chyrsophanol may exert anti-depressant effect by inhibiting P2X7/NFkappaB signaling pathway. Zhang K et al, *Neurosci Lett* 2016 613:60-5.

Trifolin induces apoptosis via death receptor dependent and mitochondria dependent pathways in human lung (NCl0H460) cancer cell lines. Kim MJ et al, *Phytomedicine* 2016 23(10):998-1004.

Kuduk-Jaworska et al, *Z Naturoforsch C* 2004 59(7-8): 485-93 found the plant contains immune modulating compounds, as well as high concentrations of selenium.

One coumarin, scoparone protects against pancreatic fibrosis by regulating the TGF-beta Smad pathway. Xu M et al, *Cell Physiol Biochem* 2016 40(1-2):277-286.

One polysaccharide from a water extract showed significant anti-inflammatory effect. The herb induces a suppressive type of dendritic cells that reduces the capacity to induce Th1 and stimulate Th17 of allogenic CD4$^+$ cells. This suggests the use in autoimmune conditions such as rheumatoid arthritis, multiple sclerosis, asthma and irritable bowel disease. Jonsdottir et al, *J Ethnopharm* 2011 136(1):88-93.

It is worthy of a trial in anorexia as well, combining well with purple-leaved bunchberry and calamus root. The former leaves are found occasionally in late summer.

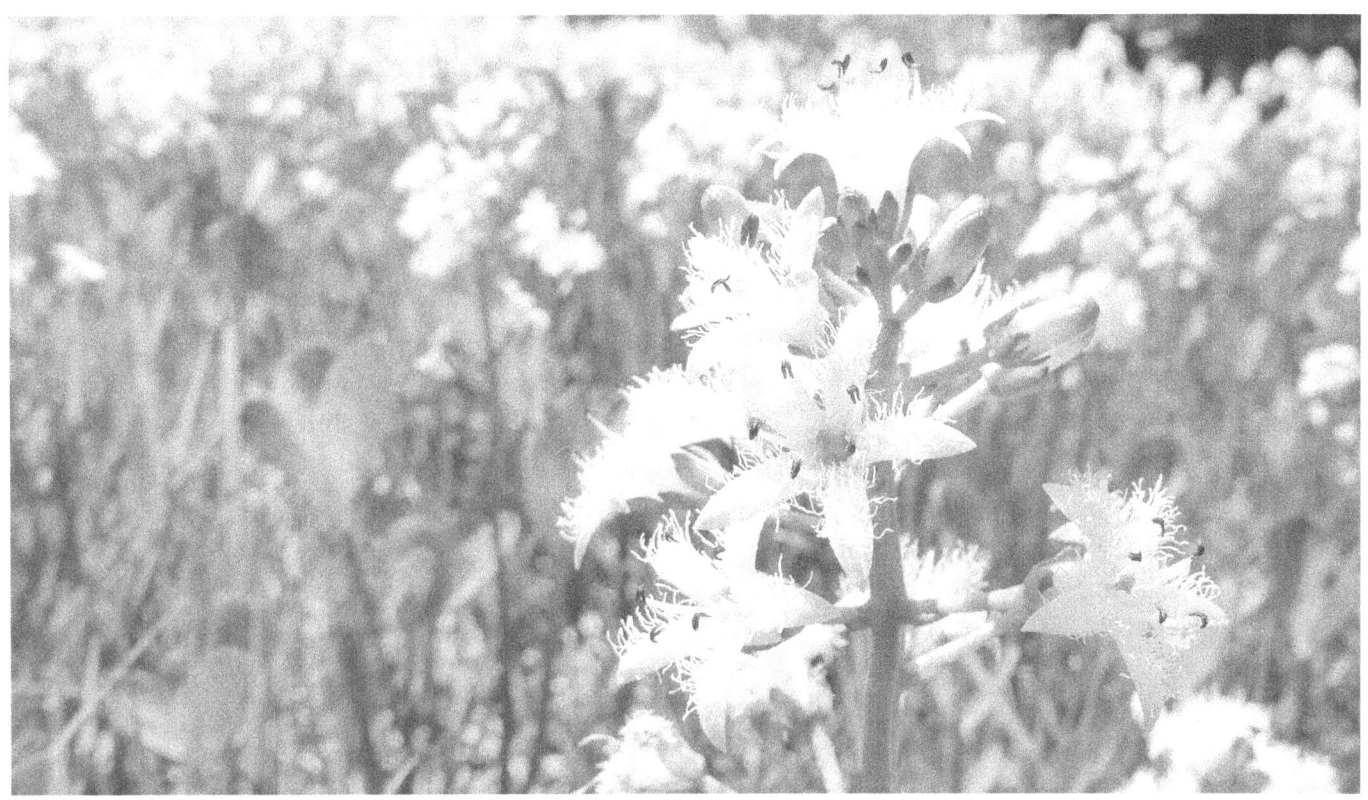

BOGBEAN

HOMEOPATHY

Buckbean is a remedy for certain headaches and intermittent fever. There may be a coldness to the abdomen, accompanied by sensations of tension and compression.

The head pain is improved by applying hard hand pressure. The symptoms are made worse by going up stairs; and improved by stooping or sitting.

There may be ravenous hunger, especially for raw meat, but no thirst. The abdomen is distended and full; and exaggerated by nicotine.

The extremities are icy cold; and the patient's legs may jerk and twitch while laying down. A cold fever may be present.

Thoughts come with difficulty, cross, ill-humored and discontented. Anxious, indifferent to amusements. Dreams of animals and dinosaurs.

DOSE- Third to thirtieth potency. The mother tincture is prepared from the whole fresh plant when coming to flower. Use 3X for pressure headaches, fever attacks, disruption of body heat regulation and trigeminal neuralgia.

First proving by Hahnemann with ten males and tincture. Teste self experimented as cited in Clarke.

He remarked. "there are few diseases where Menyanthes is indicated which could not be cured much better with Drosera. This opinion, however, is founded on my own impressions, which I am always willing to distrust."

ROOT OIL

The fresh roots are gathered and washed, and then pulverized and covered with an equal quantity of olive or canola oil. Let sit warm, in sun, for one week; shaking daily. Stain and use for arthritic/rheumatic pain. In cooler climates, it is best to use a double boiler or crock pot at low temperature for four to six hours.

FLOWER ESSENCE

BUCKBEAN (BOGBEAN)
(*Menyanthes trifoliata*)

Keywords- Calmness and detachment, focus on the present.

Buckbean flower essence helps one to maintain a calm repose in the midst of hubris and excessive activity. Learning to observe, events and responses, without becoming personally affected, takes a level of detachment.

The flower essence helps one to refrain from judgment, and accept change, including one's own point of view. At the same time, buckbean helps one avoid distraction related to the energetics of others involved in various scenarios of life. This does not mean that buckbean creates a lack of empathy, but simply helps one to develop a level of acceptance and compassion, and even a sense of humor, in the play of life.

Buckbean suggests a relationship to bogs, and becoming bogged down, on a physical, mental and emotional level. This suggests inability to see the forest for the trees. An anti-dote to being bogged down is to perceive interactions with others as an opportunity to practice compassionate detachment.

Buckbean also helps one accept that it is often unnecessary to take action on another's behalf, instead simply listen and be present. On the physical plane, this may manifest as an awareness of body language and expressions as simple as a hug. On the mental plane, it is very useful for individuals that must make quick, and accurate decisions based on their occupation. Athletes, air flight controllers, pilots, professional car drivers, police, firefighters, and emergency medical personnel may benefit from this flower essence.

Buckbean helps keep one in the present in a focused and clear manner. The essence helps one to not take on the anxiety or frustration of others, but to be present in state of detached awareness.

Buckbean flower essence may be useful to help quiet the mind, for meditation, prayer and other spiritual connections. On a mental plane, it may assist students to concentrate and attend to an intellectual exercise. Many students at a secondary and college/university level can superficially multi-task but have difficulty holding a focused attention span.

A 30-year-old mother sent this in, after her 6-year-old son chose Buckbean by himself from the photograph.

"Though he couldn't get used to a group life easily at the elementary school this first year, since he began to take the essences, he looks like he has easier time getting along with school life little by little. When I asked him what has changed, he answered. 'I have many friends now!'

Since it's a mental change, it not clearly visible to others. I think that my son's life is now more comfortable. I'd like to say thanks to the essences. As long as my son wishes, he can continue to have life with essences."

PRAIRIE DEVA

PERSONALITY TRAITS

Bogbean has a long history of use in rheumatism. The Bogbean person often has pain in the kidney region that may later affect the legs, knees and feet. There may be heat and swelling in the joints, that are improved with movement. Gouty rheumatism is a classic Bogbean!

Sciatica pain becomes worse as the body congests and stagnates with old acids and waste. Water retention is reduced, by making the lymphatic system more efficient.

In the negative state, the Bogbean person cannot climb the stairs. Repeated trips to the chiropractor only give temporary relief. They need to walk to keep the lymphatic moving and the kidneys eliminating. In this state, they crave meat and yet are not thirsty- a sure recipe for kidney damage. Pain-killers simply overload them more resulting in kidney stones, backache, sciatica and muscle pain.

In the positive state, the Bogbean type is able to start walking- and exercise like aquacize, golf and shopping take on a quality of enjoyment.
PRAIRIE DEVA

SPIRITUAL PROPERTIES

The Russian name for Bogbean is ***VAHTA***. An old folk legend tells about a girl of that name. When Vahta was little, she would play in the forest with gnomes and listen to their stories about herbs and other plants. But one day her spiteful stepmother, who was a witch, turned her into a mermaid and banished her to life at the bottom of the river.

Vahta spent many lonely months living in the river, but one day she left to play with her forest friends once more. She forgot that she had to return to the river by sundown, and when she finally returned late in the evening, the Queen of the Underwater Kingdom punished her severely. She made Vahta stand guard at the entrances of all rivers and lakes, never to venture into the forest again. Since that time, local people began to notice a plant with a beautiful white and rose flower that looked like a weeping mermaid.

The flowers were so brilliant they could be seen even at night and were always a sign that a river, lake or swamp was nearby.
ZEVIN

The Buckbean stands for change. All the species of buckbean are marsh plants. They serve to decorate the lakes upon which they float.

The buckbean stands for change in situation or sentiment. A gentle, painless change in the order of things, natural and inevitable.
GRIMAUD

RECIPES

FRESH PLANT TINCTURE- Up to four ml. four times daily. Use a 50% alcohol extract for maximum benefit of a 1:2 fresh plant extract. For dry plant use a 1:5 ratio. For hypertension, 15 drops 3x daily. Collect leaves in late spring, early summer.

POWDERED ROOT OR LEAF- 1-3 grams as a tonic. Small doses tone and larger amounts begin drainage. Go slow!

COLD INFUSION- One fluid oz. repeated every 3-4 hours. Prepare by putting one teaspoon of dried leaf in warm water overnight. Combine with mint or pineapple weed if necessary. The fresh plant can cause vomiting in some individuals.

WINE- roots can be infused in wine for treating gouty arthritis.

FRESH JUICE- One tbsp three times daily for gouty rheumatism.

FLUID EXTRACT- Ten to forty drops as needed.

BUCKBEAN ALE- Take five pounds of malted barley and mash in four gallons of water at 150° F for ninety minutes. Take the four gallons (add more boiling water if needed) and add 45 grams of dried bogbean. Boil one hour. Strain and add two pounds of brown sugar, stir to dissolve.

Cool to 70°F and pour into fermenter with yeast. Ferment one week or until complete. Siphon into bottles, add 1/2 tsp of sugar and cap. Ready in two weeks. **BUHNER**

CAUTION- Bogbean is contra-indicated in diarrhea, dysentery, biliary obstruction and colitis. It should also be avoided while taking anti-coagulants and anti-platelets like warfarin, heparin or aspirin. It is to be avoided during pregnancy and lactation.

COMMON BUGLE
BLUE BUGLE
SICKLEWORT
CARPENTER'S HERB
(***Ajuga reptans*** L.)
YELLOW BUGLE
GROUND PINE
(***A. chamaepitys*** [L.] Schreb.)
PARTS USED- aerial parts in flower

He that has bugle and sanicle thumbs his nose at the surgeon.   **OLD SAYING**

Ajuga is of obscure origin, but probably means, "not yoked", from the Greek **ZUGON**, meaning yoke; referring to the un-equal and un-divided calyx lobes.

Both Ajuga and Bugle appear to be corruptions of the plants earlier names, including abuga, abija, and Bugula; a name used in apothecaries. It may be a corruption of the Latin, **ABIGO**, to dispel (disease).

Reptans means creeping, and refers to the plants manner of spreading, similar to strawberry plants. Bugle is from the Latin **BUGILLO**, which is from Gaul. One obscure source believes the name bugle comes from **BUGULUS**, a thin glass pipe used in embroidery that resembles a bugle flower in shape. Ground Pine is so named due to the strong pine-like scent from the crushed fresh plant.

Carpenter's Herb is related to its ability to staunch bleeding and heal cuts, due in part to its content of tannins.

Bugle, the introduced plant, has escaped and now is found commonly across the prairies. It is frost resistant and hardy to zone 3. It should not be confused with Bugleweed (*Lycopus* species). This evergreen can resist low temperatures by changing its carbohydrate metabolism. High amounts of raffinose protect the chloroplast membranes during freezing.

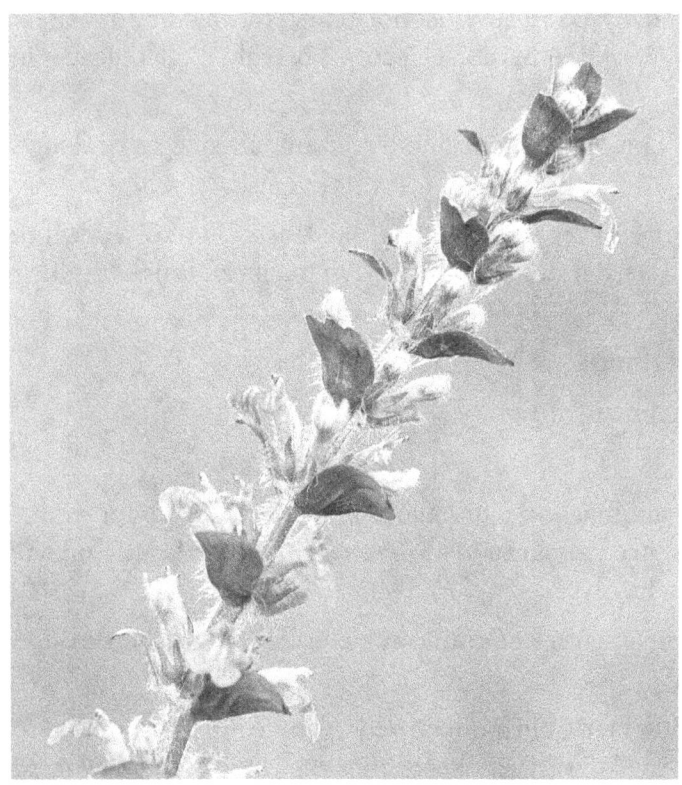

AJUGA REPTANS

It was used on the fields of battle by Romans legions to congeal wounds.

Cooks learned to spread the macerated leaves over roast meats to congeal the flesh and keep in the flavor.

The leaves are bitter, but add nice variety to a salad. In Japan, a related species is boiled and the water changed several times before eating.

It has been used traditionally in folk medicine as a tonic and stimulant due to the presence of ecdysteroids. In some countries, where plentiful, it is gathered for cattle forage.

Culpepper wrote, (it) "is so efficacious for all sorts of hurts in the body, that none should be without it." He used it to treat alcoholics suffering from hallucinations, or delirium tremens.

"Many times such as give themselves to drinking are troubled by strange fancies, strange sights in the night and some with voices...Those I have known cured by taking only two spoonfuls of the syrup of this herb after supper two hours, when you go to bed".

He continues. "An herb for all inward wounds, exulcerated lungs, or other parts, either by itself, or boiled with other similar herbs…It speedily helps green wounds, if bruised and bound thereto."

Infusions were used to treat tuberculosis, or the spitting of blood.

It was part of the *Traumatick Decoction* available from the London Dispensatory of 1694.

Mrs. Grieve reported that it lowers the pulse rate and equalizes circulation.

An old German folk tale, still persistent, associates the flowers with causing fires, if they are brought into a house.

The Eclectic physicians used it for its tonic and astringent properties, and was formerly used in hemorrhagic conditions, consumption and biliary disorders.

Bugle is used today in Tuscany as an anti-hemorrhagic, vulnerary and cicatrizant agent.

The root is used as a black dye for wool. Raffinose in the leaves appears to act as a cryo-protectant, allowing the frost hardy plant to protect itself against severe cold weather.

White fly larvae are killed when they eat bugle. Research into the plant's use for insect control continues. The scentless flowers contain nectar, that bees have no trouble in finding.

The closely related Yellow Bugle, or Ground Pine (*A. chamaepitys*) is an introduced, annual, or short-lived perennial. When walked upon, it releases a turpentine and resin-like scent, hence the reference to pine.

The herb was traditionally used to treat gout and rheumatism, but also possesses diuretic, menstruation inducing and stimulating properties. It is recorded that Emperor Charles V was cured of gout after only eight weeks of ground pine infusions.

It was at one time called Arthritic Ivy, due to its reputation in curing joint ailments. The herb was recommended internally for abdomen pain.

The plant makes a refreshing mouthwash and gargle, and has been used successfully for some forms of dropsy. It has an antiseptic, terpene odour.

The leaves are stimulating and diuretic, acting mainly on the uro-genital system.

It was part of the once famous, Porland Powder.

Culpepper also praised this herb for use in expelling afterbirth, suggesting it is strongly forbidden in cases of pregnancy. He also felt it was a "special remedy for the poison of the aconites". I'm not sure I would risk my life on that statement!

Joseph Piton De Tournefort was a late 17th century French botanist, and director of the botanical gardens in Paris. Ground pine, according to his writings, "expels a dead foetus and the afterbirth and operates so powerfully that the use of it is forbid wholly to such as are with child because it causes miscarriage".

The Eclectics used the leaves as an excitant with influence on the urinary system. According to Dr. King, "they have proved efficient in menstrual derangements and arthritic affections; and are said to be of service in dropsy, jaundice, stranguary, and visceral obstructions."

Veterinarians use Ground Pine for swollen limbs of lambs, mixing a handful finely cut to some wheat bran and gently simmered. In North Africa, the herb has been used to cure paralyzed animals, and hysteria in horses.

The related *A. decumbens* shows significant anti-inflammatory activity as well as bone resorption and bone formation potential. Ono et al, *Biol Pharm Bull* 2008 31:8.

It also inhibits NO production. Sun ZP et al, *Planta Medica* 78:14 1579-93.

Other Ajuga species used around the world are *A. australis* as a wound herb, for treating sores and boils in Australia; *A. remota* from Africa is used to treat high blood pressure, and contains compounds with potential for cancer therapy and biological pest control, *A. iva* from the Mediterranean region reveals anti-malarial properties and 4.5 mg/gram dry weight of ecdysteroids. *A. alba* is both abortifacient and oxytocic; and applied externally to treat psoriasis, and sciatica pain.

MEDICINAL

CONSTITUENTS- *A. reptans* contains iridoid glycosides including 8-0-acetylharpagide and harpagide, one of the active principles in Devil's Claw; terpenoids, teupolioside, phytoecdysones and sterols.
It appears that the more northern varieties of this species are richer in the prized ecdysteroids. These include polypodine B, 20-hydroxyecdysone, 29-norcyasterone, 20-norsengosterone, sengosterone, ajugalactone, ajugasterone B, and vitocosterone E (20-hydroxyecdysone-25-acetate); as well as reptanslactone A & B, 24-dehydroprecyasterone, breviflorasterone, ajugatansins, and sendreisterone.
The hairy roots produce clerosterol, 22-hydroxyecdysone, cyasterone, iso-cyasterone, and 29-norcyasterone.
leaves- raffinose oligosaccharides (winter), stachyose, verbascone.
flowers- four anthocyanins- delphinidin and cyanidin glucosides acylated with two cinnamic acids.
A. chamaepitys- diterpene bitter principles, ajugoside, reptoside, 8-O-acetyl harpagide, harpagide, 5-O-beta-d-glucopyranosyl-harpagide, 5-O-beta-d-glycopyranosyl-8-O-acetylharpagide, asperulosidic acid, deaceytl asperulosidic acid, caffeic acid derivatives including rosmarinic acid; iridoid glycosides, including acetyl harpagide, phyto-ecdysterols, ajugalactone C, cyasterone, makisterone and beta ecdysone.

Blue Bugle is a bitter, astringent and aromatic. It possesses mild analgesic properties and is certainly effective for healing wounds, and stopping bleeding.

In Europe, it is used as an astringent for inflammation of the throat and larynx. Simply take one or two ml tincture in a small amount of water and gargle for half a minute or so. For gingivitis make the mixture somewhat stronger and retain for several minutes at a time.

The plant is mildly laxative and has been used traditionally as a liver cleanser, and for gall bladder complaints. It has been widely used by those prone to excessive alcohol ingestion.

The herb is quite valuable in soothing coughs, and has vaso-dilating effects that require more study. Work by Breschi et al in Pisa, Italy investigated the vasoconstriction activity of the 8-0-acetylharpagide portion of the plant. *Journal of Natural Products* 1992 55. It combines well with marshmallow or hollyhock for irritating coughs.

The activity is probably due to some form of activation of beta adrenoceptors.

Bugle contains digitalis-like constituents useful as a heart tonic, according to Malcolm Stewart. It acts in a similar manner to Foxglove, lowering the pulse rate and equalizing circulation.

Some authors believe the herb to be one of the mildest and best narcotics.

Tincture of aerial parts showed strong inhibition of tumors. Yildirim AB et al, *Asian Pacific Journal Trop Med* 2013 6(8):616-24.

Harpagide is immune modulating via facilitation cell migration into inflamed tissue, and promoting the anti-inflammatory activity of resident macrophages. Schopohl P et al, *Fitoterapia* 2016 110:157-65.

The compound has potential for the prevention of bone loss by stimulating osteoblast differentiation and suppression of osteoclast formation. Chung HJ et al, *Journal of Ethnopharmacol* 2016 179:66-75.

Harpagide is well-known for its presence in Devil's Claw (*Harpagophytum procumbens*) and Figwort (Scrophularia species).

Yellow Bugle is used for gouty and rheumatic conditions. The herb also possesses emmenagogue properties that help stimulate menstruation whenever absent or delayed.

It is seldom prescribed alone, but as a part of combinations.

Both Bugles contain phyto-ecdysteroids that are involved in hormonal and endocrine activity. They are used in nature as an insect molting hormone, but have been studied for years in Eastern Europe for maximizing athletic performance, and promotion of natural testosterone release. The compound 20-hydroxyecdysone is cited in more than 2279 studies on PubMed, at last count.

It may be useful in conditions like plantar fasciitis, muscle atrophy, and the like.

One rat study, suggests it plays a protective role in counteracting memory deficit in diabetes. Xia X et al, *Eur J Pharmacol* 2014 740:45-52.

A 2.5% cream may be helpful in promoting wound healing. The presence this compound may be associated with severe pathological conditions, and considered a clinical marker of interest.

They stimulate anti-ponasterone A activity. Cyasterone, for example, stimulates protein anabolic activity in mouse livers. The compound is a natural EGFR inhibitor, inhibiting growth of A549 and MGC823 cancer cell lines. Lu X et al, *Biomed Pharmacother* 2016 84:330-39.

Teupolioside is a significant wound healer and anti-inflammatory compound. It is an effective inhibitor of chemokine and growth factor expression. Work by Pastore S et al, Ann N Y Acad Sci 2009 1171:305-13 found it suppressed oxidative stress in keratinocytes, suggesting benefit in skin inflammation.

When given orally to rats, it reduced inflamed colon tissue, suggesting use in IBD, colitis and other related conditions. Di Paola R et al, *Biochem Pharmacol* 2009 77(5):845-57.

The compound inhibits calcineurin, an important regulator of T-cell mediated inflammation. Prescott TA et al, *J Ethnopharm* 2011 137(3):1306-10.

Regenerants from *A. reptans* hairy root with high productivity of 20-hydroxy-ecdysone, up to 0.085%, as compared to 0.03% in normal roots, were obtained by Matsumato and Tanaka in 1991. When scaled up in an airlift type bioreactor for 45 days the weight of the root tissue was found to increase by 230 times (four times normal) and the content of 20-hydroxyecdysone reached 0.12% on a dry weight basis.

A thorough review, up to that point, of the genus Ajuga was written by Isiaili et al, *Pak J Pharm Sci* 2009 22:4.

HOMEOPATHY

Ajuga reptans is used for throat irritations and mouth ulcers.

DOSE- Tincture and lower potencies. The mother tincture is prepared from the fresh plant in flowers.

ESSENTIAL OIL

Ajuga chamaepitys has been steam distilled and found to contain 40% gamma muurolene, 20% limonene, and 7.8% germacrene D in one study.

In another study, the essential oil was 13.7% ethyl linoleate, 13% germacrene D, 8.4% kaurene, 6.8% beta pinene and 5.3% (E)-phytol.

The oil is moderately toxic on MDA-MB 231 and HCT116 cancer cell lines. Venditti A et al, *Fitoterapia* 2016 113:35-43.

HYDROSOL

The distilled water of (Ground Pine) hath the same effects [as Bugle], but more weakly.   **CULPEPPER**

FLOWER ESSENCE

Ajuga is about communication, bringing clarity and focus to the mind. I use this essence to help verbal communication, allow compromise, and reach an acceptable outcome for all. With the intricate throat chakra cleared, Ajuga then allows energy to flow through the shoulders and arms so it can be helpful for problems such as a frozen shoulder. **OLIVE**

Bugle (A. reptans) flower essence enhances communication skills, using the power of the spoken word to change and heal, rather than defy or condemn. Refines ranting, nagging, pedantics, etc. **HUMMINGBIRD**

Ajuga helps one to feel protected, capable and safe. It promotes clarity, discernment and decisiveness. **CHARISSA'S CAULDRON**

RECIPES

TINCTURE- 10-20 drops as needed. A 1:5 dry plant tincture is made at 40%.

POWDER- 30-60 grains of the powdered leaves every 2-3 hours.

GROUND PINE ALE- A recipe will be found in Buhner's book, *Sacred Herbal Healing Beers*.

AMERICAN BULRUSH
THREE SQUARE BULRUSH
(*Schoenoplectus pungens var. pungens* [Vahl] Palla)
TULE/ GREAT BULRUSH
VISCID BULRUSH
HARDSTEM BULRUSH
(*S. acutus var. acutus* [Muhl. ex Bigelow] A. & D. Love)
COMMON GREAT BULRUSH
SOFT STEM BULRUSH
(*S. tabernaemontani* [K.C. Gmel.] Palla)
PRAIRIE BULRUSH
ALKALI BULRUSH
(*Bolboschoenus maritimus ssp. paludosus* [A. Nels.] A. Love & D Love)
SMALL FRUIT BULRUSH
RED TINGE BULRUSH
(*Scirpus microcarpus* J. Presl & C. Presl)
HUDSON BAY BULRUSH
ALPINE COTTONGRASS
(*Trichophorum alpinum* [L.] Pers.)
RIVER BULRUSH
(*Bolboschoenus fluviatilis* [Torr.] Sojak)
BAKANA
DARK GREEN BULRUSH
(*Scirpus pallidus* [Britt.] Fern)
(*S. atrovirens* var. *pallidus* Britton)
TUFTED CLUB RUSH
(*Trichophorum cespitosum* [L.] Hartm.)
PARTS USED- root, stem and seeds

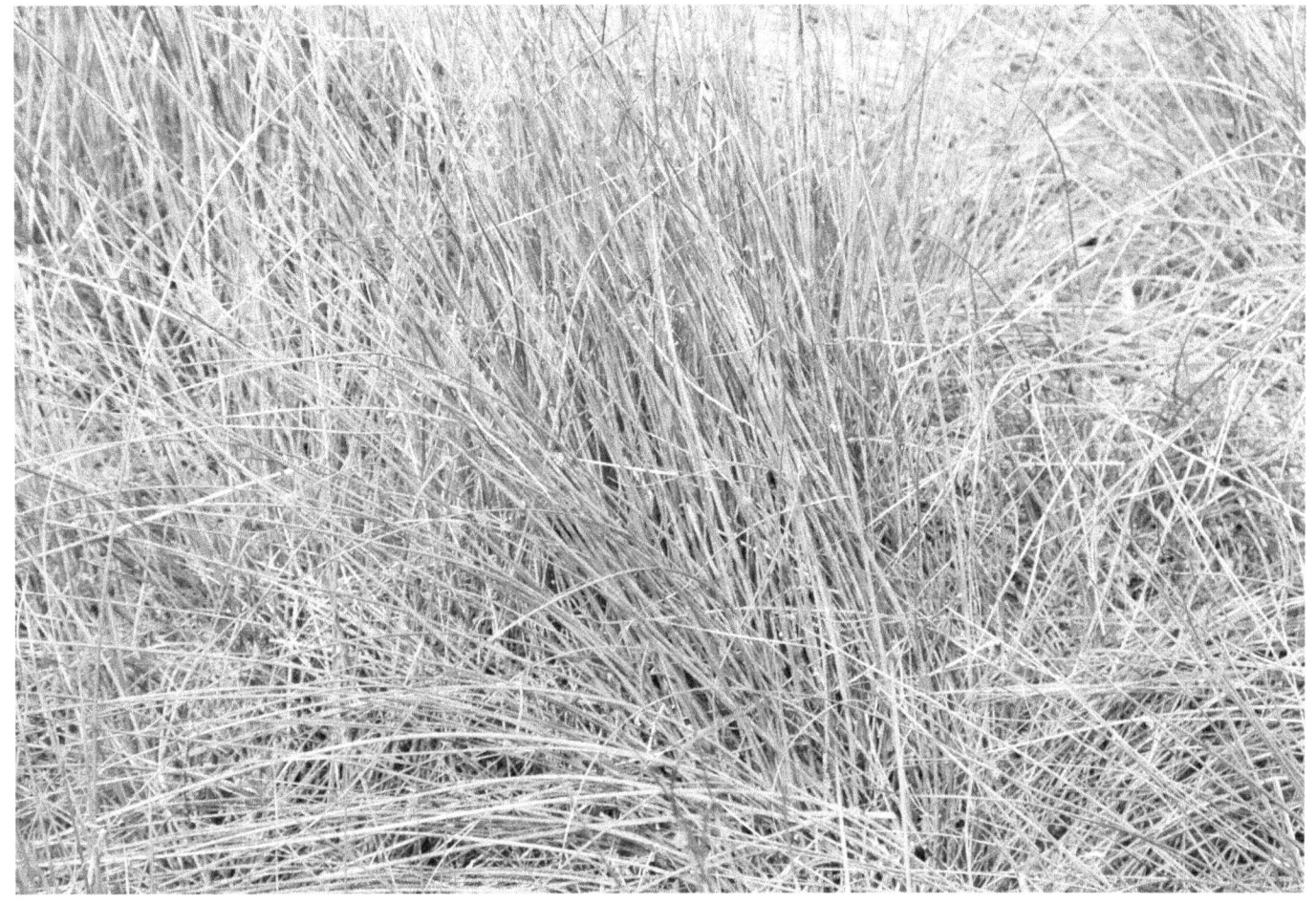

BULRUSH

Bulrush is a corruption of pole rush, or pool rush, due to where it grows. Tule is Spanish, and derived from the Nahuartl word **TOLLIN**, meaning a rush. Fluviatilis is Latin for "of rivers". Scirpus is a classic Latin name for rush, and may derive from the ancient Celtic **SIRS**, meaning rushes. You may note that none of these plants are any long in the Scirpus genus, due to taxonomic re-classification.

When you visit a lake in the boreal forest, it will often be surrounded with rush-like vegetation. Bulrush, cattail, calamus, carex and burreed all appear similar from distance.

There is an old belief that anyone who braids rushes into a ring, and looks through it, will be able to see fairies. The only catch is that whichever eye looks, will go blind after. Therefore, it has been little tested, and still survives.

The ancient Latin proverb, *Nodum in scirpo quaerere*- To seek a knot in a bulrush, means looking for problems where there are none.

Dioscorides, Galen and Pliny all recommended the raw or roasted seed in wine to slow down profuse menstruation, but to use caution as it can cause headaches. They also recommended root decoctions for coughs.

English herbalists, like Gerard, recommended the seeds for their sedative and astringent properties. "So soporiferous that care must be had in the administration thereof, lest in provoking sleep you induce a drowsiness, or dead sleep".

For the wild-crafter, the bulrush leaves are used for weaving mats, baskets and fluff for stuffing. It also makes a useful binding material in mortar and emergency absorptive in surgery.

Tule has stems that are not easily crushed, and are used for making baskets and mats that are used as walls for temporary shelters, floor mats, seat and door covers.

Mats were made by laying the stems side-by-side, alternating top and bottom, after they have dried. They were traditionally sewn together with either the fibre of stinging nettle or dogbane.

The stem and leaf base, can be eaten similarly, either raw or steamed. The roots can be dug out, wrapped in green leaves and roasted over hot coals.

Like cattail, the root can be pounded to extract nourishing flour. The roots can be boiled into a gruel, and fibres later removed.

The young, smaller roots are very rich in sugars, and can be used to make a sweet syrup by bruising and boiling them down in water for several hours.

In midsummer, a small bulb has developed where the root turns, and can be gathered and eaten raw.

The dried, sweet sap on the stems was collected by some native tribes and rolled into balls, for storage.

The leaves of small-fruited bulrush were often used for weaving, as well as wrapping foods for pit cooking.

The seeds can be gathered from fall onward through winter, and ground into a mush, or scorched on a cookie tray in the oven and eaten like tiny nuts. They also can be used as a thickener for stews.

The American Bulrush is found on every continent except Antarctica. The stems were used by indigenous people as the foundation material for wrapped twine baskets, as well as lids and handles.

To the Cree of Saskatchewan it is known as **OKIHCIKAMIWASK**, or ocean plant, perhaps to signify the universal water connection. Alberta Cree called it Ocean Grass, **KEHCIKAMEWASKWAH**, or Straight Stem Plant, **WECHAHK-AMEWUSKWA.**

The stems can be boiled to make medicine for coughs and fevers. The pith of the stem is sometimes used as a wound dressing to stop bleeding.

The northern Chipewyan call Bulrush, **TLH'OGH CHOGH**, meaning "Big Grass".

The pollen can be made into edible patties, or added to other flours.

The Kwakiutl used American Bulrush grass and fish or seal oil on a child's head to make the hair grow long and thick.

The Blackfoot ate the roots of Prairie Bulrush, common to southern sloughs that are salty or alkaline. The Navaho-Ramah used the plant as a ceremonial emetic. Prairie Bulrush (*B. maritimus*) roots are black and were used by tribes of California for basket designs.

Bulrush was traditionally used to make candles, by first soaking the stem in hot fat, allowing it to dry and then stored until needed.

Tule (*S. acutus*) root was chewed by members, of the Montana tribe, as a prevention for thirst. The burnt ashes were applied to a newborn's umbilical cord by the Chumash of California. A good read, and rich source of information on various Scirpus species is *Chumash Ethnobotany* by Jan Timbrook.

Common Great Bulrush (*S. tabernaemontani*) was used as part of a compound decoction for "spoiled saliva" by the Cherokee. The Iroquois used it in compound poultices for snakebite; and another compound decoction for consumption with water lily.

Small-fruited Bulrush (*S. microcarpus*) roots were used by the Mik'maq to treat abscesses, and the upper leaves to treat sore throats.

In British Columbia, the Thompson call *S. microcarpus*, Cut Grass, due to its sharp edges. Their mythology tells of young women using the cut grass to remove Coyote's penis. The Haida Gwaii have a similar theme and refer to the plant as Raven's Knife, or **XUYA SGAWGA**.

In some areas of the former Soviet Union, the plant, when plentiful, is processed and made into cardboard paper.

Bakana (*S. atrovirens*) is one of the most powerful herbs of the Tarahumara of Mexico. They fear to cultivate Bakana, or Bakanowa in that it might cause them to become insane. The Medicine men carry the tuberous dried root to relieve pain, and cure insanity. The whole plant is a protector of those suffering from mental ills, as an amulet. Eating the root is said to induce a long deep sleep.

The intoxication enables Indians to travel far and wide, talk with dead ancestors, and see brilliantly colored visions. The ethnobotanist Robert Bye says that this bulrush is the most important hallucinogen of this area, even more important than peyote!

While living in Peru, I had the opportunity to visit Lake Titicaca, and live on one of the floating bulrush (*S. californicus*) villages for several days. The houses, churches (two, on an island of 14 families) and boats are all made of the totora reed. The children chewed the high protein, easily digested roots, and even potatoes were planted in the decaying layers of the island.

And in Trujillo, where I spent some great time with a famous curandero, Eduardo Calderon, totora reed has used since pre-Columbian times to make sea-going fishing boats. Early in life, he was a fisherman in the cold Peruvian current.

The related *S. riparius* has been shown to reduce tumour formation; and potent binding activity of thymus DNA.

In areas of Ecuador, totora stands may be the single most important source of income for a whole family.

Scirpus species may have a role to play in bioremediation of petroleum-contaminated sites. Lin Q et al, *Ecol Engineering* 1998:10. They show ability to hyper-accumulate manganese, nickel, copper, zinc and lead.

MEDICINAL

CONSTITUENTS- *B. fluviatilis*- root- scirpusin A and B, betulin, betulinaldehyde, resveratrol, lupeol, and betulinic acid.
S. americanus- 0.1% alkaloids and 0.02% essential oils.
B. maritimus seeds- resveratrol (3',4,5'-trihydroxystilbene); piceatannol (3,3',4,5'-tetrahydroxystilbene; E-viniferin; scirpusin A and B.

The stem pith makes a handy compress for stopping bleeding. The roots can be decocted for their astringent and diuretic properties.

The Chinese call the dried rhizome of *B. fluviatilis*, **SAN-LENG** and use it for the bitter flavour and neutral energy. Its main action is on the liver and spleen meridians; and it's action is to disperse stagnant blood, move stagnant ch'i, disperse mass in the abdomen, initiate menses and control pain in the chest, abdomen and costal region.

San Leng is also obtained from the root of various Bur-Reed species.

Three plant patents have been obtained related to the root's betulinic acid. The Japanese have done extensive research and isolated hyroxystilbene compounds from the root; as anti-allergenic and anti-inflammatory agents and acetylcholine esterase inhibitors.

The rhizome is dried and then decocted for its strong blood moving properties including epigastric and abdominal distention and pain. Care must be taken that the patient has a strong enough constitution to tolerate aggressive treatment.

Scirpusin A and B inhibits alpha glucosidase, associated with breakdown and utilization of sugars in the small intestine. This makes them useful anti-hyperglycemia compounds.

Scirpusin A, along with resveratrol, show strong inhibition of amyloid-beta peptide aggregation. Riviere C et al, *Bioorg Med Chem Lett* 2010 20(11):3441-3.

Studies have found it also is active against HIV. Yang GX et al, *Planta Medica* 2005 71(6):569-71.

Scipusin B, is also found in passion fruit seeds. In work by Sanos S et al, *J Agric Food Chem* 2011 59(11):6209-13, the compound exerted great anti-oxidant and vaso-dilation benefit, suggestive of use in cardiovascular disease.

River Bulrush (*B. fluviatilis*) seeds show activity against *Staphylococcus aureus* and *Candida albicans*, with an anti-oxidant level of 8,034 TE/100 grams. Borchardt et al, *J Med Plants Res* 2008 2:4.

The influence of *S. lacustris* has been studied in Germany by A. H. Koridon. In a paper published in *Zentralbi Bakteriol Parasit Infektion Hyg* 1972 127(2):203-9, it was found the plant influenced the death of *E. coli* and the breakdown of phenols.

S. americanus leaf extracts inhibit *Staphyloccus aureus* strongly, and *E. coli and Pseudomonas aeruginosa* in a moderate manner. Borchardt et al, *J Med Plants Research* 2008 2:5.

The roots of *B. maritimus* are used in China as an astringent and diuretic. The seeds, have been studied by Powell et al, and found in a alcohol extract to contain stilbenes active in vivo against P-388 murine leukemia cells. Note the content of resveratrol, a potent anti-oxidant also present in Fleece Flower (*Polygonum cuspidatum*).

The related *S. grossus (S. kysoor)* is used in India to promote spermatogenesis and lactation, and as cardiac tonic. The tubers show the presence of steroids including small amounts of progesterone, and exhibit hypotensive and anti-spasmodic activity. Mujumdar AM et al, *J Pharm Pharmacol* 1980 32(4):308.

ESSENTIAL OIL

From *S. americanus*, an essential oil is steam distilled that contains 4 methyl benzaldehyde, cuminyl alcohol, prenylcycohexadiene carboxaldehyde and phenols. Yield is 0.02%.

FLOWER ESSENCE

Hard stem Bulrush essence helps to detoxify all types of poisons and toxins from body. It brings balance to rhythms, cycles and reactions.   **CHOMING**

Tufted Club rush helps perspective, and brings opposites into balance. It helps us see what can appear as polarities as part of a continuum. We may appear to be many but we are one. Precise order and chaos are actually different aspects of the cycle of life.   **NETTLES AND MORE**

SPIRITUAL PROPERTIES

Bulrush stems were made into the basket in which the infant Moses was set adrift on the Nile. The Moses tale was originally that of an Egyptian hero, Ra-Harakhti, the reborn Sun God of Canopus, whose life story was copied by biblical scribes.

The same story was told of the sun hero fathered by Apollo on the virgin Creusa; of Sargon, king of Akkad in 2242 B.C.; and of the mythological twin founders of Rome, among many other baby heroes set adrift in bulrush baskets.

It was a common theme. Another Egyptian version of the bulrush basket made it a dense mass of plants growing out of the water, where Isis placed the infant Horus.

In India, the Goddess Cunti gave birth to a hero child and set him adrift in a similar basket of rushes on the river Ganges.   **WALKER**

Bakanowa is another medicinal plant used in rituals. A ceremony known as simse is associated with and named after the plant simse. It is regarded as a source of vigor and is ritually venerated, especially by older women and men, who nourish it with offerings. Bakanowa is a kind of counterpoint to Hikuri (peyote). The plant is sought for in the western Sierra Tarahuama.

The ceremonial circle with the offering altar also faces to the west, while the ritual sematics depict the hikuri to the east. The bakanowa root is clearly a potent drug that is not ingested in most cases but [is] merely ritually venerated. Here, some healers use a notched piece of wood, as in the hikuri rites. **CLAUS DEIMEL**

RECIPES

DECOCTION- 3-9 grams of the stem

BUR-REED
(*Sparganium* species)
PARTS USED- roots

To me, there is spirit in a reed. It's a living thing, a weed, really, and it does contain spirit of a sort. It's really an ancient vibration. **STEVE LACY**

Sparganium is from the Greek **SPARGANION**, meaning, "a swaddling band" in reference, to the long narrow leaves. *Angustifolium* means narrow-leafed.

Bur-reed is so-named because of the bur-like fruit and reed-like leaves.

The seed heads are food for birds and ducks; while deer and muskrats go after the roots. Humans can eat the roots as well, but only in areas of clear running water is it recommended.

Dioscorides recorded the seeds and roots soaked in wine, helped to neutralize snake bites.

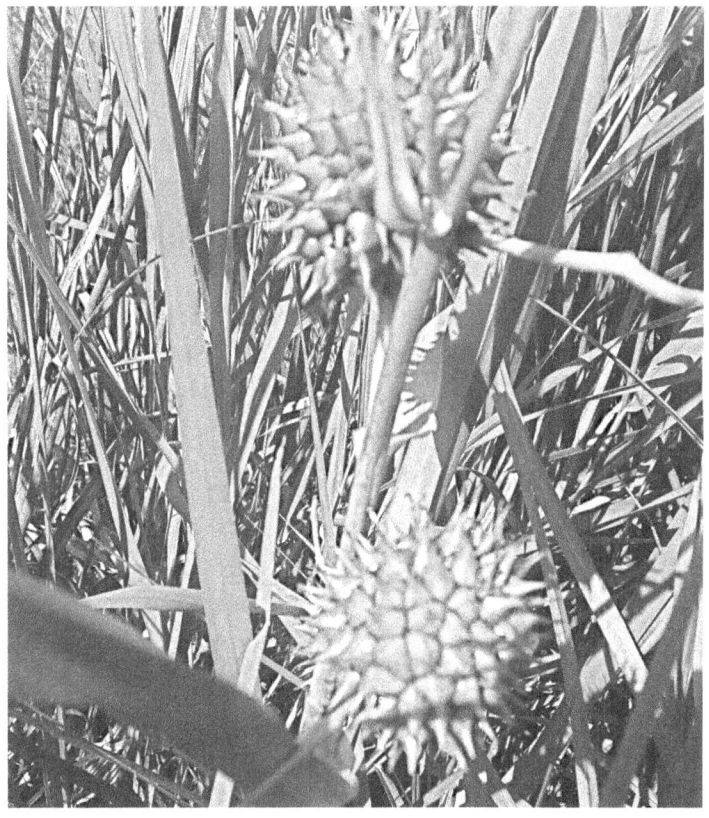
BUR-REED SEED HEADS

Narrow-leaved bur-reed (*S. angustifolium*) is the most widespread in Alberta; followed by Giant Bur-reed (*S. eurycarpum*).

The latter reed was used traditionally by the Iroquois as part of a mixture for protection medicine. The poultice was bound to ease soreness all over, in men from being witched.

Branched Bur-reed *S. erectum*) has a sweet flavoured rootstock rich in carbohydrates, and eaten by various North American natives as a famine food. Infusion of root with other plants was used to treat chills.

It was also mixed with other chopped plants with cows feed to help with a difficult calf birth.

MEDICINAL

CONSTITUENTS- *S. stoloniferum* rhizome/tuber- various phenylpropanoid glycerides and glycosides, including sparganiaside A and 1-O-feruloyl-3-p-coumaroylglycerol, beta sitosterol, succinic acid, daucosterol, stilbene derivatives, xanthone, isocoumarins, phenolics, sparstolonin A and B, vanillic, succinic, ferulic, p-hydroxylcinnamic, p-hydroxybenzoic and p-coumaric acid, hydroxytyrosol and its acetate; 21 fatty acids, sucrose esters.
Stem- alkaloids including 3-isobutyl-tetrahydro-imidazo[1,2-a]pyridine-2,5-dione.

Various bur-reed are used medicinally in China for a number of problems. The root is known as **HEI SAN LENG** meaning three edges, and is valued for its mild but effective action. In Japanese Kampo medicine, it is called **SANYRO**, or three edges; and used in a similar manner medicinally. The Koreans call it **SAMREUNG.**

The tuber is a uterine relaxant, for spasmodic menstrual cramps, and dysmenorrhea. It is used as a pain reliever for post-partum pain, as well as abdominal pain, colic and irritable bowel syndrome. Water decoctions are analgesic, but vinegar processed rhizome is stronger and longer lasting.

The tuber acts, when needed as a uterine stimulant in amenorrhea, miscarriage, prolonged pregnancy, and retained placenta. Combine with safflower petals.

Bur-reed also disperses menstrual blood clots.

At the same time, it can be taken as a tea to increase insufficient breast milk in the nursing mother.

It is used raw for food accumulation, and stir-fried with vinegar to treat menstrual blockages and other pains associated with accumulation and concretion.

The bitter flavor helps drains blood stagnation, while the acrid nature disperses qi stagnation. For this purpose, combine with germinated barley grain.

The compound hydroxytyrosol, also found in olive fruit and oil, helps attenuate cardiovascular and liver issues associated with metabolic syndrome. Lemonakis N et al, *J Chromatogr B Analyt Technol Biomed Life Sci* 2016 1041-2:45-49.

The compound helps protect the kidneys from gentamicin-induced kidney toxicity. Chashmi NA et al, *Biochem Biophys Res Commun* 2016.12.052.

The tubers contain water-soluble polysaccharides that possess anti-oxidant capacity.

Modern clinical research has confirmed the anti-tumor activity of bur-reed, especially in cases of fibroids and endometriosis.

Work by Hu YL, found rhizome extracts enhanced transformation of human lymphocytes by Epstein Barr virus. *Zhonghua Zhong Liu Za Zhi* 1985 7:6.

The root possesses analgesic effect, proven in studies by Lu et al, *Zhong Yao Cai* 1997 20:3. The processed product in vinegar was the most powerful and lasting.

Sparstolin has been studied for non-alcohol fatty liver. It appears to be an TLR4 antagonist SsnB that mitigates inflammation, and a unique molecule that decreases nitrative stress. More research is needed. Dattaroy D et al, *Am J Physiol Gastrointest Liver Physio* 2016 310(7):G510-25.

Sparstolonin B may be useful as an adjunct therapy for neuroblastoma, inducing apoptosis. Kumar A et al, *PLoS One* 2014 9(5):e96343. The compound blocks HIV-1 transcription via a novel mechanism, and inhibits HIV production and works in synergy with AZT. Deng X et al, *Virol J* 2015 12:108.

The compound significantly inhibits vascular smooth muscle cell proliferation, migration, inflammatory responses and lipid accumulation, suggesting use in ameliorating atherosclerotic lesion formation, or treatment. Liu Q et al, *Vascul Pharmacol* 2015 67-69:59-66.

It inhibits a variety of inflammatory mediators, and may be useful for endotoxin shock (sepsis) by reduction of multiple cytokines. Liang Q et al, *Cytokine* 2015 75(2):302-9.

Sparstolonin B inhibits angiogenesis, in part by down regulating CCNE2 and CDC6, halting progression through the G1/S checkpoint. Bateman HR et al, *PLoS One* 2013 8(8):e70500.

Daucosterol protects human brain from neuroblastoma, via several mechanisms. Chung MJ et al, *Life Sci* 2016 148:173-82.

Sparganium simplex appears to reduce kidney toxicicity associated with acetaminophen. Sohn SH et al, *Environ Toxicol Pharmacol* 2009 27(2):225-30.

ESSENTIAL OIL

CONSTITUENTS-*S. simplex*, *S. stoloniferum*, *S. stenophyllum* rhizome- hexadecanoic acid, phenylethanol, benzenediol, and benzopyranone.

The essential oil is spicy bitter, and has affinity for the female reproductive system.

RECIPES

DECOCTION- 3-10 grams tuber. Simmer 15 minutes at 1:20 ratio in water.

TINCTURE- 2-4 ml. Prepare tuber 1:5 in 40% alcohol.

CAUTION- Do not use during pregnancy, or heavy menstruation.

BUTTERWORT
(***Pinguicula vulgaris*** L.)
HAIRY BUTTERWORT
(***P. villosa*** L.)
WESTERN BUTTERWORT
(***P. vulgaris*** ssp. ***macroceras*** [Link] Calder & Roy L. Taylor)
PARTS USED- leaves, flowers, root

Free speech is not to be regulated like diseased cattle and impure butter.   **WILLIAM O. DOUGLAS**

Here is a bloodthirsty little miscreant that lives by reversing the natural order of higher forms of life preying upon lower ones; an anomaly in that the vegetable actually eats the animal.   **NELTJE BLANCHAN**

Pinguicula means, "Little Fat One", from the Latin **PINGUIS**, meaning fat.

Butterwort is common to peatbogs, muskegs and rock outcroppings of the alpine and boreal forest. *P. villosa* is similar but smaller, and more common to northern sphagnum moss regions.

It has a large, rich purple flower that resembles a violet; with greasy, succulent leaves covered with hairs and a color-less fluid. If you get down close to the plant, a distinct musty, mushroom-like odor is observed. This is probably an olfactory attractant for the small mosquitoes, gnats and midges it eats.

Like Sundew, and Pitcher Plant, this small flower is carnivorous, needing to supplement its nitrogen or phosphate needs with insects.

For this purpose, it secretes an enzyme that helps it break down protein; after catching insects on the sticky leaf surface. The insect's struggle to escape seems to make the yellow-green succulent leaves curl up and begin the release of digestive enzymes.

Work by Darwin (yes, that Darwin!) found the inward curling of leaves takes up to three and a half hours. Within 24-72 hours the leaf surface is again dry and curvature is normal, awaiting the next meal.

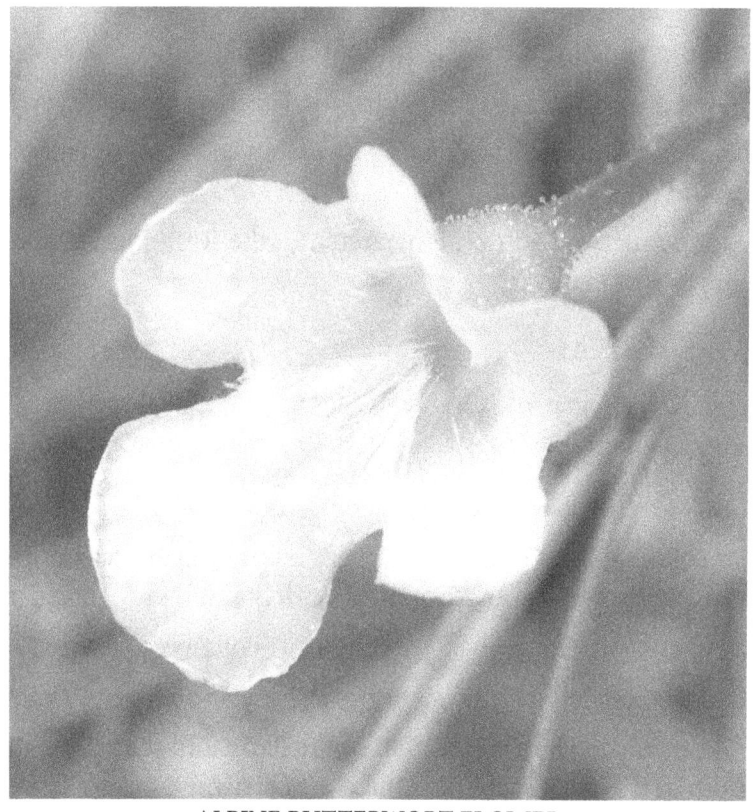

ALPINE BUTTERWORT FLOWER

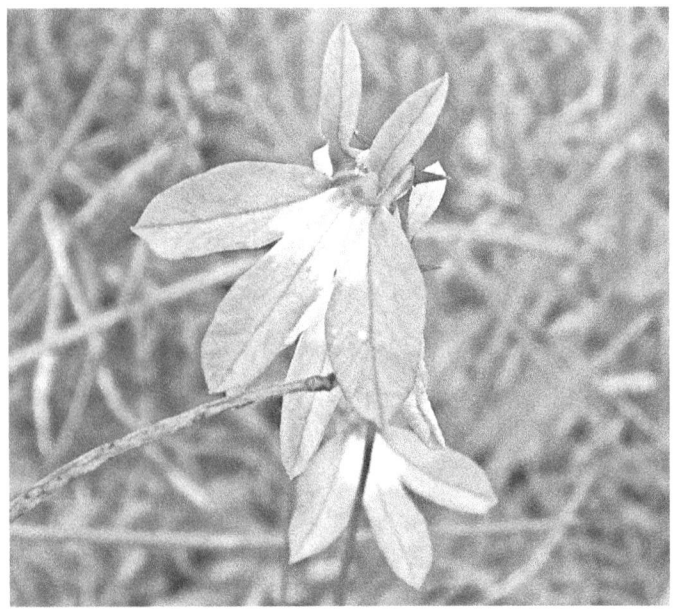

BUTTERWORT FLOWERS

Both a coloring substance and vegetable rennet for making cheese can be obtained from the leaves. Hence, the common name.

In Sweden, both Butterwort and Sundew have been used traditionally to make ropy milk known as *Tatmjolke* or *Stjir*; or *Filbunk* when the cream was not removed.

In Norway, the herb is used as a source of bacteria for a ropy fermented milk product called *Tettemelk*. Recent work indicates the plant's microbiomes are a potential source of lactic acid bacteria.

A ropy milk of pH 4.4 has been made with Butterwort, has an apple-like flavour, and lasts about three months. It has higher B vitamins than other cultured milks, especially folic acid, and the lactose content was reduced by 33%. No whey is produced so it is not strictly affecting the casein protein.

In the Hebrides of Scotland, this plant was believed to act as a charm against witchcraft. Cows that ate it were said to be safe from elfish arrows, and supernatural ailments.

Torrey, in 1894, wrote, "if you put one (butterwort flower) under your pillow and think of some one you would like to see, you will be pretty likely to dream of him".

Gerard, an English herbalist of the 17th century, says that men in Yorkshire take "the fat and oilous juice of the herbe Butterwoort, when they are bitten with any venomous worm, or chapped, rifted, and hurt by any other means."

It was applied to hands chapped by felons, and mixed with butter as an ointment for liver obstructions.

Alpine shepherds used the antiseptic, and emollient leaf juice to cure udder sores on cows.

It was often used in Welsh herbal medicine, as a purgative syrup.

Natives of Eastern Canada used the fresh leaves as an emollient for hands, and for irritated breasts of nursing mothers.

Along one twelve-kilometre stretch of the Restigouche River in New Brunswick can be found over 100,000 Butterwort plants!

MEDICINAL

CONSTITUENTS- *P. vulgaris*- a flavone, scutellarin, isoscullelarein, and various iridoids like globularin, globularicisin, and scutellarioside II; mucilage, tannins, benzoic acid, trans-cinnamic acid, valeric acid, gums, enzymes.
Glands- amylase, acid phosphatase, esterase
Leaf microbiota- proteobacteria, firmicutes, lactococcus.

Like Sundew, the Butterwort is very effective against whooping cough, and can be used as a substitute. One of the constitutents, trans-cinnamic acid, is a well known anti-spasmodic.

Both chronic and convulsive coughs will often respond to Butterwort.

Externally, a leaf poultice is very soothing and effective against various aches and pains.

Like Scullcap, the plant contains scutellarin and scutellarioside, and like Valerian and Crampbark, valeric acid. Both of these constituents exhibit anti-spasmodic activity.

FLOWER ESSENCES

Hairy Butterwort (*P. villosa*) Flower essence helps us consciously access the support and guidance we need in order to move through transitions with ease, grace and deep understanding. It also helps accomplish this, without the creation of crisis or illness.

ALASKA

Butterwort cleanses us at all energy levels, thereby removing those emotional poisons that result from negative thought patterns or excessive criticism and self-doubt.

KORTE

SPIRITUAL PROPERTIES

The flower was known as St. Patrick's Spit or Staff. One day, while crossing a wide bog, St. Patrick lost his Staff, and unable to find a tree, came upon one of these plants (butterwort), whose stem had grown so long and strong that he was able to use it as a staff. The flower on the head (which is shaped with a curve like a staff) never faded and afterwards wherever the staff touched the ground the flower sprang up. The flower is very small on a simple straight stem, the most noticeable feature being the leaves in a star shape, and very flat, touching the ground.

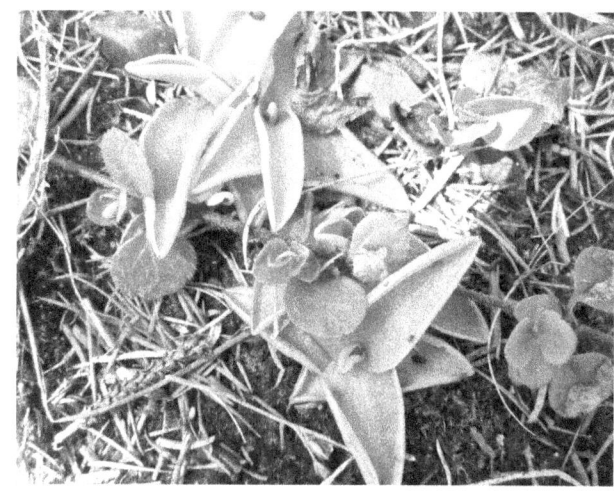
BUTTERWORT LEAVES

MYTHS AND LEGENDS

There is a story of a house on Colonsay where women were keeping watch over a new born baby to prevent fairies stealing it and leaving a changeling—a sickly, fey fairy child—in its place. Two fairies came to the cradle and, to their dismay, they could not take the child because its mother had eaten butter made from milk of a cow that had eaten butterwort.

DARWIN

CANBY'S LOVAGE
(***Ligusticum canbyi*** J.M. Coult & Rose)
PARTS USED- root

Lovage derives from love-ache, meaning love parsley in an early translation from Old French to Middle English. Ligusticum is from the Greek for a related plant used by Dioscorides. Perhaps, obscurely, it derives from Liguria, Italy, where the medicinal Lovage was first described.

Canbyi is named for William Canby, a 19th century businessman from Delaware, who enjoyed adding new plants to his extensive herbarium collection.

Canby's Lovage has not yet been found on the eastern side of the continental divide in Canada, that I am aware.

It is common west of the divide in British Columbia, Montana, and Idaho at higher elevations. At least that is where I find it.

The large perennial is a member of the carrot family and easily mistaken at first for other white flowering members like angelica, or yampa.

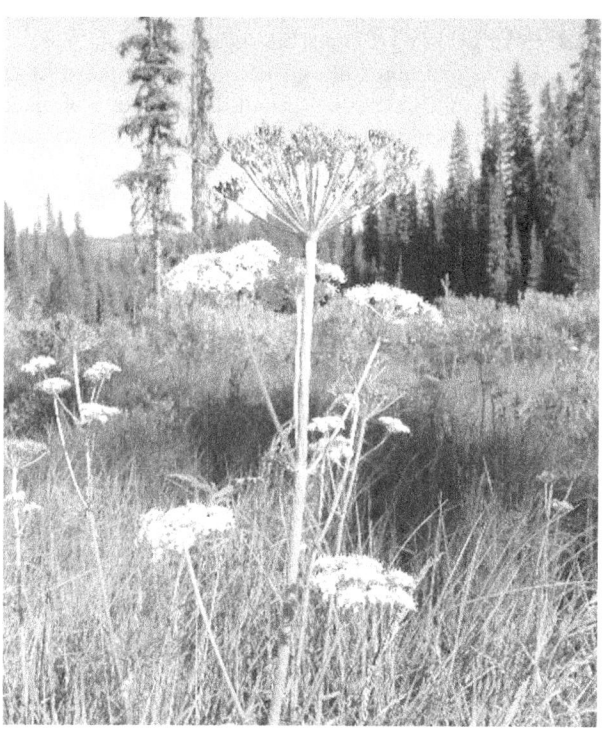
CANBY'S LOVAGE

159

One distinguishing trait, unlike other members of the Parsley family, is the dead plant material around the crown of the taproot. Another is the spicy, celery scent of the plant.

Various tribes used the dried root for sore throats and cold, either chewing on a small piece, or prepared as a tea.

For toothache, headache, stomachache, fever and heart issues, the root was chewed and the saliva slowly swallowed. The Cree traded with western Montana natives for the root, which they valued for heart problems.

Known as **QAWAQA'WS** to the Nez Perce, it was considered one of their most important medicines.

The Blackfoot, Salish and other tribes describe it as Bear Medicine, in reference to observing bears utilize the root for their own healing.

In his book on Montana native uses of plants, Jeff Hart, recalls the use of the root for seizures as told by a Flathead woman.

"We get this root. We have to chew on it and just rub it on a person's body. We also rolled cigarettes with this root in it and let the person smoke it. That calms the seizure down."

The Flathead believed that one shouldn't wash the root on site as that ensures a rainstorm. Considering the plant grows in moist, wet meadows and boggy slopes, the chances are it is raining as you are collecting the roots!

In fact, the strong-scented root was smoked, with tobacco, by the Secewepemc and Okanagan of British Columbia. They named it **XAS̲X̲ES** meaning literally, "always good". The Okanagan-Colville people would burn roots to awaken those possessed by spirits, or ceremonially unconscious.

The Crow used the root for all the above purposes, as well as use by singers to ensure vocal cords and throats did not give out during long ceremonies.

The root was shaved and added to boiling water as a steam treatment for sinus congestion and infection.

A few shavings make a pleasant-scented incense when added to some live coals.

MEDICINAL

CONSTITUENTS The roots and shoots contain melatonin (N-acetyl-5-methoxytryptamine) and serotinin (5-hydroxytryptamine), like Osha. The shoots and roots also contain Z-ligustilide, E-butylidenephthalide and ferulic acid. Other compounds include Z/E-ligustilide, 3-butyl-phthalide, senkyunolide A, (A)-iso-validene-3a, 4-dihydrophthalide, minor amounts of neocnidilide, isocnidilide, cnidilide, senkyunolides, D H I J and N, cis-E-3-butylidene-6,7-dihydroxy-4,5,6,7-tetrahydrophthalide, ligustilidiol, trans-E-3-butylidene-6,7-dihydroxy-4,5,6,6-tetra-hydrophthalide, cis-6,7-dihydroxy-ligustilide. A metabolomic analysis detected 34K compounds in each *L. canbyi* extract, and the presence of more than 82 phthalide metabolites, including Z-ligustilide, Z-3-butylidenephthalide, and senkyunolide A.
The concentration of 5HT is significantly greater in leaf than root. More melatonin is found in the root tissue of Osha than Canby's lovage, but similar amounts in the shoots.
The concentration of E-3-butylidenephthalide is higher in leaves. Ferulic acid is highest in stems. An excellent identification of compounds by Christina Turi and Susan Murch is found in *Planta Medica* 2003 79: 1370-9. This metabolomics work was conducted in Kelowna, at the University of British Columbia, Okanagan campus.

It is often compared, in an unfavorable light, to its more famous cousin Osha (*L. porteri*). This is quite unfair, as the root, although smaller, is useful for many of the same diaphoretic and stimulating qualities.

The root, like Calamus, is rich in volatile oils that rapidly disperse in heat. Cold infusions or tinctures of the fresh root make the best medicine for treating various cold, flu and respiratory conditions, similar in some ways, to Wild Ginger root.

It combines well with pleurisy root for inflamed lungs with thick yellow mucous, and you may add mallow root, or yerba santa if too thick.

Canby's Lovage root is mildly anti-viral, and analgesic, and best chewed, in the traditional manner, for sore throats and bronchial problems.

It may be a mild uterine stimulant, so caution is advised during pregnancy, at least completely in first trimester. It is probably an immune modulator, like its cousin Osha. Nguyen K et al, *J Integr Med* 2016 14(6):465-72.

A constituent analysis, at least to determine levels of tetramethylpyrazine, would be helpful. The root is said to attract bears and repel rattlesnakes. It works for me, so far!

Ferulic acid reduces serum lactic acid, and ligustilide reduces serum free fatty acid elevation in a canine model of acute myocardial ischemia. Liu X et al, *Cell Physiol Biochem* 2016 40(3):770-80. Dilustigide appears to protect the gastrointestinal tract.

Z-ligustilide may reduce ischemia/reperfusion induced increase in brain iron by regulating the expression of iron transport proteins. Zhang YT et al, *Eur J Pharmacol* 2016 792:48-53.

Both Z-ligustilide and senkyunolide I have a protective effect on PC 12 cells, suggestive of neuron protection. Tang J et al, *Sichuan Da Xue Xue Bao Yi Xue Ban* 2009 40(5):839-42.

Ligustilide and senkyunolide A exhibit vasorelaxant effects on aorta contraction. Chan SS et al, *J Ethnopharm* 2007 111(3):677-80.

Senkyunolide I has a potent effect against stroke-induced neuro-inflammation by suppressing the TLR4/NF-kappa B pathway through up-regulationing Hsp70, dependent on HSF-1. It reduced oxygen and glucose deprivation in microglial cells. Hu YY et al, *Brain Res* 2016 1649 (Pt A):123-31.

The compound may be useful in migraines, by adjusting the levels of MAO neurotransmitters and their turnover rate, as well as decreasing nitric oxide levels in the blood and brain. Wang YH et al, *J Pharm Pharmacol* 2011 63(2):261-6.

Senkyunolides H and I reduce hydrogen peroxide induced oxidative damage in human liver HepG2 cells via induction of heme oxygenase-1. Qi H et al, *Chem Biol Interact* 2010 183(3):380-9.

Senkyunolide O is a selective inhibitor of COX-2 inflammation, with IC(50) of 5 microM. Cao H et al, *Pharmacol Res* 2010 61(6):519-24.

Senkyunolide A, N-butylidenephthalide and Z-ligustilide all exhibits anti-proliferative effects against HT-29 colon cancer cell lines. Kan WL et al, *J Ethnopharm* 2008 120(1):36-43.

The compound (Z)-3-butylidenephthalide shows significant hypoglycemic effect, probably due in part to inhibition of alpha glucosidase. Brindis F et al, *J Nat Prod* 2011 74(3):314-20. Ferulic acid has been found, in previous studies, to stimulate insulin secretion.

Neocnidilide inhibits the growth of myco-toxin producing fungi. Jiao XZ et al, *J Asian Nat Prod Res* 2003 5(3):165-9.

Cnidilide is anti-inflammatory, via inhibition of p38 MAPK, JNK, AP-1 and the NF-kappa B pathway. Lee WS et al, *Int Immunopharmacol* 2016 40:146-55.

This compound, along with ligustilide and senkyunolide, induces a muscle relaxing effect, through the central nervous system pathway. Ozaki Y et al, *Yakugaku Zasshi* 1989 109(6):402-6.

A number of compounds in this plant, including Z-ligustilide, Z-butyliddenephthalide, senkyunolide and others exhibit affinity for serotonin (5-HT) receptors. Deng S et al, *J Nat Prod* 2006 69(4):536-41.

The content of melatonin and serotonin, in this plant, is most intriguing. An entire paper could be written on the possible health benefits of this plant, related to these two important compounds. Pubmed lists nearly twenty thousand citations on the former, and one hundred and thirty-five thousand on the latter.

The herb shares a phytochemical profile, similar in some ways to Dang Quai (*Angelica sinensis*). But, not exactly. More like peppermint and spearmint are similar, but different.

RECIPES

Gather the roots in fall when foliage has died back. Slice and make a fresh root tincture at 1:3 and 60% alcohol. Dosage is from 1-5 ml as needed.

You can also dry the sliced root and decoct at 1:20 ratio over low heat. 4-6 ounces as required.

CARAGANA
SIBERIAN PEA TREE
(*Caragana arborescens* Lam.)
(*C. fruticosa* [Pall.] Besser)- not accepted
RUSSIAN CARAGANA
(*C. frutex* [L.] K. Koch)
PYGMY CARAGANA
(*C. pygmaea* [L.] DC)
CHINESE CARAGANA
(*C. sinica* [Buc'hoz] Rehder)
(*C. chamlagu* Lam.)
LITTLE PEA SHRUB
(*C. microphylla* Lam.)
ROSE FLOWERED CARAGANA
(*C. rosea* Turcz. ex Kom)
(*C. intermedia* Kuang & H.C. Fu)
(*C. korshinskii* Kom.)
PARTS USED- flowers, seeds, root, aerial

The trees in Siberia are miles apart; that is why the dogs are so fast.   **BOB HOPE**

Caragana is from the Latinized version of **KARAGHAN**, the Mongolian name for a species of the genus. Arborescens means growing in a tree-like form, while frutex is Latin meaning shrubby.

Caragana, or Siberian Pea Tree, was introduced to the Canadian Prairies as a windbreak tree, for erosion control, nearly a century ago.

Like Sea Buckthorn, it is hardy and drought tolerant. Being a legume, it helps fix nitrogen and enrich poor soils. It has invaded native aspen parkland and boreal forests in northern Alberta and elsewhere.

We are all familiar with the sweet tasting yellow flowers that later form pods that loudly shatter in fall.

Six reddish-brown ripe seeds are in each pod, with about 19,000 seeds per pound.

The leaves produce a blue dye, while the bark makes suitable cordage.

The green seeds are nutritious, but somewhat bland to taste. They can be eaten raw, or better yet cooked alone, or in pods like domestic peas.

They are excellent for chickens, containing 36% protein.

The numerous, sweet flowers are an important source of nectar for honey production. The species *C. chamlagu* (*C. sinica*) has yellow red flowers with a treacle smell. They are edible. The blossoms of this species, as well as *C. microphylla* and *C. intermedia* are regularly consumed in China, as a vegetable. They can be stewed with chicken or pork, along with bamboo shoots for dizziness, tinnitus, fatigue and general lack of vital energy.

About ten species have a long history of use in traditional Chinese, Mongolian and Tibetan medicine. They nourish yin, invigorate the spleen, temper the blood and promote blood flow; and have been used for fevers, inflammation, wounds and infections, dizziness, headaches, hypertension, female disorders, arthritis and cancer.

Fourteen species are recorded in *The Compendium of New China (Xinhua) Herbal Medicine.*

The shrub, *C. microphylla*, hardy to zone 3, has been found to be one of the most drought resistant species.

The flexible stems were used for cordage, in a manner similar to willow.

Pygmy caragana roots are also edible, after considerable cooking.

Perhaps because we have grown up with the plant and been told it has no commercial or medicinal properties, that common folk misconception exists. Nothing could be further from the truth.

In Russian folk medicine, *C. arborescens* is used as an anti-phlogistic, meaning it reduces inflammation.

In Nepal, a decoction of the related *C. brevispina* is taken internally for joint aches. The young buds are a choice edible.

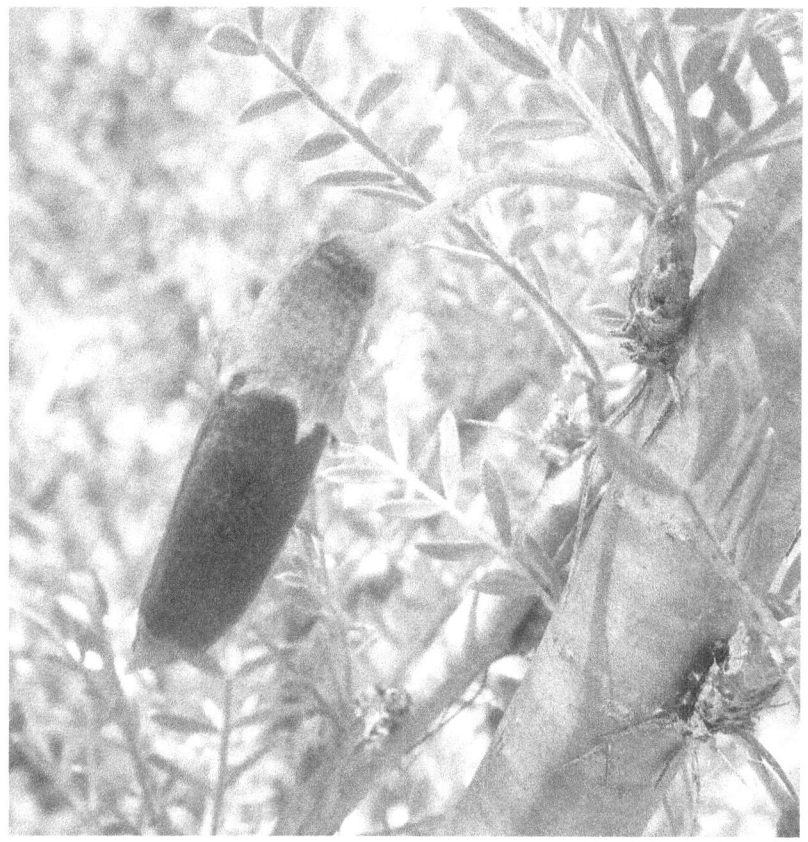

CARAGANA MICROPHYLLA

Rose flowered Caragana has purple red flowers. It is hardy in protected areas.

MEDICINAL

CONSTITUENTS- *C. sinica/chamlagu*- roots and aerial- alkaloids, flavonoids, coumarin lactones, phytosterols, a variety of oligomeric stilbenes, including caraganaphenol A, (+)-alpha-viniferin, miyabenol C, kobophenol A, carasinol B, tilanin, apigetrin, kampferol-3-O-rhamnosyl-(1>6)galactoside, rutin, pseudobaptigenin, formmononetin, various flavones and flavone glucosides, flemichapparin B, trifolirhizin, carasinaurone, miyabenol C, caraganphenol A, pallidol, cararosinol A, steophyllol B, carisinol A-D, leachinol C, Carasiphenol A-D, ampelopsin F, (+)isoampelopsin F, miyabenol C, caasinaurone, caraphenol B.
The content of carasinol B and kobophenol A in roots, is highest in winter. Alpha viniferin is highest in summer.
C. arborescens- leaves and flowers- rutin, isoquercitin, quercitin, (-)-maakiain, (-)-viriabilin, (+)pisatin, dimethylhomo-pterocarpin.
seeds- contain 35% protein, and interesting lectins that bind with N-acetyl galactomasine and L-canavanine (6%)
C. pygmaea- aerial parts during flowering- narcissin, rutin, quercitin-3'-glucoside and galactoside, 3-methylquercitin, quercitin, isorhamnetin-3-O-galactoside,
C. frutex- aerial parts during flowering- bergapten, xanthotoxin, umbelliferone, esculetin, scopoletin (coumarins); acacetin, isohamnetin, kaempferol, quercetin, and myricetin (flavanoids),
C. intermedia- eudesmanes, various dimethoxyflavones, quercitin, limocitrin, 2S,3',5-trihydroxyflavone, pseudobaptigenin, 3',4'-dimethoxy-7-O-glycosylisoflavone, ononin, rothindin, formononetin-7-O-glycoside, pseudobaptigenin-7-O-glucoside, butein, caraganoside A-B, (-)-spathulenol, various eudesmene diols, lariciresinol, carainterol A,
C. microphylla- roots contain beta sitosterol, pseudo-baptigenin, pentacosanylferulates, heptadecanyl-ferulates, ferulic acid, daucosterol, trifolirhizin, ononin, formononetin-7-O-glucoside, formononetin, calycosin-7-O-glucoside, 3'-hydroxy-4'-7-O-glycosylisoflavone, (-)-6aR,11aR)-maackianin, trifolifhrizin.
Seeds- caraganins A-B, caraganoside C-D.
C. rosea- aerial parts- myricetin, mearnsetin, p-hydroxy cinnamic acid, cararosinol A-D, scirpusin A-B, cis-scirpusin A, maackin, 7alpha-hydroxysitosterol, 7beta-hydroxysitosterol, 5alpha-stigmastane-3beta, 6alpha-diol, beta sitosterol, daucosterol, oleanolic acid, cararosinol A-D (resveratrol tetramer), rutin, myricetin, caraphenol A-C, cararosin A, lariciresinol, lyoniresinol, pinoresinol, syringaresinol.

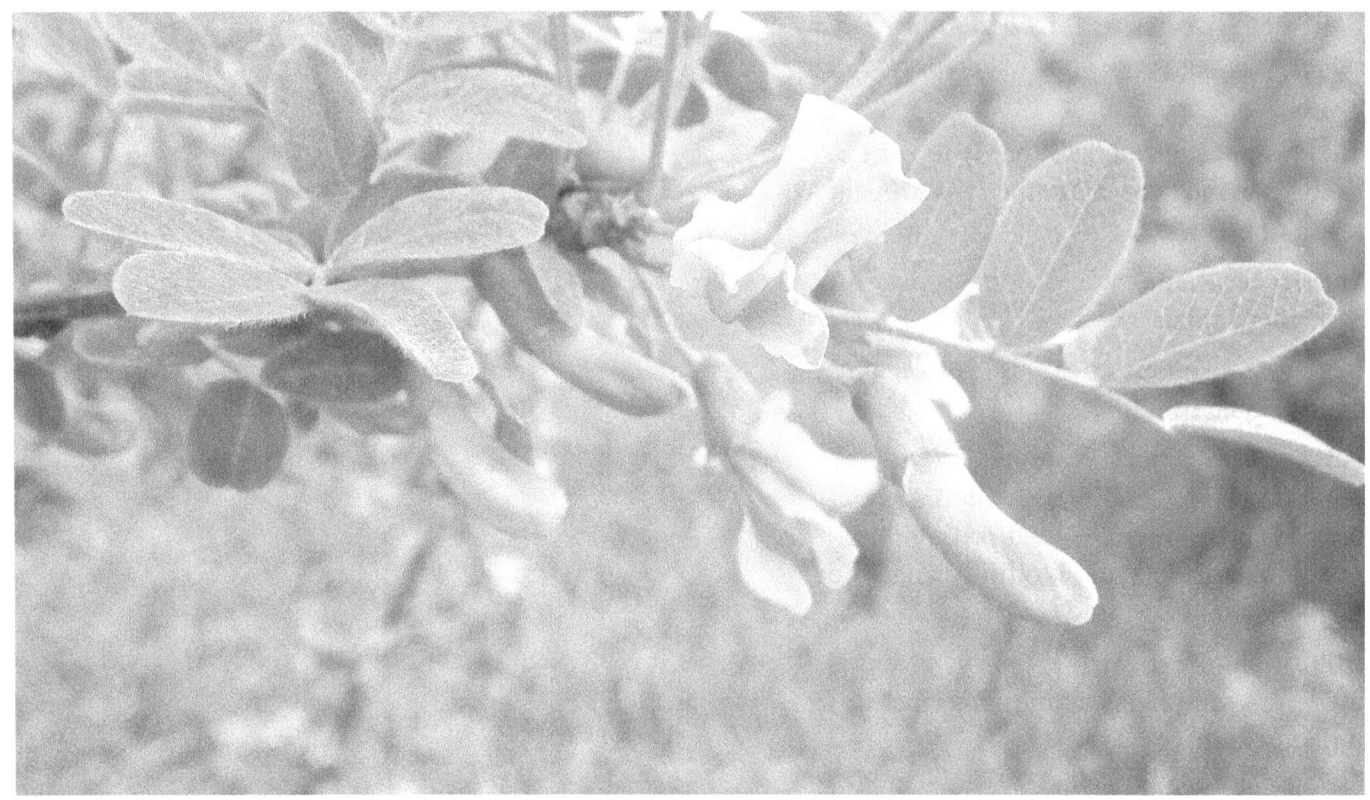

CARAGANA (*C. ARBORESCENS*) LEAVES AND FLOWERS

Siberian caragana is known in TCM as **NING TIAO**, and often used as a substitute for *C. microphylla*.

It is considered warm and sweet, nourishing the yin and blood. It is traditionally used for menoxenia, cervical, uterine and breast cancer, fatigue and asthenia.

Five patents exist for *C. arborescens*, all involving the use of lectins for testing blood and cholesterol.

Researchers have found lectins useful as markers of myoepithelioma in salivary glands. Two lectins from the seed were isolated from the glycoprotein fraction by Bloch et al, *J Biol Chem* 1976 251:19. One compound showed a high hemagglutinating activity, while the second component was low.

L-canavanine has been implicated in lupus aggravation associated with ingestion of alfalfa seeds. This compound is destroyed by heating.

Chinese caragana root (**TU HUANG QI**), or Local Huang Qi, is the name given, due to its popular usage as substitute for Astragalus root. That is, the root is used for raising Qi, as an energy tonic. It is also known as **JIN QUE GEN**, **BAI XIN PI**.

The root is neutral in nature, but bitter and salty, helping expel heat from lungs, invigorate the spleen and promote blood circulation.

It is useful for a wide variety of conditions including asthenia, hypertension, leucorrhea, bruising and contusions, asthma, dizziness, tinnitus and weakened vision.

The dried roots have been used in Korean and Chinese traditional medicine for neuralgia, rheumatism and arthritis. In the former country, the root is also used for migraines.

It is indicated for wheezing associated with bronchial asthma or bronchitis. It also helps lower blood pressure and heart palpitations. The hypertensive effect is due to a centrally mediated action on the sympathetic nervous system.

164

Caragana root is a draining remedy for water retention (edema), and stagnant conditions like rheumatism. In this regard, it is a specific for lupus erythematosus, acting as an immuno-suppressive agent.

In clinical trials, a marked hypotensive action was obtained from the root.

Out of 81 cases of second and third stage hypertension treated with an ethanol extract, 66 patients benefited, including 42 with marked improvement. Li WT et al, *Shenzhen J Integrat Trad Med & Western Med* 1995 5:37-8 (in Chinese).

In cases of hypertension with myocardial damage, caragana not only lowered blood pressure, but also improved or corrected ECG aberration. It combined well in clinical trials with ginkgo leaf.

In 36 cases of lupus erythematosus, 120 gram decoctions were given in three doses, with 14 cases of complete remission, 16 showing amelioration, and one case ineffective.

It has very low toxicity, with an LD50 of its ethanol content at 10.4 g/Kg in mice that was the equivalent of 310 grams/Kg of the crude drug.

In Korean traditional medicine, the dried root is used for hypertension, neuralgia, rheumatism and arthritis.

In a clinical trial, decoctions of *C. sinica* or *C. arborescens* (400 mls per person per day), were found effective in rheumatoid arthritis, with shorter durations of morning stiffness, less tender joints and improved grip strength compared to control. Du XW et al, *Chinese Ethnopharmacology Journal* 1998 4:11-13 (in Chinese).

Other studies found decreased T lymphocytes in mice, and inhibition of hemolytic antibodies by B cells in the spleen. In Du's study (above) the complement component 3, IgG, IgA and IgM decreased after oral human ingestion. This suggests the water extracts are immuno-suppressive, advising caution and correct usage.

Studies conducted by Kitanaka et al, *Chem Pharm Bull* 1990 38:2 identified an anti-inflammatory compound from the root as a stilbene oligomer, (+)-alpha viniferin. This compound is three to four fold stronger than resveratrol. Chung EY et al, *Planta Medica* 2003 69:710-14.

This compound shows anticholinesterase inhibition, suggestive of benefit in senile dementia and Alzheimer's disease. Kulanthaivel P et al, *Planta Med* 1995 61(1):41-44; Howes M et al, *Phytotherapy Research* 2003 17:1-18.

Recent work found the herb and alpha viniferin may be useful for Alzheimer's disease, by increasing ADAM 10 gene expression. It appears able to cross the blood-brain barrier and not only prevent formation of toxic amyloid beta peptides, but also provide a neuro-protective fragment of the amyloid precursor protein- sAPPalpha. Schuck F et al, *Phytomedicine* 2015 22(11):1027-36.

Alpha viniferin, miyabenol C and pallilol inhibit the 5-hydroxytryptamine$_6$ receptor. Kim DH et al, *Biol Pharm Bull* 2010 33(12):2024-8.

The same compound inhibits the proliferation of NHEK cells and breast tumor MCF-7 cells, in vitro. Liu HX, *Chin Acad Med Sci and Peking Union Med College*, Beijing 2004 (in Chinese).

Kulanthaivel identified this compound as well as miyabenol C and kobophenol A from the roots. The first two exhibit protein kinase C inhibitory activity at very low concentrations.

They concluded the root decoctions may be useful in treating hyper-proliferative or inflammatory skin diseases, such as psoriasis.

Miyabenol C is active against two lung cancer cell lines. Sheng Z et al, *Acta Acad Med* Shanghai 1999 26:395-9 (in Chinese).

Extracts of root show, in vitro, activity against herpes simplex virus 1 and 2. Woo ER et al, *Archives of Pharmacal Research* 1997 20:58-67.

The roots have been found to stimulate the proliferation of osteoblasts, in vitro. Ma DY et al, *Chin J Chem* 2004 22:207-11. The compound kobophenol A is phyto-estrogenic, and may play a role in stimulating osteoblast proliferation. Liang GL et al, *J Ethnopharm* 2005 101:324-9.

Kobophenol A may protect against sodium nitroprusside (which releases nitric oxide) induce cardiac cell death. Lee SR et al, *Chem Pharm Bull* (Tokyo) 2014 62(7):713-8.

Pallidol, from roots of *C. sinica*, also shows relatively strong estrogenic activity, in vitro. Sun ZH et al (mentioned elsewhere). At least ten isoflavones have so far been identified in this herb.

The caragana flower (**JIN QUE HUA**) is a popular remedy for dizziness and vertigo.

Simonot reports, according to the Dictionary of Chinese Traditional Medicine, the whole plant of *C. arborescens*, known as **NING TIAO**, is used for cancer of the breast, dysmenorrhea and other menstrual problems. This term is also used for *C. intermedia* and *C. microphylla* in practice.

Russian Caragana (*C. frutex*) leaf has been studied, and water extracts reveal activity against gram-positive bacteria.

Sun et al, *J Nat Prod* 2004 67:12 identified four new eudesmanes, one of which shows in mice models to be the equivalent of metformin on glucose activity, and blood sugar control.

Stilbenes and eudesmanes from *C. sinica, C. intermedia,* and *C. microphylla* show anti-cancer activity in a number of studies.

The flavonoids of the related *C. spinosa* possess anti-inflammatory, analgesic, anti-pyretic and wound healing properties. Large amounts of galacturonic acid have been found in the plant.

More commonly, *C. intermedia* it is known as **NING TIAO JIN JI ER**, or simply **NING TIAO**. The blossoms (NING TIA HUA) are warm and sweet, and nourish the blood and yin. They are infused for dizziness and hypertension.

The seeds of *C. intermedia* **NING TIAO ZI**, possess analgesic benefit. Huo et al, Journal Phytomedicine 14:2-3. They are decocted, and oil on top is used to alleviate itch and kill skin fungi, psoriasis and neurodermatitis. Shi et al, *Yao Xue Xue Bao* 2003 38:8 has identified ten flavonoid constituents of *C. intermedia*.

The roots (**NING TIAO GEN**) are warm and salty, and used for hypertension, dizziness, cardiac arrhythmia, shortness of breath, debility and fatigue.

Even the inner cortex of stems is used, rubbed onto skin affected by psoriasis.

The whole plant is decocted and taken orally for irregular menstruation. In the case of uterine, cervical and breast cancer from 100-200 grams of dried plant are decocted and taken orally once a day, and the cooled decoction used as vaginal wash for former issues.

Eudesmanes from *C. intermedia* show anti-diabetic and anti-obesity activity. Hu CQ et al CN 2004 1554626 (in Chinese). The hypoglycemic effect of 4(15)-eudesmene-1beta, 5alpha-diol is equivalent to the effect of metformin in diabetic mice.

A specific eudesmane sesquiterpenoid, carainterol A, shows potent glucose consumption in muscle cells and diabetic mice. It increases the protein levels of IRS-1 and the downstream protein kinase AKT phosphorylation at low micromolar levels, suggesting the ability to sensitize insulin signaling pathways. Ma K et al, *Molecules* 2016 21(10).

Crude extracts show anti-tumor activity, inhibiting cervical and breast cancer cell lines. Sun ZH et al, *Chinese Journal of Pharmaceuticals* 2004 35:197-99.

The fruit of *C. microphylla* (**NING JIER GUO**) is cold and bitter. It helps to clear pathogenic heat (anti-pyretic) and detoxify.

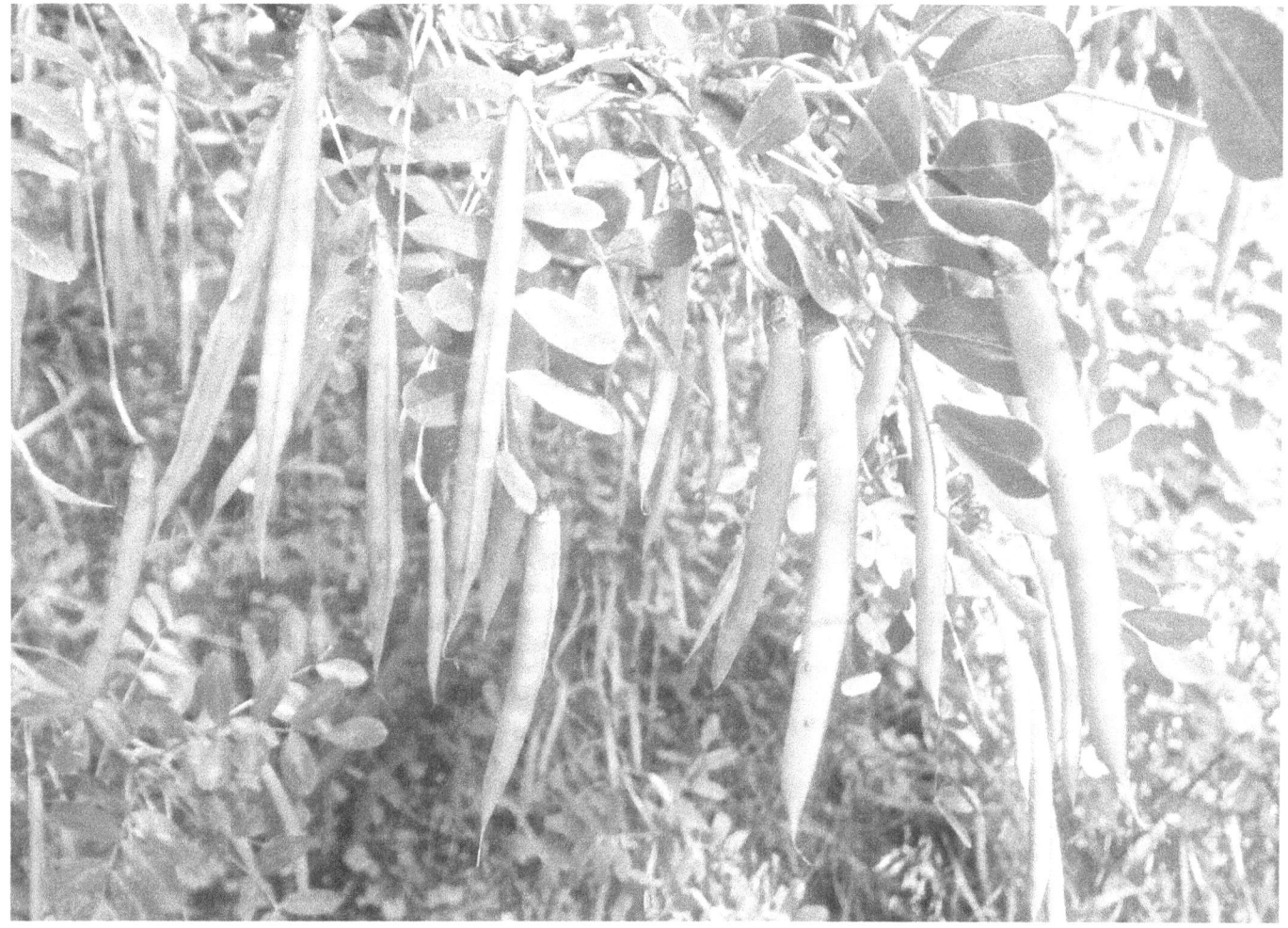

CARAGANA SEED PODS

Extracts of the aerial parts inhibit sarcoma 180. Piao HS et al, *Yanbian Univ J of Med Sci* 2004 27:16-18 (in Chinese).

The seeds contain caraganoside C, that shows weak cytotoxicity against MCF-7, HL-60, HCT 116 and A549 cancer cell lines. Jin GL et al, *Arch Pharm Res* 2011 34(6):869-73.

Various studies suggest plant extracts reduce inflammation via several mechanisms. Jin ZN et al, *Lam J Chin Material* 1994 17:267-70 (in Chinese).

The related *C. conferta* appears to possess significant anti-inflammatory activity. Khan et al, *Chem Pharm Bull* 2009 57:4.

Scirpusin A & B, isolated from *C. rosea* show activity against HIV. Yang GX et al, *Planta Medica* 2005 71(6):569-71.

The roots, known as **JIN QU ER** or **HUANG ZHI TAO** are warming and bitter. They are decocted to invigorate the spleen and stomach, to promote blood circulation, as a diuretic, and emmenagogue and lactogenetic.

It is used for tuberculosis, yin asthenia, fevers associated with fatigue, and various female reproductive conditions. For metrorrhagia, the dried cortex is decocted with unripe raspberry fruit in wine.

Pygmy Caragana (*C. pygmaea*) roots are cold, sweet and slightly bitter. They are prized for treatment of tinea, helping clear pathogenic dampness, in the form of a lotion.

A good review of caragana pharmacology and use was written by Meng et al, *Journal of Ethnopharmacology* 2009 124:3.

ESSENTIAL OIL

Caragana arborescens aerial parts have been steam distilled and yield very small amounts of a yellow essential oil. It is complex oil with approximately 6% each of alpha bergamotene, alpha humulene, and germacrene D-4-ol. Other interesting components include 2.6% beta bourbonene, 5% germacrene D, 2.6% gamma cadinene, 3.6% carophyllene oxide, and 1.4% beta selinene.

This oil was distilled in the Peace Country by Linda Prudhomme-Warrior, and analyzed with the help of the Alberta New Crops Network in 2002. It has a most unique odor that would lend itself to perfumery.

The flower essential oil of *C. sinica* contains 35% torreyol, 7.2% viridifloral, 9% germacrone, and 7.2% 1,10-di-epi cubenol.

SEED OIL

The seeds of Common Caragana (*C. arborescens)* contain about 12.5% oil, with rutin, quercitin, and quercitrin present.

The saponification value is 190.6; iodine value 128.9. Solid fatty acids were found to be palmitic, stearic and erucic acids.

The liquid fatty acids are mainly oleic and linoleic.

In southern Russia, the plant is called Yellow Acacia, and cultivated widely.

RECIPES

TINCTURE- 2-5 ml. Prepare 1:5 dried bark or seeds at 40% alcohol.

DECOCTION- 10-40 grams of root bark 2-3 times daily as needed. The chronic use of caragana for hypertension or chronic asthma, may create allergic conditions such as itchy skin, rashes, dermatitis, thirst, drowsiness, dizziness and nausea in some people. The symptoms abate upon stopping the herb. Caution is advised.

A water extraction of ground dried caragana (*C. arborescens*) leaves, twigs and pods produces a clear, yellow extract with a slight orange tinge; a faint acrid, pea smell and yielded 28.5%.

An ethanol extract was dark green, and clear; with a yield of 13.9%. The solids have a sweet, autumn smell.

CATCHFLY
BLADDER CAMPION
(***Silene vulgaris*** [Moench] Garcke.*)*
WHITE COCKLE
WHITE CAMPION
EVENING LYCHNIS
(*S. latifolia* Poir.)
MOSS CAMPION
CARPET PINK
(*S. acaulis* [L. Jaq.)
NIGHT FLOWERING CAMPION
(*S. noctiflora* L.*)*
NODDING COCKLE
MOUNTAIN CAMPION
(*S. uralensis*[Rupr.] Bocquet)

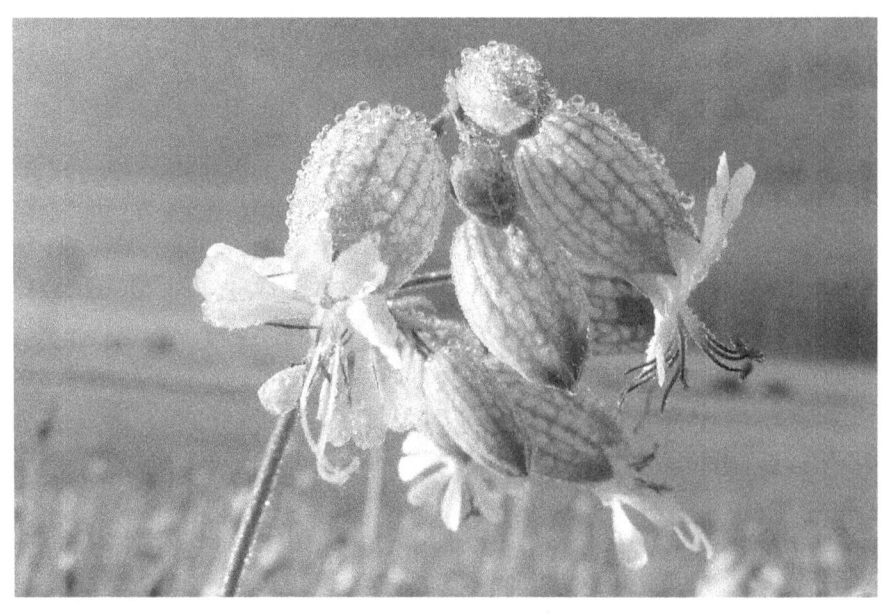

BLADDER CAMPION

INDIAN PINK
MEXICAN CATCHFLY
(**S. laciniata** Cav.)
GERMAN CATCHFLY
SWEET WILLIAM SILENE
(**S. armeria** L.)
MALTESE CROSS
(**S. chalcedonica** [L.] E.H.L. Krause)
PURPLE CORN COCKLE
(**Agrostemma githago** L.)
PARTS USED- leaf, root, seed, flower

You must lose a fly to catch a trout.   **GEORGE HERBERT**

Sow'd cockle rep'd no corn.   **SHAKESPEARE**

Silene is named for Silenus, an attendant or wise old satyr of Bacchus, whom the Greeks represented as an old man in a highly intoxicated condition. He is usually represented in a human form with ears and tail of a horse, and often covered in foam. The plural term Sileni refers to a notorious group of old satyrs famed for drunken, lecherous behaviour.

Silene may come from the Latin **SILENE**, meaning to be silent; most species blooming at night when it is quiet.

Or it could come from the Greek **SIALON**, a name given to many plants with viscid moisture, or saliva on their stalks.

Lychnis is from the Greek **LYCHNOS** meaning "lamp", probably referring to the bright coloured flowers, or **LEUKOS**, meaning white bright. The dry leaf of Campion was formerly used as a candle wick in Poland. Campion is from the Latin **CAMPUS**, meaning field, or may have derived from champion, for their use in victory garlands at sporting events.

The name catchfly is for the sticky juice on leaves and stems used as a defense against small insects attempting to steal the nectar without carrying pollen.

Agrostemma githago is from the latin meaning Field Chaplet. Cockle is from the Old English name **COCCUL**, possibly derived from the Latin **COCCUM**, a seed or grain. Early herbalist called it Nigelle, for the black seeds, but it is not to be confused with *Nigella sativa*, Black Cumin.

Carpet Pink is not related to the flower color, but to the cut and scalloped margin on the petals. To pink, in early English, was to cut, or slash, as in pinking shears. The flowers are pink, but that is not the origin of their name.

Various Silene, both native and introduced, are common throughout the region, although a few are restricted to the mountain regions.

In Northern Italy, the bladder campion (*S. vulgare*) has long been used as a pot herb, eaten raw or stewed, tasting similar to peas, with a bitter, soapy residue. In 1685, the crops on Minorca failed, and survival was due, in part, to dining on bladder campion.

To the south, the more tender leaves, known as **SCUPLIT** are picked and fried as an aromatic, with olive oil and eggs. It is even grown as an ornamental plant in areas. It is best before flower and has a mild taste similar to mangetouts. It is often served in restaurants in Slovenia and other Mediterranean countries.

Some authors suggest the root is edible, but they are very woody. I wouldn't bother.

Gerard called the plant Behen and prescribed the root decoctions for strangury and pains in the neck and hucklebone. Gypsies applied the leaves as a poultice to erysipelas.

An unusual name, White Flowers of Hell, was given to the plant in Dorset, England.

Bladder campion has evolved a resistance to copper, which usually injures plant roots.

Bladder campion was investigated in Germany, for it's abilities to bind heavy metals. Work by Grill et al in 1988, indicated Bladder Campion should be further investigated.

It may be useful for phyto-remediation in chromium polluted soils. Pradas Del Real AE et al, *Environ Sci Pollut Res Int* 2017 doi:10.1007. It collects more mercury in roots than in shoot, and makes it great for phytostabilization technology. The related *S. gallica* hyper-accumulates selenium.

Red Campion (*S. dioica*) is also an important edible green.

Various species of Silene genus are used in China for treating fevers.

White Campion (*S. latifolia*) was introduced from Europe, but now widely naturalized. It was believed that Red, White and Evening Campion would bring storms if picked, and hence known as thunder plants.

White Cockle or Campion roots were traditionally decocted and used for constipation. The Ojibwa used the root tea of White Campion, or **BASI'BUGUK**, as a physic.

The Thompson, according to ethnobotanist Teit used a "kind of Bladder Campion or Catch Fly, one kind with white flower used as a charm to obtain wealth and women".

Night flowering Catchfly (*S. noctiflora*) looks similar but has sticky hairy leaves and only three styles, while White Campion has five on the female flower. It was introduced to Alberta in 1883.

Maltese Cross, Jerusalem Cross, Scarlet Lightning and Soldier's Coat, are some of the common names of *S. chaldedonica*. It is a common perennial of the prairies, with its brilliant red blooms that go on all summer. It is available from nurseries in a white or pink form of hybrid.

German Catchfly flower smells exactly like fresh raspberries, and is the colour of raspberry ice.

Ecdysterone (see below) has been shown to improve productivity of domestic animals fed plants rich in this compound, increasing quantity of both meat and milk.

White cockle leaf and root extracts have been found highly toxic to mosquito larvae, perhaps a new source for safer insecticides (Lloydia 38).

Traditionally, several species of Silene were utilized as anthelmintics, with the Fire Pink (*S. virginiaca*) the most noted.

German Catchfly is an introduced annual that is often found in rock gardens.

Indian Pink, zone 4 perennial, is a red, ragged flowered Silene that grows from west Texas to southern British Columbia. The flowers are rich in nectar much prized by hummingbirds. The flowers have downturned petals and a sticky secretion just below them to discourage crawling insects trying to steal the same nectar.

Apetalous Campion, or Alpine Lanterns grows on calcareous soils in the subalpine and alpine regions of the mountains. The calyxes of all campions are distinctive, but this one is a translucent shell, which acts as a miniature greenhouse. The air temperature inside these protective balloons can be over 5 degrees Celsius higher than outside temperature; helping mature seeds more quickly in a short growing season.

Dioscorides noted Corn Cockle and wrote, "the seed of it being drunk in the quantity of two drams doth expel by the belly colerick matter and helpth the scorpion smitten. They say also that when this herb is laid by scorpions they become benumbed and not able to hurt." The seeds were a common laxative in the Middle Ages.

Purple Corn cockle is an introduced annual, found occasionally on prairies fields. It has interesting pink-purple flowers that remind you it is a member of the carnation family. They contain seeds at maturity that are considered poisonous to all livestock, especially chickens. They contain saponins that do not dissolve in water, but give a frothy, lathering activity.

Unfortunately it mixes well with wheat seeds and when ground as flour leaves an unpleasant and toxic residue.

Githagism, caused when the seeds contaminate grain, is a chronic form of poisoning with symptoms including drowsiness, weakness, weight loss, digestive disturbance and even death if continued long enough.

Acute poisoning is rare due to the bitter seed taste. As githagenin enters the bloodstream it causes the breakdown of red blood cells.

Japanese patents for a virus inhibitor from the callus were applied for over twenty-five years ago.

It contains saponins, similar to Soapwort and Baby's Breath. According to Millspaugh, "the plants in which this principle exists are deemed nearly equal to Sarsaparilla as cleansers of the blood in syphilis and similar affections when the skin is involved".

The related and domesticated *L. viscaria* has been investigated for anti-viral and anti-fungal activity. Studies by Roth et al, in Bonn, Germany, found that water dilutions of the plant extract resulted in enhanced resistance of tobacco, cucumber and tomato to viral and fungal pathogens up to 36% better than controls. Brassinosteroids in the plant are believed involved in the effect.

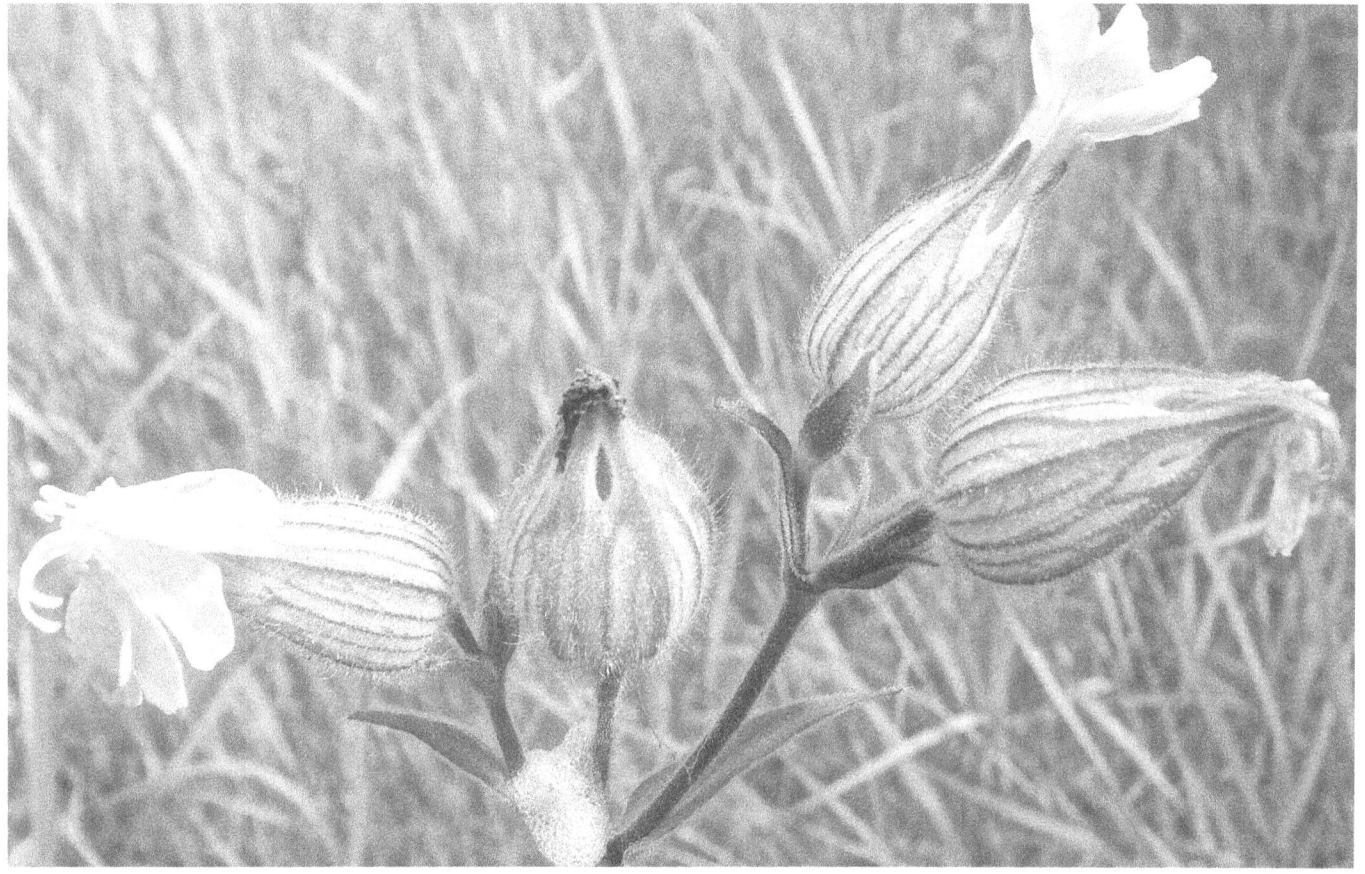

WHITE COCKLE

The related *S. undulata* (*S. capensis*) root is ingested by the Xhosa of South Africa to induce vivid, prophetic, and lucid dreams. It is known as Undela Ziimhlophe or "white paths." Other names include African Dearm Herb or **UBULAWA**. The herb is an acetylcholinesterase inhibitor, similar to huperzine-A in clubmoss. One ceremony involves a three day journey during the full moon, consuming and bathing in the frothy mixture, giving intense and symbolic dreams. The effect is often compared to going underwater by the Xhosa. The root is widely available and legal.

Moss Campion is a small flowered plant of the sub-alpine and montane regions of the mountains. It looks like a mound of moss, until it flowers.

MEDICINAL

CONSTITUENTS-*S. chalcedonia*-ecdysterone, polydine B, alpha-ecdysone, integristerone A, viticosterone E, 24(28)-dehydromakisterone A, and stachysterone D. Various alkaloids, triterpene saponins, coumarins and flavanoids. Lysozyme activity has been found in the plant as well.

ihydrospinasterol, 2-(6'-cinnamoyl)glucosido-methyl-4H-pyran-4-one, various saponins, arabinogalactan, silenin (pectin)

S. pratensis- 4-hydroxybenzoic acid, gentisic acid, (Z,E)-ferulic acid, vanillic and protocatechuic acids, (Z,E)-4-hydroxycinnamic acid.

A. githago-seed githagin, agrostemmic acid, agrostemma saponins, allantoin, githagoside, githagenin, agrostin.

Saponins from Bladder Campion (*S. vulgaris*) exhibit immunosuppressive, anti-inflammatory and immuno-modulatory effects at low concentrations and cytotoxic properties at larger concentrations, on in vitro human lymphocytes and granulocytes. Gasiorowski K et al, *Pharmazie* 1999 54(11): 864-7.

The polysaccharides and arabinogalactans appear to stimulate macrophages through different mechanism. Popov SV et al, *Int J Immunopharmacol* 1999 21(9):617-24.

Studies by Misharina et al, in Russia discovered an acidic arabinogalactan and pectic polysaccharide, silenan in the plant, possibly responsible for immuno-modulatory activity. *Silene conoidea*, an introduced plant, has shown confirmed anti-cancer activity in an astrocytoma inhibition assay.

Alpha spinasterol antagonizes TRPV1 (transient receptor potential vanilloid1) receptors, and may have benefit in treating depression. Socala K et al, *Behav Brain Res* 2016 303:19-25.

The stem and leaves of *S. latifolia* are active against *Staphylococcus aureus*.

The most interesting possibilities for Silene and Lychnis are in the production of ecdysterones. These are plant hormones that are the same, or similar to insect molting hormones.

S. chalcedonica has the highest ecdysterone content in three year-old plants (aerial 0.79%, root 0.33%) and lesser in fourth year. Ecdysterone content from the buds of latter were 0.690% with slightly less in shoots and ripe seeds.

These are now being investigated for their natural anabolic, tonic and adaptogenic effects. They appear to hasten the protein synthesizing process, as well as enhancing protein utilization.

No androgenic activity, or other negative hormonal side effects have been observed, with not toxic effects or hazard having been recorded.

At the present time, a company out of Israel, called Phytogal, is extracting ecdysterone from a Siberian plant, *Rhaponticum/Leuza carthamoides*. They then supply this tasteless, odorless, and colorless extract to companies for sports beverages, clear or sparkling drinks, as well as bars, capsules etc.

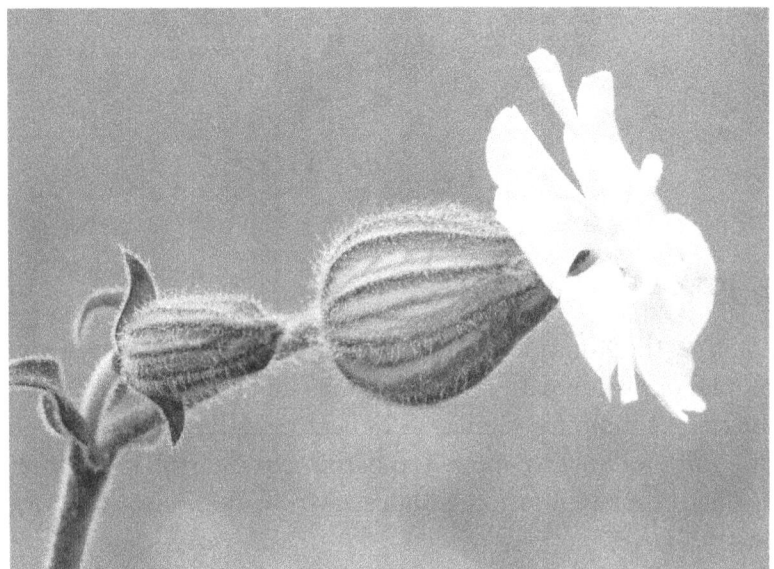

SILENE LATIFOLIA

The product easily dissolves in water, and has a long shelf life.

More study would be helpful, considering that b-ecdysone and related compounds have also been found in Lamb's quarters, and related Chenopodium species.

Integristerone, derived from *L. carthamoides* and *S. chaledonica* exhibits pronounced hypoglycemia, induced by glucose, adrenalin and alloxan. The action is comparable with steranabol on carbohydrate metabolism. Syrov VN et al, *Eksp Klin Farmakol* 2012 75(5):28-31.

Work by Matsuda et al, found that ecdysterone blocks glucagon induced hyperglycemia in laboratory animals.

Plotnikov et al, *Rastitel'nye-Resursy* 1999 35:1 looked at the above ground extracts of Maltese Cross (*S. chaledonica*) and *L. carthamoides*. They found that in lab rats with acute myocardial infarction, that the extracts (150 mg/kg p.o. daily for five days showed improved hemorrheological indices, including whole blood viscosity, plasma viscosity, aggregation of erythrocytes and fibrinogen concentration, as well as an increase in erythrocyte deformability.

Compounds, other than ecdysterone, contribute anti-oxidant and free-radical quenching properties.

This plant and *S. viridiflora* exhibit anti-ulcer activity and gastroprotective effects comparable to famotidine. Krylova SG et al, *Bull Exp Biol Med* 2014 158(2):225-8.

Ecdysterone preparations have been found useful in beekeeping. The preparations have a definite effect on the healing of bees, improvement of wintering, their spring and summer growth and development of colonies.

And spraying a 0.0005% solution of ecdysterone resulted in the death of 40% of leaf aphid larvae in one study.

Related species such as *S. fortunei*, contain 20-hydroxyecdysone in the roots. An alcohol extract of *S. aprica* protected liver cells from acetominophen in work by Ko et al, *Am J Chin Med* 2002 30:2-3.

Agrostin with agrostemma saponins possess cytotoxic effects, possibly applicable in tumor therapy. The seeds contain a triterpenoid saponin and ribosome-inactivating protein that synergistically are cytotoxic.

Water extracts of *A. githago* seeds are cytotoxic on gastric cancer cells mainly via apoptosis and cell cycle arrest at G1 checkpoint. Bohlooli S et al, *J Ethnopharm* 2015 175:295-300. Alcohol extracts of seeds show potent hyopcholesterolaemic activity, in a mouse study with high cholesterol diet. Avci G et al, *J Ethnopharm* 2006 107(3):418-23.

HOMEOPATHY

Corn Cockle (*Agrostemma githago*) is used for burning sensations in the stomach, through the esophagus, and into the throat, lower abdomen and anus.

It helps give relief to nausea and bitter vomiting.

There may be impaired locomotion, and difficulty remaining erect.

Vertigo, and headache may accompany a burning from the lower jaw to vertex.

Mouth hot and dry. Burning in bowels and rectum.

DOSE- 3rd potency. The first testing of corn cockle was by Lehmann and Mori in 1889. They mixed 20% corn cockle powder with wheat flour. At less than 2-3 grams it had no effect save some neck tickling. Four grams caused vomiting and on following day a headache, vomiting and dyspepsia. Increased to 4.7 grams there were similar symptoms as well as increased salivation, increased temperature and cough.

SEED OIL

The seeds of Purple Corn Cockle contains up to 7% oil composed of sapotoxin A, githagin, githagenin, and agrostemmic acid; and 3.4% unsaponifiable matter.

Spinasterol, an esterified triterpene, and a acylic isoprenoid ketone have been isolated from this matter.

Unsaturated fatty acids compose 41.4% of total fatty acids.

Silene vulgaris seed oil contains 17 fatty acids and shows activity against gram negative bacterium such as *Klebsiella pneumoniae*, and yeast like *Candida albicans*. Kucukboyaci et al, *Chem Nat Comp* 46:1.

FLOWER ESSENCES

Maltese Cross (*L. chaledonica*) flower essence is related to transformation and transmutation. It is used for spiritual and psychic expansion and awareness.   **PRAIRIE DEVA**

Indian Pink (*S. californica*) is for helping retain a centered and focused approach, even under stress and amongst diverse forms of activity.   **FLOWER ESSENCE SOCIETY**

German Catchfly (*S. armeria*) is for the weak individual identity, and people who constantly change their opinions. They have a tendency to agree on everything and lie.   **FLORAIS DE MINAS**

Night Flowering Catchfly essence helps one deal with division of sexes on raunchy or bawdy behavior.   **ROCKY MTN**

Bladder Campion flower essence is for those who have withdrawn into isolation because of hurts and abuse.   **CHOMING**

Silene diocia essence is for those individuals that are constantly distracted and never reach destination in conversations.   **MIRIANA**

Night flowering Campion essence helps one breathe again, and relieves anxiety that affects the respiratory system.   **MIRIANA**

SPIRITUAL PROPERTIES

When Minerva lived on earth she had for pets a score of owls that lived on flies. She used to send a small boy named Campion to entrap the insects, and in the morning he would set forth, carrying a big bladder bag in which to place his captives.

Campion used to seek the shadiest corner and sleep throughout the stillness of the day, his bladder bag lying empty by his side. Days passed and the owls lanquished and grew thinner. Finally Minerva turned Campion into a flower as punishment, and to this day we see him with the bladder wherein he was supposed to keep the flies while wandering in the sunshine. And still his head droops with shame by night when the hooting of the owls reminds him of his laziness.   **A. BROWN**

The perfect pink Corn cockle flower spirit brings us the gift of spontaneity. This message encourages you strongly now, in this moment to change. It is easy to become safe and comfortable in a daily routine that lacks spontaneity.   **ECLARE**

The Lychnis flower spirit is enticing you to let go a little and be wild and wicked in an exuberant manner. It expresses its spirit in an impish, prankish, lighthearted way. There is a palpable vibration of joy emanating from its flowers- even the bee is feasting on its delectable nectar.

Drink in the essence of the Lychnis flower spirit and feel the vitality and urge to have some fun beginning to course through your veins again.   **ECLARE**

PERSONALITY TRAITS

It is doubtful there would be as many people familiar with the campion flower as there are now if it were not for the hero of Margery Allingham's detective novels, Albert Campion. Unassuming, thin and wearing glasses, Campion is affable, inoffensive and bland, with a deceptively blank and unintelligent expression. As his name would suggest, one of Campion's characteristic affections is that he always wears a fresh Silene boutonnière. Despite appearances, he is useful. As a fictional hero rather than an unwanted weed, he considers himself to be helpful and comforting, solving mysteries and saving he occasional damsel in distress.   **VERMEULEN**

COMMON CATTAIL
(*Typha latifolia* L.)
NARROW LEAF CATTAIL
(*T. angustifolia* L.)
PARTS USED- root, leaves, stems, flowers, and pollen

I want to see with Mary's eyes:
How the cattails turn to ermine
Then shed their white fur.
LINDA N. REISING

Straight-backed sentinels in high crowned busbies rise in crowded companies from river bank and marsh.

Grown old and fluffed with a thousand florets gone to seed, the heads make fine torches for skaters on the pond.
PRENTICE & SARGENT

If you hold a cat by the tail you learn things you cannot learn any other way.
MARK TWAIN

TYPHA is from the Greek **TYPHO** meaning "of the bog". **TYPHE** is Greek for a cat's tail, while **THYPHOS or TYPHEIN** is smoke or cloud. Other words linguistically are Typhon, typhoon and typhus.

Theophrastus called them **TIPHE** and Dioscorides, the similar **TIPHES**.

To Native Americans, the cattail represents Peace and Prosperity. To Europeans, cattail symbolizes docility, and is related to the birth date of February 29th, the extra day in Leap Year.

Cattail is a valuable, nutritive food largely ignored by northern residents. The tender, inner core of the stem can be eaten raw or steamed; sometimes called Cossack asparagus. The Chipewyan of Northern Alberta call the cattail **TLH'OGHK'A,** or grass fat, due to the shoots having fat-like texture. The Cree call it "plant of the middle of the water", **OSAWÎYOWASKWA**, or **WATOTAHUK**, or various derivations. The Blackfoot call the whole plant **AAPAIAI**.

They can be gathered when up to a foot tall in spring and cut off at ground level. Within two weeks, another shoot will appear. To me, the taste when raw is like cucumber, and when boiled or steamed more slimy, like okra.

Cattail hearts are trimmed like leeks and marinated in a manner similar to heart of palm. Gerald Le Gal, of Gourmet Sauvage in Quebec, describes cattail hearts as "the caviar of all plants, subtle and refined...it takes 80 kilos of organic matter to produce a pound of cattail hearts".

The small corms that form next year's shoots can also be eaten like a potato, either raw or cooked.

The immature green "cobs" or heads can be boiled and eaten like fresh corn. Do not attempt to eat the pithy, wood centre.

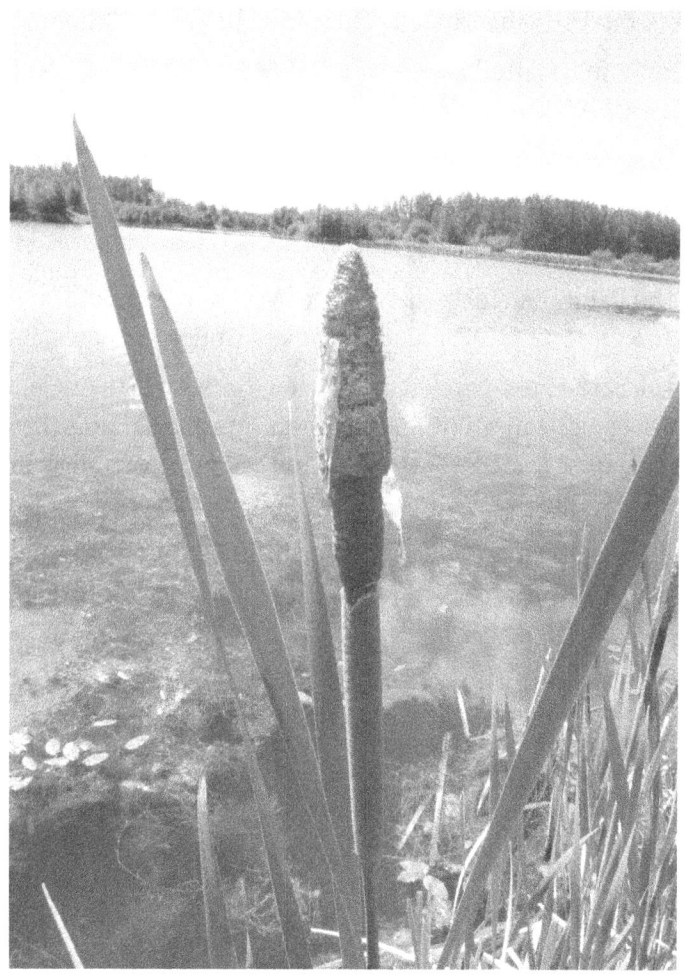

COMMON CATTAIL

The rootstocks can be collected, and ground in flour; or roasted over a fire. The roots are intertwined and difficult to collect. They have a coat that needs to be removed before it dries out, and a pithy woody centre that you cannot eat. In between, however, is a starchy layer that can be eaten, or made into flour.

This flour is nearly 7% protein and the sugar and starches (over 30%) are an excellent corn or wheat flour substitute. Only potato flour contains more minerals.

It is estimated that one hectare of cattails yield over 2265 kilograms of flour, from 7000 kilograms of root. Leland Marsh, who headed the Cattail Research Centre at Syracuse University, found that cultivating the cattail gives larger crops.

He could harvest 140 tons of rhizomes per acre, roughly ten times the average yield of potatoes. The dry weight of cattail flour from 140 tons was approximately 32 tons!

Someday this will be a commercially viable enterprise, like wild rice. The roots can also be fermented to produce organic anti-freeze (ethyl alcohol).

The seed heads produce oil rich in GLA, that can be extracted; leaving a nutritious meal for cattle or chickens.

The male flowers produce abundant pollen that when well dried makes an excellent thickening, flour substitute. In southern Iraq, the pollen is mixed with honey and sold as a candy. It is estimated that one flower head contains between 280 and 420 million grains of pollen. When living in the north, I would combine 50/50 with wheat flour for pancakes and waffles.

The Maori of New Zealand moistened the pollen and baked small cakes, described by early British explorers as tasting like gingerbread. They must have been hungry!

In China, Cattail is known as **HSIANG P'U**, broad leaf fragrant typha, **MAO LA CHU**, hairy candle, or **SHUI LA CHU**, water candle.

The Apache used this bright yellow pollen in ceremonial rites for adolescent girls called the Sunrise Ceremony.

It was known as *HADENTIN*, cattail powder, and carried in medicine bundles, as a source of energy, and brewed as a refreshing beverage.

The Paiute call the pollen **TOITSMA**, and combine it with water and knead it into dough. The formed flat cakes, or **KOSINO'HOP,** are then cooked under hot coals.

The Navajo used pollen to bless the Mother Earth or Changing Woman. She is the diety of bounty and fruitfulness. It was used in a number of ceremonies including the Striped Windway, Deer Windway, Talking God, Earth Song, and Male Shootingway. In the latter ceremony not only is pollen used, but necklaces and wristbands are made of the leaves.

Among the Apache, a Christian influenced event called **DAHGODIYAH** utilized cattail pollen. And of course, both Apache and Navajo used the pollen as part of sand paintings.

Cattail pollen (*T. domingensis*) is consumed in large amounts by various native groups of the Gran Chaco of central South America. The Quechua name is Tortora, the same name given to the reeds growing on the shore of Lake Titicaca. The male flowers are also consumed, and often separated from the pollen for separate use.

The pollen is soaked in a little water to make small biscuits that are eaten raw, or fried in oil. The flowers may also be ground in a mortar and used in the same way. One tribe gathers the powder and lightly roast it before consumption, or the inflorescence is slightly roasted, and the male flowers separated and eaten. The Maká may boil the pollen in a pan until almost evaporated, and the resultant paste cooled down and prepared into little cakes.

The seed down was applied to old wounds and ulcerated sores. Soak the down in wild bergamot (*Monarda fistulosa*), yarrow (*Achillea millefolium*) or mint plant juice and apply to wounds.

Both the Maori of New Zealand and the Zulu of Africa boiled the rhizome to help expel the placenta after birth. The pollen can be sprinkled on babies as a talcum powder substitute.

The Iroquois macerated and boiled down the roots to make sweet syrup. They also burned the roots producing ash as a salt substitute.

The Ojibwa call the plant **PUKAWAYAUSHKAWI**, or the common reed that splits, in reference to the use of split leaves for weaving. Another Chippewan name is **APUK'WE**.

The Cheyenne made a hot drink out of the pulverized root and white base of leaves to relieve abdominal cramps; while the Malecite infused the roots as a vermifuge.

The raw root can be crushed and used as a poultice for slivers, or splinters from wood; as well as the poison from insect bites. For boils or carbuncles, the root is warmed and applied to affected area.

The root has been pickled in vinegar in both Europe and China; and served in salads.

The female "tails" or seed heads can be spread and torched. All that remains after a quick fire are the delicious nut-like seeds.

Of course, other parts of cattail are also valuable. The leaves were boiled and used as skin wash for rashes. The leaves make useful weaving material for baskets, bedding and chair bottoms. The Paiute of Nevada used the leaves to make tables, floor mats, even boats.

In northern Venezuela, a small factory, "*VIVEROS LA PICA*", is set beside a cattail marsh, and the leaves are dried and made into tablemats, baskets, carpeting. On a trip to Caracas many years ago, one taxi I was in had seat covers woven from cattail leaves.

In northern Peru, the dried stems are made into a tea for prostate problems.

The Gaelic name translates as Fairy Wives' Spindle. It was gathered at Midsummer midnight and wrapped in a shroud. Keeping a dead stem and root in "dead clothes" ensured freedom from every ailment for life. In the southwest Highlands, the root was used to cure epilepsy.

In Europe, coopers placed the leaves between staves of barrels to make them watertight. My grandfather worked at a cooperage in Nova Scotia, helping set the saw blades so that the staves fit together perfectly. I have fond memories of the shops, full of smoke, and steam, salt and sweat, sawdust and soul. They did not have to use cattail leaves.

Cattail leave are a high source of protein, with a fresh standing crop yield of 2650 grams/square meter.

Natives of B.C. burn their old cattail mats, mixing the resulting charcoal with herring spawn and water to paint the inside of canoes for waterproofing.

A valuable organic adhesive can also be extracted from the leaves. The stems and leaves are suitable for papermaking; and were made commercially in 1853 in New York. It has been estimated that 3-4 tons of fiber per acre can be produced. This pulp can also be made into rayon.

The down from the mature female head was used as diaper padding by the Cree, who called it *OTAWASK* meaning "Water edge Plant".

The flower spike, or *PASIHKAN,* was burned for ashes applied to a new infant's navel.

The down was also applied to burns and scalds as a dressing. It was also combined with tallow, or animal fat as a sort of chewing gum.

The pollen and tallow were combined to condition hair damaged by sun and wind. The Dene of northern Canada brew the lesser cattail tea for dysuria, or inability to pass water. The burned spike ash was smeared on skin rashes, especially those caused in young children with moss diapers.

It possesses wonderful insulating value, and pressed and sterilized makes efficient heating and sound insulation. It can also be used in quilts, life preservers, children's toys, and herbal dream pillows.

In the past, it has been used for upholster seats, baseballs, and sleeping bags. Buoyant mattresses filled with down were supplied years ago to the Italian Navy. The fact that cattail quilts were waterproof, led to their use on mattresses and for keeping babies warm.

Processing plants with the capacity to handle in excess of 1.5 million pounds of cattail heads annually were operated at one time in Minnesota and Wisconsin. The seeds represented by this quantity would yield about 50 tons of oil.

A thirteen year-old Edmontonian, Kristin Wosar, recently won a gold medal at a Canada Wide Science Fair, using cattail fluff to absorb toxic oil from surface of water.

By taking the fluff and blend it with water and making paper-like sheets that are put between plastic mesh, she has developed and applied to patent her Ecofiber.

The product absorbs the oil, which can be squeezed out and used again. It could also be used as a liner between the double hulls of oil tankers.

Krishnan investigated the absorption of heavy metals by cattail back in 1988 in Toronto. Cadmium, mercury and lead were all found to be absorbed from industrial wastewater; and varied from 1-27 mg of metal per gram of absorbent leaves. Cadmium uptake was studied by Xu Weifeng et al, *Aquatic Botany* 2011 94:1.

Lead contaminated wastewater can be soaked up efficiently by dried cattail leaves. Sharain-Liew et al, *J Serb Chem Soc* 2011 76:7.

Crowe et al, looked at the effects of oil sands effluent on cattail and clover and their ability to survive in the presence of this stress. *Environ Pollution* 2001 113:3.

Work by Nepovim et al, *Chemosphere* 2005 60:10 found cattail took up and 90% of TNT within ten days of cultivation, suggesting use in bioremediation.

It may be a useful source of biofuel. Zhang et al, *J Int Microbio Biotech* 2011 38:7.

Riley et al, *J Environ Sci Health* 2005 40:6-7 found cattail useful in removing ammonia from contaminated wetlands.

Atrazine, a dangerous pesticide, is fully metabolized and destroyed in a cattail environment.

The down can also be mixed with ashes and lime, and is said to produce cement that is hard and smooth like marble.

The immature spikes are soaked in kerosene and lit for evening picnics, to keep insects away and to fumigate old shelters.

After removing the down, the fuzzy thin stalk can be used as a toothbrush- using the rootstock powder!

Experiments in Australia with cattail pollen have shown dusting on bean plants improved the population of *Amblyseius victoriensis* by supplying a food source.

In Utah, studies with fruit trees have shown cattail pollen to be a reliable means of disseminating bacteria to apple and pear flowers for fire blight control.

The pollen is said to produce bright flashes of light, like club moss. I will have to try this.

Narrow-leaved Cattail (*T. angustifolia*) has male and female flowers somewhat separate; and narrower leaves. It is rare in Alberta. This may be good, as studies have shown it to decrease arbuscular mycorrhizal fungi colonization of roots of neighboring vegetation, and increase in functional diversity of bacteria in invaded areas.

A hybrid of *T. latifolia* and *T. angustifolia* is found in parts of North America and known as *Typha X glauca*. White grubs found amongst the roots are a very good survival food, either popped into the mouth raw, or better yet, cooked over some campfire coals on a platform made from the woven leaves.

MEDICINAL

CONSTITUENTS-root- flavonol glycosides like quercitin, vitamin A, zinc.

pollen- various flavonoids(0.1-0.6%) including naringenin, typhaneoside, kaempferol rutinoside, 2 neo-hesperidosides, rhamnosyl-glucoside, isothamnetin, isorhamnetin 3-rutinoside-7-rhamnoside, quercitin, proline, abscisic acid; and unusual sterols like alpha typhasterol, various alkaloids, alanine, leucine, valine and aminopurine, sterols, flavones, terpenoids, long chain hydrocarbons, cerebrosides, isorhamnetin, pentacosane, alpha sitosterol, palmitic acid, alpha-typhasterol, quercitin, kaempferol 3-glucosides, hentriacontanol, nonacosanediol, arachadonic acid.

Also fatty oils, including stearic acid, sitosterol glucoside, palmitic acid, triacontanol, pentascosane, and oligosaccharide, calcium (1.3 mg/g) iron (0.063mg/g) and vitamin C (1.7 mg/gram)

The total lipid content of *T. latifolia* pollen is 123 mg/gram of dry weight, of which 37% is a polar lipid (see below). The most bioactive compounds appear to be typhaneoside, vanillic acid and p-coumaric acid.

leaves- flavanol glucosides including isorhamnetin 3-0-glucoside, 3-0-neohesperidoside, and 3,3'-di-0-methylquercitin 4'-0-glucoside. Also an unusual anti-algal sterol–(20S)-4alpha-methyl-24-methylenecholest-7-en-3beta-ol, (20-epi-24-methylenelophenol).

The sticky juice found between the leaves has pain-relieving properties that rival Novocaine and could be further investigated.

The Chinese use cattail pollen for it's drawing effect in external bleeding.

The mature pod is traditionally mashed and formulated into salves for cuts and burns.

Recent work by Gescher & Deters, *J Ethnopharm* 2011 June 6 found polysaccharides from the fruit of *T. latifolia* are water soluble and have strong stimulating effect on keratinocyte proliferation (skin) and early differentiation.

The root is boiled in milk for summer complaint and diarrhea in children. Tea of the root is used for breaking down kidney stones.

Studies from China assessing renal damage in rats show cattail extracts reduce serum creatinine, urinary NAGase, and increase creatinine clearance.

The stamen without pollen is used as an astringent in dysentery and bowel hemorrhage; while the stamen with pollen is astringent and styptic. When used fresh the pollen is dispersant, preventing blood from coagulating internally. When fried, the same pollen arrests bleeding.

An isorhamnetin compound has been shown to possess anti-hemorrhagic activity.

Work by Gibbs et al in 1983, showed that polysaccharides from cattail pollen showed pro-coagulant effects due to activation of Hageman factor; and anti-coagulant effect that was mainly directed towards fibrinogen. It was shown that the addition of cattail pollen inhibited the release of fibrinopeptides by thrombin and also the aggregation of fibrin monomers.

The fruit polysaccharides inititate keratinocyte formation, suggesting skin healing properties. Gescher et al, *J of Ethnopharmacology* 137:1.

In one study of abnormal uterine bleeding with blood clots in 31 postpartum women, the pollen taken as three grams three times daily for 3 consecutive days showed satisfactory results. *Shanghai J Chin Med Herb* 1963 9:1.

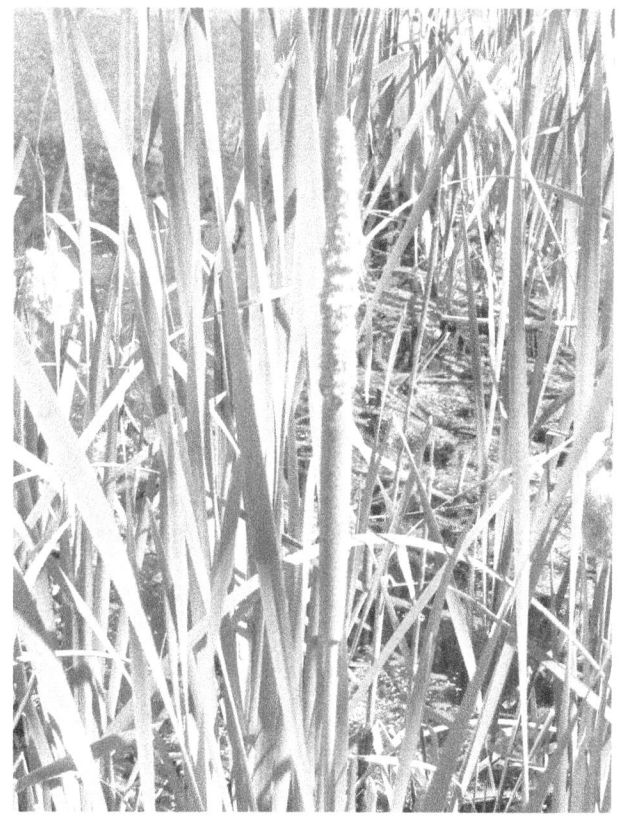

CATTAIL

The pollen extract is also used for coronary heart diseases, hyperlipidemia, and atherosclerosis.

In one clinical trial, 285 high cholesterol patients complicated with hypertension or coronary disease, pollen infusions showed a pronounced anti-cholesterol effect. It appears to lower blood plasma cholesterol by inhibiting the intestinal absorption of dietary, or re-absorption of biliary cholesterol.

Another study of 200 hypercholesterolemic patients treated with 30 grams in three equally divided doses daily showed marked reduction in total cholesterol and triglyceride levels. *J Integrat Chin & West Med* 1985 5:3 141.

Sixty-six patients with coronary heart disorder were treated for two months and showed 89% decrease in angina, 48% showed improvement on EKG, 58% had lower blood pressure as well as lowered cholesterol and triglyceride levels. *Human Journal of Med & Herb* 1982 9:3.

Angina pain in the chest or arm due to lack of oxygen to the heart muscle also calls for pollen. It has a direct effect on slowing heart rate, increasing coronary circulation, and lowering peripheral blood pressure.

It is used for irregular menstruation, acute pain in the lower abdomen and sore throats.

Cattail pollen is known as **GAN PU** in Mandarin, **PU HUANG** in Cantonese. It is used to treat cold and heat related to the heart, abdomen and urinary bladder.

The pollen also acts as a uterine stimulant, and is therefore contra-indicated in pregnancy. However, it can be successfully used for removing a retained placenta. It will relieve uterine pain associated with congealed blood and clots during menstruation and in postpartum. It combines well with elk antler and angelica root for uterine bleeding associated with liver and kidney exhaustion or injury.

When taken raw, it is slippery in nature, and able to move the blood, disperse stasis, and improve urination. It also is used to treat falls and knocks, sores, nodes, swellings, damp itch of the scrotum, tongue sores and rectal prolapse.

One interesting study involved enteric-coated capsules of pollen given orally as three doses of 1.5 grams to 17 colitis patients. Additionally, a rectal instillation of 100 ml of 5% solution was given daily. Four patients reported satisfactory results, 10 reported slight improvement. *J Chin Herbology* 1987 12:8.

When charred it is more astringent and sluggish and used to stop bleeding, including uterine and hemorrhoid afflictions. The pollen may be mixed with wine and then dry fried over low heat.

This is said to enhance the ability to promote blood movement, stop pain and reduce swelling. This is known as **JIU CHAO PU HUANG**.

Cattail pollen, combined with Chinese Thuja (*Biota orientalis*) leaf is used for excessive uterine bleeding; with Motherwort for postpartum bleeding, and with Thistle and Woolly Grass root for bloody and painful urination associated with damp heat in the bladder.

It may be sprinkled externally on mouth and tongue ulcers, damp itching skin diseases to congeal and regenerate tissue.

Cattail pollen is rich in vitamin C, four times higher than citrus fruit, and keeps for six months in a dry environment. The pollen has a higher nutrient content than the bee pollen sold in health food stores, and is quite rich in calcium and iron.

Cattail pollen ameliorates insulin resistance and dyslipidemia in diabetic rats. Feng XT et al, *Biosci Biotech Biochem* 2014 78(10):1738-42.

Both ethanol and water extracts of pollen exhibit anti-oxidant capacity. Chen P et al, *Pharm Biol* 2017 55(1): 1283-88.

In a previous study, the pollen improved insulin-induced glucose uptake via the beta-arrestin-2-mediated signaling in C2C12 myotubes. Feng XT et al, *Int J Mol Med* 2012 30(4):914-22.

The pollen, with its function as an insulin sensitizer, enhanced PPARgamma expression in 3T3-L1 adipocytes. He YM et al, *Zhong Xi Yi Jie He Xue Bao* 2008 9:939-41.

Earlier work by same research team found increased insulin sensitivity by increasing glucose transport and consumption in 3T3-L1 adipocytes and decreased free fatty acid efflux from cells.

It also inhibits the IL-6 mRNA expression and IL-6 protein secretion via NFkappaB pathway in skeletal muscle cells. This suggests one mechanism of relieving inflammation, and improving insulin resistance. Lou SY et al, *Zhong Xi Yi Jie He Xue Bao* 2008 6(5):488-92.

Sprinkled on 30 patients with eczema, all reported complete recovery in 6-15 days. Twenty-five of them reported relief from itching after first day. *New Journal of Med and Herb* 1977 9:22.

Ethanol extracts of pollen possess immuno-suppressive activity, raise cAMP levels, lower cholesterol and are anti-coagulant. Qin et al, *J Ethnopharm* 2005 102; Gibbs et al, *Thromb Res* 1983 32; Wang et al, *J TCM Res* 1998 9.

Work by Feng Qin et al, *J Ethnopharm* 102:3 found ethanol extractions of the pollen suppressed cellular and humoral immune regulation in mice. This may be useful or simply a case of too large an amount in the study suppressing immune function as is typical of many plant substances.

Two cerebrosides extracted from pollen of *T. angustifolia* inhibit proliferation of vascular smooth muscle cells, suggesting a role in prevention of atherosclerosis. Tao et al, *Fitoterapia* 2009 August 26.

The cattail seeds show significant anti-oxidant and anti-elastase activity. Kim et al, *Int J Cosm Sci* 2007 29:6.

In Argentina, one or two teaspoons full, mixed with honey are given to those suffering tuberculosis, or recovering from a debilitating illness.

Decoctions of the root are used in Argentina and Chile for treating tumours.

Externally, the grated root is a poultice for swellings, tumours, and indolent ulcers. Bruised, until it is the consistency of jelly, it forms an excellent application for burns, scalds, and skin infections.

Decoctions of the root have been combined with other plants in the treatment of various sexually transmitted disease (STD), and urethritis.

The roots decocted in milk have increased astringency useful for dysentery, diarrhea and infant summer complaint.

Recent studies in China by Yan et al studied the effect of cattail pollen on de- mineralized bone matrix in rats, and showed the pollen enhanced the osteoinductive potential. *Clinical Orthopedics* 1994 Sept: 306.

The pollen can be used externally to relieve irritated skin and genital conditions. One study of 30 eczema cases treated locally with a dressing of the crude powder, showed 100% improvement in 6-15 days.

Decoctions of the leaves stop uterine hemorrhages and relieve bloody diarrhea. An infusion of the leaves, taken hot, helps relieve fevers, pain and headaches and promotes a restful sleep.

Studies conducted by Rozycki et al in Argentina in 1997, found pollen from local cattails (*T. domingensis*) has an energetic value of 287.7 Kcal/100 grams.

The rhizomes of *T. latifolia subsp. capensis,* are decocted in Africa to increase blood circulation, dilate veins, promote female fertility, and male virility, ease childbirth, and treat intestinal and kidney problems. For dysmenorrhea, the root infusion is taken in porridge.

Typhaneoside, present in cattail pollen, is also found in calendula, gingko and meadowfoam. Its activity is uncertain.

Cattail stalks possess significant anti-oxidant activity, showing 80% inhibition at 500 ppm, and 90% at 5000 ppm. Kähkönen et al, *Journal Agric Food Chem* 2003 47:10.

HOMEOPATHY

Typha is used for diarrhea, dysentery, and various summer complaints of children.

DOSE- Tincture to 1st potency as needed.

SEED OIL

The oil has a high linoleic acid content (69.9%) with an iodine value of 141.6.

Six kilos of seed yield one kilo of oil rich in omega three, the same as seeds from evening primrose, rosehip, black currant, and borage. The yield is significant (17.9%) given the relative abundance, and reliability of supply.

The oil contains lesser amounts of linolenic, oleic and stearic acid.

The polar lipid fraction consists of phosphatidylcholine, phosphatidyl-ethanolamine, and phosphatidic acid, with minor amounts of phosphatidyl glycerol, and phosphatidyllinositol.

ESSENTIAL OILS

Concretes of the leaves, stems and root of *T. latifolia* have been produced by Salmon et al, and results published in *Rivista Italiana-EPPOS* 1998. Over 100 compounds have been identified by gas chromatography. If I can track down the article, in English, I will pass on the information.

FLOWER ESSENCES

Cattail pollen flower essence is for those who need courage during emergence. It is for standing tall in one's truth; connecting to the power of one's destiny; finding the courage to follow one's highest path.   **ALASKA**

Cattail essence helps protect from harmful influences as well as supports mental and physical ailments associated with parasites, viruses, bacteria and fungi. It helps bring suppressed feelings to the surface.   **MIRIANA**

SPIRITUAL PROPERTIES

Want to liven up your sex life? Place a large bunch of cattails in the bedroom; their presence will also help you to have multiple orgasms.

If you want to attract joy, happiness, and abundance into your life, dry the leaves, weave them into a mat, and use them as a covering for your altar.

Using the fluffy innards of cattails to make a small dream pillow will make it easier to remember your dreams and use them to find solutions to any issues in your life.   **SUSAN GREGG**

The fact that the Greeks called cat-tail **typhe** indicated that they connected it with the nadir. That relationship was through comparison to an important supernatural being who showed his presence by sending smoke to the surface through volcanoes and in storms. The Greeks called him Typhon, and he was visualized as a serpent-like dragon.   **DANIEL F. AUSTIN**

PERSONALITY TRAITS

Semen is Latin for a dormant, fertilized plant ovum- a seed. Men's ejaculate is chemically more akin to plant pollen. See, it is really more accurate to call it mammal pollen. To call it semen is to thrust an insanity deep inside our culture: that men plow women and plant their seed when, in fact, what they are doing is pollinating flowers. Now. Doesn't that change everything between us?   **BUHNER**

MYTHS AND LEGENDS

Typhaon, typhoeus and typhos all variants of typhoon refer to a giant monster.

Zeus battled Typhon and killed him by burying him under Mount Edna. Thus Typhon symbolizes volcanic forces.

Typhon, as father of the Winds, causes dangerous storms, thus related to typhoon from the Arabic **TUFAN** to turn around. Typhoon also came from the Cantonese **TAI FUNG**, meaning big wind.

The other spelling is Latin typhus. In English, typhus originally meant pride, haughtiness, or conceit, but by 1785 was applied to an infectious fever caused by Rickettsia. English-speakers call that fever "typhoid" (typhos=smoke and oid=resembling) because of the smoky or lazy state of mind of those affected.   **DANIEL F. AUSTIN**

RECIPES

INFUSION- Add one small palmful of root powder to one cup of hot water for diarrhea remedy.

DOSE- one to two cups.

LEAF DECOCTION- One part leaves to ten parts water.

DOSE- 3-4 cups daily

POLLEN DECOCTION-4-12 grams for twenty minutes in muslin cloth.

POLLEN TINCTURE- 1-4 ml. Cattail pollen, in animal studies, stimulates uterine contractions. The tincture is made 1:4 with 95% alcohol. Crush the pollen immediately before process. An optimal ethanol extraction is done three times, with eight fold the amount of 60% alcohol (1:8) for one hour each time.

Raw pollen is contraindicated during pregnancy.

FLOUR FROM ROOTSTOCK- Peel off the outer covering of root and break up in water. The flower will settle to bottom, pour water off and repeat. Dry on cookie sheets in the sun. Put any large pieces through a food or coffee grinder. Then store like regular flour.

Those interested in commercial potential of cattail are directed to the work of Leland Marsh, who published work on the subject as far back as 1947.

Those interested in mythology and sacred connections with cat-tail-dragons, water-serpents and reed-maces are referred to an excellent article by Daniel F. Austin in *Ethnobotany Res & Appl* 2007 5.

CENTAUREA SPECIES

CORNFLOWER
BACHELOR'S BUTTONS
(*Centaurea cyanus* L.)
SWEET SULTAN
(*Amberboa moschata* [L.] DC)
(*C. moschata* L.)- no longer accepted
PERENNIAL CORNFLOWER
MOUNTAIN KNAPWEED
(*C. montana* L.)
YELLOW STAR THISTLE
(*C. solstitialis* L.)
PURPLE STAR THISTLE
(*C. calcitrapa* L.)
RUSSIAN KNAPWEED
TURKESTAN THISTLE
(*Rhaponticum repens* [L.] Hidalgo)
(*C. repens* L.) no longer accepted
DIFFUSE KNAPWEED
WHITE KNAPWEED
(*C. diffusa* Lam.)
(*Acosta diffusa* [Lam.] Sojak)
SPOTTED KNAPWEED
(*C. stoebe* ssp. *microanthos* [Gugler] Hayek)
(*C. maculosa*) no longer accepted
GLOBE KNAPWEED
(*C. macrocephala* Puschk. ex Willd.)
GREATER KNAPWEED
(*C. scabiosa* L.)
CENTAURY
(*C. erythraea* Rafn.)
PARTS USED- roots, leaves, flowers

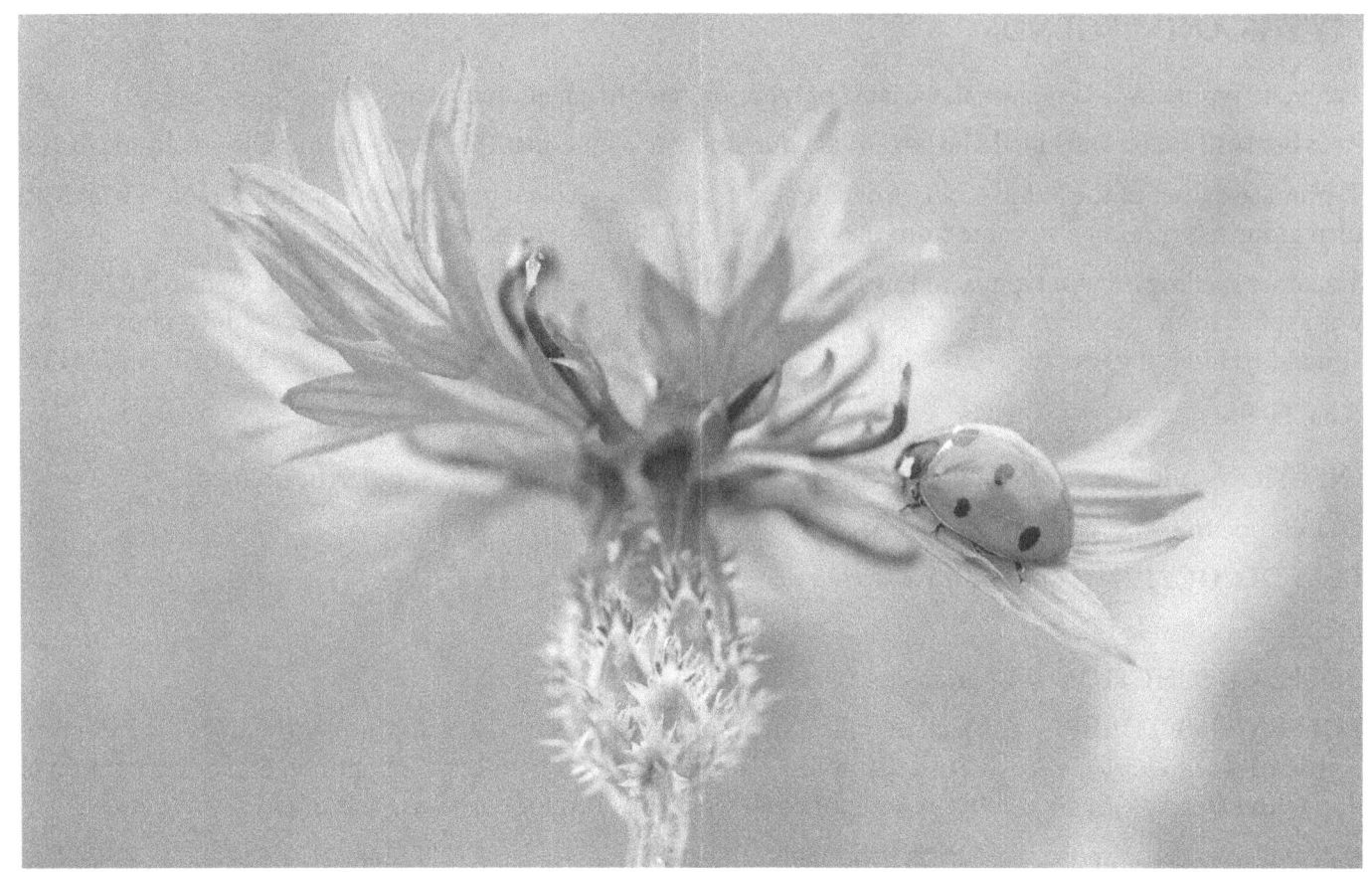

CORNFLOWER

Wormwood and Centaury, their bitter juice
To aid digestion's sickly powers, refine.   **DODSLEY**

"They pull the little blossom threads
From out the Knapweed's button heads,
And put the husk with many a smile
In their white bosoms for a while;
Then, if they guess aright the swain
Their love's sweet fancies try to gain,
"Tis said that ere it lies an hour
"T'will blossom with a second flower".   **JOHN CLARE**

While the scentless star that summer mingles with the blond corn-stalks,
Spangles with its lapis blue
The furrows that the crops turn to gold
Before its flowers are lost, and the fields have felt the sickles,
Go, go, young girls, pick Cornflowers in the field.   **VICTOR HUGO**

Why do we give flowers to the dead?...Fifty thousand years ago, the Neanderthals, too, buried their relatives
with hyacinth and knapweed.   **SHARMAN RUSSELL**

Centaurea is derived from Centaur, the mythical half-man, half-beast, that probably originated from the Greek
KENTRON meaning, spur. Therefore the original name for centaurs, **KENTAUROI** meant, "he who spurs
horses on, or breaks wild horses."

When Centaurs were feeling poorly, they were said to feed on cornflowers and suddenly restore their vigor.

Chiron who was famed for his gift of healing with herbs, was a prominent member of this race. It is said he was healed by this plant, and passed his knowledge of medicinal plants to Aesclepius, Ulysses and Achilles.

In Germany, they translated the Latin name into **CENTUM** meaning hundred; and **AURUM** meaning gold, which makes no sense at all.

Cyanus is from the Greek **KYANOS** meaning, dark blue. Cyanus from the Latin is named after Cyranus, a youthful devotee of the goddess Flora. Flora or Chloris, as she was known, occupied his time in gathering flowers for her altar, and when he died, he was transformed into a cornflower. A version of the legend finds him dead in a cornfield, in a bed of cornflowers, wearing a robe of cornflower blue.

In one Russian tale, Vassili was changed into a cornflower after falling for the siren call of the nymph Russalka. The Russian name is basilek.

In Belgium, it is known as the Blue Baron, based on the legend of a baron who constantly wore the flower, and married a young girl of low degree after watching her place a flower at the statue of the Virgin.

The German Kaiser William I chose the flower as a personal emblem, as it epitomized "Prussian Blue".

Solstitialis means happening or appearing on the summer solstice, June 21st.

Knap is from the Old English **KNAP**, and in turn from the Anglo Saxon, **CNAEPP** meaning knob or button, referring to the knob like flower heads.

Calcitrapa is named after the metal traps with four spikes, called caltrops, used long ago on European battlefields to injure horses. Nasty!

Sweet Sultan is named in honor of the Sultan of Constantinople. The flowers have a distinct honey-like aroma. Erythraea means red.

Centaurea genus includes the introduced Centaury and Cornflower, from Europe, as well as a number of invasive plants considered obnoxious or prohibited weeds. The latter are of particular interest, as they are under-utilized in northern materia medica, and plentiful for harvest by the innovative herbalist/wild crafter.

Yellow Star Thistle is an annual or biennial that has been introduced to the prairies, probably with other flower seeds.

Yellow star thistle has been found responsible for a Parkinson-like disease in horses called nigropallidal encephalomalacia, or "chewing disease". Repin is toxic to neurons in vitro and rats in vivo, suggesting it is the agent responsible for brain lesions in horses.

Work by Craig et al, 1994 suggests that ninhydrin is neurotoxic to mouse brain tissue. Or it may be the carboxy-atractyloside and derivatives. Who knows? These compounds are being researched for potential treatment of Parkinson's disease, albeit in small doses.

Solstitialin A 13-acetate and cynaropicrin are cytotoxic to cells from the substantia nigra in rat's brains. This may be contributing factor to chewing disease.

According to Grieve, the yellow star thistle seeds were made into a powder and drunk, in wine for treating stones. The powdered root was considered also a cure for stones and anal fistula.

I was in California, while editing this chapter; and the next day found Star Thistle Honey in the deli section of a store.

In that state alone, Star Thistle covers over 8 million acres. Recently, a weevil (*Bangasternus orientalis*; and a peacock fly (*Chaetorellia australis*) have been introduced to try and keep Yellow Star Thistle under control. It is considered one of the most ecologically and economically damaging invasive species in western United States.

Experiments have shown that a single peacock fly can tunnel into and eat more than 90% of the developing seeds in a flower head. Recently, it has been discovered that a False Peacock Fly (*C. succinea*) was accidentally released, and appears even more effective. Since it was not approved, there is some concern it may attack safflower and native Cirsium thistles.

The herb has historical usage for medicinal purpose. A Neanderthal grave of Shanidar IV in Iraq, contained this herb and others of medicinal value.

Purple Star Thistle is an introduced annual/biennial that can reach over six feet in height.

Culpepper says the powdered seed taken in wine "provokes urine and helps to break the stone and drive it forth".

The powdered root, taken in wine is "very profitable for fistulas in any part of the body.

Purple Star Thistle has been studied as a milk rennet substitute. Work conducted by Tavaria et al in Portugal (1997), showed that protease extracts from Purple Star Thistle had the highest generalized proteolytic activity per milligram of protein compared with animal rennet. It also exhibited higher specificity toward sheep and goat caseinates, suggesting it could be used as an alternative rennet to produce high quality cheeses, when high proteolysis rates are required in initial stages of ripening.

This is great news, since many plant rennets used in the past, either resulted in bitterness in final product or low cheese yield due to low clotting power. There is no commercial product presently available.

In Egyptian folk medicine, the plant is considered astringent, vulnerary, anti-ophthalmic, febrifuge, stomachic, diuretic, and used for intermittent fevers, eye disease and headaches.

The seeds are used to treat kidney stones and accompanying pain.

The young scales of the flower head can be steamed like artichoke. One botanist noted in the 19th century that the plants were used for nephritis and kidney stones.

Bachelor's Buttons are an annual commonly grown in gardens, and a very successful escapee. The flower heads range from white to pink, purple to blue.

It is the most widely grown annual/biennial in the world, and the national flower of Germany.

Its honey is medium bright, with an intense yellow-green color. The honey was used on digital dermatitis, on an organic dairy farm, and showed significant faster healing than control group. Oelschlaegel S et al, *J Agric Food Chem* 2012 60(47):11811-20.

In ancient Egypt, mummies were decorated with garlands of cornflowers, as it was said that they were a sign of Horus and Osiris victory over God's enemies. King Tut had such a floral necklace.

Cornflower, or Bachelor's Buttons were once cultivated for the making of inks and blue dyes, more permanent when mixed with alum.

Even today, they are a delightful addition of colour to potpourri.

It is considered a magical herb related to Venus, water, and of course, love.

Women wear this flower on their breast to attract the love of a man.

Or, the flower is put in a pocket and it will lose or retain its freshness in accordance with good or bad success in amorous pursuits.

In Victorian times, the flower became an emblem of that delicacy which marks the devotion of an inferior, feeding upon hope, the realization of which he does not look for. It symbolizes purity, and has a birth date of August 3rd.

In Austria, it is a political symbol of neo-Nazi and right wing politics. In Poland, it is the national flower.

The famous French eyewash Eau de Casse lunettes, was made from cornflower.

The famed herbalist Parkinson (1629) reported that they were used "as a cooling cordial, and commended by some to be a remedy, not only against the plague and pestilential diseases, but against the poison of scorpions and spiders."

Grieve, in her famous herbal, says "the cornflower, with its star-like blossoms of brilliant blue, is one of our most striking wild-flowers, though it is always looked on as an unwelcome weed by the farmer, for not only does it by its presence withdraw nourishment from the ground that is needed by the corn, but its tough stems in former days of hand-reaping were wont to blunt the reaper's sickle, earning it the name of Hurt-Sickle".

Russian peasants understood the value of cornflower in their rye fields. They observed that it grew better with some of this "weed" scattered throughout the crop. And to honour this companionship, they decorated the first sheaf of rye harvest with a cornflower wreath and placed it before their icons.

In Poland, the juice from the petals was used as a blue dye for wool and paints; and the dry flower as an additive to incense. Infused flower hair rinses were said to cure dandruff. Cornflower extract is found in skin creams like Revlon Moon Drops Extra Gentle Cleanser for sensitive, delicate skin.

Various artists used cornflowers on the head of angels and saints.

Cornflower has blue blossoms when growing on limestone or alkaline soil, and pink flowers in acidic. The redder the flower, in fact, the more acidic the soil.

Cornflower is the floral symbol of the ALS society, which is searching for a cause or cure for sufferers of amyotrophic lateral sclerosis, or Lou Gehrig's disease.

In Jamaica, the plant is part of a headache cure.

Hildegard de Bingen, in the 12th century, recommended the root and leaves be mixed with deer tallow for those with failing limbs and paralysis of speech. And "if one has a broken bone… he should often drink cornflower or its root mixed in wine or water, and the broken bone will become firmly united."

The wildflower is becoming an endangered species in England, due to intensive agricultural practices.

Recent initiatives to re-introduce the plant into wild meadows are showing some success. Cornflower seeds escape from the parent plant by "crawling", as if equipped by a hydraulic motor. They have a coronet of bristles at one end, with short, stiff thorns pointing forward. In dry weather the bristles spread out, and in damp weather they close up, and in this way the seeds are pulled along the ground as the pointed hairs dig into the dirt.

It is a hyper-accumulator of nickel, and moderate gatherer of iron, copper, zinc and aluminum.

Twining's tea blend Lady Gray uses bachelor button as an herbal ingredient.

Perennial Cornflower is larger than its more famous cousin, and well suited to prairie conditions. The showy flowers bloom in June and sporadically for the rest of the summer. They tend to self-sow easily.

Russian Knapweed is a troublesome, introduced perennial weed to the prairies. A nematode, *Paranguina picridis,* is being utilized as a biological control and is artificially spread by spraying suspensions containing the nematode. It seems to be working in areas introduced, with plant galls developing on plants.

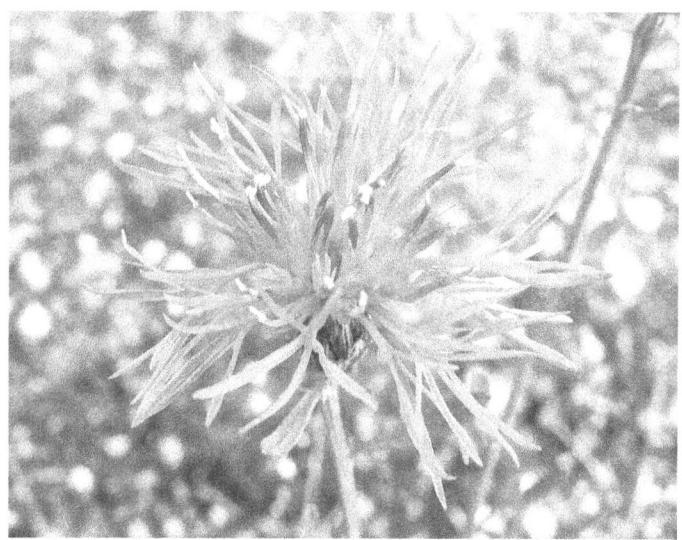

SPOTTED KNAPWEED

Spotted Knapweed has bright purple flowers, and is often found beside railways. An anti-bacterial substance was isolated from the plant by Cavallito CJ and Bailey JH, *J Bacteriol* 1949 57(2):207-12

More recently, Bais et al, *Plant Physiol* 2002 128 identified the anti-microbial activity of catechin from a rhizo-secreted racemic mixture from Spotted Knapweed.

This is probably the Knapweed written upon by Culpepper. He describes the herb as being "singularly good in all running sores, cancerous and fistulous, drying up of the moisture and healing them up so gently, without sharpness; it doth the like to running sores or scabs of the head or other parts.

It is of special use for the soreness of the throat, swelling of the uvula and jaws, and excellently good to stay bleeding, and heal up all green wounds".

Spotted Knapweed root contains catechin and has been blamed for causing oxidative stress against other plants. A USDA study found, however, that the plant acts as a potent anti-oxidant to the soil, helping restore microbial life and cleansing free radicals and toxicity. The compound may be useful as natural herbicide.

Diffuse Knapweed contains phytotoxins that help facilitate nutrient uptake for the plant particularly iron, bringing this valuable mineral to the surface of alkaline soils this plant favors.

Diffuse Knapweed is smaller, with white or creamy flowers. It has been used for Amara (bitters), according to Racz et al, 1963.

Both Diffuse and Spotted Knapweed are controlled biologically with the gallfly (*Urophora* sp.), or the root-boring beetle, *Sphenoptera jugoslavica*.

Introduction of the gallfly has created another, unexpected, problem. The insects lay eggs in the seed head, and the plant forms a gall around them. When the larvae hatch, they eat the seeds. Deer mice have learned to climb the stalk above snow levels and eat the resting larvae. This has resulting in a tripling of mice numbers and with them the level of hanta-virus that leads to a nasty respiratory viral infection.

In Alberta, about 370 acres of rangeland are overrun with these two plants, which can produce up to one thousand seeds per plant. In Montana, it covers some 1.6 million hectares.

Sweet Sultan is an introduced purple flowering annual. It has a lovely musky fragrance, with Parkinson writing, "it surpasses the best civet that ever is" and may have some future in perfume and aromatherapy work.

Greater Knapweed has been used in traditional medicine for centuries, for coughs, diuretic and diaphoretic purposes, cancer, and eye inflammation.

Giant Knapweed (*C. gigantea*) is rich in chlorogenic acid, believed responsible for anti-cancer benefit in colon carcinoma. Shoeb et al, *J Nat Med* 2007 61:2.

Centaury was considered a plant of luck by the Celts. It is used in vermouth and has similar properties as gentian. It is widely produced in Europe and North Africa as a commercial cultivated crop. It is an annual/biennial that could be grown on the prairies. Wild populations are becoming rare in Europe.

The flower opens only in fine weather and closes after noon, in cool or rainy weather or when touched. It readily self sows.

It is sometimes known as Red Gentian, and prized in Britain for promoting appetite, strengthening the nerves, colic, bilious and kidney problems and stopping hemorrhage.

A large quantity of charred remains were discovered in an excavated Roman army hospital on the Rhine river. The Romans called the herb "bile of the earth" or **FEL TERRAE** in reference to its extreme bitterness.

Lonicerus writes, "the herb, drunk each day morning and evening, kills and drives out the worm".

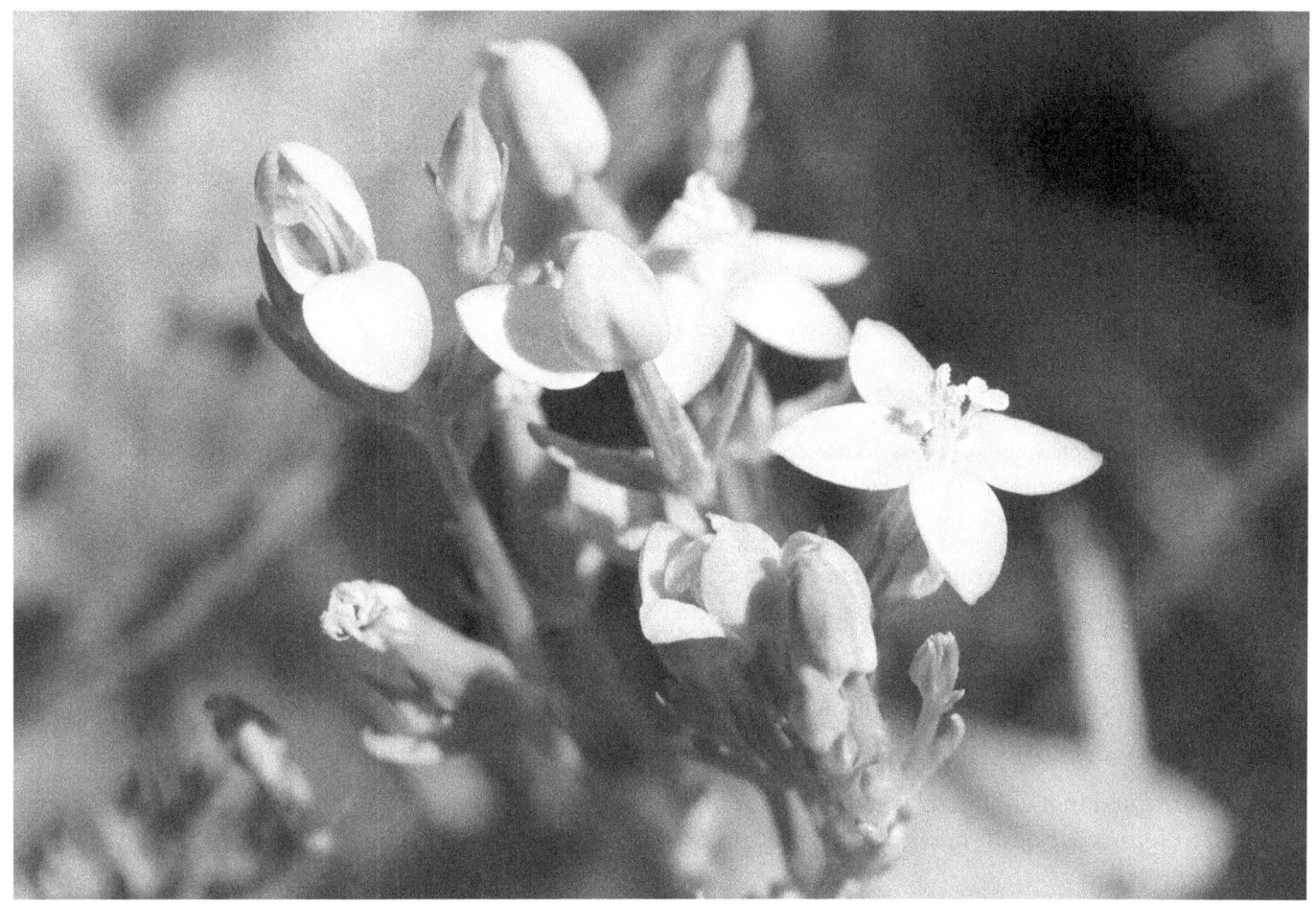

CENTAURY

MEDICINAL

CONSTITUENTS- *C. solstilatis*- aerial parts- orientin, homoorientin, and schaftoside (flavonoid C-glycosides), calcitrapic acid, cenaturin, acroptilin, repin (sesquiterpene lactone), centaurepensin (chlorohyssopifolin A, chlorojanerin and 13-acetyl solstitialin A), solstitialin A and its 13-acetate, cynaropicrin, diol monoacetate and aquerin B (guaianolides); guaianolide diol monoacetate; arctigenin and matairesinol (lignans); chlorinated sesquiterpenes; scopoletin and umbelliferone (coumarins); two chromenes, eupatoriochromene and encecalin, asparitic and glutamic acid; tyramine. Also contains subluteolide, janerin, stizolicin, solstitiolide, epi-solstitiolide, epi-centaurepensin, elegin, chlorohydrin of cynaropicrin, desacylcynaropicrin, 8-hydroxyzaluzanin C, 8-desacylsauprin, deacylaguerin A, 15-deoxyrepin, salograviolide C, cynaropicrin, sauprin, linichlorin B, linochlorin A, 8-desacylrepin, chlorohyssopifolin A, acroptilin, elegin, 19-deoxychlorojanerin, chlorojanerin, cebellin C, 17,18-epoxy-19-deoxy-chlorojanerin, solstiziolide, epi-solstiziolide, hyrcanin, centaurepensin, cebellin D,

C. cyanus- flowers- caffeic and D-quinic acids; centaurine, chlorogenic, polygalacturonic and neocholorogenic acids, coumarins including chichoriin, scopoletin and umbelliferone; six flavonoid aglycones, eight flavonoid glycosides, including quercimetrin; 4 hydroxycinnamic acid; apigenin and cyanidin glucosides, anthocyanins pelargonin and cyanin; polysaccharides such as galacturonic acid, arabinose, glucose, rhamnose and galactose, sesquiterpene lactones including cnicin; and numerous amino acids. Clanin, a blue colouring material is found in the flowers as well.

Seeds- indole alkaloids moschamine, cis-moschamine, centcyamine, and cis-centcyamine

C. calcitrapa- calcitrapin, centaurin (cnicin–a bitter principle), isocnicin, gums, resins, calcitrapic acid, 11beta,14-dehydrosalonitenolide, 11alpha, 13-dihydrosalonitenolide, aplotaxene, salonitenolide, scabiolide, squalene, phytol, taraxasterol, 5,7,-dihydroxy-6,3',4'-trimethoxyflavone, bisabalone derivatives. Alkaloids total 0.08%, with a total of ten, including stizolphine, and choline. Sugars include stachyose, raffinose, melibiose, sucrose, glucose and fructose.

Various lipids are also present in the plant, consisting of 37.78% linolenic acid, 34.28% linoleic acid, 15.3% palmitic acid and traces of myristic, oleic and stearic acids. Unsaponifiables include beta sitosterol and beta amyrin.

Flowers- aspartic proteinase.

C. repens- polyacetylenes, taraxasterol, thiophenes, repdiolide, epoxyrepdiolide, repin, repinsolide, solstitiolide, guaianolides, chlororepdiolide, cynaro-picrin, cnicin or centaurine (a bitter), centaurepensin, elegin, janerin, aguerin, and acroptilin.

flowers- cyanidine (a glycoside)

root— thiophene derivatives

C. montana- flowers- contain glucosyl-3-cyanidine and diglycosyl 1-3-5-cyanidine (anthocyanins)

whole plant- 35 acetylenes, 3 monothiophenes, and 4 tetraenic aldehydes, aplotaxene, agigenin, apigenin 3-methyl ether and arctigenin (lignan).

C. macrocephala leaf- apigenin, apigenin-4'-methyl ether, scutellarein-6.7-dimethyl ether, scutellarein-6,7,4'-trimethyl ether, luteolin, luteolin-3'-methyl ether and several methyl derivatives of 6-hydroxyluteolin,

Seeds- arctiin, lappaol A, malairesinol, malairesinoside.

C. scabiosa aerial parts- flavonoids and their glycosides, glucuronic acid, poly-acetylenes

seeds- four lignans including matairesinol and matairesinoside.

C. nigra- seeds- two serotonin conjugates, N-(trans-p-coumaroyl)-serotonin, and N- (trans-feruloyl)-serotonin (maoschamine).

C. erythraea herb- secoiridoids including gentiopicroside, sweroside and swertiamarin; various alkaloids including gentianine, gentianidine, and gentioflavine; xanthol derivatives, phenolic acids, ferulic and sinapic acids, triterpenes including alpha and beta amyrin, maslinic acid as well as erythrodiol and sitosterols, including brassicasterol and stigmasterol.

C. gigantea- salonitenolide, cynarosides,

Centaurea species contain a vast array of anthocyanins and flavonoids as flower pigments. Mishio T et al, *Nat Prod Commun* 2015 10(3):447-50 have teased out the entire range of eleven species, for those with interest in these compounds.

Yellow Star thistle is an unrecognized, and yet useful medicinal plant.

Studies conducted by Akbar et al, at the University of the Pacific, California in 1995, showed that isolated repin from yellow star thistle produced highly significant hypothermia in laboratory studies.

The hypothermia was long lasting, peaking at three hours and returning to normal temperature after eight.

It was determined that cholinergic, serotonergic, histaminergic and dopaminergic receptors were not actively involved in repin's action. Propranolol, a beta adrengenic agent, accentuated its effects. More study would be useful.

Water extracts of yellow star thistle also showed significant anti-ulcer activity in studies by Yesilada et al, *J Ethnopharm* 2004 95(2-3):213-9 at Gazi University in Ankara, Turkey.

In September of 1999, the same author published information showing both flowers and herb destroy *Helicobacter pylori*, the bacteria believed responsible for many cases of gastric ulcers. *Journal of Ethnopharmacology* 66:3.

Akkol et al, in same journal, 2009 122(2):210-15 found antinociceptive and antipyretic activity in the plant. Gurbez & Yesilada, *J Ethnopharm* 2007 112(2):284-91, identified the compounds as chlorojanerin, 13-acetyl solstitialin A, and solstitialin A.

Centaurepensin has been found to possess cytotoxic activity.

Solstitialin exhibits very high anti-proliferative activity on C6 (rat brain tumor cells), and HeLa (human uterine carcinoma) cell lines. Erenier R et al, *Comb Chem High Throughput Screen* 2016 19(1):66-72. The content of this compound is highest in stems.

Ozcelik et al, *Microbiol Res* 2009 164(5):545-52 found 13-acetyl solstitialin A showed remarkable antibiotic effect against *E. faecalis* at just 1 microg/ml; very similar to ampicillin. Anti-viral activity against DNA virus from same compound was as potent as acyclovir.

Both solstitialin A 13-acetate and cynaropicrin, however, have been shown to be toxic to horses and rats. The latter shows potent activity on acute lymphoblastic leukemia and its multidrug-resistant subline. Formisano C et al, *Fitoterapia* 2017 June 1.

Acetone extracts of the flower inhibit glutathione peroxidase, and glutathione S-transferase, suggestive of strong anti-oxidant capacity. Koc S et al, *Pharm Biol* 2015 53(5):746-51.

Star Thistle was considered by early Eclectic physicians to be similar in usage to Blessed Thistle for the treatment of intermittent fevers, inflammation, hepatitis, jaundice arthritis, and epilepsy. External applications were used for shingles (herpes zoster) pain.

Some early herbalists consider it more similar to gentian, with bitter tonic effect on digestion. Both are probably correct.

This herb and cornflower release a volatile oil that attracts the weevil, *Ceratapion basicorne.*

Cornflower, or Bachelor's Button is an excellent nervine herb. According to Juliette De Bairacli Levy, it should be grown in every pasture as it "strengthens the nerves to a degree not excelled by any other plant".

It is a valuable tonic and digestive aid; with mildly laxative properties. It is also useful for a variety of eye problems including chronic inflammation weak eyes and dimness of sight. For this purpose the hydrosol left over from distillation is best.

The herbal extract can be used in hair tonics.

The flowers are diuretic, as well as anti-inflammatory, anti-microbial, and slightly cholagogue in action. They help to improve digestion and support the liver by improving resistance to infection. This is due, in part to the content of centaurine, a bitter compound also found in Centaury. Cnicin is weakly antibiotic.

Research by Garbacki et al, *Journal of Ethnopharmacology* 1999 68:1-3 confirmed polysaccharides in flower heads exhibit anti-inflammatory activity, and interfere with complement.

The leaves are more powerful than the flowers against human acute T leukemia cell lines. Wegiera et al, *Acta Pol Pharm* 2012 69:2.

Moschamine, from seeds, may suppress cAMP formation via binding to two 5-HT1 receptors, and exhibits serotoninergic activity. It also inhibits COX-1 and COX-2. Park JB et al, *Nat Prod Res* 2012 26(16):1465-72.

This compound is also moderately active against cervical, breast and skin cancer cell lines. Csapi B et al, *Phytother Research* 2010 24(11): 16664-9. Cnicin, in flowers also exerted anti-tumor activity in same study.

Cornflower is a reliable bitter and diuretic, found in many recipes for cosmetic purpose. The flower, in action, may be thought of as similar to blessed thistle.

The flowers are often added to tisanes and herbal teas, for their colour.

The seeds have been used as a mild laxative tea for children.

Decoctions of the leaves have been used to treat rheumatism and nerve disorders.

Flower infusions are a traditional remedy for tired eyes, using a cool, well-strained infusion in an eye cup.

Under the Doctrine of signatures, cornflower was for blue eyes, and plantain for brown.

Purple Star Thistle flowers have been used for reducing fevers, the root as a diuretic; both similar to Milk Thistle.

It may be used as a substitute for Blessed Thistle.

I don't know if the seed has been analyzed for any similarity, but is worthy of investigation. In Europe, the seed is listed as a diuretic, and made palatable by crushing and adding to white wine.

Infusions of the leaves and flowering tops help relieve fevers and general debility. The roots and seed are diuretic, the leaves and flowers a better febrifuge.

For a more potent blend, combine with the leaves of angelica, wormwood and willow bark.

There is some experimental evidence that the leaves and flowers are anti-diabetic. Work by Pieroni et al, found the whorls of Purple Knapweed both anti-oxidant and inhibit xanthine oxidase, implicated in gout and other age related disease. *Phytother Res* 2002 16:5.

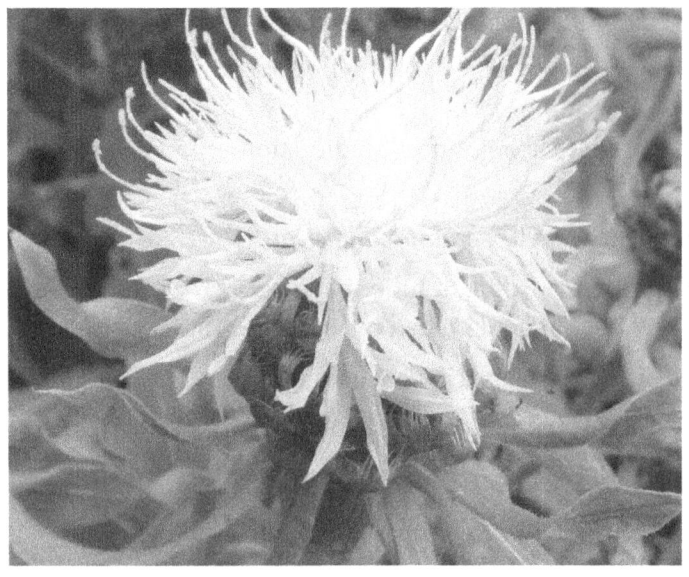
GLOBE KNAPWEED

Chickweed was also found to exhibit XO inhibiting activity in same study.

Russian Knapweed (*R. repens*) contains centaurepensin, a known cytotoxic compound. The closely related *C. nigra* has been used as a substitute for gentian as a general tonic in the past. It contains both centaurein and jacein that exhibit anti-viral activity against herpes and poliovirus. Kaij-Kamb et al, 1992.

Cnicin, from Centaurea species, shows strong activity against prostate cancer cell lines (PC-3). Sen A et al, *Pharm Biol* 2017 55(1):541-546.

Ethanol and water extracts of *C. nigra* show activity against *Staphylococcus aureus*, including methicillin resistant strains, and *Bacillus cereus*. Kenny O et al, *Food Chem* 2014 161:79-86.

C. montana is used for the same purposes as Cornflower. Sweet Sultan is anti-spasmodic, tonic and stimulates the circulation of the blood.

Greater Knapweed seeds contain lignans with anti-bacterial, anti-oxidant and ecdysteroid agonist/antagonist activity. Maitairesinoside is most active against *Pseudomonas aeruginosa, as well as E. coli,* and *Bacillus cereus;* whereas matairesinol was effective against methacillin resistant *Staphylococcus aureus* at 1 mg/mL. Kumarasamy et al, *Pharm Bio* 2003 41:3.

The seeds also contain lappaol A and arctiin, the latter also present in burdock seed. Shoeb et al, *DARU* 2004 12:3.

Both *C. macrocephala and C. scabiosa* show mild activity against *S. aureus*. Osborn et al, Br J Exp Path 1943 24.

The related *C. gigantea* contains chlorogenic acid that has been shown to possess activity against cancer of the colon.

Globe Knapweed seeds contain various lignans with anti-oxidant activity. Notable is the presence of arctiin, also found in burdock seeds.

Spotted Knapweed (*C. maculosa*) leaf extracts show activity against *Staphylococcus aureus, E. coli, Pseudomonas aeruginosa* and *Candida albicans*. Borchardt et al, *J Med Plants Res* 2008 2:5.

Sweet Sultan (*C. moschata*) contains 20-hydroxy-ecdysterones. It is easily grown and could be a medicinal source of this valuable compound.

Work at the U. of New Brunswick found that the related *C. sonchifolia* showed in vitro cytotoxic activity against carcinoma cell line KB, and antibacterial activity against *Staphylococcus aureus*.

Diffuse Knapweed shows activity against 12 different microbial organisms. Skliar et al, Fitotherapia 2005 76:7-8.

Centaury is used as a reliable bitter digestive and stimulant in the manner of Gentian. The flowering top of the biennial is used, instead of the root. Centaury aids weak stomach function, poor appetite and liver gall bladder insufficiency. It can be useful, like Calamus or Angelica root, for anorexia nervosa, combining well for specific indications.

It is worth noting that bitters do not appear to increase digestive secretions in healthy patients with normal appetite and whose reflex secretion is already optimal.

It has a bitter number of 1:4,000,000, meaning that one drop of centapicrin (secoiridoid glucoside) in four million parts of water is detectable to taste.

Still, its relative bitterness is only half of gentian and one third of wormwood.

Kumarasamy et al, *J Ethnopharm* 2002 83:1-2 showed anti-bacterial activity of seeds against three of 11 pathogenic bacteria using methanol extracts, including activity against methicillin resistant *Staphylococcus aureus*.

Work by Mroueh et al, *Phytotherapy Research* 18:5 has found alcohol extracts of the herb help prevent acetaminophen induced liver damage.

In rats fed a high fat diet to induce diabetes, the herb showed significant benefit. Hamza et al, *J Ethnopharm* 2010 128:2.

Leaf extracts appear to prevent beta cell damage in the pancreas. Sefi et al, *J Ethnopharmacology* 135:2.

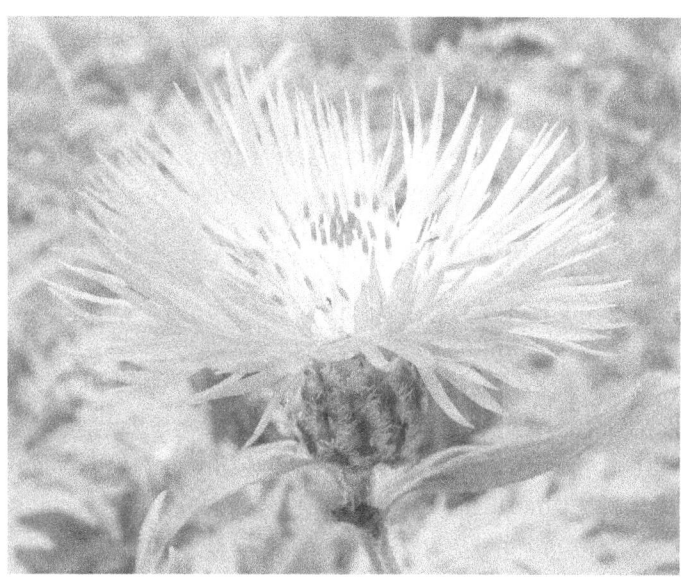

SPOTTED KNAPWEED

An herbal combination (Canephron N) of centaury, lovage root and rosemary was given to 59 patients with diabetic nephropathy. After six months the level of microalbuminaria decreased significantly compared to control. End stage renal disease occurs in up to 30% of diabetic patients, making this a significant finding. Martynyuk L et al, *J Altern Complement Med* 2014 20(6):472-8.

Intestinal bacteria convert swertiamarin into erythcentaurin and its reduced product 5-hydroxymethyl-isochroman-1-one. Some species convert it into gentianine, thus its comparison to Gentian species.

The herb contains maslinic acid that ameliorates NMDA receptor blockage-induced schizophrenia-like behaviors in mice. Kim H et al, *Planta Medica* 2016 81 (S01):S1-S381. Maslinic acid is found in olive fruit.

Swertiamarin shows activity against *Proteus mirabilis, Serratia marcescens, Bacillus cernus, B. subtilis, E. coli* and *Citrobactor freundii*. Sweroside also showed activity against last five bacteria above and *Staphylococcus epidermidis*. Kumarasamy et al, *Phytomed* 2003 10.

Centaury protects against ASA induced damage, in an animal study. Tuluce Y et al, *Toxicol Ind Health* 2011 27(8):760-8.

The related *C. ainetensis* contains salogravolide A, which has been found to possess activity against epidermal squamous cell carcinogenesis. Ghantous et al, *Int J Oncol* 2008 32:4.

The related *C. jacea* contains centaureidin, that shows activity against HeLa, MCF7 and A431 cancer cell lines. Forgo et al, *Fitoterapia* 2012 April 17. Centaureidin is also present in *Bidens pilosa*, mentioned earlier.

HOMEOPATHY

Centaurea solstitialis is used for surging of blood, homesickness, and intermittent fever.

It is used for mistakes in writing, misnaming things, difficulty spelling.

There is a desire to talk, not write. Desire to whisper. Word play, sing song, witty and mesmerizing sounds.

Feeling comfortable in group, collective ancestry, missing family, dreams of family.

Ears feel stopped up, tight throat, lump in esophagus, difficulty swallowing.

Vision watery when first focusing, allergies involved nose, sinus, eyes, watery puffy, congested, worse from cats.

Right shoulder joint sore, as if punched, better from massage.

DOSE- 5C to 30C. Proving by Osner and Quinn on three females and three males at up to 5C. Seven provers at 30C and 40C in 2007.

Canchalagua (*Erythraea venusta*), also known as Centaury is used extensively for fever and a bitter tonic. It is used in severe types of intermittent fever in hot countries. Sensation of drops, falling from and upon different spots. The skin is wrinkled like a washerwoman's. Scalp feels tight as if drawn together by India rubber.

DOSE- Tincture in drop dose. Must be made from the fresh plant, as its medicinal properties are lost in the dry.

ESSENTIAL OIL

Centaury has no scent but if the stems are cut and immersed in warm water for twenty-four hours and then distilled, a thin green oil is produced. It has a most penetrating odour that is quite agreeable.

Star Thistle (*C. solstitialis*) essential oil contains over 30% hexadecanoic acid and 25% carophyllene oxide, as well as alpha linolenic acid, germacrene D and heptacosane. The oil shows good inhibition potential against *Pseudomonas aeruginosa, E. coli* and all tested fungi. Carev I et al, *Chem Biodivers* 2016 August 23.

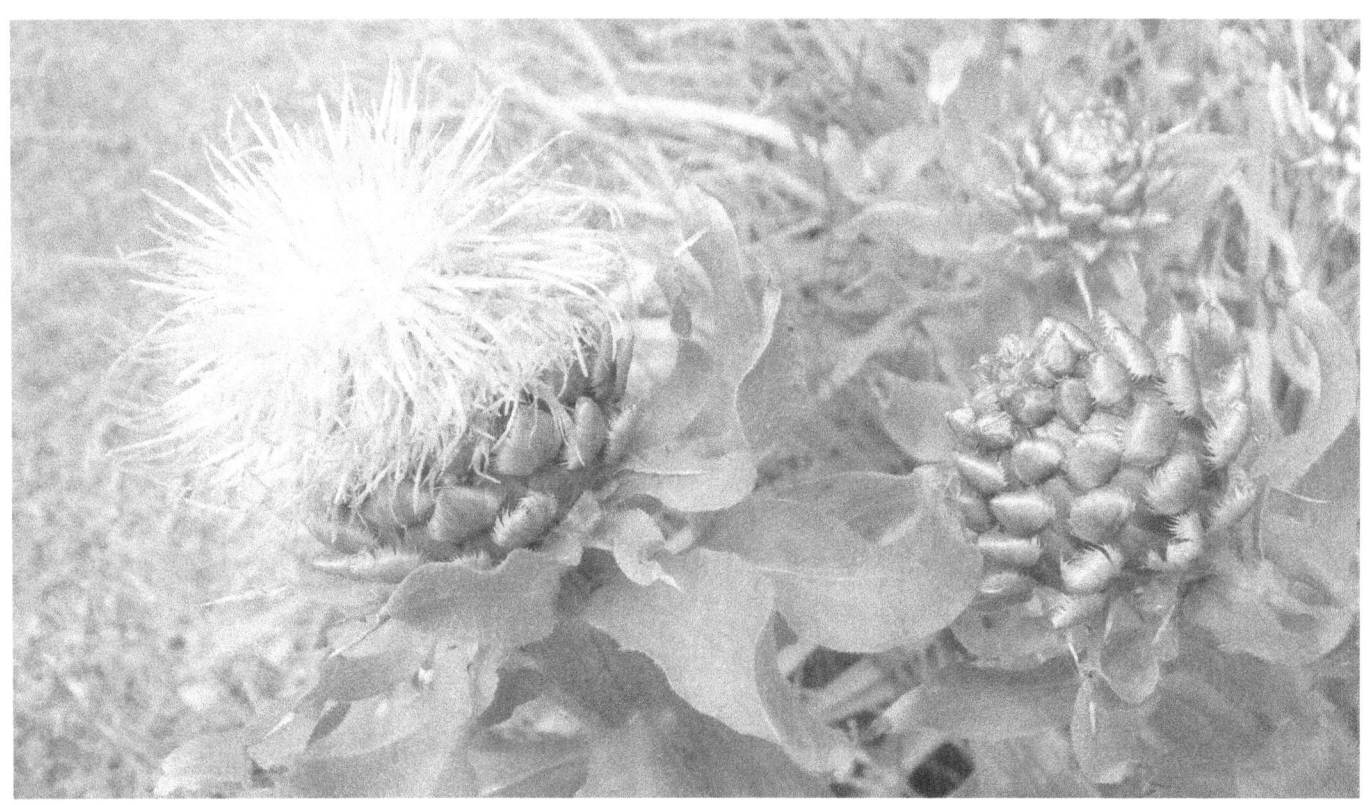

GLOBE KNAPWEED

HYDROSOLS

CONSTITUENTS- linalool 16-61%, terpinen-4-ol 5-6%, alpha terpineol 7-11%, eucalypol 4%, borneol up to 4%, camphor 4% and minor components.

Cornflower hydrosol scent goes from none when cold to faintly floral when warm. It tastes slightly green with a mild bitter aftertaste.

Cornflower water has been used for centuries as eyewash and for dry and delicate skin types. The famous French eyewash, Eau de casse lunettes, is simply Cornflower hydrolat.

It is often combined with oils and emulsifiers in a wide range of creams and lotions as a moisturizer.

It can be used as a douche for urinary tract infections.

For young infants, a tsp at a time can be tried for reducing fevers.

Suzanne Catty recommends it not be taken internally in the first trimester due to hormonal constituents, as well a mild diuretic and douche for reproductive and urinary infections.

Brunschwig, in his Book of Distillation published in 1530, suggested the water for spots in the eye, skin cankers, and such.

Jeanne Rose suggests the hydrolat to tone creped skin, and is the esthetician's choice for dry, devitalized and mature or bruised skin.

Caroline Ingraham writes, "Cornflower aromatic water is especially popular with dogs but also frequently selected by horses and inhaled (sometimes licked) by cats. Since cornflowers are renowned for their therapeutic effectiveness with eye problems, they could then be attributed to opening the inner (third) eye [?], which is perhaps why animals select this remedy if they are 'shut down'.

Animals also often select cornflower water after surgery, perhaps for its soporific effect".

The pH ranges from 4.7 to 5.

Star Thistle distilled water, being drank, doth help the French disease (syphilis), to open the obstructions of the liver, and cleanse the blood from corrupted humours, and is profitable against the quotidian or tertian ague.
BAPTISTA SARDAS

Centaury water is distilled from leaves and flowers. It warms the stomach, and removes worms from the belly. It helps heal broken bones, increases appetite, especially of choleric and phlegmatic temperaments, gout in the bowel, podagra and sciatica. It also removes dead fetus from the womb. **BRUNSCHWIG**

The distilled water of Centaury comforts a cold stomach, helps in fever of choler, it kills worms and provokes appetite. **CULPEPPER**

FLOWER ESSENCES

Star Thistle is for those individuals basing their actions on a fear of lack, with an inability to give freely and openly, or to trust a higher providence.

The positive qualities include a generous and inclusive personality, with a giving and sharing a nature, and feeling an inner sense of abundance. **FLOWER ESSENCE SOCIETY**

Russian Centaurea (*C. repens*) flower essence teaches the strong hearted that there are times to keep your flame alight but hidden. For those one might bring undue attention from forces seeking to destroy you. With resolute calmness, one waits for the right moment. **LIVING ESSENCES**

Bachelor's Button (*C. cyanus*) flower essence is about conscious expression. It is about bringing into form a sense of gentleness and quiet, and at the same time a clear ability to express ideas. It is very useful for writers to bring into form ideas that might be controversial and have them more easily accepted. It is about understanding the truth about something. **PEGASUS**

Star Thistle (*C. solstitialis*) flower essence is about spiritual awakening.

It assists individuals in radiating energy. Energies of the 9th and 10th chakras are activated (especially with the visualization of gold and silver colours). **PEGASUS**

Centaury is indicated for kind, gentle people who are over-anxious to serve others. They become servants rather than willing helpers, thus neglecting their own mission in life. Meek, submissive and imposed upon because of their good nature. **BACH**

"These people, in their striving for power, have lost their sense of proportion of their own relative position and importance in the world. They are noisy in speech and movement; demanding of attention; impatient; and particular over the details of their own wants and comfort. They are overbearing and full of their own achievements. Usually big of physique; high colour; tend to suffer from high blood pressure and its companion ills.

BACH (initial indications in 1930).

The flower essence has indications for servility and lack of courage to say no and stand up for oneself. These are analogous to its action on the gallbladder, the organ associated with the will and courage in traditional Chinese medicine.

JULIA GRAVES

Centaurea (*C. montana*) essence allow you to deal with the truth, flipping energy from negative to positive.

OLIVE

SPIRITUAL PROPERTIES

Cornflower represents idealism. Always the ideal beckoned from afar, awakened by the touch of the Unseen, Deserting the boundary of things achieved, aspired the strong discoverer, timeless thought, revealing at each step a luminous world.

Delicate and harmonious, it gives elegance to life.

THE MOTHER

PERSONALITY TRAITS

The dead—spectres of guilt, weedy bestowers of a profound grace—find you in a dream. They chose you and you throw up glass. Now you brush flowers from your hair—centaury, storksbill, pyramidal orchid, mallow—which fall onto a grassy hill where moths fasten on their sweetness. This 'now' you're dreaming comes without the permanence the dead have planned for you; instead summer breathes in your face.

PAUL EVANS

MYTHS AND LEGENDS

Cornflower is named after a melancholy youth who, according to classical mythology, loved flowers so much that he passed all his time in making wreaths of them. He especially admired the cornflower and longed to clothe himself in the garments of the same vivid blue. One day, Cyanus was found dead in a field, lying among the cornflowers he had gathered, and Flora, the goddess of flowers, transformed him into a cornflower as a graceful acknowledgment of his veneration for her.

POWELL

Centaurea is named after the Centaurs, whose image expressed to the early Greeks an awe of horse riding tribes.

The Centaurs were also known as Magnetes, or Great Ones.

Greek myth made the centaurs to be wild, shaggy, anarchists who battled the Lapiths, who used weapons fashioned from chipped stone.

But Centaurs were also great wizards, or shape shifters and fountainheads of ancient lore.

The centaur Cheiron of Magnesia was a teacher to Achilles, Jason, Heracles and others; and known as the son of a god "renowned for his skill in hunting, medicine, music, gymnastics and divination".

When killed by Heracles, Cheiron was made the Bowman of the Greek Zodiac.

WALKER

Chiron was the first centaur, but different than all others that were mortal or unrelated to him by blood. The "wild centaurs" were uncivilized, violent, and prone to drunkenness, rape and destruction.

Chiron was the bastard son of the immortal Greek God, Chronos, and a mortal sea-nymph, Philyra. Zeus was his half brother. The god Apollo and his sister, the goddess Artemis were his tutors. He spent much of his life in a cave on Mount Pelion. He married a water nymph, Chariclo, and fathered a daughter Euippe.

Later in life, Chiron and Hercules, his friend and former student, attended a wedding feast. Wild centaurs crashed the party and began drinking wine and raping women. Hercules fought them off, killing them with arrows dipped in a poison provided by Chiron. He was accidentally wound by one of the arrows, but because of his immortal lines did not die, but because of mortal blood, he was not immune to the poison. He developed a wound that would not heal. This led to the sacrifice of his immortality, his descent to the underworld, where he changed places with Prometheus. After nine days, Zeus raised his half brother Chiron from the underworld and transformed him into the constellation, Centaurus.

Crotus was the son of Pan the Woodland god who, like his father, loved the forests and hunting. However, through the influence of his mother Eupheme, nurse to the Muses who were his playfellows, Crotus became a skilled artist and poet.

EASON

ASTROLOGY

The knapweed proved an interesting case…In the course of their long budding season (over two months) these cases undergo considerable changes of shape, but remain the whole time as almost perfect path curve spirals… What in fact eventuates is a curve increasing in a series of fourteen day leaps…Experience in subsequent years went to show that the soli-lunar relationships are irrelevant to this phenomenon, but the peaks in the curve continued to coincide with the Moon Jupiter alignment very closely.

LAWRENCE EDWARDS

RECIPES

CORN FLOWER DECOCTION-One handful of herb to a pint of water. Gently simmer, strain, and use as eyewash or eye compress.

Two Tbsp of crushed seeds act as a laxative.

TINCTURE- Centaury is prepared, dry herb at 1:5 and 25% alcohol. It is given in doses of 20 or more drops in water before meals to stimulate appetite and digestion.

CHUFA
YELLOW NUT GRASS
YELLOW NUTSEDGE
(*Cyperus esculentus* L.)
(*C. esculentus var. sativus* Boeckler)
PURPLE NUT SEDGE
(*C. rotundus* L.)
PARTS USED- tubers, leaves

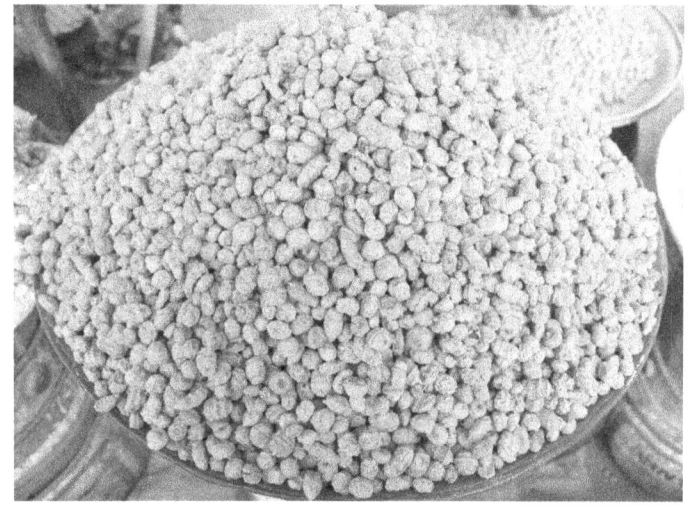

CHUFA IN MARKET PLACE

No more the grassy brook reflects the day,
But choked with sedges, works its weedy way.

OLIVER GOLDSMITH

Cyperus is from the Greek **KYPEIROS**, meaning a rush or sedge. Pliny referred to the sedges as **CYPEROS**.

Esculentus is from the Latin **ESCA**, meaning food, and **ULENTUS**, meaning abundance. Esculent also means edible, or good to eat. Rotundus means round.

Yellow nutgrass is a perennial herb found mainly in ditches, low, wet soils, and the edges of marshes and ponds. They are often confused with grasses, but are distinguished by a triangular cross section, with leaves in three rows.

It is confined to the extreme south of the prairies, mainly in Saskatchewan, Manitoba and then across Northern Ontario all the way to Newfoundland.

The Ancient Egyptians developed cultivated strains over 7000 years ago.

They called it **GYW**, and it was the third most cultivated food, after Emmer Wheat and Barley. A beverage from the tuber was drunk in Egypt around 2400 B.C. Evidence of the drink were found in Pharaoh's tombs.

The tubers were used medicinally taken orally, or smashed into an ointment, decocted as an enema, or simply fumigated for a pleasant odor. Chufa tubers are found illustrated in tombs, and archeology sites. It is probably the unnamed sweet root eaten by Abba Or during his years of asceticism in the Theban Desert.

The root was also made into a drink in a region of South Sudan, called Chut. It is locally known in Arabic as **HAB ELAZIZ**. When the Roman Empire conquered Egypt around 30 B.C., they introduced the drink into their culture and named it hordeata, hordiate or orzata. In the early 700s, the Moorish traders introduced cultivation to the Mediterranean region, including Spain. Horchata derived from the Latin hordeata in the 1200 in Valencia. The drink was offered to King Jaime I in Alboraya as "leche de chufa", or tiger nut milk.

The tuber oil was used in ancient times for soaps, perfumes and a lubricant.

The cultivated form rarely flowers, is not frost tolerant and is less aggressive in growth; but has higher starch and oil content than its wild cousin.

The tubers can be collected anytime the ground is not frozen and used raw, baked or boiled. They are very crisp when raw, and do not soften appreciably when cooked.

They taste like hazelnuts or almonds, combined with coconut, but are not crunchy like a nut. When chewed, the tubers exude sweet white milk.

Production is 7-9 tubers per plant. In experiments one tuber in the field produced 36 plants and 332 tubers in 16 weeks; in one year 1918 new plants and 6864 tubers.

Tubers grown on peat averaged 823 per square foot, or 8.9 tons per acre; compared to potatoes at 12 tons per acre. They range in size from one centimeter to 1.3 cm.

Care must be taken in digging, as the small tubers easily break off. In light, sandy soil the whole plant can be tugged up, bringing most of the tubers with it.

They can also be ground into flour by drying the tubers slowly, until they break apart instead of mash when hammered lightly. Then grind them in a blender or food mill.

The flour can be combined with wheat flour 50/50 for baking, bannock, and biscuits.

For beverage use, soak two cups of tubers in water for two days. Drain and then blend with one quart of water and 1/4 cup of honey. Let stand one hour. Strain, and drink.

Or after soaking, dry for one day, and eat like peanuts. If the tubers are soaked for a day, and then simmered with sugar and water, they become clear and tender. Remove from syrup, dry and enjoy.

In Cuba and Spain, the tubers are substituted for Almonds in making Orgeat, a syrupy drink prepared with orange flower water. When combined with sugar it is a popular soft drink called Horchata de Chufas. In West Africa, a white, jelly-like tiger-nut milk is used as a famine food.

The Zulu chew the roots for indigestion accompanied by halitosis. Zulu girls eat a porridge containing mashed roots to bring on menstruation, while in North Africa, the tubers are used as aphrodisiac spermatogens, and increase sperm count.

For a coffee substitute, roast the tubers until dark brown, grind and brew using one tablespoon per cup. It is pleasant and similar to roasted cereal drinks.

Dioscorides mentioned their use in comforting the stomach; and in fact the tubers are a great digestive aid.

Gerard, the English herbalist mentioned they help respiratory complaints, coughs, and the "heate and sharpnesse of the urine".

After their introduction to North America, the Navaho-Ramah began using the plant as a ceremonial emetic. The Pima tribe chewed the roots for coughs and colds.

They poulticed the roots to apply to snake bites, and placed the chewed root in their horse's nostrils as a stimulant.

The Paiute crushed the tubers and combined them with tobacco leaves as a wet dressing to help treat athlete's foot. It is believed the Paiute cultivated it on a large scale.

Remains of several hundred charred nut grass tubers, were found in two pit ovens during archeological excavations at San Antonio Terrace. Miksicek, *Plant Processing on the San Antonio Tracce* 1998.

The Spanish make a refreshing cold drink, as is, or used as part of a more potent concoction. One popular alcoholic drink is made by partially freezing the beverage and then, adding equal rum as a sort of wild daiquiri. I'll have to try that!

The Russians have studied Chufa (*C. esculentus*) extensively for their cultivation requirements, and biochemical composition (especially lipids).

With continuous illumination, chufa yields a high total of productivity and economic effectiveness. The tubers have the optimal ratio of proteins, carbohydrates, and fats containing essential fatty acids to meet human daily requirements.

The tubers are sometimes called Tiger Nuts, or Earth Almonds.

The best-known food use is the production of Milk of Chufa. It has been used successfully in flavoring ice cream.

In order to do this, a daily production of 150-200 grams of dry chufa tubers is necessary for sustenance. This could be used in sealed life support systems like outer space, or the Biosphere in Arizona.

Work by Adebajo at Ogun State University in Nigeria, investigated the levels of invert sugars in the tubers. It was found that at 10 to 20 degrees Celsius, the invert sugar count increased during the forty day test. Yeasts were found to increase the hydrolysis of sucrose from juice extracts.

At the present time, Yellow Nut sedge is not grown commercially in Canada, because of some harvesting problems, but mostly due to economics.

In fact, it is considered a weed in Manitoba, and has been ranked as the 16th worst weed in the world.

Both the tubers and seeds are enjoyed by waterfowl and other birds, and ranked one of the top ten most important waterfowl foods.

Recently, it is undergoing a revival in several European countries, Israel and the United States. It is grown in the southeastern states as an animal feed.

The tops are rich in salts, and have been traditionally gathered, dried and burned into ash, as a salt substitute; or used to cover dried meat for storage as both a surface sealant and fly repellent.

The tubers have been studied and during trans-esterification produce methyl and ethyl esters, suggesting biofuel potential. Barminas et al, 2001.

Recent work suggests waste hydrolysate is better fuel for *Chlorella vulgaris*, suggesting use as potential feedstock for biodiesel production. Wang W et al, *Bioresour Technol* 2013 136:24-9. This algae is a prized nutraceutical for the health industry, as well.

The related annual *C. squarrosus* and perennial *C. schweinitzii* are rare in southern Alberta.

The related Purple or Red Nut sedge, *C. rotundus,* is a well known medicinal, and found from Florida to New York and west to Minnesota and Oregon. It has long been prized for edibility, despite its bitter taste. It was used as an aromatic in ancient Egypt, Greece as a perfume and medicine.

Dioscorides, Galen, Serapion, Avicenna and Rhazes have described its health benefits as stomachic, emmenagogue and de-obstruent.

The rhizome is known as **SUO CAO** in Mandarin, **HEUNG FU** in Cantonese, and **KOBU** in Kampo medicine of Japan.

The tubers were eaten and present in dental calculus from central Sudan, dating before 6700 BCE. Recent studies suggest its inhibition of *Streptococcus mutans*, helped maintain good dental hygiene and caries. Buckley S et al, *PLoS ONE* 2014 9(7): e100808.

It is considered an invasive weed, like its cousin. The plant may be useful in phytoremediation of crude oil spills.

In Ecuador, various Cyperus species including *C. articulatus, C. odoratus* and *C. prolixus*, are used by Shaman and known as Piri-Piri. The former plant is known in Venezuala as Borrachera, or inebriating agent, due to its psychoactivity. In El Salvador, the plant is used as an analgesic for tooth pain. The black tubers have a lavender-like odor.

The roots are decocted by Shuar shaman and used in place of ayahuasca in making medical diagnosis. The tea helps them enter a trance and communicate with the dead. The neighboring Secoya use the root to induce labour, while the Jivaro add the root extract to their drinking tobacco.

An ergot-type fungus, *Balansia cyperi*, infects the seed head of this genus. I can find no record of native use of this fungus for medical purpose.

MEDICINAL

CONSTITUENTS- *C. esculenta* tuber- the amino acids alanine, arginine, aspartic, uronic and glutamic acid. Also contains lauric acid, myristic acid, oleic acid, palmitic acid stigmasterol, beta sitosterol and stearic acid. Fructose, glucose, melibiose, sucrose, mannose, xylose, arabinose, galactose and lipase also present. Tocopherols and beta carotene also preset with sources of calcium, copper, manganese, zinc and potassium.
Protein content averages 50.5 grams per 100 grams dry weight. Reducing sugars are 154 total sugar and 130 sucrose.
Leaves- flavonoids.
C. rotundus rhizomes- alpha cyperone, isocyperol, rotunduside, loganic acid, 10-O-p-hydroxybenzoyltheviridoside, 10-O-vanilloytheviridoside, cassigarol E, scirpusin A & B, nootkatone, patchoulane-type sesquiterpenoids including cyperene-3,8-dione, 14-acetoxy cyperotundone, 3 beta-hydroxycyperenoic acid, and sugetriol-3,9-diacetate; luteolin, 6'-acetyl-3,6-diferuloylsucrose, p-coumaric acid, ferulic acid, pinellic acid, fulgidic acid, cyprotusides A and B (cycloartane glycosides), valencene, rotunduside G-H, negundoside, nishindaside, isooleuropein, neonuezhenide, kobusone, cardiac glycosides, epoxyguaine, copadiene, cyperolone, kotundone.
leaf- orientin

The dried roots of yellow nut sedge are used in medicine as a digestive tonic. The root is chewed for the relief of indigestion, or a handful of roots is boiled and mixed with porridge to hasten the inception of menstruation. For polymenorrhea, a powder of the dried roots is wrapped in cotton and inserted into the vagina three times daily.

The tubers can be eaten whole by children in place of sweets, to enhance resilience of the immune system; or mixed with honey and milk to treat colic.

Decoctions have also been used for various stomach troubles, including flatulence; as well as promoting urine production.

The root juice is given to relieve canker sores of the mouth and gums.

The roots are eaten to increase breast milk production in nursing mothers.

In Ayurvedic medicine, the roots are used in colic, diarrhea, and conditions of excessive thirst.

In clinical trials with rats and mice, the water extract have shown pronounced uterine stimulating properties.

The tuber is claimed to have anti-implantation effect on female rats.

The tubers stimulated sexual motivation in both highly and moderately active rats. It improved their sexual performance and increased serum testosterone. Allouh MZ et al, *BMC Complement Altern Med* 2015 15:331.

Water extracts of the root, stem, leaves and flowers exhibit anti-tumour effect on sarcoma 180 and adenocarcinoma 755.

Alcoholic extracts are anti-bacterial against *Bacillus subtilis and Staphylococcus aureus.*

The leaf flavonoids exhibit inhibition against gram negative and gram positive bacteria, and have anti-oxidant activity. Jing S et al, *Food Chem* 2016 192:319-27.

Purple Nut Sedge has been used traditionally for diarrhea, diabetes, inflammation, malaria and various stomach and bowel disorders. Ethnobotanical uses for atherosclerosis, aging, apoptosis, cancer, cystitis, epilepsy, hirsutism, prostatitis and other conditions abound. A review on the herb by Pirzada AM et al, *J Ethnopharm* 2015 174:540-60 is useful for those wishing to look further into this valuable plant.

The traditional use of the root as galactogogue, appears warranted, based on the work of Badgujar SB & Bandivdekar AH, *J Ethnopharm* 2015 163:39-42.

In Ayurvedic medicine, the plant is known as **MUSTA**.

In China, the herb ranks 8th among 250 anti-fertility plants.

It is a used to treat irregular, prolonged or light menstruation, spasmodic dysmenorrhea, over-due periods and depression, during menstruation.

The root is pungent, slightly bitter and sweet, warming and drying, relaxing, calming and slightly astringent. It is a good Qi circulator, and release restraint in the digestive and cardiovascular systems.

It is an estrogen stimulant, useful for breast tenderness, abnormal PAP smears and infertility.

The rhizome is useful for restlessness, irritability and a cardiovascular relaxant for issues such as palpitations, arrhythmia, angina, and hypertension.

Liver Yang rising issues such as dizziness, ringing in ears, moodiness and stress are relieved.

Purple Nut Sedge is used in TCM with *Astragalus membranaceus* and *Andrographis paniculata*, in the formula Xiang Qi Tang.

Together these herbs appear useful in cardiac issues associated with inflammation and coagulation. He CL et al, *Immunopharmacol Immunotoxicol* 2013 35(2):215-24.

The rhizome is used in China for hepatitis. It appears that the eudesmane-type sesquiterpenoids contribute to the anti-hepatitis B activity. Xu HB et al, *Journal of Ethnopharmacology* 2015 171:131-40.

It may also be useful for non-alcoholic fatty liver through selective inhibition of the lipogenic pathway. Oh GS et al, *Am J Chin Med* 2015 43(3):477-94.

The rhizome extract appears to be preventative against induced neurotoxicity against human neuroblastoma cells. Hermanth KK et al, *Neurotoxicity* 2013 34:150-9.

Scirpusin A and B exhibit anti-oxidative, neuroprotective, anti-inflammatory and anti- amyloid B activity, suggestive of benefit in neurodegenerative disease. Sim Y et al, *Biomol Ther* (Seoul) 2016 24(4):438-45.

Alpha cyperone binds and interacts with tubulin and could reduce inflammation that would benefit inflammatory conditions such as Alzheimer's disease. Azimi A et al, *Journal of Ethnopharmacology* 2016 194:219-227.

Alpha cyperone down regulates COX-2 and IL-6, explaining in part, the benefit of rhizome decoctions in reducing inflammation. Jung SH et al, *J Ethnopharm* 2013 147(1): 208-14. The mechanism is mediated by both peripheral and central analgesic action.

Isocyperol increased survival rate in septic shocked mice, via suppression of NFkappaB, STAT3 pathways and reduction of reactive oxygen species. Seo YJ et al, *Int Immunopharmacol* 2016 38:61-9.

The rhizome may be useful in hyperglycemia, due to its inhibition of alpha amylase and alpha glucosidase. Tran HH et al, *Pharm Biol* 2014 52(1):74-7.

Ethanol extracts showed significant anti-diabetic activity in mice study. Singh P et al, *J Pharm Bioallied Sci* 2015 7(4):289-92.

A combination of rhizomes of purple nut sedge, ginger root and mint was used in an eight week study of irritable bowel syndrome on forty patients in Iraq. Significant improvement was noted. Sahib AS, *J Ethnopharm* 2013 148(3):1008-12.

The rhizomes act as a molecular brake and down-regulate pro-inflammatory cytokines, reducing the severity of IBD. Johari S et al *Iran J Med Sci* 2016 41(5):391-8.

The rhizome has long been used for gastric problems in Ayurveda medicine. It shows significant inhibition of aspirin-induced gastric ulcer, comparable to the drug ranitidine. Thomas D et al, *J Basic Clin Physiol Pharmacol* 2015 26(5):485-90.

Alcohol extracts of the aerial parts inhibit xanthine oxidase activity, suggestive of benefit in gout and rheumatic conditions. Soumaya KJ et al, *Asian Pac J Trop Med* 2014 7(2):105-12.

An ethanol extract showed protective effect against hypoxia, in a rat study. Hypoxia injury is one of the leading causes of morbidity and death on the planet. Jebasingh D et al, *Pharm Biol* 2014 52(12): 1558-69.

Cyprotusides A and B, from rhizomes, showed significant anti-depressant activity in a mice study by Zhou ZL et al, *J Asian Nat Prod Res* 2016 18(7):662-8. The same year, the same research group identified rotunduside G and H, and attributed anti-depressant activity to these two compounds. *Chem Pharm Bull* 2016 64(1):73-7. Nothing like double dipping to fulfill your research paper requirements for the year!

In another study, an ethanol extract of rhizomes induced potent anti-proliferation and apoptosis of MDA-MB-231 human breast cancer cell lines. Park SE et al, *Oncol Rep* 2014 32(6):2461-70.

The patchoulane sesquiterpen 6-acetoxy cyerene is cytotoxic to human ovarian cancer cells lines (A2780, SKOV3 and OVCAR3). Ahn JH et al, *Phytother Res* 2015 June 10.

The rhizomes may have potential therapeutic benefit on UV-induced photo-aging, with cosmetic application. The compound valencene reduced melanin content in work by Nam JH et al, *J Nat Prod* 2016 79(4): 1091-6. It may also be useful for treatment of atopic dermatitis. Yang IJ et al, *Evid Based Complement Altern Med* 2016:9370893.

TUBER OIL

The tuber of chufa contains 23% oil consisting of arachidic acid, linoleic acid (33.3%), oleic acid (50.2%), palmitic acid, stearic acid; as well as vitamin C, and alpha and gamma tocopherols.

As oleic acid constitutes the major part of the acids, over 60% triolein, 33.7% diolein, and 5.6% monoolein were found.

The oil is not dissimilar to hazelnut oil, and has a golden yellow colour, with neutral taste. Cold pressed Chufa oil can be used for edible purposes without any refining.

Enzymatic treatment will yield up to 33% oil.

Yang Z et al, *Plant Cell Physiol* 2016 57(12): 2519-40 has studied the biosynthesis involved in fatty acid production.

Oleanolic acid, from rhizomes of *C. rotundus*, inhibits transient receptor potential vanilloid 1 channel, suggests of analgesic and UV-induced photo-aging benefit. Nam JH & Lee DU, *Planta Medica* 2015 81(1):20-5.

ESSENTIAL OILS

CONSTITUENTS- *C. rotundus*- cyperine, pinene, cyperol, cyperone, isocyperol, patchouleneone, rotundene, nootkatone, cyperotundene, kobusone, alpha-cyperone, isokobusone, sugeonol, and beta selinene. CO_2 extraction yields 1.82%.

The essential oil has a spicy, woody, earthy, smoky and camphorous scent.

Purple Nut Sedge essential oil, known as Nagarmotha, in Hindi, has been found as effective as laser for decreasing the growth of axillary hair (dark and white), in an open-label pilot study. Sixty-five clients were enrolled in one of three groups. The benefit from oil may derive from its anti-androgenic activity. Mohammed GF, *Aesthet Surg Journal* 2014 34(2):298-305.

The rhizome contains up to 30 µg/10 grams of nootkatone, a commercially important sesquiterpenoid.

Nootkatone inhibits TNFalpha and interferon gamma-induced production of cytokines, suggesting its benefit in inflammatory skin conditions such as atopic dermatitis. Choi HJ et al, *Biochem Biophys Res Commun* 2014 447(2):278-84.

The oil can be put in a bath, four drops in little cream, to calm nervous digestion, relieve menstrual pain, reduce arthritis and rheumatism and treat anorexia.

It alleviates stress, nervous tension and respiratory congestion in form of a steam.

The oil is used in creams, lotions and perfumery, and massage oil, all in diluted form.

In India, it is used in the production of soap, incense, attars, hair products and to flavour tobacco.

The related *C. longus* is known in England as English Galingale. The roots, when broken, are said to smell like violets.

PERSONALITY TRAITS

The cleaned roots are stored by the meadow mouse and these are also gathered. The caches of roots are found by looking for small mounds of dirt with grass growing on top.

When a woman gathers these roots, the meadow mouse helps her. When she takes the roots from the cache, he pushes more out to her. If a woman chases a meadow mouse or makes remarks about the mouse she will not be lucky. She will not find the mouse's caches of roots or any seed.

A good woman says good things to the meadow mice. She asks them to be good to her and to help her find the roots and seeds. When a woman hear the chuckling sound made by the meadow mouse she knows it wants her to find his cache of roots or seeds. The roots...are not eaten by a pregnant woman or her husband. If either were to eat these roots the meadow mouse would eat the fetus just as he eats the roots.   **WILLARD Z PARK**

RECIPES

SPANISH DRINK- Take 500 grams of well-rinsed tubers and soak in water for two days. Then drain, and blend them with four cups of water and one-third cup of sugar. Strain and drink.

TINCTURE- both species- 2-4 ml. The tincture is produced from dried, crushed tubers or rhizomes 1:5 at 40% alcohol.

DECOCTION- 6-14 grams. 1:20 slow simmer for fifteen minutes.

CAUTION- Do not use during pregnancy or constipation. Do not use in Qi deficiency without signs of stagnation, Yin deficiency and Blood heat.

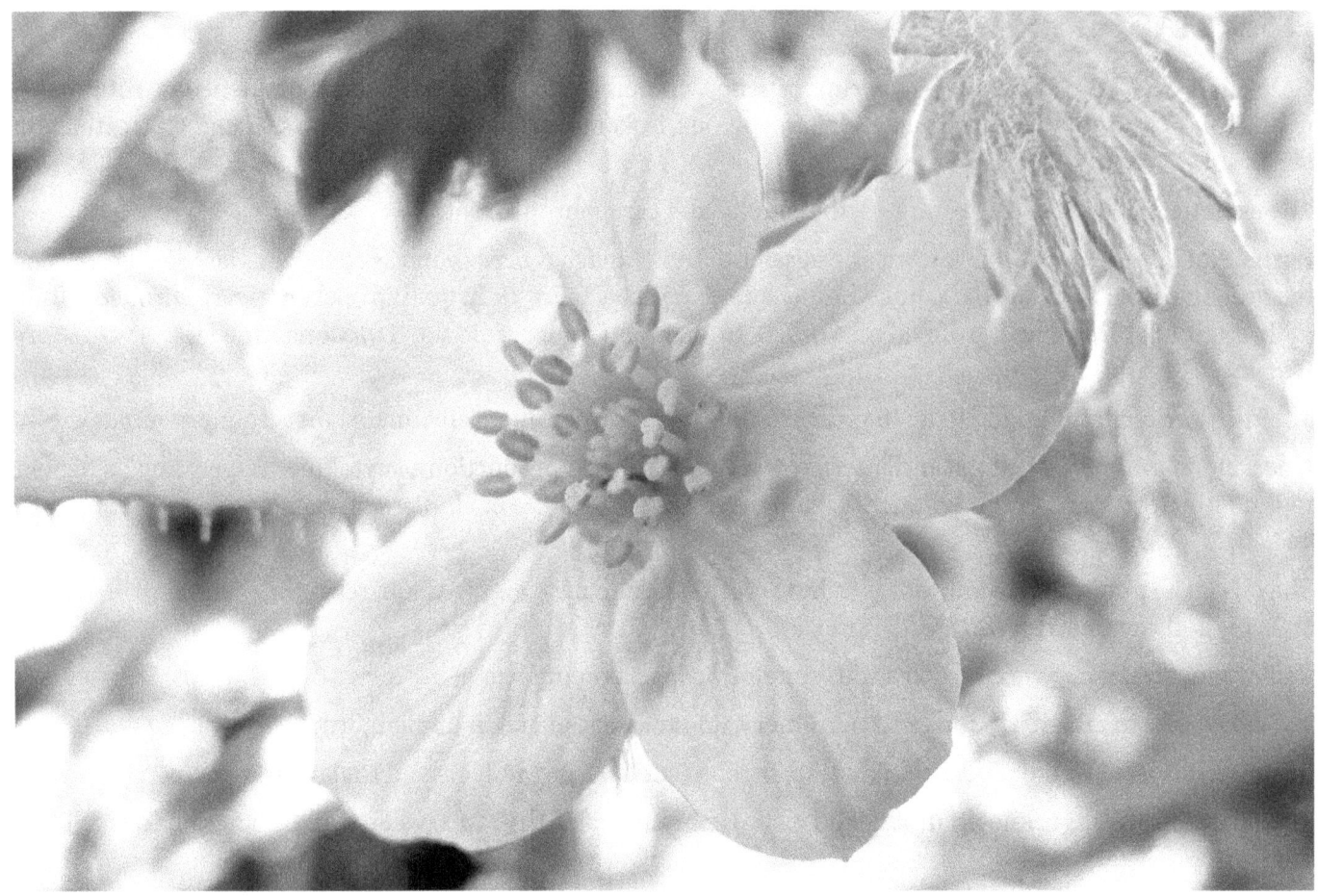

SILVERWEED

CINQUEFOIL
SILVERWEED
CRAMPWEED
GOOSEWORT
(*Potentilla anserina* L.)
(*Argentina anserina* [L.] Rydb.) not accepted
(*P. anserina ssp. yukonensis* [Hulten] Sojak ex
Elven & D. F. Murray)
SHRUBBY CINQUEFOIL
BUSH CINQUEFOIL
TUNDRA ROSE
(*P. fruticosa* auct. non L.) not accepted
(*P. floribunda* Pursh.) not accepted
(*Pentaphylloides floribunda* [Pursh] A. Löve)
not accepted
(*Dasiphora fruticosa* [L.] Rydb.)
ROUGH CINQUEFOIL
NORWEGIAN CINQUEFOIL
(*P. norvegica* L.)
(*P. monspeliensis* L.) not accepted

STICKY CINQUEFOIL
(*P. glandulosa* Lindl.) not accepted
(*Drymocallis glandulosa var. glandulosa*
[Lindl.] Rydb.)
GRACEFUL CINQUEFOIL
CUTLEAF CINQUEFOIL
(*P. gracilis* Douglas ex Hook.)
SILVERY CINQUEFOIL
(*P. argentea* L.)
EARLY CINQUEFOIL
RED CINQUEFOIL
(*P. concinna* Richardson)
WHITE CINQUEFOIL
TALL CINQUEFOIL
GLANDULAR CINQUEFOIL
(*P. arguta* Pursh.) not accepted
(*D. arguta* [Pursh.] Rydb.)
MARSH CINQUEFOIL
MARSHLOCKS
(*P. palustris* [L.] Scop.) not accepted
(*Comarum palustre* L.)

PRAIRIE CINQUEFOIL
(*P. pennsylvanica* L.)
THREE-TOOTHED CINQUEFOIL
(*P. tridentata* Ait.) not accepted
(*Sibbaldiopsis tridentata* [Ait] Rydb.)
SIBBALDIA
(*P. sibbaldii* Haller f.) not accepted
(*Sibbaldia procumbens* L.)
SNOW CINQUEFOIL
(*P. nivea* L.)
VILLOUS CINQUEFOIL
(*P. villosa* Pall. ex Pursh)
WOOLLY CINQUEFOIL
HORSE CINQUEFOIL
(*P. hippiana* Lehm.)

SULPHUR CINQUEFOIL
ROUGH FRUITED CINQUEFOIL
(*P. recta* L.)
(*P. sulphurea* Lam.) not accepted
NEPAL POTENTILLA
NEPAL CINQUEFOIL
(*C. nepalensis* Hook.)
FALSE STRAWBERRY
MOCK STRAWBERRY
(*Duchesnea indica* [Turcz] Baill.)
(*P. indica* [Andr.] T. Wolf)
PARTS USED- root, flower and leaves

Honey under ground,
Silverweed of spring.
Honey and condiment
Wisked whey of summer.
Honey and fruitage
Carrot of autumn.
Honey and crunching
Nuts of winter.

ALEXANDER CARMICHAEL

The lovely cinquefoil is a rose,
A fact that any botanist knows,
Though it seems to me a mystery
How such a lowly plant can be
Sibling to a flower that grows
As glorious as garden rose.
The bigger question does remain:
How you pronounce the funny name?
Does it "sink" or does it "sank"
As it wanders up the bank?
And as it creeps across the soil
What, pray tell, does it foil?

JACK SANDERS

Potentilla is from the Latin **POTENS** meaning powerful, alluding to its medicinal qualities. Pentaphylloides is from the Greek meaning five like leaves. This genus was recently separated from Potentilla, which is now reserved for herbaceous species.

Anserina may be translated as "goose" in honour of the fondness they have for the plant; or more likely from the Latin **ARGENT** for silver, referring to the underside colour of the leaves. Cinquefoil, another common name for this genus, is named for the five-fingered leaves. This is derived as a corruption from the French **CINQUE FEUILLES**.

Villous means hairy. Recta means upright. Nivea means snow, and concinna means elegant and well kept.

Argentea is named after silver, and is a fairly new designation by taxonomists looking for something to do.

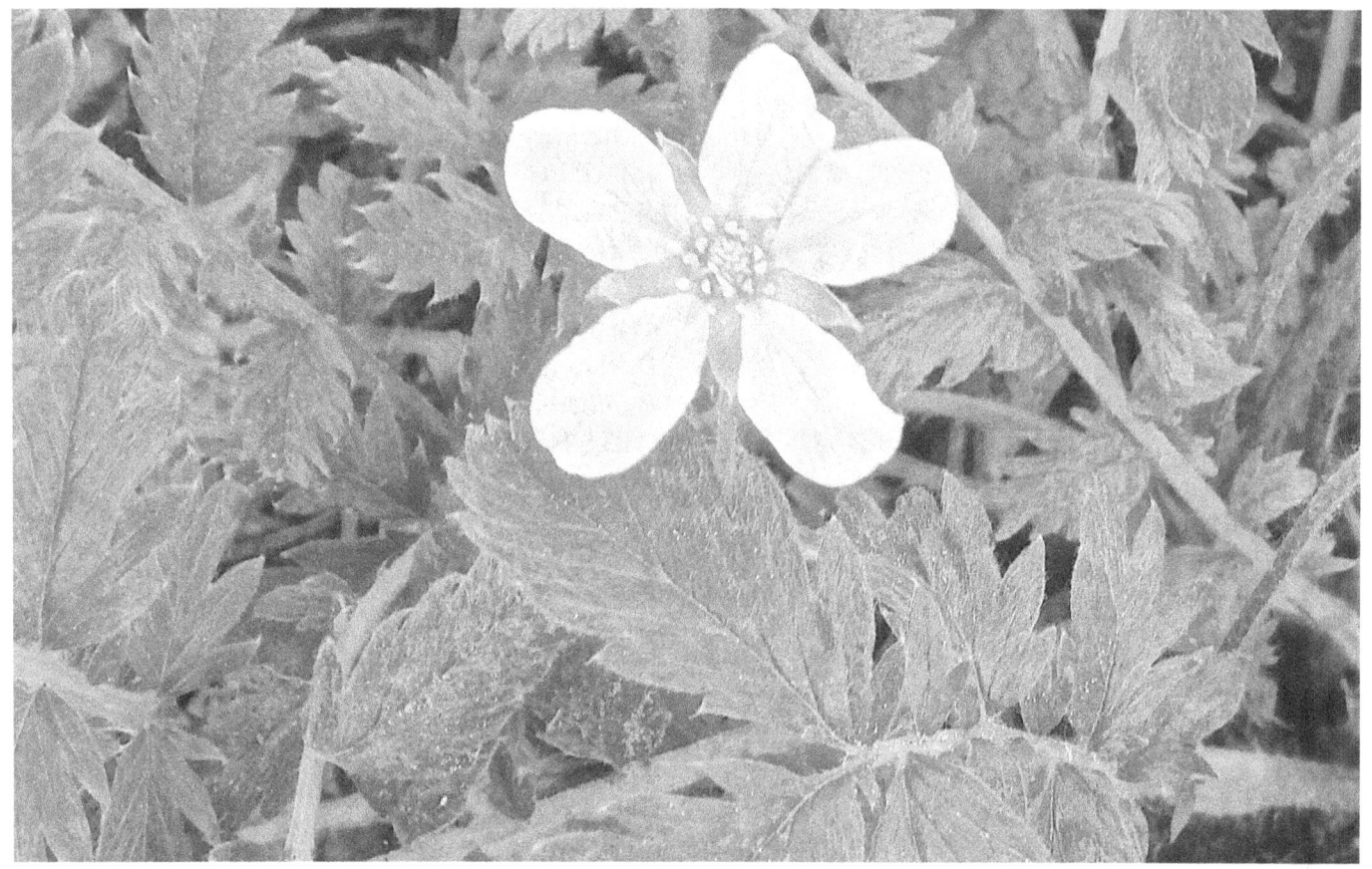

SILVERWEED FLOWER AND LEAVES

Duchesnea is named for Antoine Nicolas Duchesne (1747-1827), a French horticulturalist who published a book on the history of strawberries, and worked at hybridizing and improving cultivated strains. Ironically, the Indian or Mock Strawberry is tasteless. It has recently been classified in the genus *Potentilla*.

Silverweed infusions have traditionally been added to ritual baths for purification; or protection from evil. It is said to bestow eloquence and protection to the wearer; it's five fingered leaves symbolizing love, power, wisdom, health and abundance.

According to legend, fairies and plant spirits use silverweed, on which to congregate and dance in the moonlight. Maybe that is why many young people find smoking silverweed leaves gives them a "marijuana type" high.

One superstition from Scotland is the use of brisgein (brittle) or silverweed root as part of a fairy banquet. It was used extensively as a survival food both roasted and boiled. It is known as **AN SEACHDAMH ARAN** in Gaelic, meaning the seventh bread, due to its importance in the diet before potatoes.

The plant is widespread throughout Alberta, preferring sandy soil. It grows/spreads in the manner of wild strawberries sending out runners, in all directions. In bad weather, the furry leaves curve up over the flowers to protect them.

Many drier meadows of the Peace Athabasca delta, which are no longer flooded annually due to the Bennett dam, are completely taken over by Silverweed.

The plant has an almond-like fragrance and dry taste.

The Blackfoot called silverweed either garter root (**KITA-KOP-SIM**); or dry root (**PASHI**).

The Blood and Blackfoot roasted or boiled the root as an "Indian sweet potato" . The longer roots were ripped from the sand and used as rope.

The astringent tannins were put to benefit by boiling the roots and drinking it for chest pains and to alleviate diarrhea. For wounds and cuts, the root was simply chewed and the juice spit on the affected area to heal and prevent infection.

Native people of British Columbia bestowed the largest, straightest and most prized silverweed roots on the Chief. The smaller, curly roots near the surface were for commoners, but all enjoyed their addition to wedding feasts. The Pacific Silverweed (*P. anersina ssp. pacifica*) is known as Wild Sweet Potato, to the Haida, with the roots known as Salmonberry shoots, or **TS'a7aal**.

The Alaskan Haida word for the roots represents an interesting case of potential homonymy, as reported by Nancy Turner in her book on plants of Haida Gwaii.

The roots were then cooked in fist-like bundles and dried for the winter. They have a hazelnut like flavour, after drying, while the young spring roots are more like parsnips, but a bit tougher.

The fresh root contains 31% assimilable starch, more than cultivated potato, and comparable to burdock root.

They can be gathered in fall, or in early spring when the new white to purple roots grow from the central stock.

The root was also used as a famine food in the Scottish Highlands, and it was said that a man could sustain himself on a square of ground of his own length.

Highlanders gathered the roots and ate them in a similar manner; calling them *AN SEACHDAMH ARAN* meaning the seventh bread.

They were a favorite of the Tanguts from northeastern Tibet, as well as eastern Turkmenistan and Zinijang, China.

Dioscorides called the plant **MYRIOPHYLLON**, and suggested nearly 2000 years ago, boiling the plant in salted water to treat hemorrhages.

Bullherb, an ancient name, reminds us that the herb was once used for infertility in bulls. Another name, Scurfweed, refers to veterinary use for injury and infection. Farmers simmer the root in milk for internal and external use for above as well as colic and whenever cattle stop ruminating.

The root was also ground and used as fodder for domestic animals like geese.

In Medieval Europe, it was said that the best cinquefoil was gathered under a full moon. This was burned as incense and said to bring dreams of one's perfect partner. Full five-fingered leaves were pressed and dried, and sent in pages of personal books between friends.

The right to bear Cinquefoil was at one time considered an honorable distinction to those who mastered their senses and conquered their passions. Knights painted the plant on their shields to symbolize the five senses.

Silverweed leaf has an exquisite shape that is used in Church and Cathedral woodcarvings.

The leaves were worn in footware to prevent over sweating and soreness, keeping feet cool and dry, hence the Old English names of Traveler's Joy and Chafe Grass. The bruised leaves, mixed with salt and vinegar, were applied to soles of feet to allay heat of fevers.

It was said to be one of the ingredients in Witches Flying Ointment, and was said to increase their power, focus and desire. Today, fishermen use the root as part of a recipe with the juice of houseleek and stinging nettles to enhance their bait.

The roots, due to their extremely high tannin content, were used for tanning leather.

The French used Silverweed traditionally as a cure for tetany. William Wethering, the 18th century physician who discovered from a female herbalist the cardiotonic benefits of foxglove, recommended a teaspoon of dried leaves every three hours for bouts of malarial fever.

The infusion was used for tetanus infections, but I cannot vouch for the efficacy of this application.

Dr. Fernie writes, "silverweed tea is excellent to relieve cramps of the belly; and compresses, wrung out of a hot decoction of the herb, may at the same time be helpfully applied over the seat of the cramps."

Father Johann Kunzle (a 19th century Swiss herbalist pastor) wrote. "Every woman should know this herb because there hardly exists a better remedy against menstrual cramps and haemorrhages. Numerous women have found relief by drinking two cups of Potentilla decoction on the ten days preceding their menstruation".

The Shrubby Cinquefoil is a small bush, unlike its crawling cousin, but with the small yellow flowers. It is often planted on the prairies for ornamental purpose, due to its hardiness, freedom from pests and disease and minimal caretaking. It is the ancestor of all other cultivated Cinquefoils.

Shrubby Cinquefoil leaves were used by the Blackfoot for deodorizing and spicing their dried meat; and by the Slave, who made a beverage tea of the leaf and stem.

The dry, flaky bark was used for tinder by the Blackfoot, when using a bow drill to make fire. They called it Deer Seat, because the animals were often found resting where it grows.

The Slave of the northern boreal forest know the shrub as **TLINTE DEDZHINE**. They boil the leaves, stems and root together as a remedy for fevers accompanied by body aches and a cough. The northern Dene made decoctions of the stems, leaves and roots for fever accompanied by sore chest, arms, legs, with a cough.

The Cheyenne drank a tea of the leaves, and used strong decoctions as a medicine against the enemy. Arrow tips were dipped into leaf decoctions, and the poison was thought to go directly to the heart. The poison was also put into porcupine quills and shot into the mouth. Only holy people could use it.

They also claimed that the leaves protected them from severe, but temporary, heat. They call it Sage Mint Soup, **VANO?E-MOXESHE-HOHPE** , or **O NUHK'IS E' EYO**, meaning contrary medicine.

The dried, powdered leaves were rubbed over the hands, or an infusion of the powder made by soaking in cold water and rubbed over the whole body during the Contrary Dance. The coated hands were thrust into a kettle of boiling soup with no apparent injury.

Russians used the fresh, young leaves in salads, and soups. The mashed leaves were added to various fish and meat dishes.

Natives of Siberia used the dried leaves as tea, known as **KURIL CHAI**. This gives it another common name Tea bush. In both appearance and taste it is much like green tea, but not stimulating.

The Chinese called it **JIN LU MEI**, or Golden Dew Plum. In Nepal, the leaves are also used as a tea substitute, and the root juice used for indigestion. The powdered plant is also added to incense.

Marsh Cinquefoil has a reddish purple flower with unpleasant odour that attracts carrion flies and other insects. The Haida, and other native tribes, used the plant stem for treating tuberculosis. It is called **SANIXILA**.

The leaves have been used as a popular tea throughout the Arctic. The roots taste like parsnips or sweet potatoes with a bit of imagination, either boiled or roasted.

The roots have been used medicinally to treat stomach cramps and dysentery, or for washing cuts and burns by various Native tribes, including the Chippewa, who call it Prairie Chicken or Grouse Leaf, **BINE'BUG**.

The Dena'ina of Alaska call it **KENGGITS'A** meaning "the flat's hard one", in reference to the hard fruit.

Decoctions are useful for dysentery and stomach cramps.

The rhizome is widely available as a dietary supplement in Russia.

The whole plant of Rough cinquefoil was steeped and used for cramps of the stomach by the Fox and other native tribes. Chippewa natives used root decoctions to soothe sore throats. The Navaho smoldered the plant in attempts to treat sexual infection; and used cold infusion of the whole plant for pain.

Work by Towers et al, at UBC found the whole plant active against a broad spectrum of fungal species.

White Cinquefoil (*P. arguta*) root was dried and pulverized into a powder by the Chippewa to either prick into the temple or snuffed up the nostril for headaches. A small amount of the powder was moistened and applied to cuts; as was the fresh cut root.

Blood-letting was performed by the Ojibwa, and later checked with the prepared root, either wet or dry on soft duck down over the incision.

Root decoctions of Big Heart Berry Root, or **GI-TCIODE' IMINIDJI'BIK** were used for dysentery, and the root powder for convulsions.

The Slave, of northern Canada, call it **KOTHENTELI NAYDI**.

Sticky Cinquefoil is used by the Gosiute as a poultice for swollen parts of the body.

The Okanagan used infusions of the whole plant, without roots as a stimulant and tonic; as did the neighboring Thompson. It is called **SNU'KAS A XI'LAXIL**, meaning friend of silverweed.

The leaves were boiled in water, as a thirst quenching drink by the Blackfoot.

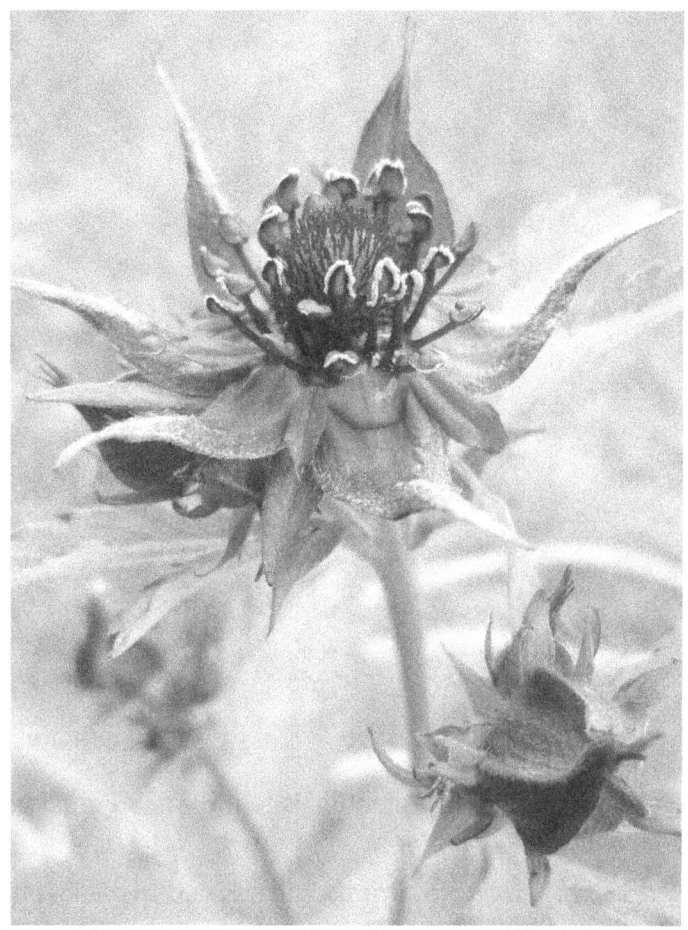

MARSH CINQUEFOIL

Graceful or Cut-leaf Cinquefoil leaves and roots were crushed and mixed with Alpine Fir pitch, as a salve for drawing out pain. The Chehalis mention that the plant has both white and yellow flowers. If a woman wished to bear a girl she drank a tea of yellow flowers; and for a boy they would brew up white.

Sticky Cinquefoil root may have been used by the Chumash, for blood purifying, fever and Spanish flu. Known as Tabardillo in Spanish, this may be a case of mistaken identity.

Villous Cinquefoil is a mountainous or alpine perennial that is low growing but has relatively large yellow flowers. As the name suggests, it is hairy.

Rough fruited or Sulphur Cinquefoil (*P. recta*) is an introduced plant found all over the prairie region. In some areas, including Alberta, it is considered a noxious weed.

Woolly Cinquefoil is fairly common in the southwestern parts of the prairie. The Navaho used the plant as a burn lotion, or to expedite childbirth. Cold infusions of the root were taken as a "life medicine".

Graceful Cinquefoil root was used, by the Okanagan tribe as a blood purifier, and tonic and to treat diarrhea and gonorrhea. Externally, a wash was used for sores, and treating aches and pains.

The Thompson macerated the roots, but combined them with tree pitch as a wound salve.

The leaf tea infusion is quite mild, and less astringent than rest of genus.

Potentilla paradoxa is found on moist flats and shores throughout the prairies, east to Ontario and south to Texas.

In Nepal, it is known as **BAJRA DANTI**. Pieces of the root are kept in the mouth for relieving toothaches, while the juice, at 3 teaspoons three times daily, is given for indigestion.

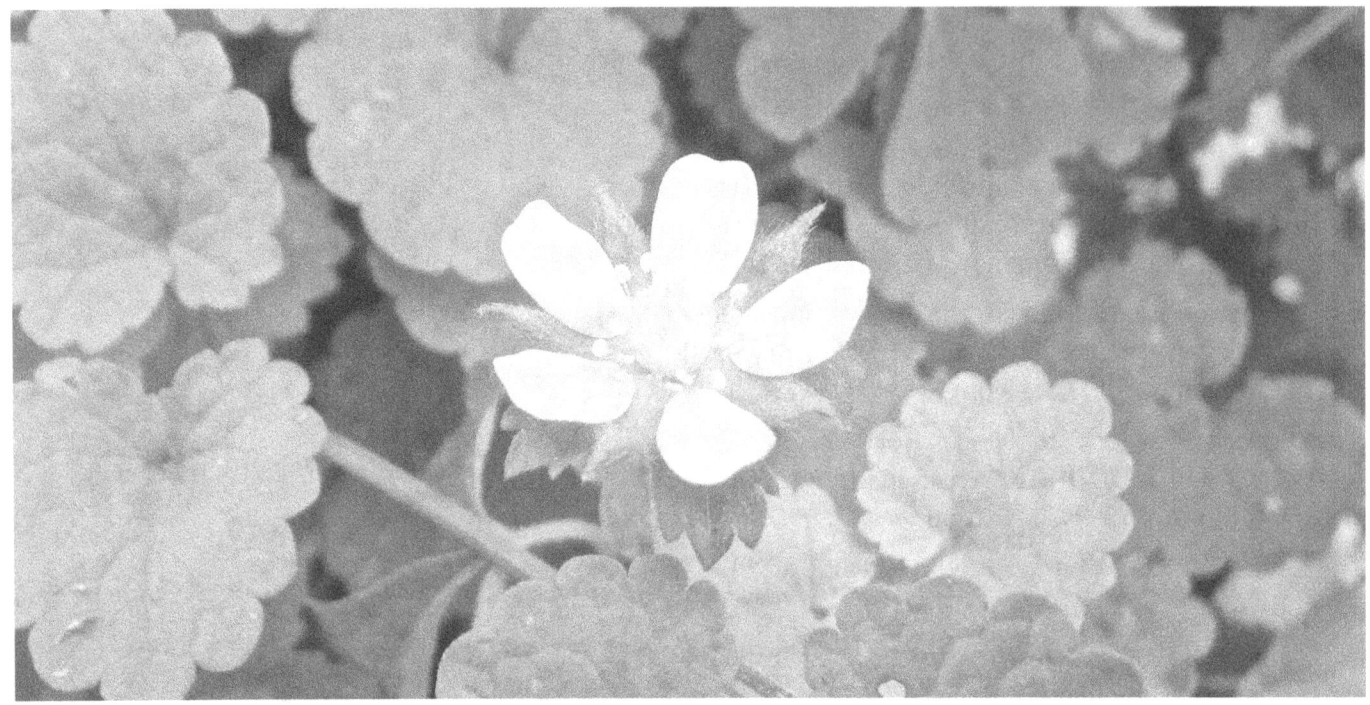

FALSE STRAWBERRY FLOWER AND LEAF

Nepal Cinquefoil or Potentilla is found in perennial gardens, making a fine, hardy ground cover with warm, cherry flowers that bloom all summer.

The leaf of *P. davurica*, from China, is said to possess the odour of roses.

False Strawberry (*Duchesnea indica*) is cultivated as a hardy, dense ground cover, especially beneath shrubs. It has decorative yellow flowers, that later develop red strawberry-like fruit.

In China, the herb is known as **SHE-MEI,** and serves as a snake nest from which it derives the name. It has long been used in Asia to treat cancer.

It has a number of interesting synonyms including **TI CHIN,** ground tapestry, **SAN HSIEN TS'AO,** three fairy grass, **WU CHAO LUNG,** five claw dragon, **SHE PAO TS'AO,** snake bubble grass; and **WU CHIH HU,** meaning five fingered tiger.

Natives of Argentina call it "*Frutilla sylvestre*", and prefer to eat the berries with sauce or oil.

MEDICINAL

CONSTITUENTS- *P. anserina* root- catechin, tannins (17-25%), tormentoside, gallocatechin, glycosides, calcium oxalate, various triterpenes such as potentillanosides A-F, six triterpene 28-O-monoglucopyranosyl esters, pomolic acid, rosamutin, kaji-ichigoside F1, genistein, chlorogenic acid, acacetin 7-O-rutinoside, organic acids, resins, gums and essential oils.
Leaf and flowers- bisabolol, farnesene, various flavonoids including gentisic acid, 4-hydrocinnamic acid, vanillic and salicylic acids, umbelliferone, syringic acid, ellagic acid (216mg/g), scopolin, potentilin A, 19 flavonol glycosides, including the important querctin-3-0-beta-D-glucuronide. The leaves also contain vitamin E (198 ppm) and 2-pyrone-4, 6-dicarboxylic acid, as well as a number of phenolics including caffeic acid, myricetin-3-O-glucuronide, agrimoniin, ellagic acid, miquelianin, isorhamnetin-3-O-glucuronide, and kaempferol-3-O-rhamnoside. Polyphronols (0.3% fresh weight).
Flowers- above, as well as herbacetin 8-methyl ether-3-O-beta-D- sophoroside (8-methoxykaempferol 3-sophoroside.
D. fruticosa flower and young shoots–quercitin, epi-ursolic acid, 3-0-alpha-L- arabinopyranoside, quercitin 3-O-beta-D-galactopyranoside, 3',4',7-trimethyl-quercitin, 2 alpha-hydroxyrsolic acid, hyperoside (8.86 mg/gram), termentic acid, terniflorin, tribuloside beta-sisosterol, stigmasterol, campesterol and various catechins including (+)-catechin, epicatechingallate, epictechin, ellagic acid and epigallocatechin.

P. argentea- scopoletin, umbelliferone, beta-sitosterol, alpha and beta-carotene, tannins, flavonoids, cholines, histidine and glycobetaine compounds.

P. nivea-leaves- 314 mg Vitamin C/100 grams dry weight

P. pennsylvanica-leaf- various flavonoids including glucosides, rutinosides and galactosides of apigenin, kaempferol, and quercitin. Nothing unusual really.

P. pacifica- 68 grams of root contain 234 kilojoules of energy, 28 grams of calcium and 6.2 grams of iron.

P. indica leaves- ellagic glycosides (ducheside A and B); and four glucopyranosides, 27 phenolic compounds including hydroxybenzoic and hydroxycinnamic acid derivatives, and flavonols.

whole plant- emodin, chrysophanic acid, phytosterol, calcium, volatile oil.

Fruit- anthocyanins including cyaniding 3-O-rutinoside (61%), peonidin 3-O-rutinoside (34%) and petunidin 3-O-rutinoside.

Silverweed, due to cool, drying and astringent nature is a specific for all types of inflammation and fever caused by infection. It can be safely used by those who do not tolerate, or are allergic, to sulfa drugs.

A plant patent from Germany contains silverweed for the treatment of uro-liathisis (urinary stones and gravel).

The root may be boiled in milk for astringent and anti-hemorrhage activity. Boiled in vinegar or wine, it is a specific for shingle pain, taken internally, and applied externally to the affected areas. Hemorrhoids also are relieved with compresses of the root externally.

Decoctions of the root are an excellent gargle for spongy, bleeding gums, and ulcerated mouth and throat sores. A stronger decoction is also used for healing esophageal and stomach ulcers. Even alternating diarrhea and constipation is soothed and regulated.

It should be noted silverweed extracts may antagonize the laxative effects of senna, buckthorn and rhubarb. Vogel G et al, *Arzneimittelforschung* 1975 25(9): 1356-65.

Silverweed, *P. argentea* and *P. erecta* have all been analyzed and found that water extracts of aerial parts, modulate cytokine production in colon cells. Paduch R et al, *Curr Drug Targets* 2015 16(13): 495-502.

It can be combined with other herbs like couch grass to dissolve stones in the bladder.

Fresh leaf infusions are used in Russia, to help regulate the body's metabolism, in cases of diabetes, goiter, and obesity. Infusions are also used for menstrual cramping, while stronger decoctions are used for uterine hemorrhage, and excessive menstrual bleeding.

Aerial infusion of nine species were investigated by Tomczyk M et al, *Fitoterapia* 2008 79(7-8): 592-4, and found strongly active against *Helicobacter pylori*.

Cooled decoctions can be used as a vaginal douche for yeast or bacterial infections. Skin blemishes and acne, as well as skin pigmentation mask will over time respond to cooled decoctions. Distilled water from the plant is used cosmetically for soothing reddened, and delicate baby's skin.

A unique Russian remedy for dysentery is combining silverweed powdered leaves with fried eggs.

The fresh root juice gives rapid relief in cases of nervous stomach and spastic cramping of the intestine. It's anti-spasmodic nature also relieves menstrual pain, headache, and neuralgia, combining well 4:1 with valerian root.

Dysmenorrhea of a spastic nature may be one of its great applications. Bliss et al, *J Am Pharm Assoc* 1940 29.

The isoflavone genistein may play a role in PMS. Mari A et al, *Metabolomics* 2013 9(3): 599-607.

Herbal use in Germany includes nervous restlessness, and psycho-sexual problems associated with andropause.

Combined with honey, Silverweed is an excellent remedy for clearing hoarseness of the throat and lungs. Work by Guo T et al, *Pharm Biol* 2016 54(5): 807-11 found polysaccharides from the herb bioactive for antitussive and expectorant use.

The fresh leaf juice can be taken internally for chronic gallbladder inflammation; or apply to wounds, eczema, and even to external hemorrhoids.

Silverweed is an excellent detoxifying herb, helping wean individuals from nicotine and cocaine; as well as removing traces from the blood in a short period of time. This may be due, in part, to the significant organic sulphur content of the herb.

The dried root powder can be sprinkled on skin and leg ulcers.

Studies at the Univeristy of Innsbruck, Austria have confirmed the anti-spasmodic effect of silverweed on the uterus and intestines. It shares with shepherd's purse, and a few other herbs, the unusual attribute of being slightly radioactive, and exhibits local analgesia being placed over the painful area.

Juliette de Bairacli Levy suggests in one of her books that a white wine tincture of silverweed may help epilepsy; an attribute suggested by Culpepper.

Of course, the dried leaf may also be infused for diarrhea and general spring tonic, but is much milder in action.

The compound, 2-pyrone-4, 6-dicarboxylic acid, isolated from Silverweed, was previously only found in bacteria, until work by Wilkes and Glasi in Germany. *Phytochemistry* 2001 58:3.

Silverweed, despite low phenolic content, possesses moderate anti-oxidant activity, according to work by Kähkönen et al, *J Agric Food Chem* 2003 47:10.

Polysaccharides exhibit immune modulating activity in mice studies. Chen JR et al, *Fitoterapia* 2010 81(8): 1117-24.

A root polysaccharide reduces oxidative damage and is potential anti-apoptotic agent. Hu et al, *Carbo Polymers* 79:2.

Anserine increases the anti-tumor activity of doxorubicin without changing its metabolism, suggestive of a herb/drug benefit. Sadzuka et al, *Food Chem Tox* 45:6.

A triterpenoid saponin from the plant has been found to inhibit the hepatitis B virus from replicating, in a duck study. Zhao et al, *Phytomed* 2008 15(4): 253-8.

Alcohol extracts of the root, containing triterpenes, appear to protect the liver from chemical injury. Morikawa T et al, *Phytochemistry* 2014 102:169-81.

Polysaccharides reduce oxidative damage and are anti-apoptotic. Hu et al, *Carbo Polymers* 79:2.

Alcohol extracts were found to protect myocardial tissue from apoptosis after an acute mycocardial ischemia and reperfusion injury in rats, and inhibition of the expressions of caspase-9 and 3 mRNA and proteins. Qin X et al, *Zhongguo Zhong Yao Zhi* 2012 37(9): 1279-84. Earlier work by Li JY et al, found this herb and Salvia militorrhiza significantly diminish cardiac muscle damage from ischemia, in high and medium doses. *Zhong Xi Yi Jie He Xue Bao* 2009 7(1): 48-52.

Silvery Cinquefoil was recommended by Starostenko and Starostenko as among the active agents used for treating cirrhosis in human livers, especially associated with edema and ascites. *Zdravook-hranenie* 1971 14:6.

Both acetone and water extracts are active against Gram positive bacteria.

Silvery Cinquefoil (*P. argentea*) aerial extracts during flowering were examined by the showed biologically active ingredients worthy of further study.

Tiliroside from this herb shows activity against human endometrial carcinoma cell lines. Tomczyk et al, *Planta Medica* 2010 76:10 963-8.

The aerial parts contain methyl brevifolin carboxylate, a compound that shows activity against MCF-7 breast cancer cell lines. Tomczyk et al, *Pharmazie* 2008 63(5): 389-93.

Further work by the same author, *Fitoterapia* 2008 79 found water extracts of *P. anserina*, *P. argentea*, *P. fruticosa* and *P. recta* inhibit *Helicobacter pylori* associated with gastric ulcers. Growth of *Micrococcus luteus, Staphylococcus aureus and Bacillus subtilis* was inhibited, but Gram negative bacteria were not affected.

Chinese Silverweed (*P. chinensis*) **WEI LING CAI** is used for almost the exact purposes; as a febrifuge and detoxifying agent that removes heat from the blood for treating diarrhea, dysentery, bleeding hemorrhoids, carbuncles and furuncles.

Liu et al, *Zhongguo Zhong Yao Za Zhi* 2006 31:22 found strong anti-cancer activity in this plant, including significant effect from corosolic acid and another compound. Coroslic acid has been found to play a role in blood sugar regulation.

Shrubby Cinquefoil shows promise for the high content of flavanols in the flowers and leaves. These compounds are both anti-microbial and have thrombo-clastic activity.

Leaf catechins inhibit platelet aggregation and inhibit net glycogen synthesis in rat hepatocytes, suggesting need for further study.

Aerial parts of nine Potentilla species were tested, and this one showed the highest concentrations of tannins, proanthocyanidins, phenolic acids and flavonoids. It also shows the highest anti-biofilm activity for Streptococcus strains associated with dental caries. Tomczyk M et al, *Molecules* 2010 15(7): 4639-51.

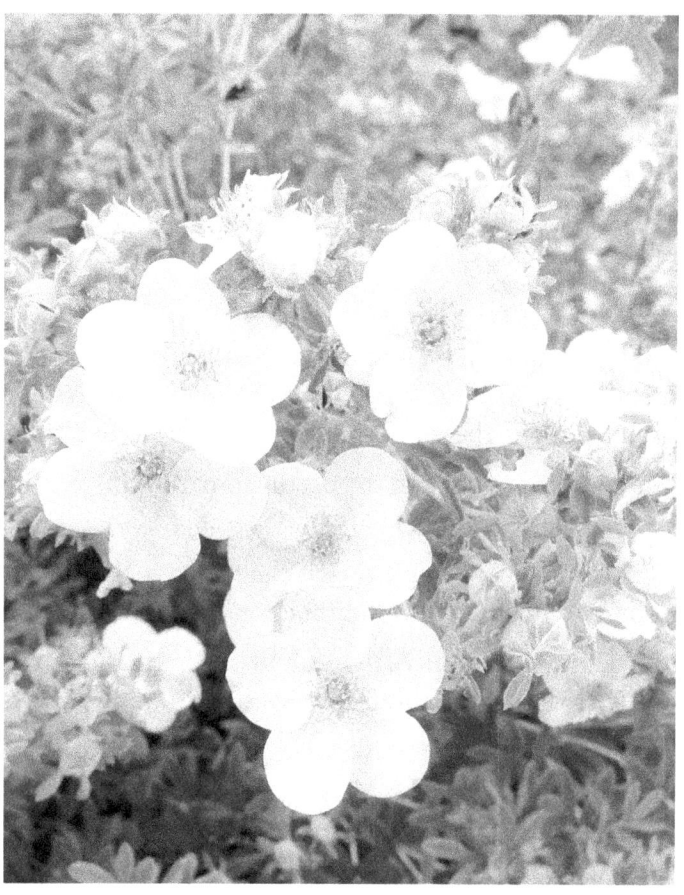

SHRUBBY CINQUEFOIL

The herb shows strong inhibition of bacteria, including *Pseudomonas aeruginosa* and the fungi *Candida albicans*. Wang SS et al, *BMC Complement Altern Med* 2013 13:231.

Earlier work found ethanol extracts active against gram positive bacteria such as *Staphylococcus aureus* and *Enterococcus faecalis*, as well as gram negative bacteria such as *E. coli, P. aeruginosa, Klebsiella pneumoniae* and *Proteus mirabilis*, as well as spore forming bacteria *Bacillus subtilis* and *B. cereus*. Jurkstiene V et al, *Medicina* (Kaunas) 2011 47(3): 174-9.

Khobrakova et al, *Rastitel'ney-Resursy* 2000 36:1 reported on the immune modulating properties of the shoots of *D. fruticosa*. Cellular and humoural pathways of immune response, and stimulating effect on phagocytosis are described.

In fact, the immuno-modulatory effects of the dry plant extract were greater than those of the liquid extract of Siberian Ginseng (*Eleutherococcus senticosus*) used for comparison.

Work by Khramova the year before discovered that the highest flavono-glycone and glycoside content is found in the leaves at bud stage, and in flowers when fully open. It is also rich in calcium. It was a traditional cancer herb.

A water soluble extract showed immune modulation, and increased survival rates, in new born mice infected with Coxsackie B3 virus. Evstropov AN et al, *Zh Mikrobiol Epidemiol Immunobiol* 2005 3:102-4.

In China, the leaf tea is used for dizziness caused by summer heat, blurred vision, disorders of stomach qi, and irregular menstruation. It is known as **JIN LAO MEI** or **GE SANG HUA**, and used for inflammation, cancers, and diabetes.

The herb is synergistic with *Ginkgo biloba* and green tea for antioxidant properties. Liu ZH et al, *BMC Complement Altern Med* 2016 16(1): 495; *J Food Sci* 2016 81(5): C1091-101.

White Cinquefoil (*P. arguta*) root extracts have been examined for anti-viral activity by McCutcheon et al, at UBC, and found it completely inhibited bovine respiratory syncytial virus. *J Ethnopharm* 1995 49(2): 101-10.

Inhibition of eight of ten bacterial strains from root extracts was noted by same author. *J Ethnopharm* 1992 37 213-223.

Leaf and seed extracts show activity against *Candida albicans*. Borchardt et al, *J Med Plants Res* 2008 2:4-5.

The seeds possess significant anti-oxidant activity, nearly 20 times that of blueberries.

More research is warranted.

Marsh Cinquefoil is used for the treatment of various ailments including tuberculosis, dysentery, and various metabolic disorders. Russian studies conducted in 1990 indicate that the rich mineral content is highest during shoot growth. The glycoside:flavonoid aglycone ratio of the above ground parts is 63:37.

The aerial parts contain the pectin comaruman, that shows anti-inflammatory and leucocyte adhesion activity. Popov et al, *Fitoterapia* 76:3.

Comaruman is a complex sugar chain composed of two-thirds galacturonic acid. It appears to decrease adhesion of human neutrophils to fibronectin. Popov SV et al, *Biochemistry* (Moscow) 2005 70(1): 108-12.

The compound reduces neutrophil infiltration and improves mucus membrane integrity, helping protect from acetic acid induced colitis in mice study. Popov SV et al, *Dig Dis Sci* 2006 51(9): 1532-7.

The herb shows protective quality in chronic experimental glomerulonephritis. Mondodoev AG et al, *Patol Fiziol Eksp Ter* 2010(1): 24-7.

Agrimoniin exhibits anti-alpha glucosidase activity and lowers plasma glucose and glycosylated hemoglobin in diabetic rats. Kaskchenko NJ et al, *Molecules* 2017 22:73.

Agrimoniin is found in several Cinquefoil species.

The roots exhibit anti-inflammatory activity, due to proanthocyanidins. Yerschik OA et al, *Dokl Biol Sci* 2009 429:535-7. The compounds appear useful in the relief of arthritis. Buzuk GN et la, *Dokl Biochem Biophys* 2008 421: 211-13.

Prairie Cinquefoil plants extracted with water, show activity against both gram positive and mycobacterium.

In Mexico, the related *P. candicans* has been shown to increase blood flow and nerve conduction to the sciatic nerve. The plant contains potent aldose reductase inhibitors that may explain in part, its usefulness in diabetic neuropathy.

The related *P. fulgens* root has been found to significantly lower blood sugar levels, in work by Syiem et al, *J Ethnopharmacology* 2002 83:1-2.

The root shows significant inhibition of methicillin resistant *Staphylococcus aureus,* in work by Zuo et al, *J Ethnopharm* 2008 August 28.

The European *P. alba* has been cell cultured and inoculated with Agrobacterium rhizogenes to obtain hairy roots. Terpenes from the roots have been found to inhibit thyroxine levels in lab rats. Other studies suggest it has adaptogenic properties similar to rhodiola. Shikov AN et al, *Pharm Biol* 2011 49(10): 1023-8.

The related *P. simplex* shows strong anti-fungal activity against nearly all of 23 human pathogenic organisms tested. Webster et al, *J Ethnopharm* 2008 115:1.

False Strawberry, like strawberry fruit, contains ellagic acid, an anti-carcinogenic compound.

In Traditional Chinese Medicine, the whole dried plant is used for its sweet bitter flavour, cold properties and somewhat poisonous nature.

It helps dispel heat, cools the blood, disperses swelling and helps remove toxins.

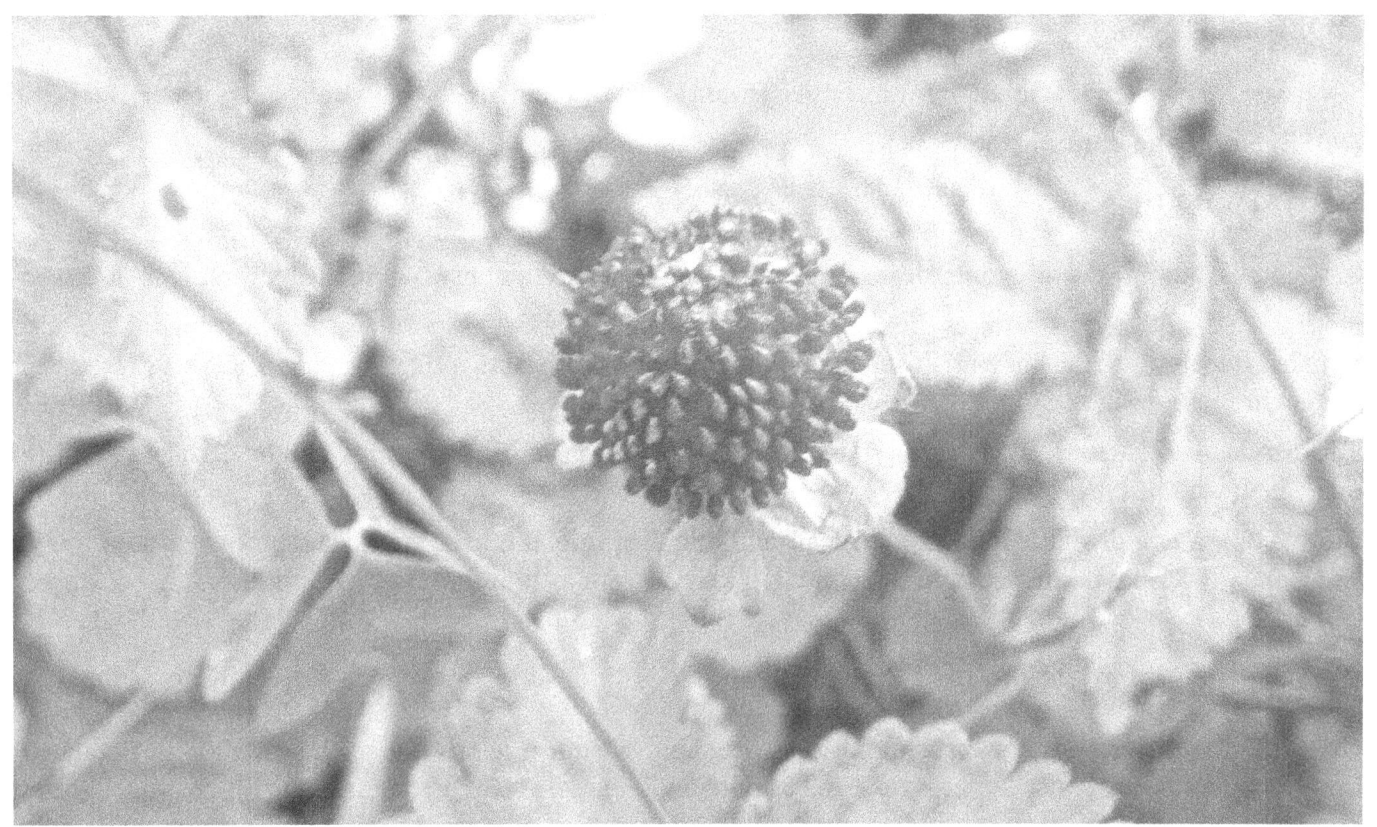

FALSE STRAWBERRY FRUIT

False Strawberry is used in fever states, epilepsy, coughs, laryngitis, dysentery, furuncles, burns, scalds and insect bites.

The plant exerts potent inhibition of neuraminidase, suggestive of benefit in preventing influenza A virus replication. Tian L et al, *J Ethnopharm* 2011 137(1): 534-42.

In TCM, it is called **SHE MEI**, or **TI CHIN**, which means Ground Tapestry. The whole plant is used for boils and abscesses, weeping eczema, and ringworm externally. For laryngitis and tonsillitis the decoction is gargled and swallowed.

Research conducted by Lee H and JY Lin, *Mutat Res* 1988 204(2): 229-34 found false strawberry water decoctions (two hour) have moderate anti-mutagenic activity.

Zhang ZX, and XS Bo found false strawberry active on extracorporeal esophageal cancer cells. *Zhong Xi Yi Jie He Za Zhi* 1988 8(4): 221-2.

The plant inhibits sarcoma 180, Ehrlich ascites cells, and treats thyroid cancer and hepatoma cancer cell lines.

Work by Peng et al, *Gynecol Oncol* 2008 108:1 found phenolic fractions of the herb cytotoxic against ovarian cancer SKOV-3 cell lines, via apoptosis and arresting cell cycle in the S phase.

Peng et al, *Exp Biol Med* (Maywood) 2009 234(1): 74-83 found it inhibits cervical cancer activity through induction of apoptosis and cell cycle arrest.

Ethanol extracts increase caspase-3 and reduced herpes simplex encephalitis, induced inflammatory injury on neurons, due to the induction of microglia apoptosis. Li XF et al, *Int J Immunopath Pharmacol* 2011 24(3): 631-8.

The leaf extract, in vitro, increased thymocyte proliferation by 41%, and splenocyte proliferation by 42%, suggesting immune stimulation, and possiblenew source of immune modulation for treatment of human immune mediated disease. Ang HY et al, *Exp Ther Med* 2014 7(6): 1733-1737.

HOMEOPATHY

Silverweed is given in low dilution for intestinal spasms and for relieving the pain of dysmenorrhea.

DOSE- mother tincture and low potencies

HYDROSOLS

Cinquefoil water breaks the stone, cleanses the reins, and is of excellent use in putrified fevers.

Silverweed distilled water cleanses the skin of all discolourings therein, as morphew, sun-burnings, etc. as also pimples, freckles, and the like; and dropped into the eyes, or cloths wet therein and applied, takes away the heat and inflammations in them.
CULPEPPER

The distilled water takes away freckles, spots, pimples in the face, and sun-burning, but the herb laid to infuse or steep in white wine is far better.
GERARD

Cinquefoil water is distilled from the herb, stalk and root in spring. It is used for old and new wounds, removes stone and gravel and cleans the kidneys, is applied to head with a cloth for nosebleed, for trembling members and hands.
BRUNSCHWIG

FLOWER ESSENCES

Cinquefoil is the remedy for discrimination, focus and wisdom. It promotes a calm, patient, detached, one-pointed state of consciousness. It helps to perceive the essence of any situation, and cut through the old patterns and attachments. It helps to reduce the dissipation of energy from excessive mental activity.
LIGHT MOUNTAIN

Tundra Rose (*P. fruticosa*) flower essence is for opening to inspiration, and letting go of resistance to the experience and expression of joy in daily life.
ALASKA

Silverweed helps us to detach from material concerns and over-indulgence, and promotes moderation and self-awareness. It speaks of the necessity of living lightly on the earth, and is useful in times when we become overly engrossed in material concerns. It allows us to get back to basics, to grass roots.
FINDHORN

Rough Cinquefoil (*P. norvegica*) flower essence is for those struggling with life, and wanting things to change, or are lonely in their struggle. It helps bring one to a place of inner nurturing and true experience of one's inner worth, where one may share from.
CANADIAN FOREST

Silverweed (*P. ansinera*) flower essence helps bring a sense of communication and awareness, combined with a maternal nature. It brings a natural energetic balance, and allow the intent to manifest. Symbolically, it is the affectionate mother shielding a beloved daughter from anticipated calamity.
PRAIRIE DEVA

Silverweed helps us to live lightly in our bodies and on the Earth, through moderation and self-awareness. When we become caught up in material concerns, we may lose contact with our higher purpose.
RAVENWORKS

Cinquefoil essence is for unhealthy relationships, whether based on filling needs, a variety of fears, possessiveness or fear of being alone.
CHOMING

Silverweed essence helps strengthen your relationship with nature, to feel and see the rhythms.
CHOMING

SPIRITUAL PROPERTIES

Congested or impacted energy may manifest spiritually in a person in many ways. Frequently, individuals not on a spiritual path will impact this energy in the emotional body. Cinquefoil will help to balance this energy by dispersing it throughout the rest of the emotional body.

Taking a tea will ease of disperse energy in a self-governing way. The plant, when used medicinally, has a self-regulating effect on the blood, thereby relieving cramps.

The plant signature shows the way in which the energy of the plant compacts, strengthens, and then moves out in all directions.

There is greater sight, impacting the third eye. Auras can be seen more easily as you remove your own filters. The throat chakra is strengthened; resulting in a willingness to express. Kidney and bladder meridians are enhanced, so that the energy may flow more readily into the physical body. Cinquefoil's primary effect is to focus energy in one part- usually the emotional or mental. This focus of energy allows greater energy transfer and dispersal. There is also some relief of the cancer and gonorrhea miasm. **GURUDAS**

These three species of Cinquefoil (including *P. fruticosa*) are able to bring into balance the inner senses and the outer senses. We mean, the inner ear and inner eye. These are not to be confused with the organs of clairvoyant sight and hearing, which are seated elsewhere within the sheaths of the lower bodies. The inner senses-those which allow one to "pick up" information, thoughts and images from higher planes-were always intended to be strongly tied to the physical senses, as indeed they were thousands of years ago when man was more in touch with the higher realities. However, man's increasing materiality and his tendency to focus attention only on physical phenomena have led to atrophying of the links that once united the higher and lower senses.

The Cinquefoils have the ability, when used to make a tea by steeping the flowers for ten minutes in near boiling water, to re-establish the connections that all men were intended to have as their birthright. The tea should be drunk twice a day. **HILARION**

Used with awareness, cinquefoil magnetizes appropriate energies. It is considered an ally for movement through astral realms, a household protector, and an aid to prophetic dreaming. **CRUDEN**

Cinquefoil is uplifting and empowering for those who need it, as well as protective.
DEBORAH FRANCES ND

ASTROLOGY

Only the marsh cinquefoil grows on marshland and peat pastures. Its creeping, rhizome-like shoot develops in the water-saturated soil. On the upwardly expanding shoots, a few dark, dull blossoms develop above the digitate, divided leaves. The perianth consists essentially of the calyx only. The petals are extremely small. The moistness and the moon-related form of the shoot allow the full development of the flower bud up to the calyx only. The metamorphosis into the perianth and the other organs of the flower is hardly able to overcome these influences. **KRANICH**

RECIPES

INFUSION- Pour one cup of boiling water on three teaspoons of dried leaf and flower. Cover and steep for ten minutes. Drink up to three cups.

In wild plants, the optimal tannin content of roots is highest in May-June when the plant buds just appear.

DECOCTION- Take two Tbsp of dried, chopped root to one pint of water. Simmer for twenty minutes. You may then add leaf and flower as above after moving the container off heat. Drink 1-2 ounces cool, up to three times daily. A good decoction for children's diarrhea is equal parts of blueberry leaves, silverweed root and Irish moss.

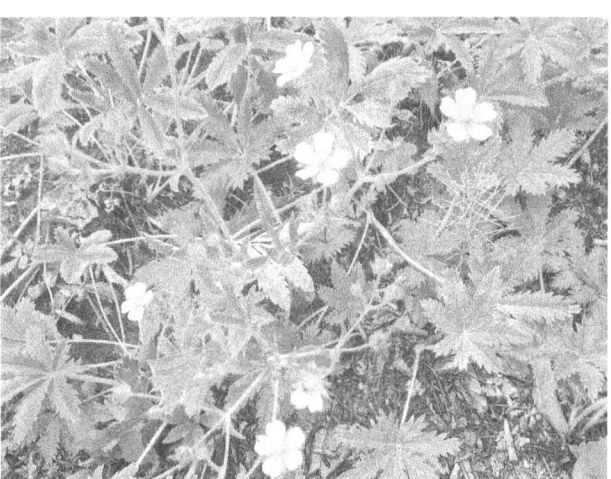

POTENTILLA GRACILIS

For adults try four parts silverweed, three parts plantain, and two parts Knotgrass (*Polygonum periscaria*) decocted for twenty minutes.

COMPRESS- Strain above decoction and soak cotton cloth. Wring out and apply to affected area. Replace as needed.

DECOCTION- False Strawberry- 9-15 grams as needed.

TINCTURE- 2-4 ml three times daily. Make a 1:4 with whole Potentilla plant including root at 60% alcohol and 10% glycerine. This will ensure tannins remain in solution.

EXTRACT- An extract is made by boiling one part of bruised root with eight parts water by weight for twenty minutes. Strain and repeat with another equal part of water. Mix the two together and evaporate slowly to extract consistency. Preserve with vegetable glycerine.

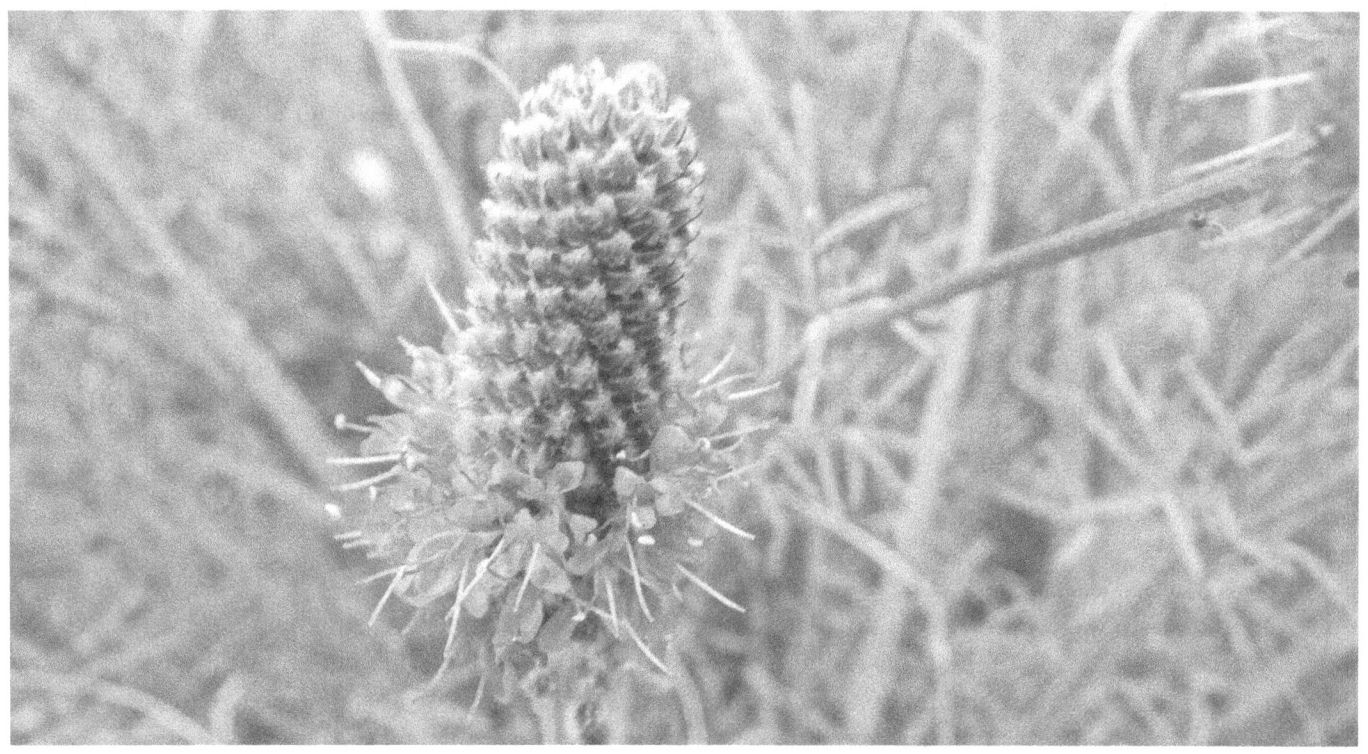

PURPLE PRAIRIE CLOVER

CLOVER, WHITE PRAIRIE
(***Dalea candida*** Michx. ex Willd.)
CLOVER, PURPLE PRAIRIE
(***P. purpureum*** [Vent] Rydb.)
(***D. purpurea*** Vent.)
CLOVER, HAIRY PRAIRIE
CLOVER, SILKY PRAIRIE
(***D. villosa*** [Nutt.] Spreng.)
PARTS USED- flowers, leaves, roots

To make a prairie it takes a clover and one bee,
One clover, and a bee, and revery.
The revery alone will do, if bees are few.   **EMILY DICKINSON**

What a miserable thing life is: you're living in clover, only the clover isn't good enough. **BERTOIT BRECHT**

The former genus name, Petalostemon or petalostemum, refers to the fact that the petal and stamen are joined. Dalea is named after Samuel Dale, an English botanist of the late 17th century. It was first noted and described by Etienne Ventenat, a French botanist in the late 18th century.

Both the white and rose-coloured prairie clovers are common to the drier, prairie grasslands.

Various native tribes used the purple prairie clover for heart conditions, diarrhea, measles, and pneumonia.

Others made a wash from the roots and leaves to clean open wounds; or just directly bruised the leaf and applied to the affected area.

The root tea was used for diarrhea and to prevent illness.

Purple Prairie Clover root tea was given, traditionally, by Fox healers for relief of measles and related fevers. They named it **KEPIA'EKIE' SHIKIKI**, meaning Thimble Top.

The flowers were mixed with white oak bark and Wild Cranesbill (*G. maculatum*) into medicine called **NESWAIYAGATWI**, meaning "three different kinds", to treat diarrhea.

The Lakota name means Kit Fox's Medicine Stem Female, and the White Clover its male equivalent due to the coarser leaves.

John Lame Deer, a Lakota healer, said, "the blossoms of the prairie clover are good for swollen throats, and its roots purge you but good."

The Navaho used the whole plant for pneumonia, and the root for measles, while the Chippewa decocted the leaves and blossoms for heart trouble. They called the plant Small leaves or **BA'SIBUGUK**.

Both the Omaha and Ponca tribe name for both Prairie Clovers is **MAKAN SKITHE**, or Sweet Medicine.

The roots are quite sweet, and can be chewed like wild licorice root.

White Prairie Clover root is an excellent tonic decoction. The Navaho used it as part of a compound for abdomen pain caused by colds and loose bowels.

It was considered analgesic and chewed for toothache, or as tea for stomach pain.

Decoctions of the plant were used for "snake infection" or fevers and a preventative life medicine,

The Pawnee call it Broom Weed, **KIHA PILIWUS HAWASTAT**, and used it traditionally to sweep out their lodges.

Kahlee Keane (Root Woman) says that she gathered some of the sturdy stalks, removed the seeds and tied them around a willow pole.

"It made a dandy broom! The end of the flower stalks, where the seeds had been attached, have a sort of 'Velcro' feel which made a dandy dust ball catcher."

The seeds can be ground into flour, or just added to cereals, breads and the like.

Hairy Prairie Clover roots were used, by Lakota as a purge, while the leaves and blossoms were eaten to relieve a swollen throat. It had two names, meaning either gray sand stem or gray weed stem.

Purple Prairie Clover is recommended by the Alberta Research Council for native restoration. It is very drought resistant, with the taproot growing several meters into the earth. Dale Lindgren, a researcher at the University of Nebraska has done considerable selection work on Purple and Hairy Prairie Clover. He can be reached at dlindgren@uni.edu.

The young shoots are nutritious and high in protein. Recent work suggests the plant reduces shedding of *E. coli* from grazing cattle, due to its anti-bacterial properties. Jin L et al, *J Food Protein* 2015 78(8):434-41.

One kilogram contains 290,000-550,000 seeds with a 98% germination rate after scarification, or placing the seeds in hot water (80° Celsius) and allowing them to soak for 24 hours.

The closely related *D. aurea*, or Golden Dalea, contains manufolin K and 3S(+)-7-methoxymanuifolin K.

These compounds exhibit significant activity against amoeba responsible for meningo-encephalitis, with activity similar to amphoreticin B, and superior inhibition after day four. Belofsky et al *Planta Medica* 2006 72(4):383-6.

Work by Patit, *J Nat Products* 60:3 found the root of *D. filiciformis* contains daleformis that inhibits endothelin-converting enzyme.

The related *D. versicolor*, potentiates berberine and prescription antibiotics. Belofsky et al, *Journal of Natural Products* 67(3):481-4.

The related Black Prairie Clover (*D. frutescens*) contains sanjuanolide, which shows cytotoxic activity against prostate cancer cells. Shaffer CV et al, *J Nat Prod* 2016 79(3):531-40. The perennial is native to New Mexico, Oklahoma and Texas.

A native of the western United States, *D. searisiae*, contains rotenoids, flavanones and isoflavones in aerial parts and root. Research has found activity against fall armyworm (*Spodoptera frugiperda*), as well as *Streptococcus mutans, Bacillus cereus* and oxacillin-sensitive and resistant strains of *Staphylococcus aureus*. Belofsky G et al, *Journal Natural Products* 2014 77(5):1140-9.

MEDICINAL

CONSTITUENTS- *D. purpurea* root-petalostemumol, petalopurpurenol, methyl ethers, benzyl ethers and acetates. Isoflavones such as 6,7,8', 4', 5'-hexamethoxyisoflavone and 7, 8, 3', 4', 5'-pentamethoxy isoflavone are found in the root and stem bark. Three geranyl stilbenes, and pawhuskins A-C are present.
flowers and bark- pterocarpans and isoflavones respectively. The pterocarpan (+)-3,4-dihydroxy-8,9-methyl enedioxy-pterocarpan is most active.
D. candidum- petalostein (an isoflavone)
D. villosum- unidentified flavonoids.
D. frutescens- sanjuanolide, sanjoseolide
D. formosa- sedonans A-F, but-2-enolide, 4'-O-methylpuerol, ent-sandwicensin.

Extracts from the Purple Prairie Clover root contain petalostemumol, a very active antibacterial and antifungal compound.

Research conducted at University of Mississippi by Hufford et al, in 1993, found petalostemumol exhibited good activity against both gram positive (*Staphlyococcus aureus, Bacillus subtilis*) bacteria, and moderate activity against gram negative bacteria like *E. coli*.

More recent work found the condensed tannins from purple prairie clover reduced growth rate of E. coli O157:H7, the organism responsible for "hamburger disease". Its activity may involve alternation in the fatty acid composition and disruption of the outer membrane of the cell. Wang Y et al, *J Food Prot* 2013 76(4):560-7. Similar findings were produced by Liu et al, *Molecules* 2013 18(2):2183-99, in another case of double-dipping on the same studies.

It showed moderate activity against *Candida albicans*, and marginal activity against *Cryptococcus neoformans*.

Huang et al, *J Nat Products* 1996 59:3 isolated petalopurpurenol, a prenylated flavanol from the root.

A 50% ethanol extract of the root showed activity against a variety of human cancer cell lines.

The pterocarpans from the flowers have shown cytotoxic activity against the KB tumour cell line.

Pawhuskin A has been found to exhibit strong activity, *in vitro*, for opioid receptor affinity. Belofsky et al, *Journal Natural Products* 2004 67:1 26-30. The compound has been synthesized. Neighbours JD et al, *J Nat Prod* 2008 71(11):1949-52.

This is incredibly important, as only two other plants on earth possess this action.

The poppy family, and the related synthetic drugs morphine, heroin, etc. are the best known, and Kratom the other.

The stilbene, pawhuskin A appears to preferentially bind to the kappa opioid receptor, and shows high selectivity as an antagonist of the delta opioid receptor. Hartung AM et al, *Bioorg Med Chem Lett* 2015 25(23):5532-5.

The related *D. elegans* root contains a preylated flavonoid, 2', 4'-dihydroxy-5'-(1'''-dimethylallyl)-6-prenylpino-cembrin (6PP).

It possesses significant anti-oxidant activity and is cytotoxic to liver cancer cell lines, suggesting possible use as an adjunct therapy. Elingold I et al, *Chem Biol Interact* 2008 171(3):294-305.

Work by Perez et al, in Pharm Bio 2003, 41:3 found it active against oxacillin sensitive and oxalic resistant *Staphylococcus aureus*, as well as *Micrococcus luteus*.

It was inhibitory against a number of opportunistic pathogens isolated from AIDS patients, such as *Candida albicans strains, C. glabrata, C. krusei, C. parapsilosis,* and *C. tropicalis,* as well as *Cryptococcus neoformans*, associated with meningitis; and *Trychophyton mentagrophytes,* a fungal disease of the skin, hair and nails.

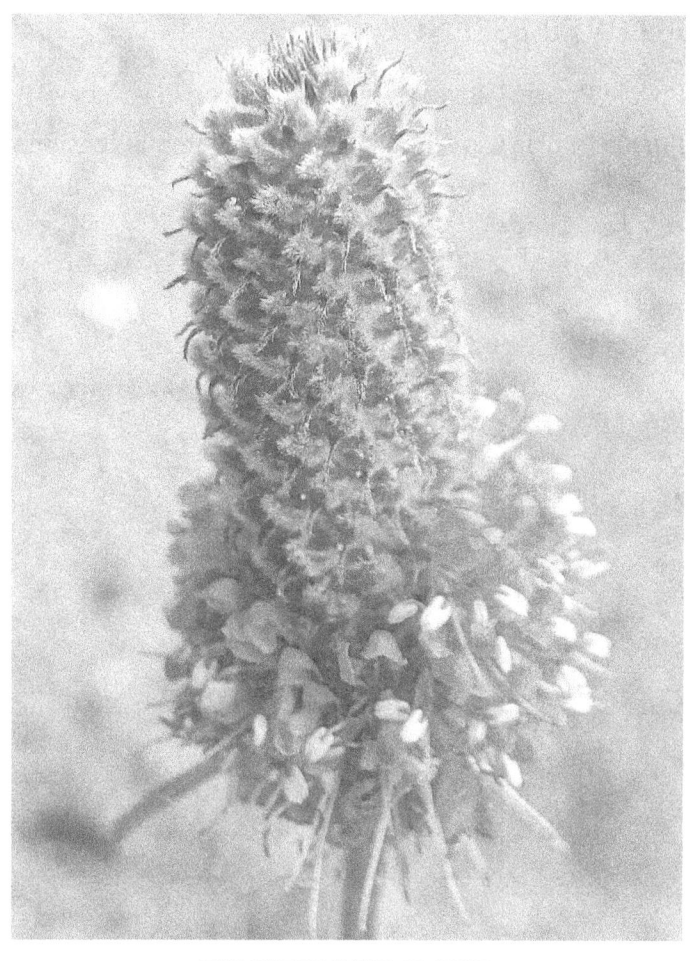

PURPLE PRAIRIE CLOVER

Work by Peralta et al, *Planta Medica* 78:10 981-7 found activity against fluconazole resistant strains of *C. albicans*. Recent work by the same research team identified the prenylflavonoid (8PP) with activity on *C. albicans* biofilms.

The flavanone dalenin is 52 and 495 times more effective a monophenolase inihibitor than either hydroquinone and kojic acid, respectively. This suggests great potential as a cosmetic agent for melanin related skin conditions. Chiari ME et al, *Bioorg Med Chem* 2011 19(11):3474-82.

The related *D. formosa* contains the isoflavonoid sedonan A, that shows anti-fungal activity against *Candida glabrata*, at levels higher than fluconazole. This is a frequent, and all too common, human fungal pathogen.

Other sedonans were active against *Saccharomyces cerevisiae*. A combination of sedonan A and ent-sandwicensin exhibits synergistic growth inhibition. Belofsky G et al, *J Nat Prod* 2013 76(5):915-25.

Natural approaches to opportunistic fungal infections, in patients suffering immune compromised conditions, should be explored more thoroughly.

The substance 8PP (formerly 6PP) impairs hepatic energy metabolism by acting as a mitochondrial un-coupler and inhibits enzymatic activities linked to respiratory chain. Elingold et al, *Chem Biol Interac* 2008 171:3.

Work by Belofsky et al, *J Nat Prod* 2004 67:3 found phenolic metabolites from *D. versicolor* enhanced the activity of berberine and antibiotics against *Staphylococcus aureus and Bacillus cereus*. A particular efflux pump (NorA) in MRSA is inhibited, as well as the Bmr efflux pump in *B. subtilis*.

The root of related *D. filiciformis* contains daleformis, that inhibits endothelin-converting enzyme. Patil AD et al, *J Nat Prod* 1997 60(3):306-8.

FLOWER ESSENCE

Purple Prairie Clover essence is for people who have it all together in all areas except one. **ROCKY MTN**
Purple Prairie Clover helps relieve the mental tension associated with opioid addiction. **PRAIRIE DEVA**

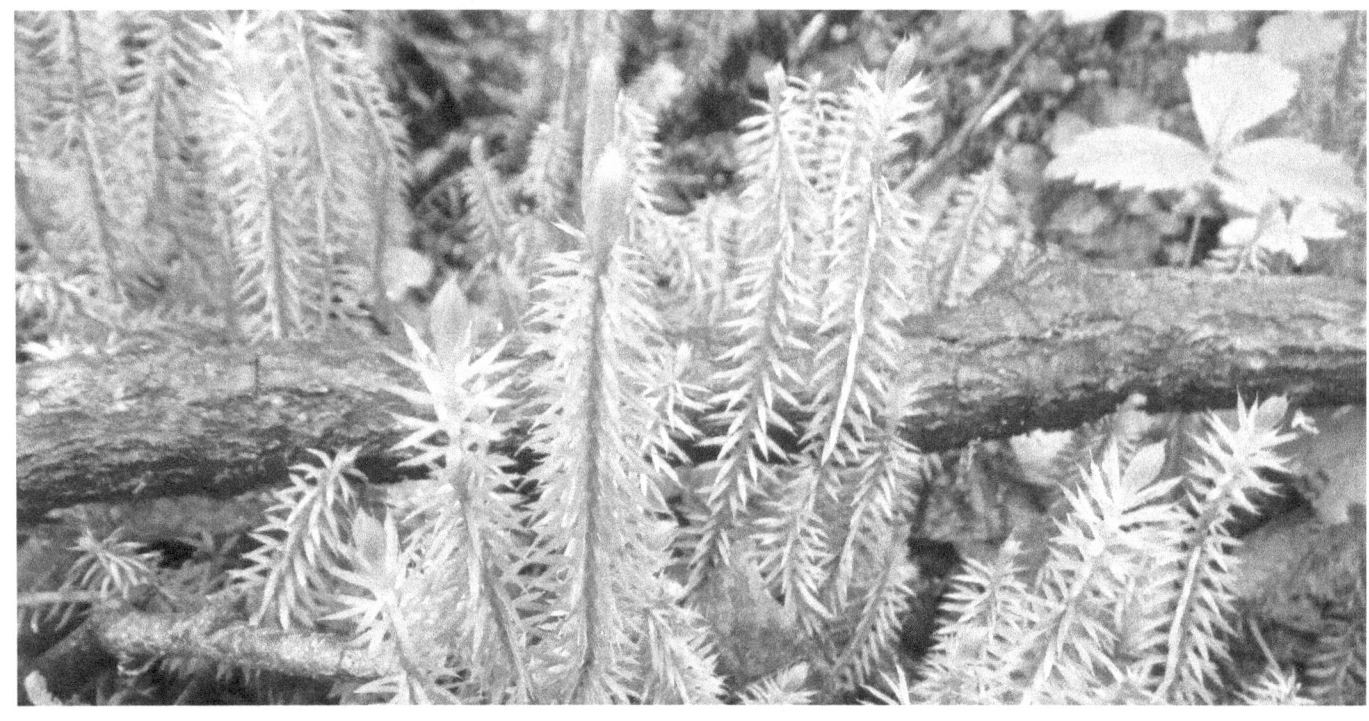

RUNNING CLUBMOSS

RUNNING CLUBMOSS
(***Lycopodium clavatum*** L.)
GROUND CEDAR
(***L. complanatum*** L.*)*
GROUND PINE
TREE CLUBMOSS
(***L. obscurum*** L.)
NORTHERN FIR CLUBMOSS
MOUNTAIN CLUBMOSS
(***L. selago*** L.) – not accepted
(***Huperzia selago*** [L.] Bernh. *ex* Schrank & Mart.)
MOUNTAIN FIR CLUBMOSS
ALPINE FIR MOSS
(***H. haleakalae*** [Brackenridge] Holub.)
STIFF CLUBMOSS
BRISTLY CLUBMOSS
INTERRUPTED CLUBMOSS
(***L. annotinum*** L.*)*
NORTHERN BOG CLUBMOSS
(***L. inundatum*** L.*)* not accepted
(***Lycopodiella inundata*** [L.] Holub.)
PARTS USED- spores, plant and root

The club-moss is on my person,
No harm or mishap can me befall;
No sprite shall slay me, no arrow shall wound me,
No fay nor dun water-nymph shall tear me.

ALEXANDER CARMICHAEL

Lycopodium is from the Greek **LYKOS**, meaning wolf, and **PODUS** for foot.

Club moss and its related genus and family are valuable medicinal plants that form fairy rings in fields and openings of the boreal forest. Inundatum means "apt to be flooded" and refers to a species that grows in bogs and moister regions of the boreal forest.

The Druids used the spores as a "cloth of gold" to protect them from black magic. Club moss is ruled over by the planets Saturn and Capricorn.

Druid nuns gathered the plant in the Loire Valley of France for their altars.

It had to be picked by a naked virgin with a newly woven cloth covering her hand and personifying the moon. She had to uproot the Selago with the tip of her little finger, after drawing a circle around it.

In some parts of Europe, club moss was believed to cause discord and argument when brought into groups. And yet, ironically, the Swedes use the stems for matting of Christmas wreaths.

While in Peru, I observed club moss species added to San Pedro cacti to enhance the hallucinogenic effect. Various species are known as Condor plant, in honor of the large bird. When added to San Pedro, the plant spirit appears to the Curandero as a Condor, which can astral travel. In this way, the healer can bring back the lost soul to a patient suffering from Susto, or fright.

I observed this ceremony on more than one occasion while living in Peru. In Trujillo, the plant is known as *Trenza Shimbe*, and used to improve visionary sight. Another name is *Trencilla Verde*. In southern Ecuador, they are used in a similar manner for Espanto, meaning to startle; and added to mixtures of plants to induce trance or hallucination.

The spores are referred to as Flour of the Witches.

In Nepal, club moss is sacred to the Hindu god Vishnu, and used in ceremonies.

The Native people of Alberta used the yellow spore powder on wounds; inhaling them for severe nosebleeds. Steaming decoctions of white spruce needles and club moss were used for stiff joints in sweat lodges.

The Cree of northern Alberta call Running Clubmoss, **ASTASKAMKWA**.

Cree medicine used the spores as a metaphysical expression of a patient's health. Spores were placed on top of water; and if they radiated towards the sun, then the patient would survive. The waterproof property of spores was put to good use in separating fish eggs from the membranes in food preparation.

The Nitinaht of Vancouver Island considered it bad luck; and touching the plant would cause one to lose their way in the forest. The Tlingit word is **KUWAKAAN SIIGI** meaning "deer's belt".

The Gitksan call it **BELANA WATSX**, meaning belt of land otter. It was traditionally used to make wreaths for graves, as the otter is a powerful, spiritual animal, but one that can be dangerous and cause madness or death.

The spore powder or "witch's flour" is highly flammable, and was put to good use by early photographers and theatre prop artists; known as "vegetable cordite".

It is source of the expression "flash in a pan". The powder was used in early stages of photocopy technology as well as forensic science.

A fun campfire trick is to quickly sprinkle some spores for a dramatic flash, something practiced by shaman from various cultures.

It has been previously used in hair powder, suppositories, surgical gloves and condoms. As many mature males are having their prostate health checked more frequently, it is best to use spore free condoms in rectal exams. These spores can cause allergic reaction in sensitive individuals; including hay fever, asthma and serious cell granuloma.

The Chinese use **SHEN JIN CAO** (*L. clavatum*) pollen as a dusting powder, to coat suppositories, and a dehumidifier to keep pills from sticking together. Decoctions of the plant are analgesic, and used for cramping, and arthritic complaints associated with painful joint movement. The herb is said to relax the tendons and circulate blood.

In the Himalayas, the whole plant and spores are taken internally for spasmodic retention of urine in infants, and externally for catarrhal cystitis.

In Africa, running clubmoss is mixed with *Selaginella rupestris* for headaches.

Ground cedar decoctions were used by Blackfoot in the treatment of lung and venereal disease; very similar to its use by the Chinese. They used ground cedar spores for athlete's foot and fungal ulcers. The roots were a mordant or fixative for natural dyes like alum root.

Ground cedar (*L. complanatum*) was used traditionally by making a tea of the dried, powdered plant for increasing urine flow, starting delayed menstruation and relieving uterine spasms. The tea was used as an aphrodisiac. Further southeast, the Ojibwa used the dried leaves as a reviver; and the Iroquois used the herb as part of a combination decoction to induce pregnancy.

The herb contains stimulating effect, as opposed to the more narcotic *L. selago*.

The spores were boiled, and used as a hair wash for lice. The plant may live up to 850 years old.

Ground Pine (*L. obscurum*) spores were traditionally used by the Chinese, as a desiccant for athlete's foot and other fungal infections. The plant was decocted for spasmodic and analgesic conditions, like arthritis, back pain and nocturnal emissions.

Ground Pine was boiled and drunk as a purgative by the Montagnais in cases of biliousness. The Iroquois used cold decoctions for weak blood and root decoctions for the menopausal change of life.

The Flambeau used it along with Northern Bush Honeysuckle (*Diervilla lonicera*) as a diuretic; while the Chippewa used it with spruce twigs to steam rheumatic joints.

Fir club moss (*H. selago*) is chewed by indigenous Alaskans, as an intoxicant that creates a mild hypnotic and narcotic state. Northern and Mountain Clubmoss are similar, with the latter somewhat smaller, and found at higher elevation. Both have been called *L. selago* in the past; and were used by the Druids of Wales as an active cathartic and de-obstruent.

Women of the Scottish Highlands used the plant as an abortifacient. This is not surprising as women in Argentina use decoctions of the related *L. saururus*, known as Cola de quirquincho, for the same purpose.

William Emboden wrote a tea from three stems will induce narcosis with small amounts both emetic and cathartic. In the Highlands of Scotland, it was taken in small doses to induce giddiness, and in larger amounts caused convulsion or miscarriage.

Fir Clubmoss was dried and ground as a dusting powder, or steeped and cooled for a softening lotion for skin.

Millspaugh wrote "it is also strongly counterirritant when applied to the skin, being used to keep blisters open, and to kill lice upon animals."

Huperzia species are without cones, and come in two forms often mistaken for two different species. One is short and thick, and another long and thinner, but neither creep on the ground.

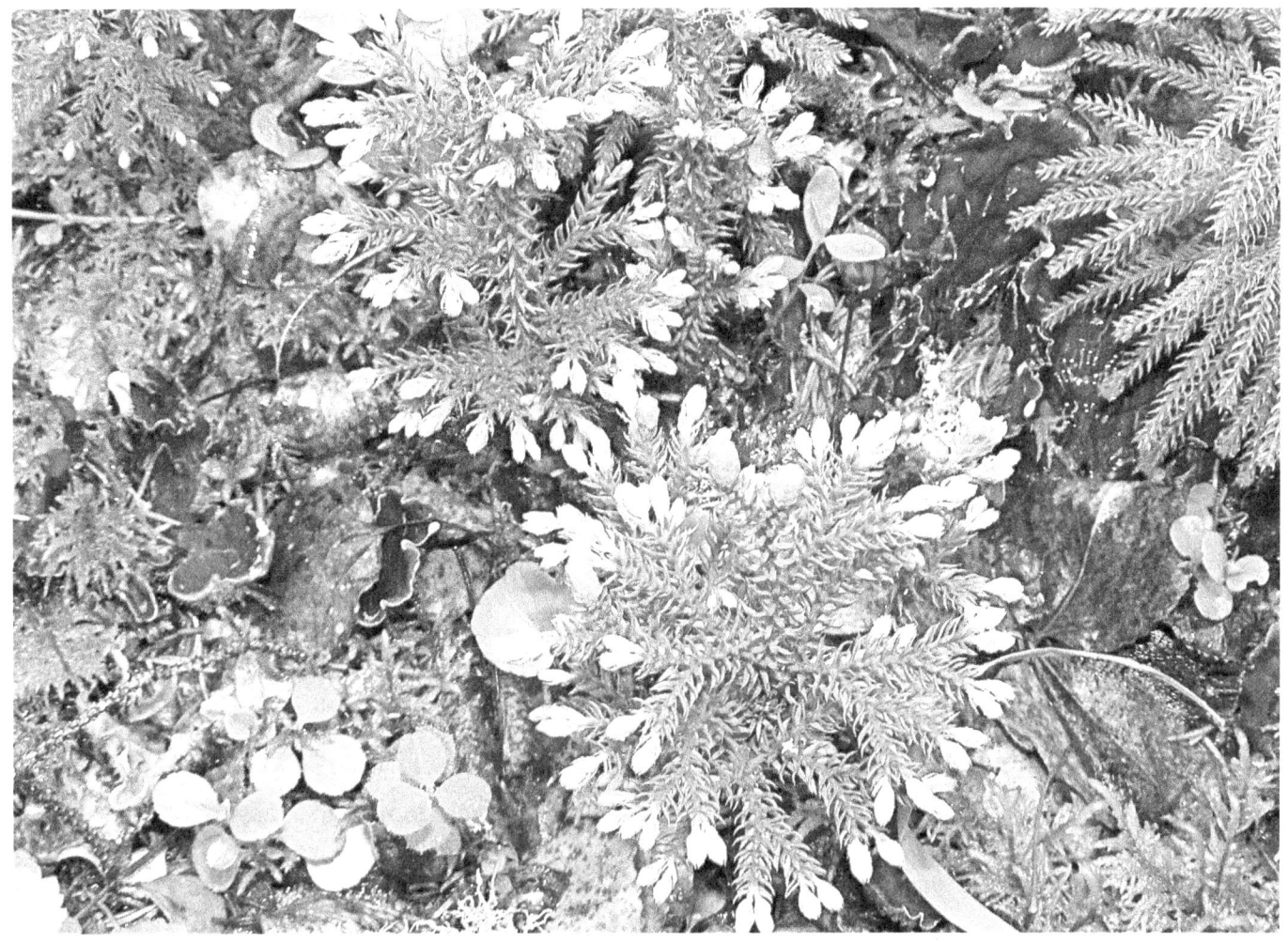

CLUBMOSS- NEW GROWTH

Pliny mentions its use in treating uterine problems, knee problems, swollen thighs, water retention, and dropsy. One German name **BÄRLAPP** means uterine ointment.

It was listed in the US Pharmacopoeia as useful in absorbing fluids from injured tissue.

Smoke from dried club moss was used to treat eye disease in Highlands of Scotland. It was given internally, to treat glaucoma by Polish physicians in the 1940s.

The Inuit of Baffin Island and other northern islands used Stiff Club Moss for eye problems. The name **SIQPIIJAUTIT** means, "that which is used to remove siqpik," or discharge from the inner corner of the eye. The tops are very soft when ripe.

Inuit elders use it as an intoxicant that makes one dizzy and a light feeling in the head. It was boiled until the water turned black.

A recent article by Black et al, *Can J Botany* 2008 86 identified a broth containing Stiff Club Moss by the Inuit of Baffin Island, and *Oxyria digyna* for general health and hallucinogenic activity.

Mountain Sorrel (*O. digyna*) is known as **QUNGULIIT** by Inuit of Baffin Island.

Sporopollenin from *L. clavatum* has been found to be capable of acting as a solid support for peptide synthesis. In work by MacKenzie et al, *Int J Pept Protein Res* 1980 15:3 it was found to have numerous important practical advantages over synthetic resins.

Several authors believe that Clubmoss takes up astonishing amounts of aluminum from the soil. The ash is said to contain up to 30% of this metal.

This content of aluminum led to its replacement of the mordant alum (potassium aluminum sulphate) in fixing dyes. The colors are soft and less bright than alum but last longer.

MEDICINAL

CONSTITUENTS- *Lycopodium clavatum* spores- pollenin (45%), sporopollenin, decyl-isopropyl-acrylic acids, myristic acid, sporonine, lycopodine, radium, resins, 50% fatty acid, various decanoic acids, and flabelline.

The plant contains flavones, beta-sitosterol, clavatine, nicotine, lycopodine, acetyldihydrolycopodine, fawcetine, fawcetimine, deactyl-fawcetine, clavatoxine, and apigenin-4'-O-beta-D-glucoside. It contains over 201 alkaloids including dihydro-lycopodine, acetyldihydrolycopodine, alpha obscurine, clavolonine, lycodine and numerous triterpenoids including alpha onocerin, lyclaninol, lyclanitin, lyclavanol, lyclavinin, lyclavatol, lycocryptol. Also contains vanillic, ferulic and azelaic acid, as well as 16-oxoseratenediol.

Ground cedar (*L. complanatum*) has similar spore composition.

The plant contains complanatine, lycopodine (60.8%), alpha-obscurine, serra-tenediol, tohogenol, lyconadins A-H, complanadine C-D, dehydroisofawcelline N-oxide, lycospidine A, lycopladines B-D, and nicotine.

Ground Pine (*L. obscurum*)- alpha & beta obscurine (diazaphenanthrene alkaloids), obscurumines H-P, various onoceranoid triterpenoids, lycobscurines A-C.

Northern Fir Clubmoss (*H. selago*)- huperzine A (selagine) alkaloids including lycopodines, arifoline, serratidine, pseudo-selagine (isolycodoline), selagoline and lycodoline.

L. annotinum- alpha and beta obscurine, and various alkaloids including annofoline, annopodine, annotine, annotinine, annotinolides A-C, isolycopodine, alpha and beta lofoline, lycodine, lycodoline, lycofawcine, lycofoline, lyconnotine, lycoposerramine M, anhydrolycodoline, gnidioidine, lannotinidine D, H-J, acrifoline, N oxide of annotine and lycopodine.

L. inundata- dehydrolycopecurine, (-)-3-dehydro-trans-9-methyl-10-ethyl-lobelidiol, inundatine, isoinun-datine, lycopodine.

Club moss spore powder was previously used as a dusting powder for condoms, and a safe pharmaceutical aid to prevent pills sticking together. It was a valuable body powder for the bedridden, known as Vegetable Sulphur, and dusted on bedsores, eczema, and herpes eruptions.

It excels for diaper rash, because it is not only soothing, but contains a waxy substance that is water repellent. If you coat your hand with spores and put it into water, your hand will remain completely dry!

Intertrigo, a dermatitis associated with moisture between skin folds, responds well to the soothing spore powder.

Fomentations of the plant, or pillows stuffed with the dry herb, relieve leg and foot cramps; and even headaches.

A tincture of the spores is recommended for extreme sensitivities of the skin. Slow, painful boils and swollen lymphatic nodes respond to the tincture.

Tinctures of the fresh plant, before it spores, sedate gastric disturbance, accompanied by blood filled urine. Painful urine retention by children and adults suffering from mucous filled, painful urination is helped.

Rheumatism and gout, with buildups of uric acid in the system and chronic kidney weakness with fevers are assisted.

Lycopine, an alkaloid of club moss, has been found to stimulate peristalsis, which encourages bowel movements. Lycopodine, however, produces uterine contractions and increases small intestinal peristalsis, so caution is advised.

Cirrhosis of the liver, accompanied by shortness of breath, responds to frequent infusions of the warm tea.

In China, the whole plant of *L. clavatum* is called **SHEN JIN CAO** meaning, "stretch the tendon herb", and is used to dispel wind and remove dampness. It relieves the rigidity of muscles, tendons and joints and dysmenorrhea. The herb is acrid, warm and dispersing.

For trauma related pain, combine with ground ivy.

When wine mix-fried, club moss is superior for dispelling wind, cold, dampness, and opening network blood vessels.

Studies by Orhan et al, in Turkey isolated alpha onocerin from *L. clavatum*, and found it to be a new acetyl-cholinesterase (AChE) inhibitor, that may be useful in the treatment of Alzheimer's disease. *Planta Medica* 2003 69:3. Alpha onocerin has an IC50 of 5.2 mcg/M.

Work by Calderon AI et al, *Nat Prod Res* 2013 27(4-5):500-5 found *L. clavatum* showed strong AChE inhibition. This was also confirmed in work by Konrath EL et al, *J Ethnopharm* 2012 139(1):58-67.

More recent work by same author, *J Ethnopharm* 109:1 found the alkaloid lycopodine, which comprises 85% of alkaloids, a powerful anti-inflammatory.

Lycopodine triggers apoptosis by depolarizing mitochondrial membranes in androgen sensitive and refractory prostate cancer cells, with modulating p53 activity. Bishayee K et al, *Eur J Pharmacol* 2013 698(1-3):110-21.

Lycopodine inhibits growth of HeLa cancer cell lines. Mandal SK et al, *Eur J Pharmacol* 2010 626(2-3):115-22.

Clubmoss extracts exhibit acetyl-cholinesterase inhibition, at least in rat brain cortex, striatum and hippocampus. Konrath et al, *J Ethnopharm* 139:1.

In the Journal *Phytochemistry* 6:1 the same author found extracts active against *Staphylococcus aureus*, various fungi, and the *Herpes simplex* virus.

Work by Orhan et al, *Phytochem Rev* 2007 6 found activity against *S. aureus, Proteus mirabilis, Klebsiella pneumoniae, Acinetobacter baumannii* and *E. faecalis*. It possesses anti-viral effect against *herpes simplex* virus, similar to acyclovir, while an alkaloid fraction shows activity against para-influenza virus similar to oseltamivir. High antioxidant activity was noted as well.

Clubmoss extracts, *in vitro*, inhibit CYP3A4 liver enzymes, suggesting caution when combinied with drugs. Tam et al, *Can J Physio Pharmacol* 2011 89:1.

Spore extracts show protective effects against various markers in mice, when given carcinogens leading to liver tumors. Reductions in glutathione reductase, hemoglobin, estradiol and testosterone, and increased blood glucose and cortisol were all normalized with administration. Pathak S et al, *Ind J Exp Biol* 2009 47(7)602-7.

Ground Cedar (*L. complanatum*) contains complanadine D that enhances mRNA expression for NGF (natural growth factor). The plant contains 61% lycopodine. Ether extracts show activity against anti-cholinesterase and butyrl-cholinesterase, as well as the *herpes simplex* virus. Orhan et al, *Nat Prod Res* 2009 23(6):514-26.

Alkaloids from this species and *H. selago* prevent oxidative damage and apoptosis in age-related neurodegenerative disorders. Lenkiewicz AM et al, *Folia Neuropathol* 2016 54(2): 156-66.

Fir club moss (*H. selago*) may be boiled and strained as effective eyewash. The spores are used in China for uterine problems, swollen knees, thighs and ankles, and water retention.

Recent research indicates it may be effective treatment for herpes, myasthenia gravis and Alzheimer's disease- an exciting possibility! This is due to the discovery that *L. selago* contains selagine- a compound chemically identical to huperzine. Work by Dr. Alan Kozikowski at the University of Pittsburgh identified selagine as identical to huperzine.

Work by Feigenhauer et al, found Fir Club Moss water extracts to contain significant anti-cholinesterase activity. They found that the amount of huperzine A and B in *L. selago* was sufficient for relevant acetyl cholinesterase inhibition. *Journal Tox Clinical Toxicology* 2000 38:7. This followed from observing two patients who drank the herb tea by mistake, and experienced excess sweating, dizziness, and slurring of speech.

The related Chinese Clubmoss, **CHIEN TSENG TA**, or **SHUANG YI PING** (*L. serratum*) contains huperzine A, which is three times more potent than phytostigmine, as an acetylcholinesterase (AChE) inhibitor.

Other names include *Huperzia serrata*, **QIAN CENG TA**, meaning "thousand layered pagoda", and **JIN BU HUAN**, "more valuable than gold". Indeed!

In clinical trials conducted by Cheng in 1986, it showed improvement in 98% of cases of myasthenia gravis; and improving memory in senile dementia. Content of huperzine A is highest in mid-fall and lowest in early spring.

It has shown in studies to decrease neuronal cell death caused by toxic levels of glutamate.

This makes huperzine A a potential medicine for reducing neuronal injury from strokes, epilepsy, and other disorders.

Huperzine A shows NMDA receptor blocking, as well as anti-cholinesterase activity, and may be useful for prevention of epileptic seizures. Schneider et al, *Epilepsy Behav* 2009 July 16.

Huperzine A is a novel cognition enhancer, inhibiting cholinesterase activity and modulating NMDA (N-methyl-D-aspartic acid) an excitatory amino acid transmitter. Both dementia and schizophrenia patients may benefit. Chiu et al, *J Compl Integr Med* 2007 4:1.

Huperzine B is reported in *Acta Pharm Sinica* 1999 20:2 to have anti-cholinesterase properties, is more selective than tacrine, and with less toxicity.

In one double-blind, randomized study, huperzine A was tested in 56 patients with senile dementia and 104 patients with senile and pre-senile simple memory disorders. The injectable form showed the most significant positive effects.

Another study of 50 Alzheimer's disease patients showed significant improvement in 58% of patients, in a multi-centre, randomized, double-blind, placebo-controlled study.

A placebo-controlled, double-blind study of 160 Alzheimer's patients found huperzine A significantly superior to placebo, tacrine and physostigmine, a cholinesterase inhibitor, with longer activity than either drug.

Huperizine A works on acetylcholine, only in the brain, giving it vast advantage over drugs such as cholinesterase inhibitors, often prescribed for Alzheimer's disease. It is non-toxic at up to 100 times human therapeutic dosage, and is an atropine antidote.

Huperizine A, when compared to tacrine, donepezil and rivastigmine, shows better penetration of the blood brain barrier, higher oral bioavailability and longer AChE inhibition.

The alkaloids isolated from *H. selago* provide a new therapeutic approach for oxidative stress-dependent disorders. Czapski GA et al, *Folia Neuropathol* 2014 52(4):394-406.

Huperzine A may be a useful adjunct therapy for improving cognitive function for patients with schizophrenia spectrum disorders. Zheng W et al, *Hum Psychopharmacol* 2016 31(4):286-95.

The compound protects against excitotoxicity and neuronal death and increases GABAergic transmission associated with anti-convulsant activity. Damar U et al, *Expert Rev Neurother* 2016 16(6): 671-80.

John Heinerman used club moss herb in an energy and stamina formula. He added the plant because it contained some compounds that cross the blood brain barrier, and positively affect the limbic centre of the brain.

Stiff Clubmoss contains annotine but does not contain alkaloids that inhibit acetylcholinesterase. Annotine increases the ability of dendritic cells to direct the differentiation of allogeneic CD4(+) T cells toward Th2. This suggests possible application for Th1 and/or Th17 mediated inflammatory disease. Hardardottir I et al, *Phytomedicine* 2015 22(2):277-82.

Ground Pine (*L. obscurum*) has been shown in clinical trials to contain anti-viral properties against the herpes simplex I implicated in cold sores.

Lycopodium spores were widely used in the 1920s as a dusting powder. If the spores found their way into surgical wounds they would cause granulation, even decades later, resembling cancerous or tuberculosis sores. The soothing, water resistant nature of the spores was put to use at one time in the treatment of intertrigo, a dermatitis caused by a build up of water between skin folds. The spores should not, however, be used externally on wounds.

The alkaloid fordine has been found in at least 14 species of *Huperzia*, and has similar action. All club moss in the boreal forest could be tested for this valuable compound.

In rat studies, fordine at 0.01-0.04 mg/kg IP speeds up conditioned avoidance responses, reverses impairment of conditioned avoidance response, and antagonizes hippocampal and cortical EEG changes induced by quinuclidinyl benilate.

Stiff club moss contains a number of alkaloids including annotine and lycodine that show activity noted above.

Recent work found novel C25 steroids derived from endophytic fungi in *H. serrata*, exhibit acetylcholinesterase activity. Fei-Xue Yu et al, *Fitoterapia* 2017 117:41-46.

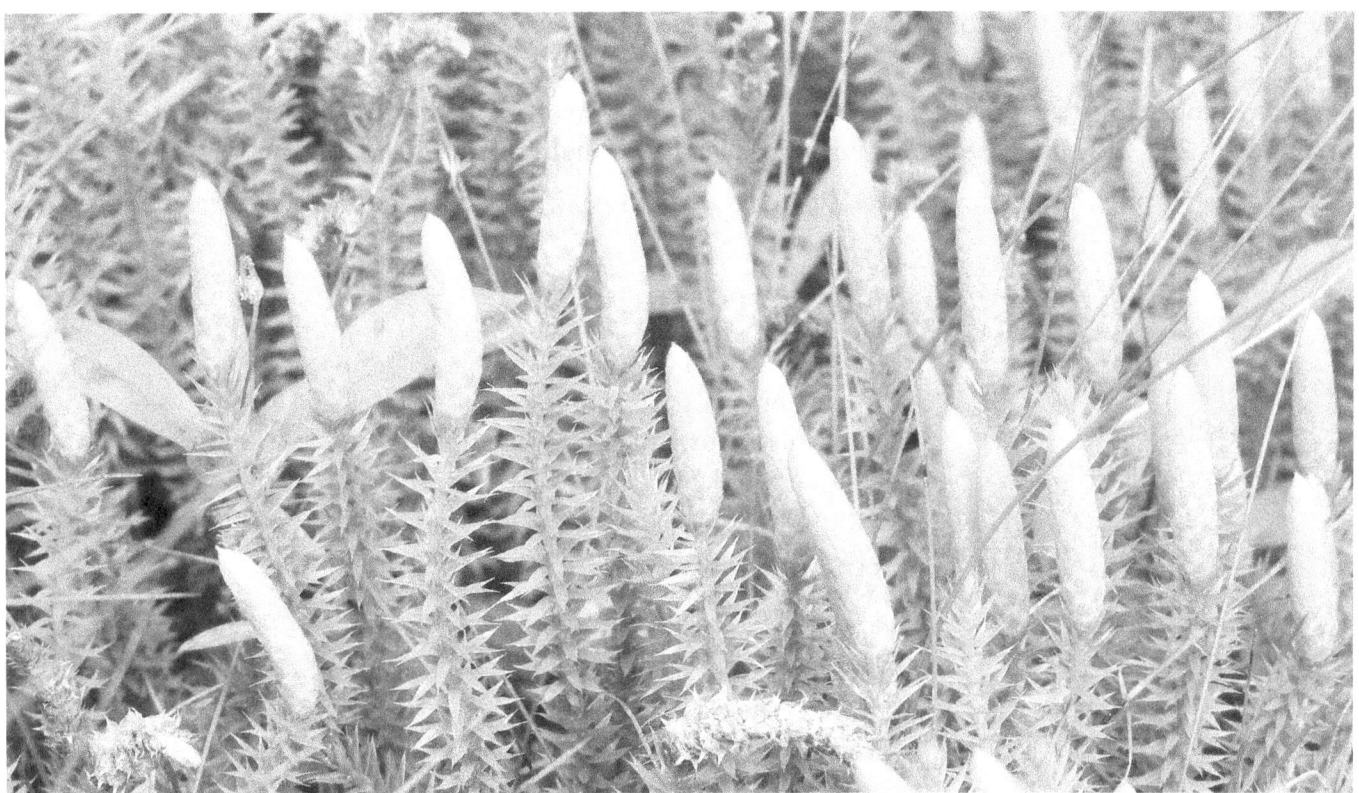

STIFF CLUBMOSS

HOMEOPATHY

Lycopodium (*L. clavatum*) is one of our most valuable remedies. Patients that can benefit are prone to disorders of the digestive system often suffering from bloating and gas. They may sit down hungry, and yet a bite or two fills them up.

They may be awakened, by hunger pains and headaches, if they don't eat when their body suggests. Meat, oysters, onions, cabbage, or milk may aggravate their symptoms.

One peculiar symptom is that one foot may be hot; but the other is cold. All symptoms are worse on the right side of the body and worse between 4 and 8 pm. A fan-like movement of the wings of the nostrils observed during breathing, suggests this remedy may be helpful in alleviating the above symptoms. There is a craving for sweets and warm drinks.

The male may be impotent, and the female have menses that are long and profuse. Vaginal dryness is irritated by sex.

Classically, the Lycopodium patient needs someone to be close, but not necessarily in the same room.

DOSE- For elimination try 2X or 3X, a few drops in water before meals. Use 4X for mood swings and desire for sweets, related to both physiological and psychological issues.

The mother tincture and 200 C showed increased cerebral blood flow in a rat study. Hanif K et al, *Homeopathy* 2015 104(1):24-8.

Higher potency is for mental and emotional symptoms. Try 30X for babies that sleep all day and cry all night. The mother tincture is prepared from the spores, gathered towards the end of summer. The powder is pale yellow, and both odorless and tasteless.

The first three attenuations are made by mixing, and grinding one grain of powder to one hundred grains of milk sugar, for 1X, and so on.

For higher potencies, the 1X powder can be diluted in alcohol. Work by Pathak et al, *Forsch Komple* 14:3 found Lycopodium 200, as alcohol extraction, possesses liver cancer fighting potential.

The 5C and 15C potencies induced apoptosis in HeLa cancer cells. Samadder A et al, *J Acupunct Meridian Stud* 2013 6(4):180-7.

MATERIA POETICA

You are bossy, so I see
Boaster, braggart, class bully
I didn't like your puffed up shirt
Treating me like I was dirt
Then I saw you acquiesce
Act so meek and kiss her feet
I wondered what was going on
First you've got an awful bark
Then you snivel in the dark
Outside big and inside small
What a split that fooled us all
Afraid of trying something new
Afraid someone is watching you
Afraid your body's on the blink
Sudden weeping when you're thanked
Your tummy rumbles full of air
Like your ego making noise
Thirsty, hungry, food's your fare
Eating sweets, life's simple joys
On your right the problem starts
Then to the left and with a fart
Lycopodium don't be a bore
Early mornings and at 4
Take your remedy today
Before your hair starts turning gray!

SYLVIA CHATROUX

SPORE OIL

The spores of *L. clavatum* contain about 50% fat. This fat is interesting, in that its fatty acids contain only a small proportion of saturated acids, and more than 90% of the liquid acids are monoethenoic acids. About 30% of the total fatty acids consist of 9-hexadecenoic acid, according to work by Reibsomer and Johnson.

Lycopodium oil has been prepared by extracting the spores with chloroform with a saponification value of 195, and iodine value of 91.8. The oil is a bright yellowish-green. It does not solidify, even at -15° Celsius.

The oil, according to Rathje, contains 81% lycopodic acid, 3.2% dihydroxystearic acid, and small amounts of stearic, myristic and palmitic acid.

Various *Lycopodium* species contain lipids in both the runners and spikelets. Here is a brief synopsis:

Total lipids- *D. complanatum* runners, 39 mg/g, with spikelets, 87; *H. selago*, 89-202 mg/g; *L. annotinum* 72-202.

In the neutral lipids, *H. selago* stands out with 29.4 % diacylglycerol (DAG), but all contain mono- di and tricylyglycerols, as well as free sterols, sterol esters, alcohols, and waxes.

Interestingly, *D. complantum* is highest in phospholipids, including phosphatidyl choline and phosphatidyl ethanolamine. *Chemistry of Natural Compounds* 2002 38:5.

LICHEN ESSENCES

Stiff Clubmoss essence teaches us to exist in spite of adversity, and gives courage in times of set backs or resignation.   **MARIANA**

Clubmoss spore essence is for those people who have great fear of being alone. They are intellectually keen, but physically slow and underdeveloped. In social circles, they worry what other may think of them. They can never be satisfied, and can be stubborn, ungrateful and dictatorial.

They try to hide their insecurity by bluff and bravado; being domineering to those younger, weaker or less intelligent. They may have fear of the dark, crowds, speaking in public, and even death.   **PRAIRIE DEVA**

PERSONALITY TRAITS

Clubmoss people are of keen intellect, with weak muscular power. They have a dry temperament with dark complexions.

The dryness results from excessive mental activity; while decreased glandular and lymphatic activity affects the liver and adrenal function.

Intellectually keen children, with high nervous tension and weak physicality, they may feel inferior and insecure. They may compensate for their weakness by exaggerating their strengths.

Carried to extreme, this is the "bookworm", or brooding introvert. And while this philosophical life may lead to highly, evolved spiritual values; it may also create neurotic, and self-centered goals. The result may be easily offended, intolerant, over-bearing and domineering personalities. They are usually smokers.

Often, sexual capacity is reduce, with incomplete erection and difficult ejaculation.

Indeed, the characteristics of the plant compare favorably with those who can use it.

Clubmoss is of dry and thin growth, creeping shyly along the ground. The spores repel water (emotion), are extremely hard; and burn with a very bright flash.

The spores germinate after 6-7 years, and the plant reaches maturity at 12-15 years.

The living dynamics of the herb are expressed as dryness, slowness, hardness with hidden, fiery qualities, and yet a great hesitance to grow and reproduce.   **PRAIRIE DEVA**

[Clubmoss types] are charming, intellectual, and ambitious, and struggle with sexuality and commitment. They are well known as dictators in their work or at home but at the other end of the scale can be very timid in all situations. They commonly display both traits in differing situations. Their love of power makes them poor team players, as they prefer to be at the top.

Being essentially ambitious academics rather than practical types, they are found in professions rather than business, often at the top of a partnership or committee. They think they are equal players, but to everyone else they act like the boss. They give the idea of a petty tyrant rather than a warlord. They exaggerate and puff up their intellectual and other abilities to make themselves look better and more capable than they are.

They can be tyrannical children and even before they speak they boss the parents around. When older they can take the lead role and tell the others what they are doing wrong.

Or they can be introverted type, cautious and fearful of normal playground behavior, and can become absorbed in safe, intellectual activities such as reading and computers.

According to their type they can be either the bullied or the bully.

Commitment is a major issue for *Lycopodium*, because they find that their passion is short lived (dry emotions); so they can thrive on affairs but not easily in marriage. The man may decide not to marry; or once the children have arrived and he is no longer top of the list in his wife's affections, he may run off with his secretary, who restores him to top place and massages his ego projections (confident at work, uncertain at home). One problem that can plague him is his anticipatory anxieties and cowardice underneath, leading to failing erections.

PETER CHAPPELL

The central theme of the *Lycopodium* remedy pattern is a lack of confidence. People in this pattern are sensitive to criticism. These stresses and anxieties can make them irritable. They tend to complain when they feel overburdened with responsibilities and sometimes they try to shirk them. They feel trapped if they have all the financial responsibility for their dependents, and they can be grudging with money as well as with time spent with their families.

Lycopodium helps you feel more confident and secure in your own power. Your experience of power was that it was imposed from the outside, which made you believe that the only way to be strong was to strive for power over others.

LORIUS

MYTHS AND LEGENDS

It was gathered with great care, no iron instrument was allowed to touch it, even bare hands were unworthy of this honor. A special covering, or "sagus" was used with the right hand. This covering had to be consecrated and secretly received from a holy personage with the left hand. It could be collected only by a white clad druid, with bare feet, that had been washed in clear water.

Before he collected this plant, he had to make an offering of bread and wine; after this, the plant was carried away from the place in which it grew in a new, clean cloth.

In the "Kadir Taliesin", selago is referred to as "the gift of god", and in modern Welsh as the "gras duw", or the "grace of god".

SCHOPF

Once when were children we stayed up late. The oldest person in our group boiled some plants over a fire at night. He made this brew. He gave us some and we drank it. After that I lay down and couldn't get up for quite a while. I was mentally aware of my surroundings but whenever I moved, I became really dizzy. When I tried to get up, I would fall forward. I think that we were drunk. Even after quite some time passed, I could not get up.

Those plants (*L. annotinum*) are intoxicating substances.

MALAIJA (OOTOOVA Et al)

RECIPES

INFUSIONS- Pour one quart of boiling water over one tbsp of dry herb. Take small sips, on empty stomach, before meals. One to two cups daily.

TINCTURE- One teaspoon every three to four hours in water. The mother tincture for homeopathy is made from the ground powder of spores gathered at summer's end at a 2:1 ratio with 95% alcohol.

The spores are considerable work to collect. The spikes are best picked in late summer and placed in a glass jar. They will mature in there and the occasional shake will have them fall to the bottom. Trying to shake a little at a time into a paper bag has never worked well for me, especially when it may be cold and snowing at the same time as sporulation in northern Alberta.

HUPERZINE A- 100-150 mcg, twice daily or 2 microgram per kilo of patient weight.

CAUTION- Do not use during pregnancy, or with hypertension, liver or kidney disease, epilepsy, asthma, IBS or irregular heart.

It may increase the effects of acetyl-cholinesterase inhibitors such as tacrine, and anti-cholinergic drugs such as bethanechol.

PILLOW- Fill a small bag with the newly dried club moss. Apply as needed.

DECOCTION- Use the entire plant including root. For dyes, combine root with the natural plant and boil together.

NORTHERN COMANDRA
NORTHERN BASTARD TOADFLAX
FALSE BASTARD TOADFLAX
(***Geocaulon lividum*** [Richardson] Fernald)
(***Comandra livida*** Rich.) not accepted
PALE COMANDRA
BASTARD TOADFLAX
(***C. umbellata*** [L.] Nutt.)
PARTS USED- whole plant in flower, including roots, seed.

I tried to drown my sorrows, but the bastards learned how to swim, and now I am overwhelmed by this decent and good feeling. **FRIDA KAHLO**

Comandra is from the Greek **KOME** for tufts of hair, and **ANDROS**, meaning man. This refers to the hairy base of the stamens. Geocaulon means a "stem that is found under the ground", in reference to the slim red rhizomes. Lividum means pale.

Umbellata refers to the flower clusters, even though they are not real umbels, but look like the framework of an umbrella. They are the only two members of the Sandalwood family in my part of the world, and like the famous essential oil bearing tree from India, are semi-parasitic.

Northern Bastard Toadflax is usually living off neighbours like bearberry, in the boreal forest. It mostly draws water from them, not acting like a true parasite.

The leaves are often streaked yellow, particularly when young and this helps to identify them. It is caused by Comandra blister rust (*Cronartium comandrae*) associated with Lodgepole pine, as an alternate host. The roots have a peculiar odour.

Pale Comandra is also semi-parasitic, and confined to the dry foothills and alpine regions. It has white funnel shaped flowers tinged in purple and green. A brown to purple drupe, with single seed, can be eaten when mature, but still slightly green, with a sweet and oily acquired taste. Various birds and rodents use the small, oily fruits for food.

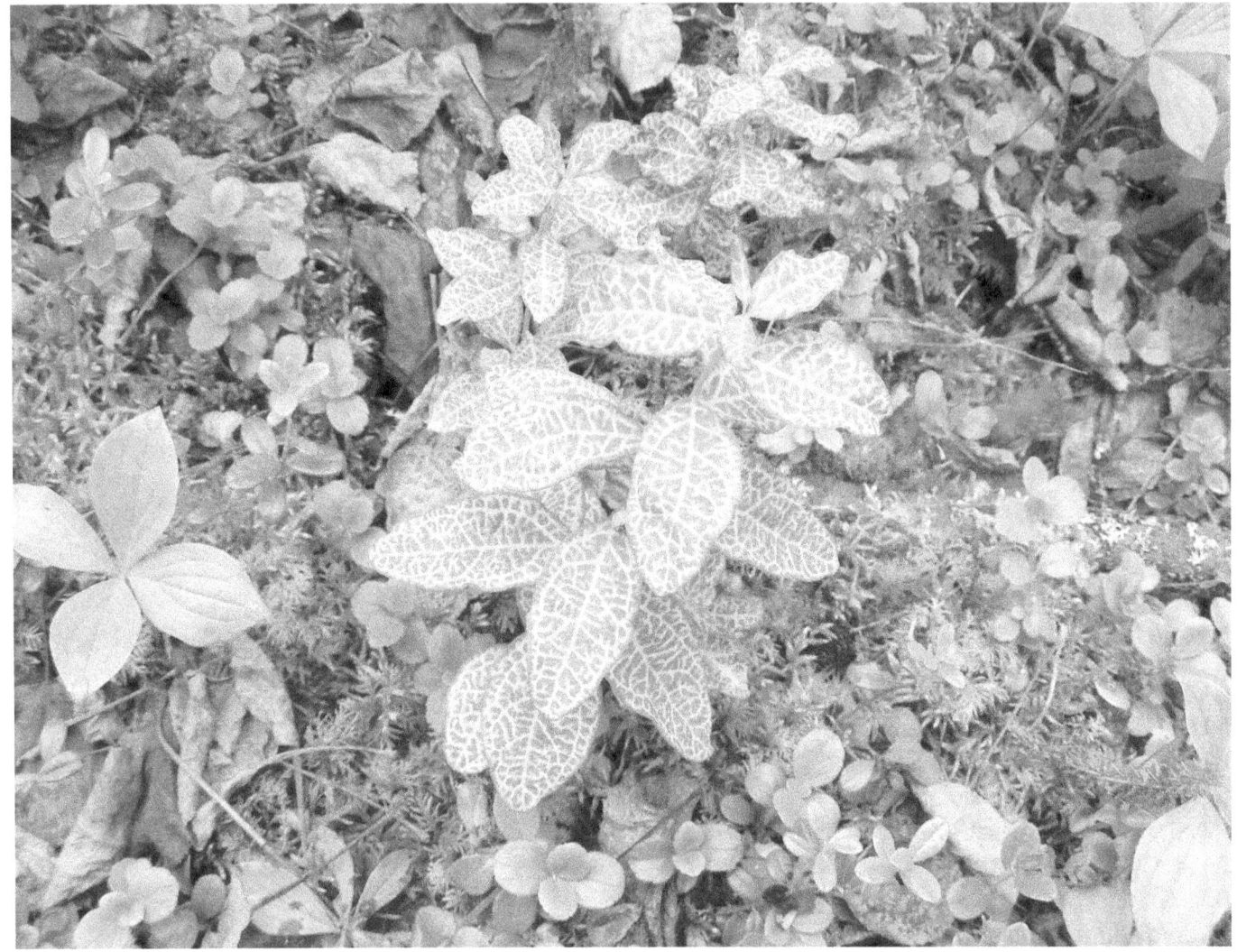

NORTHERN COMANDRA- NOTED STREAKED LEAVES

Northern Comandra berries are bright orange, and also edible but not very tasty.

The Chipewyan tribe swallowed the berries of Northern Comandra to relieve chronic lung complaints such as tuberculosis, and call them **SAS JIE** meaning, "bear berry". The Slave call it **NOTHE DZHI**, meaning Marten Berry.

The Dena'ina know it as Brown Bear's berry, Mouse's berry and Raven's Berry.

The berries were chewed raw and take a root infusion for stomach trouble, sore throat and tuberculosis. The fresh leaves were applied to sores after chewing first.

The Cree boiled the leaves and bark of the stem as a tea to purge the system.

The leaves, stems, and roots are used by indigenous medicine people for heart conditions.

The chewed leaves and stems can be used as a wound poultice.

The leaves are quite sweet tasting and can be added to salads.

Pale Comandra was traditionally used by the indigenous Thompson of British Columbia. It is known as /q'apuxʷ=éʃp meaning nut plant, as it grows near hazelnut.

The early ethnobotanist Steedman (1930) wrote that the fresh roots were washed and combined with breast milk as a wash or salve for inflammation of the eyes and sore eyes in general.

Nancy Turner interviewed a member of the group who said it was for sores. "Her mother had sores on her hands and neck that would not heal. One lady boiled up the plant…and used the decoction as a wash for the sores. 'I think they get better after…fix that up.'"

Pale Comandra was decocted by Navaho, as a footbath for corns, gargle for canker sores, wash for sore eyes, and as a narcotic. The Thompson tribe used plant decoctions for general body sores.

The Cherokee applied the fresh juice to cuts and sores on the skin. The herb is infused with pink lady slipper for kidney complaints.

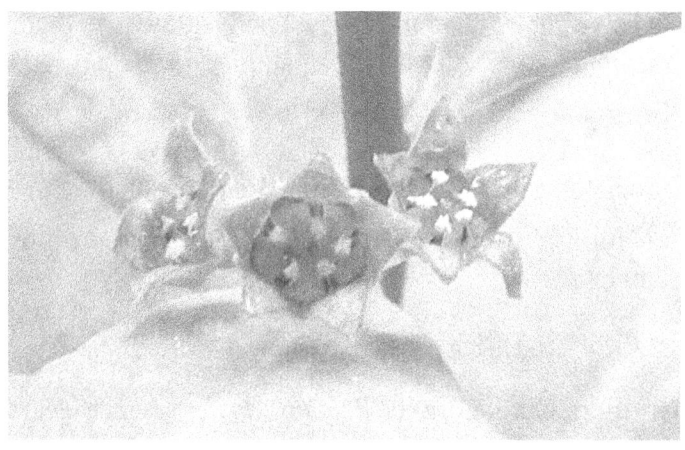

NORTHERN COMANDRA FLOWERS

The Fox used Pale Comandra as a lung medicine, taking leaf infusions for pain in the lungs; or licking the immature florets to ease labored breathing from colds.

The Kayenta Navajo used the plant as a narcotic in unspecified manner.

The Arapaho Nation is known today as Hinonoeiteen. The term Arapaho may originate from the Crow word for tattoo. The Dakota refer to this group as Blue Colored Men, or Mahpíyato, and the Lakota and Assiniboine know them as Blue Sky People or Mahpíyathó. The Blue river of Colorado is derived from an Arapaho term roughly "where we gather blue paint".

This may have significance to a dye obtained from the root. Rawhide boxes, called parfleches, (from the French word fleche for arrows) were painted with what the Arapaho call "the lost blue". The exact method is long lost, but the blue dye lies beneath the skin of the root. This was powdered, and mixed to paint thickness with the juice of a pincushion cactus, the vitreous humor liquid from an animal's eye or gall. This was used for dyeing the rawhide boxes, and perhaps the ceremonial blue as body paint.

Pale Comandra is a bio-accumulator of selenium; be careful where you pick.

MEDICINAL

Extracts from Bastard Toadflax aerial parts have shown inhibitory effect on *Cladosporium cucumerinum*, *Bacillus subtils, E. coli,* and *Biomphalaria glabrata.* This was found in work by Bergeron et al, and supported by the Swiss National Science Foundation. The seeds have been reported to possess red blood cell clumping activity.

SEED OIL

Bastard Toadflax (*C. pallida*) seed contains 43% of ximenynic acid, an 18 carbon acid with a triple bond at the 9,10 position, and a double bond at the 11, 12 position. That is, trans-11-octadecen-9-ynoic acid.

This is the first native plant of the prairies found to produce an acetylenic oil having dry oil properties. It absorbs readily into adipose tissue.

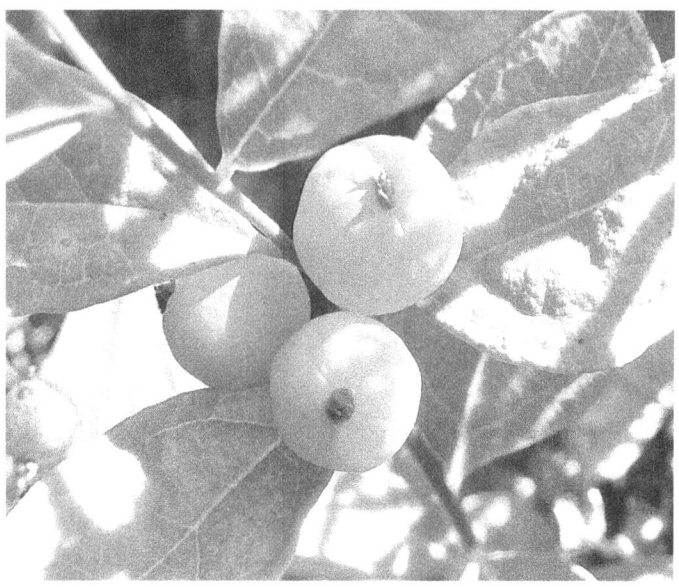

NORTHERN COMANDRA BERRIES

The oil inhibits thromboxane B2 and leukotriene B4 of stimulated leukocytes, and at higher doses may inhibit phospholipase A2. Croft KD et al, *Biochim Biophys Acta* 1987 921(3):621-4.

Ximenynic acid is a conjugated enyne fatty acid. It may inhibit growth of HepG2 (human hepatoma) cancer cell lines by selective inhibition of COX-1 expression, which leads to cell cycle arrest, apoptosis, and angiogenesis associated genes. Cai F et al, *Mol Med Rep* 2016 14(6):5667-76.

It is found in considerable amounts in the seed oil of Sandalwood (*S. album*). At one time it was known as santalbic acid.

FLOWER ESSENCE

Northern Comandra (*C. lividum*) flower essence clears disharmonious energies from the heart that limit one's ability to perceive, experience and co-create with the subtle realms of nature.   **ALASKA**

LEGENDS AND MYTHS

Among the Gitksan, according to John Fowler (August 27 1925) this plant (Northern Comandra) was of no use, but there is a long story of Wi Get, which Mr. C. Marius Barbeau collected and this story relates how Wi Get was the first man.

Wi Get liked to eat salmon and the salmon came out of the water on to the ground for him to eat them. He boiled and ate the salmon and he ate all the berries even this kind which are not eaten by the Gitksan. After eating all the berries he would move on to another place to eat.   **SMITH**

COMMON TICKSEED
PLAINS COREOPSIS
(***Coreopsis tinctoria*** Nutt.)
THREAD LEAF TICKSEED
WHORLED TICKSEED
(***C. verticillata*** L.)
LANCE LEAF TICKSEED
(***C. lanceolata*** L.)
PARTS USED- whole plant

The Coreopsis, cheerful as the smile
That brightens on the cheek of youth
And sheds a gladness o'er the aged.   **LEYEL**

Coreopsis is from the Greek **KORIS** meaning a bedbug or tick, and the Greek **OPSIS** for vision or seeing. From this Coreopsis is an attempt to form a word that is bug-like, and refers to the seed- pod.

This is a classic example of a botanist/taxonomist with no experience on how Greek words are formed. A better choice may have been **CORIOID** for bug-like, but no one asked me.

Lance leaf tickseed is a long blooming perennial, with beautiful yellow flowers. It is fairly drought resistant, and will do well in poor soil; and is a great addition to rock garden situations. It is the state wildflower of Florida and Mississippi.

Common tickseed is a native annual of the dry, southern prairies, and can be found in the extreme southeast of Alberta, around sloughs and clay flats.

It is hardy from British Columbia to Quebec, and most of the United States and down to Mexico. In the southern states it is commonly called Calliopsis.

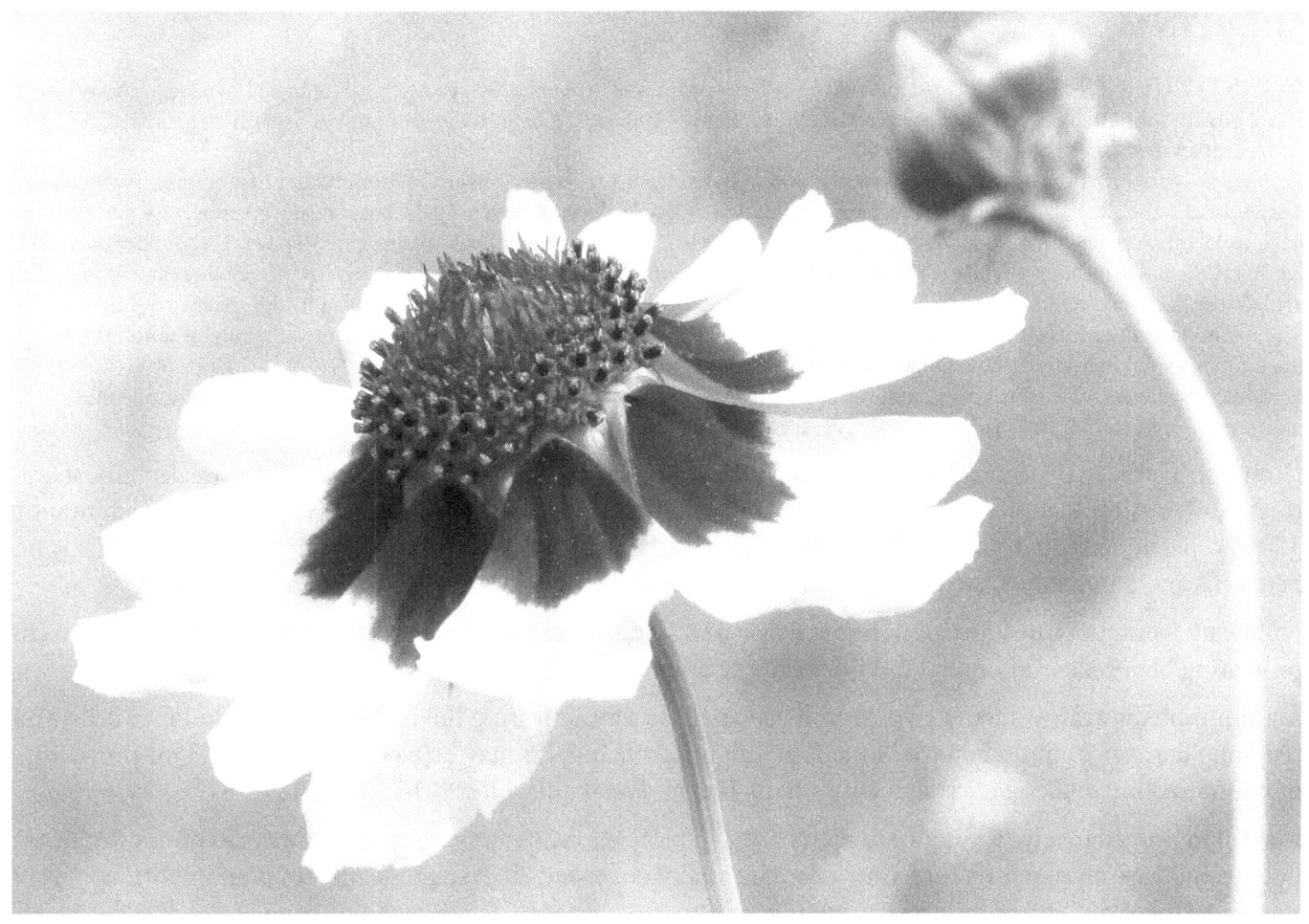

COMMON TICKSEED

Various native tribes including the Cherokee, used infusions of the root for treating bloody diarrhea. They made a ceremonial lotion that was applied to the body during singing and chanting.

The Ramah Navaho considered the root a life medicine. When burned, the smoke was directed towards skin lesions associated with sexual disease.

The aerial parts (not the roots) were infused and drunk by women seeking to increase their chances of a female baby.

The Lakota know the plant as **CANHLO'GAN WAKAL'YAPI**, meaning boiled weed.

In Portugal, the herb is used to treat diabetic conditions.

The specific "tinctoria" gives a clue as to the flower use in dyeing a bright yellow. Use three cups of flowers for every eight ounces of wool or cotton material and a pinch of cream of tartar for an even brighter result. The Zuni used the blossoms to produce a mahogany red dye.

The Navaho use a related tickseed, *C. cardaminefolia*, as a cold infusion of the dried plant with salt for "lightning infection". I'm not sure what that is, but if someone knows, I'd like to hear from you.

Thread leaf tickseed is hardy to -40° C. while its lance-leafed cousin can only tolerate minus 34° C.

Common Tickseed is known in China as Snow Chrysanthemum, due to its winter hardiness. It is also known as **KUNLUN XUEJU**. It is widely used as a daily tea, known as Juhua, since its introduction to country over a century ago. I have also seen it referred to as **SHEMUJU** in the Xinhua Herbal Scheme. It is widely used for its heat clearing, detoxifying and dampness removal.

MEDICINAL

CONSTITUENTS-*C. verticillata*- 1-phenylhepta-1,3,5-triyne and 2-phenyl-5-(1-propynyl)thiophene (ovicides); and two larval growth inhibitors (3-(4-isobutyryloxy-3-methoxyphenyl)-1-propen-3-ol and 3-(4-isobutryryl-3-methoxyphenyl)-2,3-epoxypropan-1-ol.

C. tinctoria- aerial parts (E)-1-acetoxy-7-phenlhepta-4,6-diyn-2-ene; 1'-acety-oxyeugenol 4-isobutyrate; 1'isobutyryl-oxyeugenol 4-isobutyrate; 1'-(2-methyl-butyryloxy) eugenol 4-isobutyrate; 1'iso-valeryloxyeugenol 4-isobutyrate; (1',2') epoxy-3'-isobutyrylconiferyl alcohol 4 isobutyrate; (1',2')epoxy-3'-acetyl-coniferyl alcohol 4-isobutyrate; (1',2')-epoxy-3'-(2-methylbutyryl) coniferyl alcohol 4-isobutyrate; and (1',2')-epoxy-3'-isovalerylconiferyl alcohol 4-iso-butyrate; marein, flavanomarein, chlorogenic acid, (RIS)-flavanomarein, butin-7-O-beta-D-glucopyranoside, isookanin, taxifolin, okanin, isookanin, 3,5-dicaffeoylquinic acid, taxifolin-7-O-glucoside, isocoreopsin, coreopsin, coretinterpenoid, coretinphenol, querctin, luteolin, butein, sulfuretin, linocinnamarin, coreosides A-D, beta-sitosterol

C. lanceolata- flowers- laceolin, flavanones, various chalcones, aurones, 4-methoxylanceoletin, flavanocorepsin, flavanokanin, maritimein, leptosidin, 7,3',4'-trihydroxy-8-methoxyflavanone,

Common Tickseed infusions have been used traditionally in Portugal for diabetes. In a three week study of oral treatment on streptozotocin-induced glucose intolerant rats, the extacts had no effect on insulin secretion by MIN6 cells, but a reduction of glucose intolerance was found. It is possible that anti-oxidant mechanisms on beta cells and pancreatic function are involved. Dias et al, *Phyto Res* 2010 24:5; *J Ethnopharm* 132:2.

Follow up work, in same journal by Teresa Dias 2012 139:2 identified marein and flavanomarein as involved in protecting beta cells from injury and inhibition of apoptotic pathways.

Marein protects against methylglyoxal-induced apoptosis by activating the AMPK pathway in PC12 cells, and reducing damage to mitochondrial function. This suggests marein may be a potent compound for preventing or counteracting diabetic encephalopathy. Jiang B et al, *Free Radical Res* 2016 50(11):1172-87.

Marein improved insulin resistance in high glucose in HepG2 cells via a variety of pathways to promote glucose uptake, increase glycogen synthesis and decrease gluconeogenesis. This suggests marein is an important part of this use of this plant for hyperglycemic conditions or an adjuvant for diabetes mellitus. Jiang B et al, *Phytomedicine* 23(9):891-900.

This all fits with the inclusion of this herb in a traditional Cree formulation for diabetes, shared with me by Clifford Cardinal.

Both water and alcohol flower extracts blocked an increase in fasting blood glucose, serum triglycerides, insulin, leptin and liver lipid levels, and prevented the development of insulin resistance in mice fed a high fat diet. The extracts inhibited alpha glycosidase, as one pathway of benefit. The authors suggest a flower beverage may be useful for treatment of diabetes. Cai W et al, *J Diabetes Res* 2016:2340276.

The flavonoids reduce blood lipids, without liver damage, in a manner better than Fenofibrate, by down-regulating ADRP (adipose differentiation-related protein). Li Y et al, *Lipids Health Dis* 2014 13:193.

Extracts control blood glucose, inhibit inflammatory and fibrotic process, suppress the TGF-beta1/Smad signaling pathway and activate phosphorylation of AMPKalpha in the kidneys, suggests the protection in early stages of diabetic kidney disease. Yao L et al, *BMC Complementary Altern Med* 2015 15:314.

Coreopsis flower tea improves glucose balance by inhibiting the expression of gluconeogenic pathway key proteins, glucose-6-phosphatase and phosphophoenolpyruvate; as well as regulating the mRNA or protein levels of the Krebs cycle enzymes. These include critical ones such as citrate synthase, succinate dehydrogenase complex, subunit A, flavoprotein and dihydrolipoamide S-succinyl transferase. Jiang B et al, *Endocrinology* 2015 156)6):2006-18.

Polyacetylene glucosides, isolated from capitula tincture, reduce lipid accumulation in 3T3-L1 adipocytes, suggested benefit in obesity and weight loss. Du D et al, *J Asian Nat Prod Res* 2016 18(8):784-90.

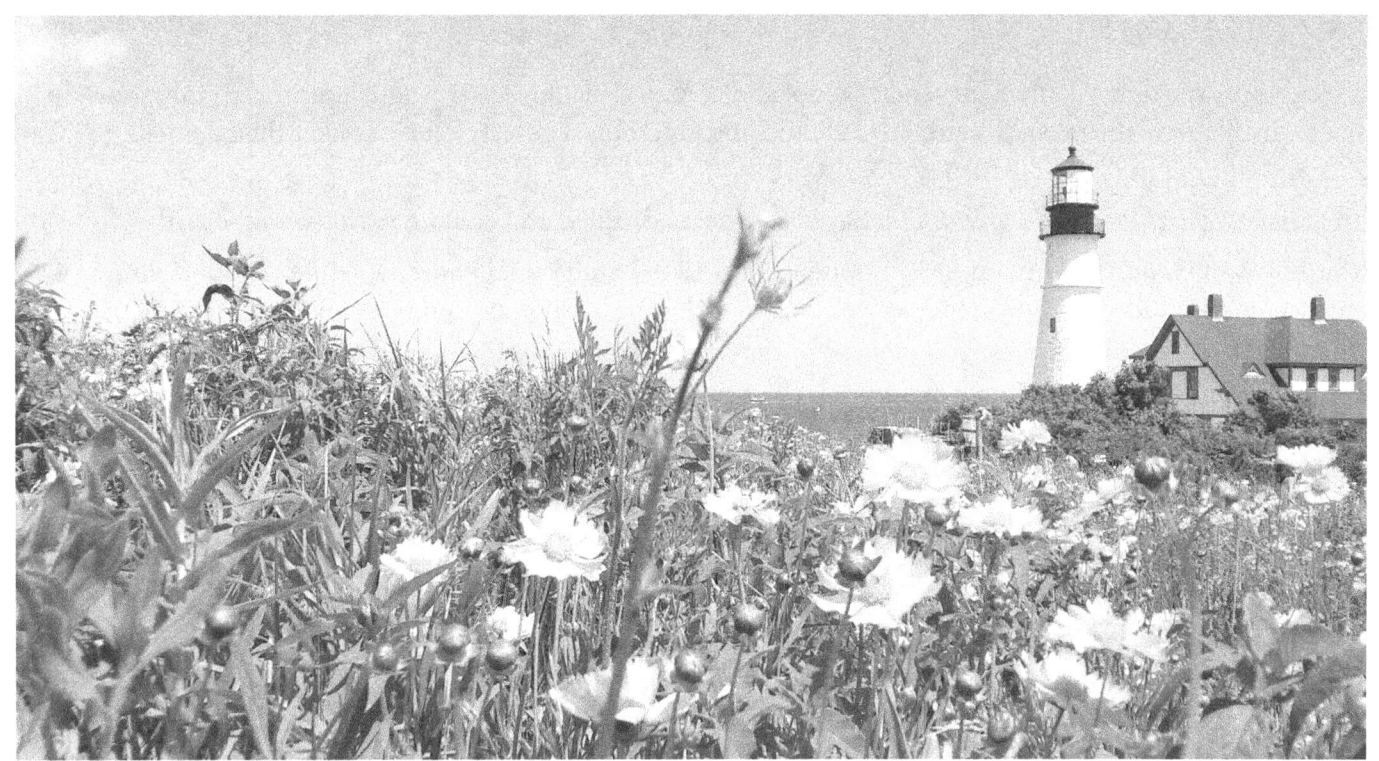

LANCE-LEAFED TICKSEED

Recent work suggests that flavonoid extracts exert cardio-protective effects against myocardial ischemia/ reperfusion injury. This can occur when the heart, after suffering an attack and lack of oxygen, is suddenly flooding with oxidative and inflammatory insult.

Work by Sun YH et al, *Pharm Biol* 2013 51(9): 1158-64 suggests the vasorelaxant effects are likely due to inhibition of calcium through cell membranes. A calcium-channel blocker if you will.

This animal experiment suggests coreopsis protects via anti-oxidant, anti-inflammatory and anti-apoptotic activity. Zhang Y et al, *Iran J Basic Med Sci* 2016 19(9):1016-1023.

The herb contains a number of compounds with anti-oxidant activity. Lam SC et al, *J Food Sci* 2016 81(9):C2218-23.

Coreosides A-D show significant inhibition of COX-2. Zhang Y et al, *Fitoterapia* 2013 87:93-7.

Tickseed (*C. verticillata*) has been studied in Japan, for it's use as a natural insecticide. Studies conducted by Nakajima and Kawazu in 1980 in Japan, showed strong insecticide and larval growth inhibitors from the plant.

Lance-leafed Tickseed was screened for nematicidal activity in the flowers. It too, proved to have pronounced activity.

The compound laceolin exhibits significant radical scavenging capacity with SC50 of 2.6 mug/mL. Tanimoto et al, *J Oleo Sci* 2009 58:3.

Various chalcones also exhibit anti-oxidant activity. Shang YF et al, *Planta Medica* 2013 79(3-4):295-300.

The dried flowers leaves and seeds can be infused in hot water as a quick pick me up without caffeine. Try it, using the plant alone or combining it with wild bergamot, or safflower petals.

Flavonoids show inhibition and possible induction of apoptosis in human leukemia HL-60 cells. Pardede A et al, *Bioorg Med Chem Lett* 2016 26(12):2784-7.

Lance Leaf Tickseed shows significant nematicidal activity. Kimura et al, *Z Naturforsch* 2008 63:11-12.

ESSENTIAL OILS

Tickseed *(C. tinctoria)* contains several eugenol and coniferyl alcohols that would almost certainly show up in steam distillation. The oil shows anti-oxidant and anti-microbial capacity, albeit weaker than penicillin G. Yao X et al, *Nat Prod Res* 2016 30(10):1170-3.

The related *C. barteri and C. grandiflora* have been steam distilled and contain various components.

The leaves of *C. barteri* contain 55% limonene, and 12.9% alpha phellandrene; while *C. grandiflora* is 42% germacrene D, and 11.7% mycrene; as well as two rather unusual compounds, 1-phenyl-1, 3, 5-heptatriyne (5.2%) and precocene I (0.9%).

FLOWER ESSENCES

Coreopsis lanceolata is a research flower essence of Flower Essence Society.

Coreopsis verticellata or Moonbeam is an excellent essence to be used in any kind of recuperation, whether it's post operative, emotional, physical, mental or spiritual. It facilitates heart rebuilding and depth of a healing process. This is an essence that energetically hugs or holds you, grounds you, and gives you a reassuring touch from the devic realms…Moonbeam Coreopsis is a wonderful strengthener for connecting with life all around you. Its beauty is that it very gently holds relationship to all these realms. **HIGH SIERRA**

Calliopsis (*C. tinctoria*) essence is a good tonic for grief and sorrow…A secondary use is in the elimination of toxins—-emotional, mental, physical and spiritual—-because sometimes toxins require different qualities of release to become active and begin moving. **HIGH SIERRA**

SPIRITUAL PROPERTIES

Coreopsis represents cheerfulness in work, for the Divine. When you work for the divine, you will feel an ineffable joy filling your being. **THE MOTHER**

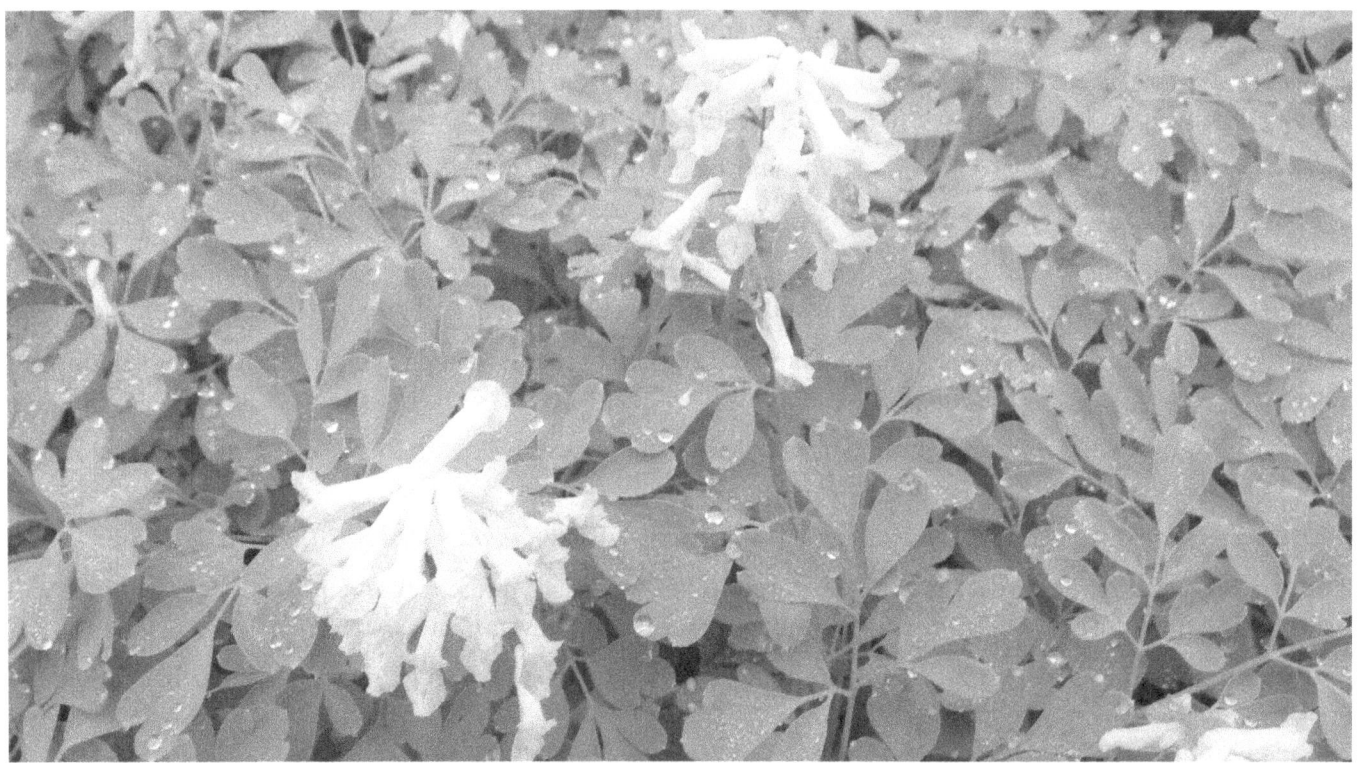

GOLDEN CORYDALIS

GOLDEN CORYDALIS
SCRAMBLED EGGS
(*Corydalis aurea* Wiild.)
(*C. washingtoniana* Fedde)
(*Capnoides aureum* [Willd.] Kuntze)
WESTERN BLEEDING HEART
(*Dicentra formosa* [Haw.] Walp.)
TURKEY CORN
SQUIRREL CORN
(*Dicentra canadensis* [Goldie] Walp.)
BLEEDING HEART
(*D. spectabilis* [L.] Lem)
(*Lamprocapnos spectabilis* [L.] Fukuhara)
PINK CORYDALIS
PALE CORYDALIS
ROCK HARLEQUIN
(*C. sempervirens* [L.] Pers.)
(*Capnoides sempervirens* [L.] Borkh.)

STEERS HEAD
(*D. uniflora* Kellogg)
SIBERIAN CORYDALIS
(*C. nobilis* [L.] Pers.)
DUTCHMAN'S BREECHES
LITTLE BLUE STAGGER
COLIC WEED
SQUIRREL CORN
(*D. cucullaria* [L.] Bernh.)
(*D. occidentalis* [Rydb.] Fedde.)
STAGGER WEED
BULBOUS CORYDALIS
BIRD IN THE BUSH
HOLLOW ROOT
(*C. cava* [L.] Sweigg. & Korte.)
(*C. tuberosa* DC.)
PARTS USED- root, leaves, flower

Why would Dutchmen wear such britches,
Bloated so their legs looked huge?
Was it so they'd not have itches-
From tight woollies, a refuge?
Or did they see the plant Dicentra
And decide its blooms looked swell,
And, with that fashion pattern, went ta
A tailor who'd cut their pants from hell.

JACK SANDERS

A bed among rocks of much-cleft silver-green foliage, set with flower-sprays of two-pointed white and yellow bloom that might be pairs of elfin trousers hung out to bleach.   **M. O. WRIGHT**

A bleeding heart is of no help to anyone if it bleeds to death.   **FREDERICK BUECHNER**

Dicentra means twice spurred; and refers to the two spurs on each flower. Formosa means beautiful. Corydalis is from the Greek, **KORUDALLIS**, meaning crested lark, due to the likeness of the upper petal appearing crested, and the spur resembling a lark's spur. Cava means hollow, and aurea means gold.

Bleeding heart originated in Chinese folklore from the resemblance of the red flowers to the heart, with a "drop of blood" between the two tiny spurs.

Turkey Corn is so named for the appearance of fall plant that looks like kernels of corn.

Corydalis and Dicentra are interesting members of the Fumitory family. They all like to grow in moist forest and woodland meadows, including up into the boreal forests.

They are biennial or, sometimes considered annual plants that are usually dismissed as poisonous. The plants all contain interesting alkaloids, but those growing on selenium soils should not be used.

Siberian Corydalis is an introduced perennial that is one of our earliest flowering plants.

Golden corydalis is all over the ravine, near my home in Edmonton, Alberta, Canada.

This species led me to investigate the related species growing in western Canada, including in backyard gardens.

In Mexico, the Golden Corydalis leaf tea is considered good for women after childbirth. There it goes by the name of **CYLANDRILLO**.

The Navaho, amongst other tribes, used the plant as a remedy for rheumatism. They also applied the fresh leaves to puerperal infections in new mothers.

Cold infusions were taken for sore throat, stomachache, and applied to backache as a lotion.

The Ojibwa tribe used the root smoke of **TIPOTIE KWASON** as a stimulant to clear the head and revive the patient.

Pink Corydalis was used as part of a decoction for hemorrhoids, the tea both drunk and applied as a wash to the piles.

In Quebec, the roots of both Pink and Golden Corydalis were considered bitter and astringent, used as an anthelmintic and emmenagogue to promote menstruation.

There have not been any cases of human fatalities recorded from eating *Dicentra* or *Corydalis* species in North America. In large quantities, however there would be symptoms of trembling, staggering and convulsions. The words blue stagger and staggerweed derive from the grazing cattle that suffer convulsions, and sometimes death, from eating too much foliage.

Watermelon seeds were soaked, at one time, in corydalis tea to increase their production.

Western Bleeding Heart (*D. formosa*) root is used as medicine by Thompson tribe of the British Columbia interior. They call it "heart flower", as did the Cowlitz.

Other tribes, including the Skagit chewed the fresh root for toothache, or decocted the root for intestinal worms. The Skagit names, in fact, translate as Toothache medicine, or medicine for worms.

The whole plant was infused and used as a hair rinse to make it grow better.

Dutchman's Breeches is rare in Manitoba, but found more plentifully further south and east. The white flowers, with bits of yellow, look like an old fashioned pair of panties, or Bloomers. The meaning of breech is buttocks or rump.

Mabel Osgood Wright (1901) wrote "set with flower-sprays of two-pointed white and yellow bloom that might be pairs of elfin trousers hung out to bleach."

The Menominee used it as a love charm. Huron Smith, an early ethnobotanist wrote. "The young swain tries to throw it at his intended and hit her with it. Another way is for him to chew the root, breathing out so that the scent will carry to her.

He then circles around the girl and when she catches the scent, she will follow him wherever he goes, even against her will."

They are an early spring flower, blooming near the same time as bloodroot.

Bleeding Heart is one of my favorite cultivated flowers; hardy to zone 2, with beautiful pink and white heart shaped flowers early in the summer.

Children of all ages love the flowers that can be hung over the ears as earrings, woven into the hair as a tiara, and gently pulled apart to reveal the lady in a bathtub or a man in a gondola. It makes a lovely pressed flower.

Staggerweed (*C. cava*) has purple or white flowers, and is a hardy addition to the prairie garden. It prefers light shade, good humus, and will go dormant during the late summer.

It has been called an "intelligent flower" as they rotate by 90 degrees, allowing only educated insects to find their opening. The stalk, and tuber become hollow in older plants.

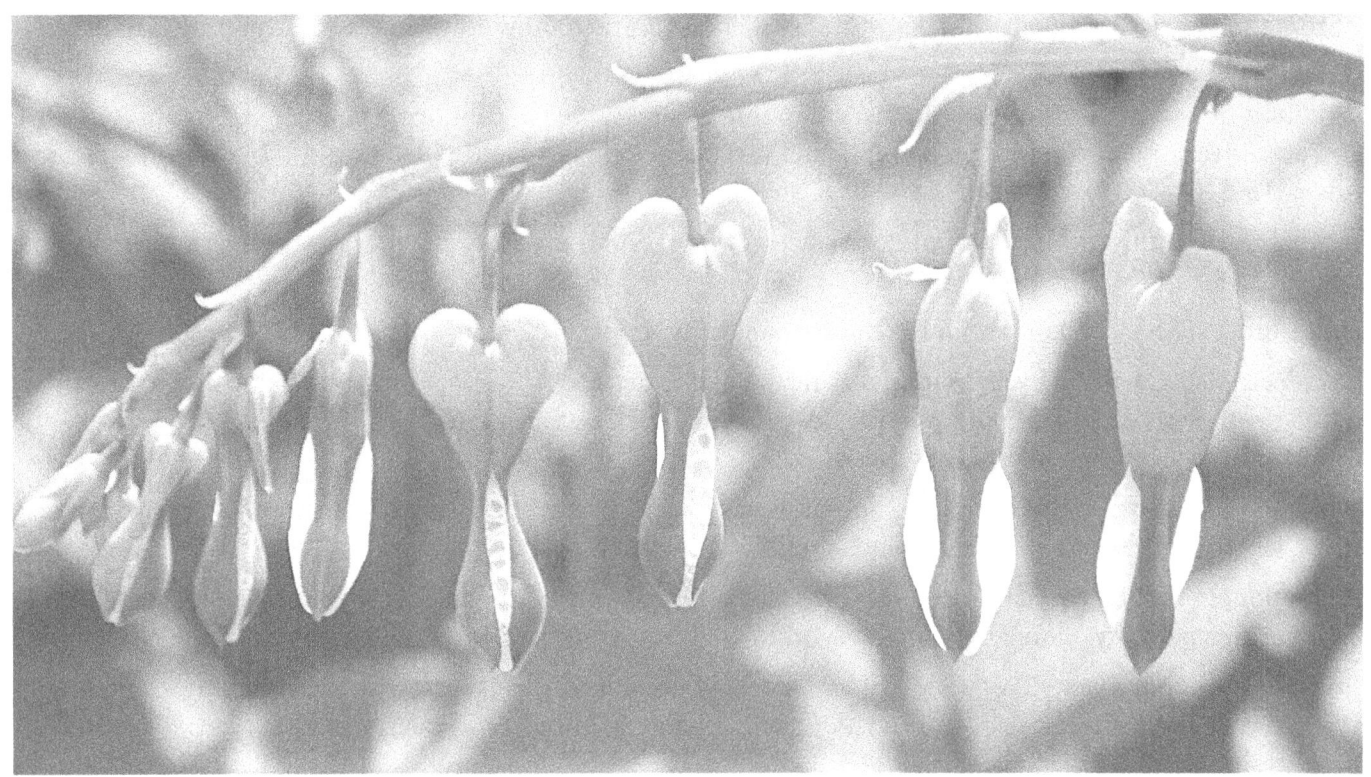

BLEEDING HEART

Many species of Corydalis and Dicentra contain alkaloids of the isoquinoline class that are toxic to livestock. Signs of poisoning include depression, uneasiness, twitching, convulsive clonic spasms, muscular rigidity, and biting movements.

MEDICINAL

CONSTITUENTS- *C. aurea-* protopine, allocrytopine, corydaline, aurotensine, bicucculine, sendaverine, bisculline, capauridine, cordrastine, corypalline, stylopine, corpaverine, levo-tetrahydropalmatine (also known as caseanine, gindarine and rotundine), capaurine.
C. sempervirens root- adlumiceine, adlumidiceine, capnoidine, protopine, cryptopine, coptisine, l-adlumine, adlumidine, hydroxysanguinarine, bicucine, bicuculline (alkaloids); chorismate synthase, and 12-oxo-phytodienoate reductase.
leaves- adlumine (0.19-0.72% of dried leaf)
D. formosa- aporphines such as corydine, isocorydine, bulbocapnine, dicentrine; protopine and other isoquinoline alkaloids.
C. cava- corydaline, bulbocapnine, corytuberine, tetrahydropalmatine, narcotine (noscapine), (+)corynoline, (-)-corycavamine, corycavadine, canadine, canadaline.
D. spectabilis- six poppy type alkaloids, bicucculine, menisdaurilide, aquilegiolide.
D. cucullaria- cularine, cularidine, protopine, cryptopine, bicuculline, corlumine, and fumaric acid.
D. canadensis- bulb- fumaric acid, alkaloids, resin, dicentrine, bulbocapnine.

Golden Corydalis is indicated for neuralgias with nervous muscular twitching, especially when tired and overworked. It combines well with Scullcap or Valerian root in cases of nervousness and trembling, shaking, and tics. Be careful with dosage, as too much may cause these symptoms to appear.

It is indicated in cases of leucorrhea, without odour, as well as pelvic atony and hemorrhoids. In Sydenham's chorea, it is an optional therapy.

It can help in cases of sluggish digestion, with hypo-secretions and blood dyscrasia. Ulcerations of the mouth and lymphadenitis are indications of use.

Chronic skin conditions that are of a low-grade, allergic nature in thin individuals with hypersensitive nervous systems are helped.

Protopine, found in this species and others mentioned here, as well as California poppy, exhibits anti-adhesive and anti-invasion effect on MDA-MB-231 breast cancer cell lines. He K & Gao JL, *Afr J Tradit Complement Altern Med* 2014 11(2):415-24.

Protopine also inhibits acetylcholinesterase activity, suggesting use in Alzheimer's disease and related senile dementia.

Pink Cordydalis has similar uses, and in fact contains a multitude of alkaloids with activity on the nervous system.

Octadecanoids are potent cyclic plant signaling molecules derived from alpha-linolenic acid. They are involved in the regulation of a number of physiological processes such as senescence, herbivore and pathogen defense, mechanical perception and morphogenesis.

Work conducted by Schaller et al, at Ruhr University in Germany, shows the enzyme in Pink Corydalis may play a key role in various enzymatic, biochemical and immunological activities.

A component of Pink corydalis is 12-oxo-phytodienoic acid, one of the first cyclic intermediates on the Vick-Zimmerman pathway of octadecanoid biosynthesis.

Both varieties combine well with Scullcap or Valerian for aiding nervousness, shaking, twitching, trembling or tics. They should be used in small doses and in combinations for best, and safest effect.

Protopine, has been shown to inhibit acetyl-cholinesterase activity. In fact, in a study by Kim et al, *Planta Medica* 1999 65:3, protopine has an efficacy almost identical to that of velnacrine, a tacrine derivative developed pharmaceutically to treat Alzheimer's disease, at an identical therapeutic concentration.

Both water and alcohol extracts of various Corydalis species show acetyl-cholineasterase inhibition. Adsersen A et al, *J Ethnopharm* 2006 104 418-22.

Bicucine and bicuculline, found in several species, may bind to specific GABA binding sites. Chiu TH & Rosenberg HC, *Eur J Pharmacol* 1979 56(4):337-45. Bicucine may mediate GABAergic effects, resulting in variable results in states of anxiety.

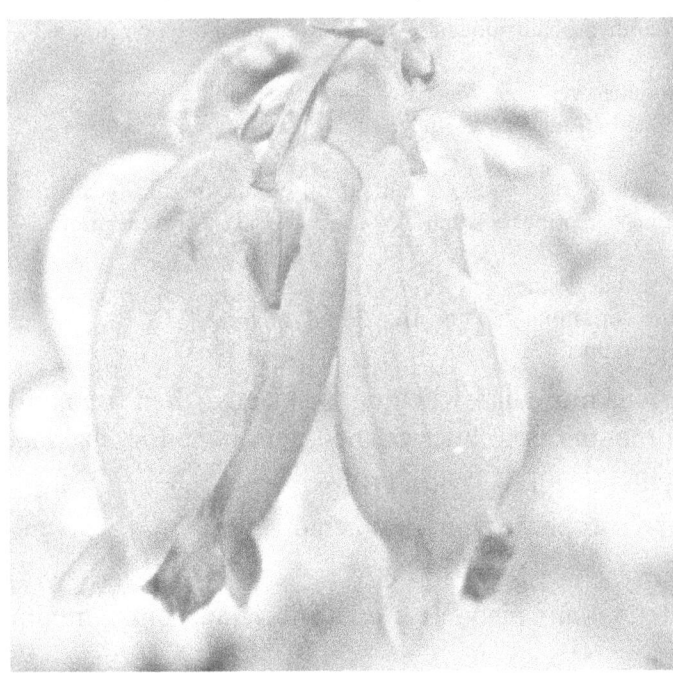

WESTERN BLEEDING HEART

Western Bleeding Heart is a general narcotic-analgesic for pain of the central nervous system, according to Michael Moore.

The root is considered the strongest part, and can be tinctured from either the fresh or dry root.

It greatly relieves dental nerve pain, from sore tooth, broken or lost fillings and other mouth trauma.

It can be combined with the more superficial nerve pain relief of cow parsnip seed/root and yarrow root; but is a much deeper acting remedy.

The fresh leaf, as well as root can be poulticed and applied to sprains, bruises and contusions. Apply the tincture to the affected area and cover with a hot towel for faster action.

Jethro Kloss recommended the root be used in combination with hot baths and salt glows for treating boils, and skin conditions.

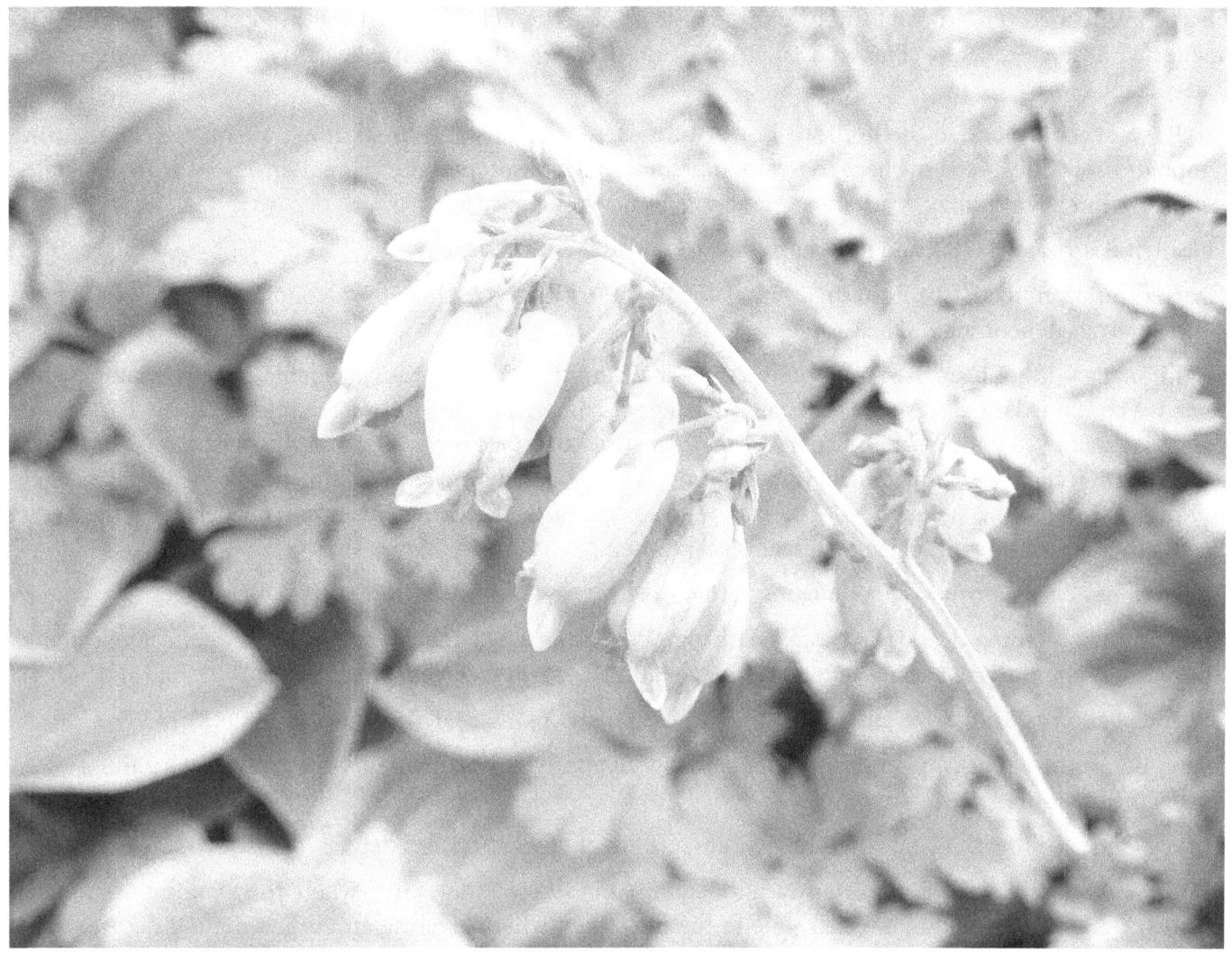

WESTERN BLEEDING HEART

He considered it one of our most valuable alteratives in the herbal kingdom; and an excellent tonic in all enfeebled conditions.

It may be considered the herbal equivalent of the Bach Rescue Remedy. Internally, the tincture helps to calm down and centre one after a trauma, fright or uncontrollable angry encounter.

The herb combines well with California Poppy, Pulsatilla or Scullcap for pain relief.

It is a tonic alterative that was used in the last century for helping strengthen those with venereal disease.

It helps to increase appetite, stimulate liver metabolism, and improve anabolic function in convalescents. It soothes those who feel weak and tired, with proneness to cold, weight loss and dry skin with eczema patches.

As a tonic, it combines well with pipsissewa for those with kidney complications and mild edema. It combines well with bittersweet for those with joint pain, and aversion to cold, damp weather.

Bleeding heart is used whenever there is generalized shakiness and nervous tiredness.

Western Bleeding Heart (*D. formosa*) is very useful for advanced cancer in patients with swollen lymphatic glands, dry and scaly skin and toxicity.

It was one of the main ingredients in Scrophularia, an Eli Jones formulation. Combined with Petasites root, it provides safe, non-toxic pain relief for those suffering cancer.

He recommended ten drops of tincture three times daily. The Eclectic physician Frederick Petersen (1905) suggested it for nodular swelling and enlarged glands. He considered it an alterative for increasing vitality and metabolism.

Dr. Bastyr recommended the herb for bone nodules, ulcerations and breakdown of soft tissue including lymphatics. He often used the herb to treat lymphatic conditions, especially vaginal infections with associated lymph swelling. It also may be used in amenorrhea, and dysmenorrhea.

Dicentrine is vaso-relaxing and may stop spasms of bladder and prostate.

Charles Garcia, noted Hispanic herbalist, makes a fresh root tincture 1:2 at 50% alcohol, "using anywhere from 10 to 30 drops depending on the case.

Traditionally this has been used in my culture internally for the after effects of accidents, attacks, trauma, when there is a continued racing heart or the beginning of grief-shock, and allows the person to function…For chronic pain triggered by skin or peripheral nerve pain…I've used this for fibromyalia and the mysterious conditions called RSDS (reflex sympathy dystrophy syndrome)…I like to combine with California Poppy tincture to help trauma victims sleep…While the root of yarrow acts much faster, Bleeding Heart goes deeper down the nerve. It can also be used on painful surgical scars as a liniment."

The herb has been shown to stimulate interferon, *in vitro*.

The cultivated Bleeding Heart (*D. spectabilis*) rhizome contains two butenolides, menisdaurilide and aquilegiolide. They induce apoptosis in various human tumor cell lines. McNulty J et al, *Planta Medica* 2007 73(15): 1543-47.

The former compound shows anti-Hepatitis B virus activity. Yi XX et al, *Molecules* 2015 20(8):14565-75.

Diana Beresford-Kroeger mentions *D. canadensis* is an aboriginal medicine for long-distance runners, in an unspecified manner.

Turkey Corn is bitter, pungent and diffusive, and useful for stagnation and depression.

Matthew Wood writes. "*Dicentra* was traditionally used in sluggish digestion, where the food in the stomach, ferments, and is delivered in a rotten state to the intestines, where bloating and inflammation occur. Toxins are absorbed into the bloodstream and lymph, giving rise to 'bad blood'. It slowly increases the circulation to provide warmth and vitalization, and opens the skin and kidneys to provide elimination.

Dr. William Cook noted that perspirations is mild and insensible, and the urine is increased in both volume and solid parts.

In *The Earthwise Herbal- New World-* Matthew Wood lists some traditional uses, written by Rafinesque, Edwin Hale, the eclectic Ellingwood and the physio-medicalist Christopher Menzies-Trull. These include:

Bad breath, tongue persistently coated, ulceration of mouth and tonsils, glands (scrofula), loss of appetite, indigestion, full, bloated feeling, catarrh in stomach and intestines.

Swelling and enlargement of abdominal structures, irregular bowels, colic, diarrhea, or constipation.

Females complaints including amenorrhea, dysmenorrheal and leucorrhea.

Relaxed ligaments of uterus, prolapsus, sometimes occurring from extreme debility, following fevers. Rheumatism.

Chronic skin disorders, with marked cachexia; eczema with great relaxation of the tissues and general plethoric fullness. Persistant ulceration with breakdown of soft tissue (i.e., syphilis, scrofula).

Malaise, digestive torpor, glandular atonicity, impairment of nutrition; following a protracted intermittent fever, ague or malaria.

Due to its relative scarcity, use only homeopathic preparations or small doses from commercial growers.

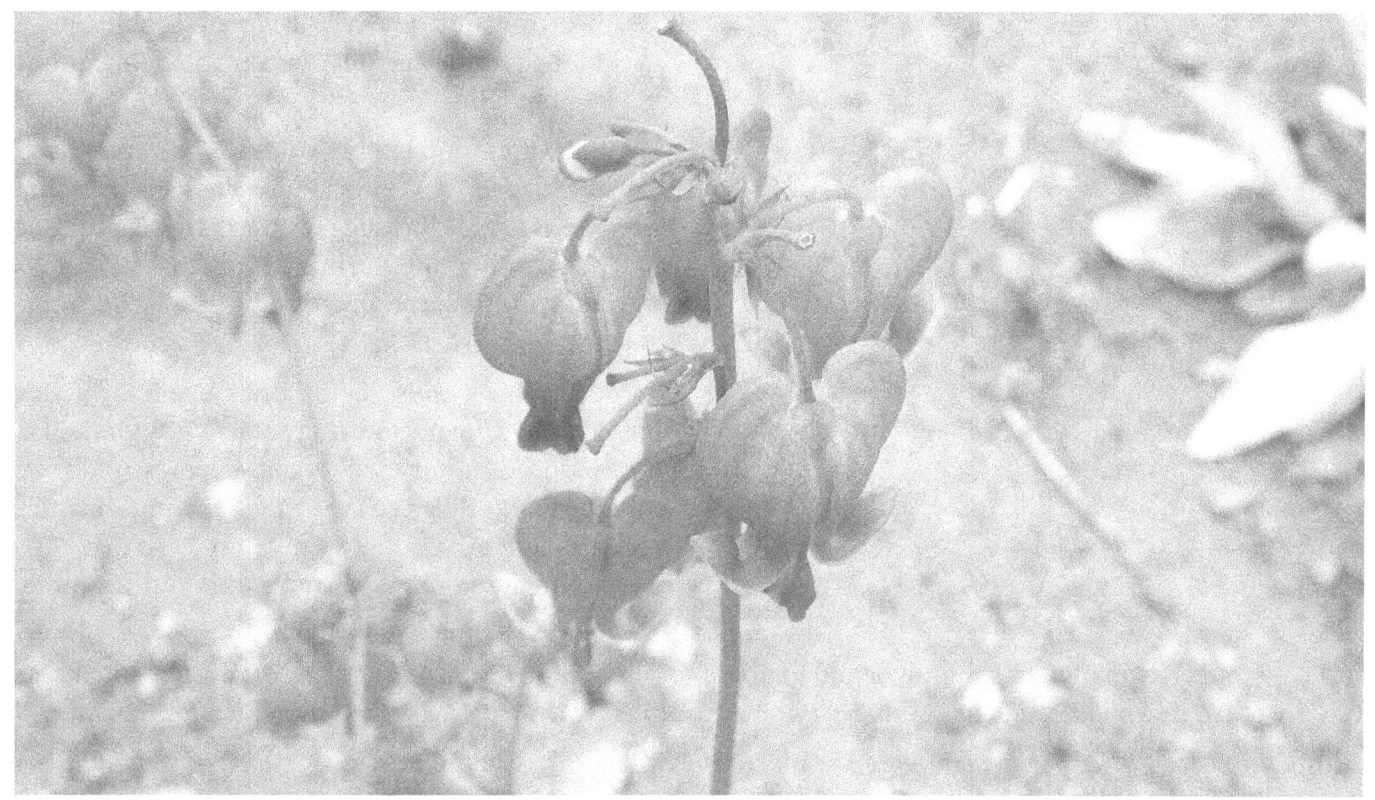

WILD BLEEDING HEART

The seeds of Wild Bleeding Heart (*D. exemia*) show significant anti-oxidant activity with TE/100 grams of over fifty-five thousand.

Because the alkaloids of the Corydalis and Dicentra species are related to those in the opium poppy, they have been intensively investigated.

Bicucculine is a cardio relaxant, protopine possesses anti-arrhythmic and anti-seizure activity, cryptopine helps lower blood pressure, and bulbocapnine is a cardiotonic, anti-spasmodic, and sedative.

Bicucculine and its quaternary methiodide have been identified as potent GABA antagonists with widespread application as pharmacological probes for convulsants acting at GABA neuro-receptors. As it blocks the inhibitory effect of GABA receptors, it mimics epilepsy. Capaurine is a uterine stimulant.

Bicucculine given in low doses to sexually exhausted rats, induced sexual behavior. Rodriguez-Manzo G & Canseco-Alba A, *Behav Brain Res* 2017 320:21-9.

Tetrahydropalmatine is of the main constituents of Corydalis and has been extensively studied.

It has been shown clinically to possess sedative and tranquilizing effect, through the inhibition of postsynaptic domaminergic receptors, while leaving the GABA receptors open. It is analgesic and hypnotic, and alters the amount of neurotransmitters in the brain, decreasing neuron firing rate in the nucleus accumbens.

Tetrahydropalmatine (THP) has been investigated for its effect on the hypothalamus-pituitary-thyroid system.

Thyroid function experiments by Ming Tseun et al, *J of Pharmacy and Pharmacology* 1996 48:9 showed THP produced significant decreases in thyroid function.

These included decreased serum thyroxine, triiodothyronine, free triiodothyronine, and free thyroxine in hyperthyroid cases after 14 days of treatment.

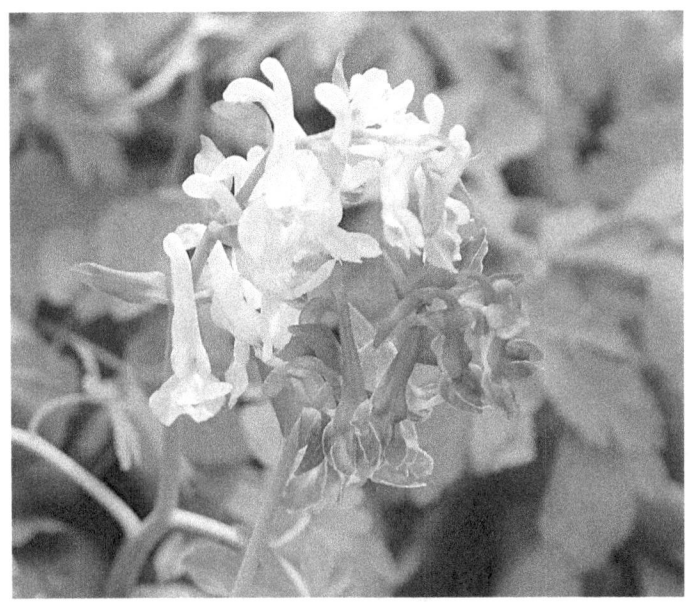
CORYDALIS CAVA

Its anti-thyroid function may be related to inhibition of TSH in the pituitary, similar in activity to Bugleweed and Lemon Balm.

Antagonism of dopamine D1 and D2 receptors and activity at dopamine D3, alpha adrenergic and serotonin receptors is noted. This suggests use in treating cocaine addiction and withdrawal from Ritalin. Rat studies suggest there may be benefit in human addiction. Wang JB et al, *Future Med Chem* 2012 4:2 177-86.

Bulbocapnine when purified has been shown in animals and humans to bring about a catatonic state with reduced motor activity and suppression of all voluntary and reflex movements. The musculature becomes quite flaccid and limbs can be moved like lead piping into bizarre postures. It is anti-psychotic and reduces perceptions of pain.

It acts as an acetylcholinesterase inhibitor and inhibits biosynthesis of dopamine. It inhibits the reflex and motor activity of striated muscle, and has been used in the treatment of muscle tremors and vestibular nystagmus.

Although it has a chemical resemble to apomorphine, it lacks the characteristic emetic action. It causes a catalepsy-like condition, that may include suppression of voluntary and reflex movements, but in contrast to true catalepsy, muscle tonus and resonse to sensory stimuli are maintained.

Willam Burroughs, in his book *Naked Lunch*, looked at all kinds of drug abuse.

"Bulbocapnine induces a state approximating schizophrenic catatonia…instances of automatic obedience have been observed. Bulbocapnine is a backbrain depressant probably putting out of action the centres of motion in the hypothalamus."

Bulbocapnine is also an effective inhibitor of butrylcholinesterase, suggestive of benefit in senile dementia and Alzheimer's disease.

Bulbocapnine may be useful in Meniere's disease and muscular tremors.

Levo-tetrahydropalmitine is used and approved in China under name Rotundine. The compound alleviates neuropathic pain and chronic inflammation in mice, by enhancing dopamine D1 receptor-mediated dopaminergic transmission. Zhou HH et al, *Neuroreport* 2016 27(7):476-80.

Two alkaloids from *C. cava* cross the blood brain barrier and target alzheimer's disease via various pathways, including prolyl oligopeptidase, cholinesterases and beta stie amyloid precursor protein cleaving enzyme. Chlebek J et al, *Fitoterapia* 2016 109:241-7.

Corylucinine shows moderate inhibition of acetylcholinesterase and butyryl-cholinesterase. Novak Z et al, *Nat Prod Commun* 2012 7(7):859-60.

There is certainly room for more study in this area; particularly in alleviating memory impairment associated with dementia.

Staggerweed (*C. cava*) is a powerful alterative and antiseptic, with additional nervine properties. It has a long history of use for ulcerations, chancre sores, sore throats related to syphilis, and the chronic nerve dystrophy that follows. It is reputed to work well in combination with Pokeroot, and is an analogue of Goldenseal.

Corydalis binds to opiate receptors for pain relief, promoting the degradation of adrenaline and the synthesis of melanin.

Bulbocarpnine is anti-spasmodic, sedative, hypotensive, and helps inhibit the contractions of striates muscles.

Corydalis and fennel relieves menstrual cramping and abdominal bloating. Do not combine Corydalis with California poppy, as uterine cramping may increase rather than decrease.

The compounds (-)corycavamine and (+)-corynoline are able to cross the blood-brain barrier, and may be useful in treatment of Alzheimer's disease. Chlebek J et al, *Fitoterapia* 2016 109:241-7. (+)Canadaline inhibits both acetylcholinesterase and butyrycholinesterase, while (+)-Canadine is a potent inhibitor of the former. Chlebek J et al, *Nat Prod Commun* 2011 6(5):607-10.

Corynoline protects cells from inflammation by suppressing cytokines via the Nrf2/ARE pathway. Yang C et al, *Molecules* 2016 21(8).

Some herbalists use it as part of combinations for Parkinson's and other severe neuro-muscular conditions including multiple sclerosis.

It combines well with Scullcap for epilepsy and vertigo. Bulbocapnine is used before and after treatment with anaesthetics, and for use during brain scans.

"Bulbocapnine was also tried as a therapy for the behavioural problems that were often more prominent than parkinsonian signs in children who had suffered encephalitis lethargia. These problems generally involved a loss of inhibition, leading to often violent and otherwise socially inappropriate responses to internal and external stimuli.

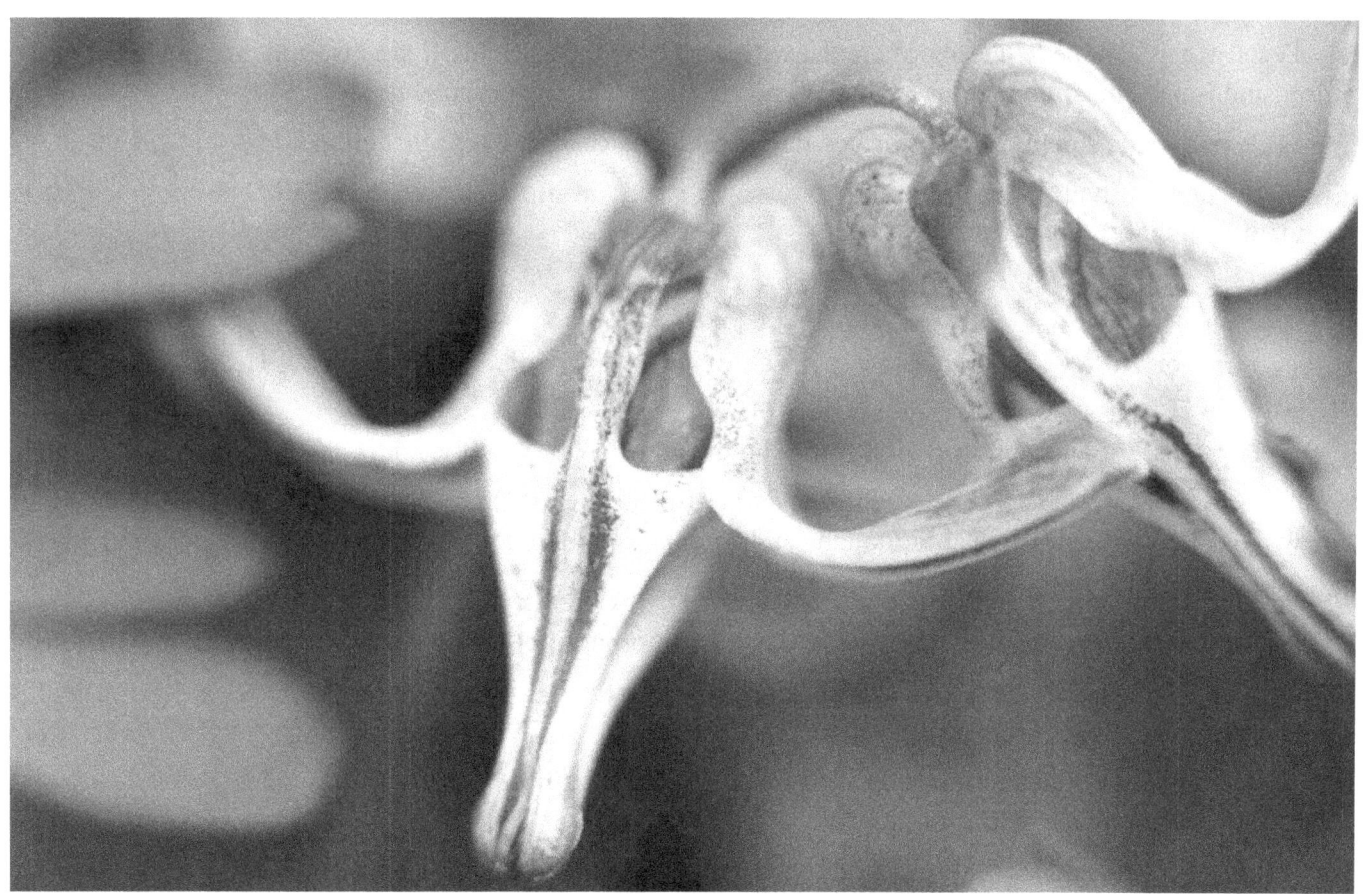

STEERS HEAD (D. UNIFLORA) - PHOTO BY ROSALEE DE LA FORET

Attempts to treat this syndrome, which in many ways resembles what is now described as 'attention deficit disorder' by psycho-therapeutic means had proved futile, and attention had turned to chemical options." **FOLEY**

The tincture is made from the root when in flower.

Dutchman's Breeches (*D. cucullaria*) was traditionally used for skin problems, digestive disorders, urinary tract infections, menstrual disorders and as anti-spasmodic and tonic. An alternate name is Colic weed, suggesting its use in the ailment.

It contains protopine (see above), also present in Black Cohosh rhizome. The two herbs, in combination, are useful for spasmodic and neuromuscular pain.

The herb combines well with crampbark (*Viburnum opulus*) for dysmenorrhea.

Cularine exhibits relaxant effect on bronchial contractions somewhere between papaverine and theophylline. Candenas ML et al, *J Pharm Pharmacol* 1990 42(2):102-7.

Other work showed relaxing effect on uterine contractions, similar to nifedipine. D'Ocon P et al, *Eur J Pharmacol* 1991 196(2):183-7.

Blue Panda (*C. flexuosa*) is a native of China that prefers cool parts of the prairie garden. In its native country, it is often substituted for *C. yanhusuo*, called **YAN HU SUO**. This is the corydalis used in TCM, which is energetically quite different.

Like other members of the poppy family it has important pain relieving properties, mainly due to blood moving ability.

It can be used for painful menstruation, or anytime nervous hyper-functioning is associated with unrest, pain, insomnia, neuralgia, anxiety and high levels of chronic, unproductive stress.

It is classed as a mild remedy, due to no cumulative toxicity from the alkaloids. It has vaso-relaxant and hypotensive action, and is used in combinations for hypertension, angina and myocardial infarct.

Epigastric pain from a peptic ulcer is helped due to both analgesic and antacid action.

It is quite different than the European *C. cava*, which is a neuromuscular sedative; and *D. formosa*, a gastric stimulant, lymphatic and diuretic.

HOMEOPATHY

Turkey Corn, or Turkey Pea *(D. canadensis)* is an eastern relative of Western Bleeding Heart, and used in a similar manner.

It is used for syphilitic affections and ulcers of the mouth and throat. Syphilitic nodes are present on skull, or tibia.

Weakness associated with cancer, and chronic diseases associated with atony. The tongue is clean, broad and full; while the body tissues are flabby, doughy and cold. Like goldenseal, it can be used for gastric catarrh.

The skin is dry, scaly and scabby in the elderly. Lymphatic glands are swollen.

DOSE- Mother tincture- 20 drops three times daily. The mother tincture is made from the fresh bulb in flower.

Hollow root, or Stagger Weed (*C. cava)* is for sadness without clear cause, for lack of joy and energy. Patient is emotionally indifferent, feeling insufficient or inadequate.

Desire for pungent, acidic and sour foods. Aversion to sweets and wine. Anxiety, dyspnoea, palpitations, and cold sweats; a sense of doom during sleep at 3 a.m.

Vertigo, right-sided headaches, number of fingers, tingling in hands in cold weather.

DOSE- lower potencies 1x-6x. Proving by Mezger and Mayer with 14 provers at tincture, 1x, 2x, 3x, and 6x in 1951.

FLOWER ESSENCES

Pink or Pale Corydalis (*C. sempervirens*) flower essence balances addictive and conditional patterns of loving. It helps us see our relationships as catalysts for spiritual growth. **ALASKA**

Pink or Pale Corydalis (*C. sempervirens*) is about receptivity opening the way to inner transformation. It assists one in surrendering to the power and intensity of the process when facing changes or new experiences in life. It is energizing, warming, and soothing to the female organs around menses. **RUNNING FOX**

Bleeding Heart (*D. formosa*) is for those who tend to form relationships based on fear or possessiveness, and emotional co-dependence. It gives one the open-hearted ability to love others unconditionally, and give emotional freedom. It helps heal broken-heartedness and the accompanied feelings of loss and pain. **FLOWER ESSENCE SOCIETY**

SPIRITUAL PROPERTIES

The spirit of the flower appears as a woman bent in sorrow, her hand cupped to her heart. A drop falls from the heart shaped flowers. As she presses its essence to her bosom, it helps soothe the burning in her own heart. The drop of the Bleeding Heart is a symbol of the tears and the suffering that we endure when are going through heartbreak. **RUDGINSKY**

Bleeding Heart represents sentimental remembrance. Only those circumstances which helped us in our seeking for the Divine, must be the object of this remembrance. **THE MOTHER**

PERSONALITY TRAITS

The plants in this family all have significant neurological effects. Everything gets slowed down, sedated, numbed and tranquilized, even to the point of what is experienced as a complete stop. It all began as a way to stop pain, the pain of living, the pain of sadness, the pain of having a will of one's own. The desired calming effect goes too far turning into an enervated inertia of mind, body and spirit…The will is immobile and receptively passive. It can't be roused into action, resulting in apathy and paralytic indifference.

The typical flat effect so characteristic of the Parkinson's patient is emblematic. Life is bland, joyless, grey, vegetative and inert. **VERMEULEN**

Dutchman's breeches are actually four-petaled flowers. Two of the petals unite to form the two legs of the pantaloons while the two others are inside, but project like lips over the stamens.

Why these flowers evolved so strange a form must be left to conjecture. The shape has its advantages.

Each "upside-down" blossom is sealed from the effects of rain and wind on the pollen. It's also sealed from invasion by most crawling or small flying insects that might steal the nectar without carrying the pollen to the next flower. In fact, only the long, strong tongue of the female bumblebee is said to be able to reach from the flower's bottom opening up into each of the two long petal-spurs to lap up the sweets. **JACK SANDERS**

Dutchman's breeches—worn not grown—could be sizable affairs, and F. Schuyler Matthews tells the story of a settler who induced some Indians to sell him for a pittance, all the land that could be enclosed by a pair of these voluminous trousers. The Indians thought they had the best of the deal until the Dutchman sliced up his ample drawers into narrow strips, sewed them together end to end, and made a ribbon that enclosed several acres! **J. SANDERS**

251

MYTHS AND LEGENDS

My favorite is the story of the beautiful Princess Dicentra who wandered away from her walled garden and became lost in the darkness of an ancient forest. The princess fell prey to an evil crone angered to have her privacy disturbed. In an instant, Di was reduced to a fraction of her normal size and entrapped in the satiny folds of an oddly shaped flower.

The old crone cackled happily and told Di that she was to remain forever imprisoned unless discovered and released by an innocent youngling.

Little did the crone know how tempting the Princess would be to any passing child! Only three days passed before a party of riders stopped for water in the forest. Drinking from a stream on bended knee, a boy glanced up, spied the dancing wand tipped by a pink and white heart, and plucked it (as innocent children will do). Short, plump fingers folded back Di's voluminous pink skirt and the lovely princess was saved!   **LOVEJOY**

RECIPES

TINCTURE- *D. formosa* fresh root (1:2) 10 to 20 drops as needed or topically. For advanced cancers use ten drops four times daily.

Dry root tincture (1:5) at 50% alcohol- 15-30 drops. Whole dried herb is processed at 1:5 and 50% alcohol. 25-50 drops 3 times daily.

C. aurea- whole fresh plant 1:2, 50% alcohol- 10-40 drops. Frequent is best. 10-30 drops three times daily.

Dry leaf tincture (1:5) at 50% alcohol- 25-50 drops- 3 times daily as needed.

The root is gathered in summer and fall until leaves yellow. The leaves are collected in summer after seedpods mature. The fresh root is dark yellow throughout and has a fracture that resembles honeycomb. The Eclectics preferred Dicentra tubers be collected in spring, when plants in flower.

Corydalis rhizome is processed with vinegar in TCM to increase its analgesic effect.

CAUTION- Do not use any of these plants with pregnancy, overt neuropathies or with a variety of prescription drugs. They may show as a false positive in drug testing for opiates, so be warned. Do not combine Corydalis and California Poppy (additive effect). In fact, the plant acts like red root (Ceanothus) and this poppy combined in some ways. It inhibits platelet aggregation so avoid with blood thinners. Use for short term only.

Protopine, (+)bulbocapnine, (+)corynoline may increase toxicity of the human ether-a-go-go-related gene. Caution is advised. Schramm A et al, *Planta Medica* 2014 80(8-9):740-6. Several drugs have been removed from the market, due to their potentially fatal adverse effects.

Chorismate synthase is a potential anti-microbial target, in bacteria like *Listeria moncytogenes*, and *Plasmodium falciparum*, associated with malaria. Its presence in rhizome of Pink Corydalis suggests avoiding this herb in various drug resistant and "regular" microbial infections. Hossain MM et al, *Ind J Biochem Biophys* 2015 52(1):45-59.

COTTON GRASS
(Eriophorum species)
PARTS USED- stems, flowers, roots

Thank God I have the seeing eye, that is to say, as I lie in bed I can walk step by step on the fells and rough land seeing every stone and flower and patch of bog and cotton pass where my old legs will never take me again.
BEATRIX POTTER

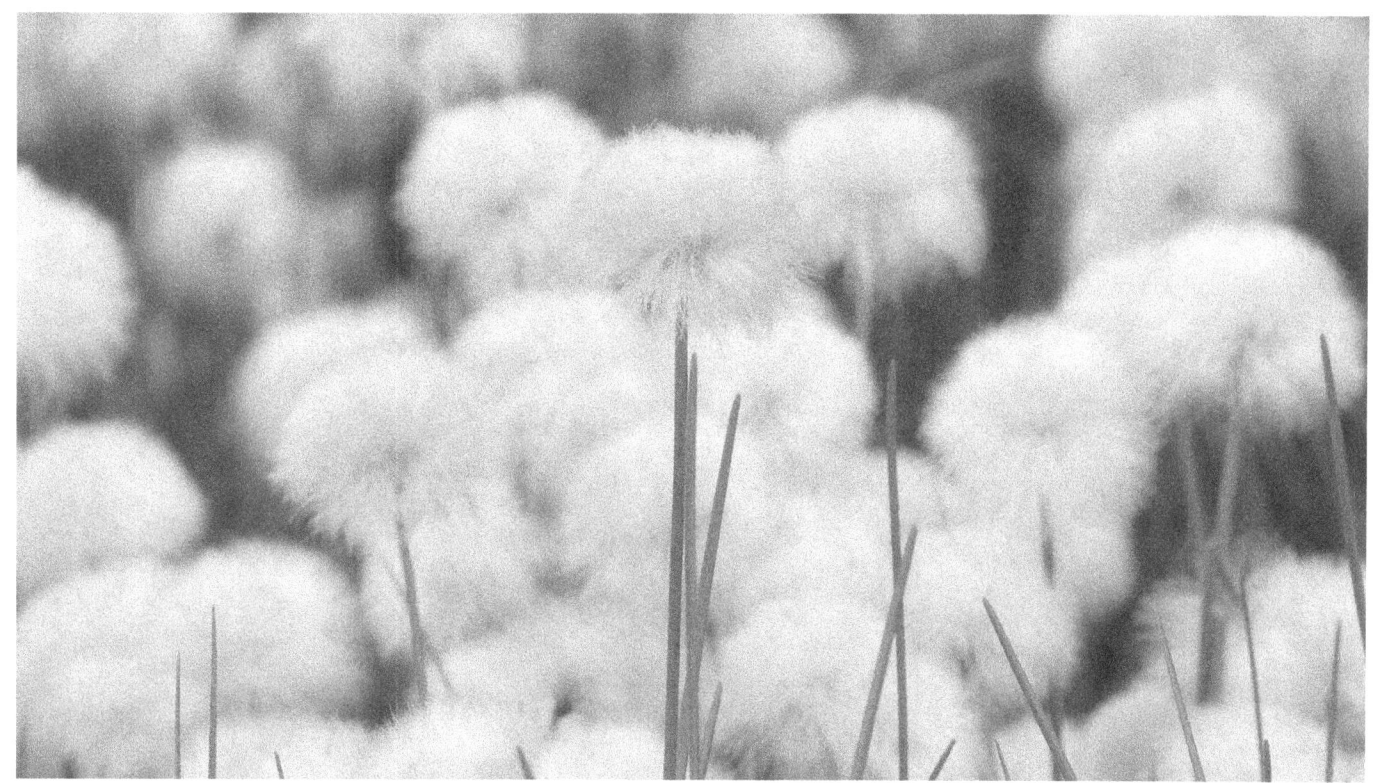

WHITE COTTON GRASS

The genus name is derived from the Greek **ERION** meaning wool, and **PHOROS** bearing, referring to the silky tails of the seed coverings.

Cotton grass is well named, and a distinctive looking addition to the boreal bog where it lives.

The cotton-like heads of the plant were once used to start fires. The heads were also called Arctic cotton and were collected as a cotton substitute. It will not spin into cloth easily, but will stuff pillows and mattresses. It has also been made into paper, and wicks for candles and oil lamps.

The wicks were traditionally stored in walrus kidney membrane containers by natives of Nunavut. The wicks needed to be gathered each year, as too old they would smoke and the flame would go out too fast.

The fleshy, pink stems and underground corm can be eaten. The natives often let mice and voles collect these roots, and then rob them from their winter caches.

Boiling water was poured over them, and the dark, thick coating removed. Boiled or eaten raw, they are sweet like water chestnut, or Jerusalem artichoke.

The leaves can also be eaten, especially the tender white base, according to Russel Willier.

The Kwakiutl in British Columbia called it **KEMXWA** or "eagle down", and it was probably used in a manner similar to fireweed down; that is, combined with mountain goat wool to soften blankets and clothing.

The Thompson decocted Narrow leaved Cotton Grass (*E. angustifolium*) as a treatment for ulcers.

The cotton grass was mixed with a little ground charcoal and applied to a newborn infant's navel. Likewise, the cotton fuzz can be applied to any bleeding wounds or sores. The Flambeau tribe also used Cotton grass fuzz as a hemostat.

In Nunavut, Cotton grass was used to clean ears, in the manner of Q-tips.

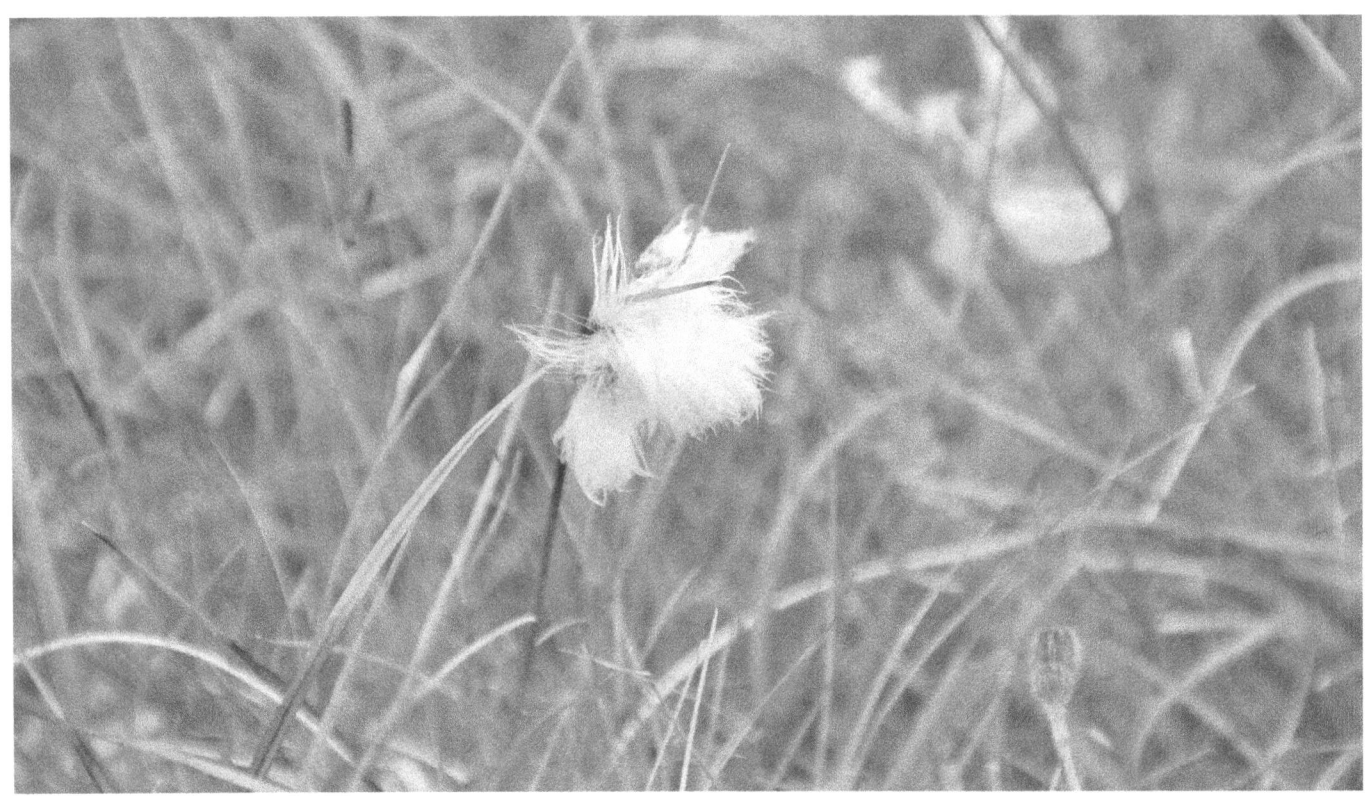

COTTONGRASS

White Cotton Grass (*E. scheuchzeri*) is known, to the Inuit as **PUALUNNGUAT** meaning, "imitation mittens". In Kinngait the name given the plant is **KUMAKSIUTINNGUAT**, meaning "an imitation object to remove lice", while on North Baffin Island the term **KANGUUJAIT** is used, meaning, "what looks like snow geese". They are used as a lamp wick, but not the first choice due to easy crushing. The fluff is often mixed with Dicranum species moss. In Western Alaska, the stems are gathered in summer and used for boot insoles. It may be mixed with rancid seal fat for aches and pains. The fresh shoots can be eaten, and quite sweet when chewed. The Dena'ina of Alaska call it **TL'EGH LITS' A** meaning "sedge fluffy".

In Poland, the species *E. vaginatum* is known locally as Lord Jesus's hair.

In Irish and Scottish folktales, the plant is considered a powerful instrument of enchantment.

On the Isle of Skye, the cotton heads were gathered by children and dried for pillows and quilts.

The stem is also collected in season and used like dandelion sap to clear up warts.

Under the name of Camel's hair, the herb was promoted by Gerard to "bring down the termes", suggesting emmenagogue activity. The unusual vascular system of this species, helps it recycle nutrients internally, giving it a competitive advantage in infertile and cold sites.

It is interesting to note that cotton grass is the first and sometimes only plant to grow on oil spills; and the sowing and planting of cotton grass species is one way to help along severely damaged ecosystems; by providing some cover and below ground biomass.

The use of Tall Cottongrass *(E. angustifolium)* and White Cottongrass *(E. scheuchzeri)* for phyto-stabilization of mine tailings, has been studied by Stoltz and Gregor in Sweden. They found cotton grass stabilized the leakage of metals, such as arsenic, and reduced the use of lime for stabilizing metals. Stoltz E & Greger M, *J of Environmental Quality* 2002 31(5):1477-83.

Tall Cottongrass tolerates elevated levels of zinc. Matthews DJ et al, *Environ Pollut* 2005 134(2):343-51.

MEDICINAL

CONSTITUENTS- all species contain sugars mainly of the xylose and galactose, and flavonoids cyanidin, kaempferol and quercitin.

E. scheuchzeri- aerial parts- eight flavonoids, including three isoflavones, eriophorin A-C, a flavanone, parvisoflavones A-B, tricin (flavone aglycone) and cajanin.

Phosphorus soil seems correlated to areas where cotton grass lives.

The cottongrass is a natural cotton ball, and can be used, as do the Eskimos, to absorb the discharge from draining boils, and sore, inflamed eyes. It is the perfect medium to apply rose water to the face for complexion.

Cotton grass is used as a medicine in northern Europe for diarrhea and relieving coughs. In large doses it can cause headaches and sleepiness.

Parvisoflavones A and B possess anti-fungal activity against *Candida albicans* and *Cladosporium cucumerinum*. Maver M et al, *J Nat Products* 2005 68:1094-8.

Parvisoflavone B inhibits the enzyme PTP1B, also known as protein tyrosine phosphatase 1B. This inhibition plays a role in the treatment of high blood sugar issues, including diabetic retinopathy. This enzyme also plays a role in promoting angiogenesis, helping spread cancer cell growth and progression. The compound tricin also exhibits potent anti-angiogenic activity, *in vitro*. Han JM et al, *Int J Oncol* 2016 49(4):1497-504.

Cajanin improved glucose uptake into peripheral cells better than rosiglitazone, a widely used anti-diabetic drug. Chen QC et al, *Planta Medica* 2010 76(1):79-81.

Cajanin increases bone mineral density, strength and formation compared to control. Bhargavan B et al, *J Cell Biochem* 2009 108(2):388-99.

PTP1B inhibition may also be useful in obesity. Jing C et al, *Arch Pharm* (Weinheim) 2017 350(1). It may play a role in inflammation associated with NF-kappa B. An interesting study by Stoney PN et al, *Brain Behav Immun* 2016 December 18, examined the role of gene expression associated with the hypothalamus and inflammatory pathways during long day summer-like conditions. A compound that inhibits PTP1B reduced this inflammation. More research is warranted, considering the abundance of cottongrass in the Arctic, and the long daylight hours of summer.

Recent work by Liu B et al, *Planta Medica* 2016 81(S01):S1-S381, examined PTP1B inhibitory effect of 45 medical plant extracts. Zinc and vanadium supplementation may be useful additions to assist inhibition of this enzyme, and promote more efficient use of insulin.

Parvisoflavone B is a potent alpha-glucosidase inhibitor (half the drug acarbose), but still notable. Dendup T et al, *Planta Medica* 2014 80(7):604-8.

The herb shows anti-oxidant properties that help protect it against strong UV radiation and other extreme climate challenges.

FLOWER ESSENCES

Cotton grass (*E. chamissonis*) flower essence is for use during cycles of unrelenting stress, feeling " strung out" and trauma of any kind. Cotton grass is for insulating our nervous system, returning us to a womb-like state of nurturing.   **CANADIAN FOREST**

Cotton grass is for letting go of pain held in the body; for restoring equilibrium after injury or trauma; and for shifting one's focus from pain to healing.   **ALASKA**

Cotton grass flower essence is for individuals that have extreme sensitivity to the destructive forces projected on their psyche. This may come from unbalanced individuals like energy "vampires", or from corporate and media projection.   **PRAIRIE DEVA**

Cotton grass (*E. angustifolium*) is for healing of injury, where we cannot move forward into healing due to preoccupation with the injury itself. It helps with understanding the nature of injury, enabling us to create the proper environment within us for healing. **NETTLES AND MORE**

MYTHS AND LEGENDS

Cotton grass appears in a number of Irish and Highland folk tales as a powerful instrument against enchantment, for example in the one called The three skirts of canach down quoted by J G McKay. There the sister had to make each of her enchanted brothers a shirt of the moorland canach which was the Highland name for the plant, ceannabhaan mona in Irish. She had to remain completely silent until she herself, after making the shirts, had put them on her brothers to free them from the spell. **WATTS**

RECIPES

ARTHRITIS BLEND- Take equal parts of cotton grass and nettle leaf juice, and combine with an equal part of walnut leaves in 1.5 litres of water. Bring to a boil, with small amount of vinegar, skim and strain.

Take in small amounts with honey for two weeks after meals. **HILDEGARD**

CRANESBILL
HERB ROBERT
ARB RABBIT
RED ROBIN
FOX GERANIUM
(*Geranium robertianum* L.)
WILD WHITE GERANIUM
(*G. richardsonii* Fisch. & Trautv.)
STICKY GERANIUM
MEADOW CRANESBILL
(*G. pratense* L.)
WOOLLY CRANESBILL
(*G. pratense* L. **var erianthum** [DC] B. Boivin)
(*G. erianthum* DC.)
STICKY PURPLE GERANIUM
(*G. viscosissimum* Fisch & CA Mey. Ex CA Mey)
AMERICAN CRANESBILL
SPOTTED CRANESBILL
OLD MAID'S NIGHTCAP
WILD GERANIUM
(*G. maculatum* L.)
BICKNELL'S GERANIUM
NORTHERN CRANE'S BILL
(*G. bicknelli* Britton)
CAROLINA GERANIUM
(*G. carolinianum* L.)
SMALL FLOWERED CRANESBILL
(*G. pusillum* L.)
ZDRAVETZ
BIG ROOT GERANIUM
MUSK GERANIUM

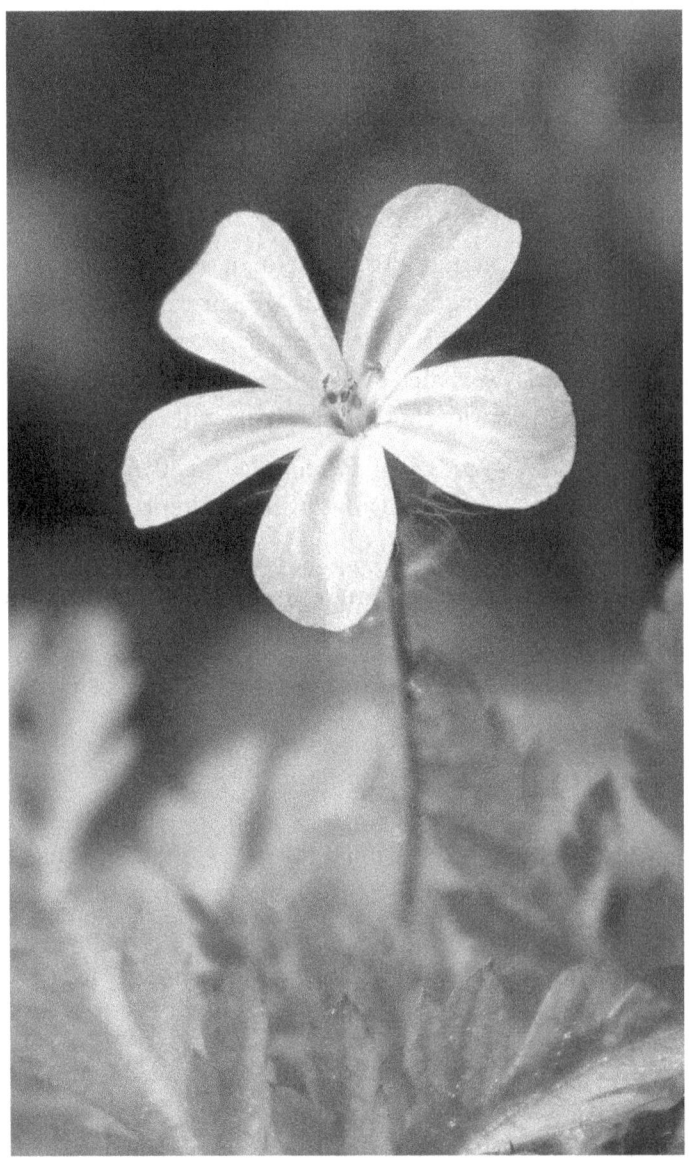

HERB ROBERT

BULGARIAN GERANIUM
(*G. macrorrhizum* L.)
BLOOD RED GERANIUM
(*G. sanguineum* L.)
HIMALAYAN CRANESBILL
(*G. himalayense* Klotzsch)
(*G. grandiflorum* L.)
PARTS USED- whole aerial plant, root

Geranium seeds are a traveling lot,
First they fly, fired like a shot,
Then they crawl in search of a spot,
A nook or a cranny in which to squat
And settle with a new geranium plot.
JACK SANDERS

Nature got it right with the cranes. They have been around since the Eocene, which ended 34 million years ago.
ALEX SHOUMATOFF

Geranium is from the Greek **GERANOS** meaning crane. This is due to the seedpod having slender beaks resembling the bills of cranes. Crane originated from the Indo-European **GRU** for the call of the crane, and later the Latin **GRUS** the Welsh **GARAN** and finally Old English **CRAN**.

Cranesbill or Stork's bill is connected to deliverance of children in a round about way. The herbal tea was often suggested to women unable to conceive, helping bring children to the home.

Richardsonii is named after Sir John Richardson, a Scottish naturalist, physician and Arctic explorer of the early 1800s.

Robert is thought to be named after Robert, the Abbot of Molesme, an 11ᵗʰ century healer. The first reference is from a manuscript written in 1265, in which it was called "Herba Roberti". His birthday of April 29 was about when the plant started flowering in Europe. Or it may be named after Robert, Duke of Normandy, for in Germany it was used to cure a disease known as Ruprechtsplage.

The older name Arb Rabbit, suggests another, unrelated origin.

It may be named after St. Rupert, the first archbishop of Salzbur, the plant at one time known as **HERBA SANCTII RUPERTI.**

Or it is simply a derivation of Rubor, which is Latin for red, the colour of the flowers. This is the most likely. It is associated with Mars and Venus, and symbolizes steadfast piety and birth date of October 26ᵗʰ.

Fox Geranium is so-named from the peculiar foxy, musky smell of the plant after a summer shower.

Macrorrhizum means big root. Zdravetz is from the Bulgarian **ZDRAVE** meaning health. *Viscosissimum* is from the Latin meaning "very sticky". *Erianthum* means with woolly flowers, and *maculatum*, spotted.

Herb Robert grows in rocky woods, cold ravines and along stream beds as far northwest as Manitoba, and is easily grown as a self-sowing annual on the prairies. It is circumpolar and more well-known herb in Europe.

In times of starvation, the root was cooked as a vegetable, like parsnips. Traditionally, it was used for melancholy and sadness. Its ability to stimulate and remove toxins from the body may have been part of its efficacy.

The crushed leaves smell most unpleasant, like a wet goat or crushed insects. This unpleasant scent led to using the freshly crushed leaves as an insect repellant. They were rubbed directly on skin or used an insecticide amongst bedding for animals, hence the name Fetid Geranium.

Another ancient name was Orvale, for the fairies ruling water and air, and the power to heal disease in animals.

257

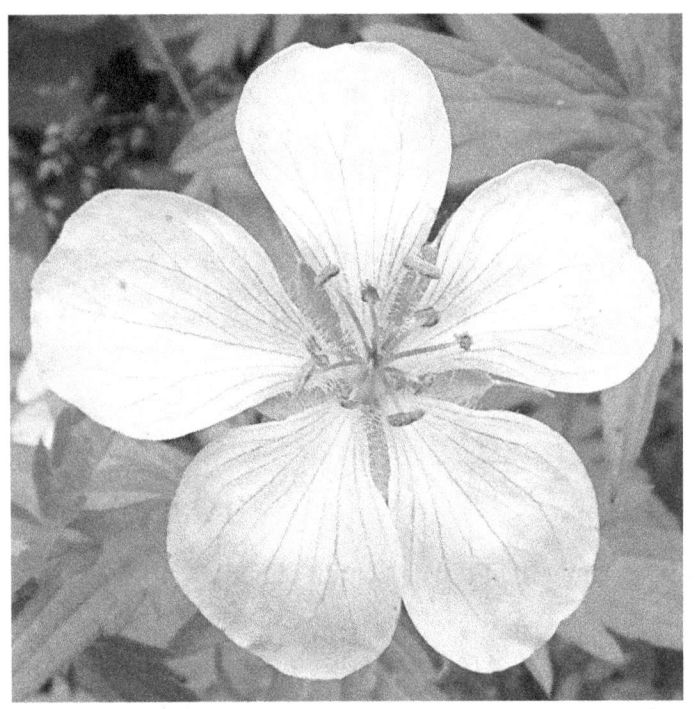

WILD WHITE GERANIUM

Tinctures were applied to the hair and combed in well, to remove lice and eggs.

It has long been used in veterinary medicine for internal hemorrhage in cattle, blood in urine (red water fever), or retained urine as well as mastitis. The fresh juice can be rubbed on skin rashes of pigs.

In Germany, the herb was called **BISWURM**, the ancient name for anthrax, and used to treat this disease in cattle. Red Flow herb was another name.

The fresh leaves are dipped in cold water and applied to bleeding wounds.

Traditional Irish uses include gallstones, diabetes, urinary gravel and retention, and rheumatic pain. The Gaelic name means "plant for hives". In England, by contrast, the herb was used for skin cancer and erysipelas.

The pollen is a bright blue, most unusual, as most pollen is orange or yellow.

In Glouchestershire, England it was believed that one side of the leaf draws out poison, and the other side heals.

Robert's Herb seed germinates best on blotting paper, in full sunlight at 20-30° Celsius and after one year of storage. Seed germination is 80% in the second and third years after harvest.

Robert's Herb (*G. robertianum*) will hyper-accumulate cadmium in its leaf, making it a useful choice for bioremediation of contaminated sites. And of course, caution if picked for medicine.

Wild White Geranium is perennial, growing in open woods. It has white flowers with purple veins.

The Cheyenne used infusions of the dried root as a hemostat, even the powdered leaves were used as a snuff for nosebleed. They call it Nosebleed Plant, or **MATOMENE-VO?ESTSE**.

The Navaho-Ramah used the plant as a "life medicine".

I can find no record of traditional use by the Northern Cree, but they call the plant **NEPIHKAN**, or **WAPIKWANIY**.

The Slave used the plant as a trap lure for fishers, and animal similar to mink or martens, and hence the name **NOØE TSO NAYDI** meaning fisher medicine.

Bicknell's Geranium is an annual, common to oil clearings and logging roads. It blooms all summer and in fall produces the characteristic crane's bill shaped seedpod.

As the pods dry, they uncurl and fling the seeds distances of up to 30 feet. Upon landing, the seeds continue to move. They have a tail, or awn, which curls when dry and straightens out when wet, allowing them to creep until they become stuck in small depressions and holes.

Small Flowered Geranium (*G. pusillum*) possesses anti-oxidant activity. Alaniia M et al, *Georgian Med News* 2013 222:69-72 (in Russian).

Sticky Purple Geranium was used by the Flathead of Montana to remove corns and warts. First the root was boiled until a cream like scum rises to top of water. This is removed and applied to affected area and kept covered. The fresh sap of the stem was used as well, but only as a second choice, and in season.

The Blackfoot simmered the leaves and inhaled the steam for colds, later drinking the cooled tea for additional relief. It was also used for headache and sore eyes. The leaves were used to wrap food and help improve the scent associated with food storage.

The Nez Perce used root poultices previously baked on various swellings and wounds.

New mothers with mastitis, or painful swollen breasts applied hot root poultices to area and covered it with buckskin or cloth.

Sores, cut and rope burns on horses were also treated with the root paste.

The Dena'ina of Alaska call it Crane's foreleg, or **NDALJADA**. The root was boiled or soaked in hot water for a gargle for sore throat, or mouth ulcers. It was swallowed for diarrhea and heart problems.

The leaves were boiled for stomach trouble and tuberculosis, and a wash for sore eyes.

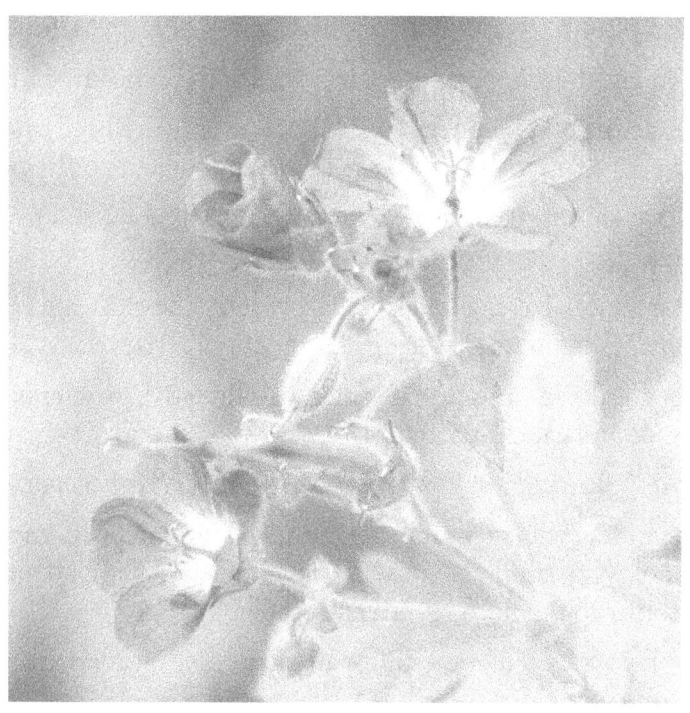

AMERICAN CRANESBILL

An infusion of the leaf and flowers was taken as a refreshing beverage.

The herb exhibits anthelmintic activity against gastrointestinal nematodes, particularly Barber Pole worm (*Haemonchus contortus*) larvae and egg hatch. This is a very common, pathogenic parasite in sheep and goats. Acharya J et al, *Vet Parasit* 2014 201(1-2):75-81.

Carolina Geranium is widespread, and only named so, because of its origin of discovery by students of Linnaeus.

Zdravetz is a hardy, introduced, perennial geranium with many natural hybrids and cultivars. It makes an excellent ground cover, because the leaves are horizontal and shade weed growth.

It does best in dry shade, and requires annual splitting and replanting for best results.

Also known as Bulgarian, or Big Foot Geranium, it is highly esteemed as an aphrodisiac in that country; young men being recommended to spend the night before marriage in a zdravetz meadow.

It is a general symbol of good luck and health; and a common custom is to offer a bunch on birthdays, in hospital, or the start of a new job.

Blood Red Geranium (*G. sanguineum*) is a heat tolerant perennial with purple to magenta to white flowers blooming all summer long.

Spotted Cranesbill was decocted by Chippewa for sore mouths. They call the plant **BE'CIGODJI'BIGUK**, meaning One Root.

American Cranesbill was prized by Dr. Eli Jones, for treating hemorrhage associated with stomach cancer. Herbal writers, such as Alma Hutchens, mention its use to alleviate mercury retention in the body. The root combines well, in a 2:1 ratio with Bloodroot, as a douche for severe leucorrhea.

Dr. Ellingwood, in his remarkable *American Materia Medica* writes "I ...esteem geranium more highly than any other vegetale astringent, where a simple tonic astringent action is needed. It is palatable, prompt, efficient and invariable in its effects, and entirely devoid of unpleasant influences".

Dr. Shook recommended root decoctions as an external astringent to reduce skin wrinkles and large pores.

Today, the whole plant extract is used in both skin and hair care products. It is a clear yellow, with pH 5.5-6.5.

One study showed that 0.1% extract stimulated cell proliferation by 155%. In an eight-week chronic use study, a 10% extract in water was used as the subject's only moisturizer.

Skin smoothness increased 24%, firmness 66%, and hydration by 22%. Also noted was a 21% reduction in fine lines.

Dr. Samuel Waggaman (1895) wrote, "The rhizome of the geranium has some tonic properties, but its main virtues lie in its powerful astringent properties, and it is highly recommended in diarrhea and dysentery."

A good and time-tested remedy for digestive problems is a combination of American cranesbill, marshmallow root and calendula petals.

American cranesbill was official in the *US Pharmacopoeia* from 1820-1916 and the *National Formulary* until 1936.

Carolina wild geranium is an annual found in open, moist meadows. Bicknell's Crane's Bill and *G. carolinianum* look very similar to me. In some books they are synonyms, but I have given each their own section to avoid confusion to both myself and reader.

Small flowered cranesbill is an introduced European escapee found here and there.

Meadow cranesbill is a native of northern Europe, Siberia and China, but often found in nurseries and backyard gardens in zones 3-4.

Studies in Japan, published in *Soil Science and Plant Nutrition* 1998 44:2 found that intercropping Meadow cranesbill with potatoes decreased the incidence of common scab. Applications of the dried root powder or alcohol extracts proved effective.

Ushiki et al, *Antiviral* 1996 42:2 found root extracts effective against a variety of soil borne pathogens, and may be useful as an antagonistic plant in mixed, organic cropping systems.

The book *Geranium and Pelargonium*, edited by Maria Lis-Balchin from Taylor & Francis 2002 is a good review of the former genus.

MEDICINAL

CONSTITUENTS-*G. macrorrhizum* leaves- four flavanols and maltol (a phenolic compound); two tricylic sesquiterpene lactones, astringent tannins, 5'hydroxymorin.
G robertianum- contains a bitter substance, geraniin (45 mg/100g), flavonoids (5.8 mg/100grams) including rutin, 3,4-dimethoxyflavone, quercitin-3-0-rhamnogalactoside, and kaempferol-3-0-rhamnoglucoside; homoeriodictyol, and hyperoside; as well as hydrolyzable tannins (149 mg/100g) such as ellagic acid, geraniin, isogeraniin, castalagin/vescalagin (49mg/100g); beta-penta-0-galloylglucose, a variety of lipophilic compounds, tocopherols, and a volatile oil.
G. pratense- aerial- various phenolics, including querticin, kaempferol and myrictin galactopyranosides and glycopyranosides.
G. sanguineum- Polyphenols (leaves 9-11%, stems 2.5-3.5%, and roots 16-18%), kaempferol, quercitin, rutin, 2-galloylglucose, 2,3-digalloylglucose, and 3-galloylglucose.
G. viscossissimum- ellagic and gallic acids upon hydrolysis; flavonoids and tannins.
G. carolinianum- geraniin (1.3%) and hyperin; tannins (2.4% in fresh leaves and stems), including gallic acid, corilagin, methyl brevifolincarboxylate, ellagic acid and rutin. Glandular trichome exudates include caroliniasides A-C (n-Alkyl glycosides).
G. maculatum-root- hydrolysable tannins (highest in spring before flowering at 28%. By October, down to less than 10%). Composed of geraniin, some starch and calcium oxalate.
Leaf- hydrolysable tannins, 27.5% of galloyl esters of which 10% ellagitannins and remainder gallotannins, probably geraniin. Also called phlobaphenetannin. Also includes gallic, caffeic and p-coumaric acids.

The roots of our native Geraniums are rich in gallic acid and tannins (gallo-tannins), and make an astringent decocted gargle for treating mouth sores, tonsillitis and sore throats.

The fresh root can be crushed and applied to gum and tooth infections directly, while the fresh leaf can be chewed for similar purpose.

Gargling with the root decoction will help firm up a relaxed or elongated uvula, associated with snoring and apnea.

It will relieve gastritis, and the vomiting caused by stomach ulcers, due to its astringent and anti-secretory activity. In the same manner, the herb will help reduce excessive lactation, or perspiration.

It is taken internally for diarrhea, excessive menstruation, post-partum bleeding, urinary complaints, and can be helpful in stomach flu.

Cooled to body temperature, it is used as a retention enema for bleeding hemorrhoids, or inflamed diverticuli. Douche with the same mixture for vaginitis.

For ulcers and Crohn's disease combine two parts root, two parts willow bark and one part Oregon grape root tincture.

The root is effective against stomach ulcers and inflammation of the uterus. The root is a powerful astringent for the treatment of cancer patients who suffer excessive bleeding that will not stop.

Dr. Rudolf Breuss, who suggested a fresh vegetable juice diet for cancer, recommends the herb tea be included in his regime.

Thomas Bartram, an accomplished herbalist in Great Britain, views Cranesbill as a vaso-compressor that increases the vital potency of living matter of the ganglionic neurons.

He suggests it is most useful in over-relaxed conditions, such as incontinence in the young and old, bed-wetting and, of course, blood in the urine.

Geraniin is a histamine receptor ligand that inhibits epinephrine induced, but increases ACTH induced, adipocyte lipolysis. ACTH or adenocorticotropic hormone is produced by the pituitary and stimulates adrenal cortex.

Geraniin reduces blood pressure, and is an ACE inhibitor, suggesting use in cardiovascular health. Lin et al, *Food Chem Tox* 2008 April 13.

It is important to note that all the species mentioned here contain geraniin.

Geraniin, comprising 15% of the root by dry weight was found to have anti-microbial activity relative to 1.25% of streptomycin.

Geraniin interacts with *Staphylococcus aureus* enterotoxin A, and inhibits toxin activity, preventing infection and staph food poisoning. Shimamura Y et al, *PLoS* 2016 11(6).

Work by Notka et al, *Antiviral Res* 2004 64 found geraniin to inhibit reverse transcriptase in HIV infections.

The compound is anti-inflammatory via various pathways determined by Wang P et al, *Chem Biol Interact* 2016 253:134-42; *Biochem Biophys Acta* 2015 1850(9):1751-61.

It protects against cisplatin-induced nephrotoxicity by inhibiting oxidative stress and inflammatory response, in a mouse study. Jiang L et al, *Free Radical Research* 2016 50(8):813-9. Other studies suggest it may help ameliorate wear particle induced osteolysis that may extend the longevity of prostheses. Xiao F et al, *Exp Cell Res* 2015 330(1):91-101.

Li et al, *Antiviral* 2008 79:2 found activity against human hepatitis virus and significant improvement in liver cell lines after exposure to plant extract.

Geraniin inhibits hepatitis B virus replication. Liu C et al, *Antiviral Res* 2016 134:97-107.

The compound exhibits strong inhibitory activity on interleukin-1beta release, in a study of cytokine release from phagocytes by Yuandani et al, *Drug Des Devel Ther* 2016 10:1935-45. Other work found geraniin inhibits inflammation associated with atherosclerosis. Liu X et al, *Inflammation* 2016 39(4):1421-33.

Herb Robert can be used internally for diarrhea, poor liver and gall bladder functioning or inflammation; as well as inflammation of the kidneys and bladder including stone formation.

It combines well with goldenrod in the treatment of acute nephritis, or obstructed urination.

Michael Moore suggests applying the crushed fresh plant or root powder made into a paste with water to pus-filled ulcers or skin abrasions. This will help remove the pyogenic membrane to allow draining and reduction of pressure. Homeopaths used the mother tincture in a similar manner.

Herb Robert has been investigated for anti-viral activity. The fresh plant extract has been shown effective against the vesicular stomatitis virus, which is in the same family as the rabies virus.

The expressed juice of the entire plant has been shown to inhibit gram-positive bacteria.

An 80% ethanol extract shows inhibitory effect on the growth of *E. coli*, *Staphylococcus aureus* and *Pseudomonas aeruginosa*. In a serial dilution test, the growth of *Microsporum canis* and *Trichophyton mentagrophytes* was completely halted. Cranesbill was highest among a number of herbs tested, inhibiting growth of *Helicobacter pylori* and *Campylobacter jejuni*. Cwikla et al, Grifith University, Australia.

Work by Corina et al, *Ofthalmologia* 1999 64:1 found the plant extract, combined with burdock and calendula, was more effective than acyclovir in treating 52 hepatic keratitis patients.

Modern research suggests Herb Robert may have benefit in lowering blood sugar levels. Leaf decoctions, over a period of four weeks, lowered blood glucose levels in diabetic rats, by improving liver mitochondrial oxidative phosphorylation. Ferreira FM et al, *Acta Biochim Pol* 2010 57(4):399-402.

The leaf decoctions have been shown to lower blood sugar and increase liver oxidative phosphorylation in rats. Ferreira et al, *Acta Biochim* Pol 2010 November 1.

Extracts have shown inhibition of enzymes including urease, alpha-chymotrypsin and acetylcholinesterase. The latter is significant, as this is an indicator of benefit in senile dementia and possibly Alzheimer's disease. Lima IS, Master's Thesis, University of Lisbon, 2009.

Water extracts of the herb show cytotoxic activity against human laryngeal carcinoma cell lines (Hep-2p). Neagu E et al, *Arabian Journal of Chem* 2013 doi:10.1016/j.arabjc.2013.09.028.

A recent paper found water and alcohol extracts show activity against human breast cancer (MCF-7), non-small lung cancer (NCI-H460), and hepatic cancer (HepG2) cell lines. Graca VC et al, *Food & Function* 2016 7:3807-14.

American Cranesbill root has similar properties but is perhaps an even more powerful astringent, useful in canker sores, to intestinal and uterine bleeding, to chronic, externally engorged hemorrhoids. For the latter, internal herbal combinations are combined with external poultices or fomentations.

It is taken internally for menorrhagia, metrorrhagia and post-partum hemorrhage, combining well with fresh shepherd's purse.

It was part of the *United States Pharmacopoeia* from 1820-1990. Its removal is questionable.

Dr. Cook suggest "it is not so intense as oak or catechu, but much stronger than rubus or hamamelis", as an astringent tonic.

Dr Fyfe wrote in *Specific Diagnosis and Specific Medication* (1909). "A very efficient medicament in all cases characterized by profuse fluxes, whether of mucus, blood or serum. These often occur in chronic or sub-acute diseases. It is most excellent remedial agent in may cases of diarrhea, especially when there is frequent watery stools and constant desire to evacuate the bowels."

It is a well-known ingredient in Roberts Formula, a well-known combination for ulcerative colitis and ulcers. It combines marshmallow root, goldenseal, echinacea and pokeroot, sometimes combined with slippery elm. I used it successfully in many obstinate cases. Ironically, Roberts Herb is not the cranesbill of choice for this formula.

The herb showed activity against *Tuberculosis mycobacterium*. Fitzpatrick, *Antibiotics and Chemotherapy* 1954 4:5.

Work by Guervara et al, *Revista de Gastroenterologia del Peru* 1994 14 looked at the positive in vitro action of the herb on the gram-negative bacteria *Vibrio cholerae* (cholera).

The herb obviously has anti-viral activity against herpes simplex. A Calgary firm has produced Dr. Krane's (after Cranesbill, no doubt) KoolLips Cold Sore formula containing a 4:1 extract at 50 mg/g from this herb.

This herb is not recommended for long-term use internally, as it may cause liver damage.

Combine with goldthread for gastrointestinal bleeding, with bloodroot 1:2 for leucorrhea, with slippery elm and/or marshmallow root for swollen tonsils, sore throat or ulcerated gums as a gargle. A warm decoction can be used with neti pot for nasal polyps, or a fomentation on bruises, black eyes, bedsores and ulcers. For the latter, you can prepare a 1:10 carrier oil with root, and apply several times daily.

Matthew Wood suggests, "It is perhaps the archetypal remedy for catarrhal gastritis." He also notes that the herb is for "children who fail to thrive due to a wet, mucusy stomach that impedes digestion; or a dampness in the stomach; swishing and watery sounds".

Meadow Crane's Bill aerial parts, extracted in water, exhibit anti-inflammatory and anti-nociceptive activity in laboratory studies. Kupeli E et al, *J Ethnopharm* 2007 114(2):234-40. The aerial parts also contain tryptophan. Akdemir ZS et al, *Phytochemistry* 2001 56(2):189-93.

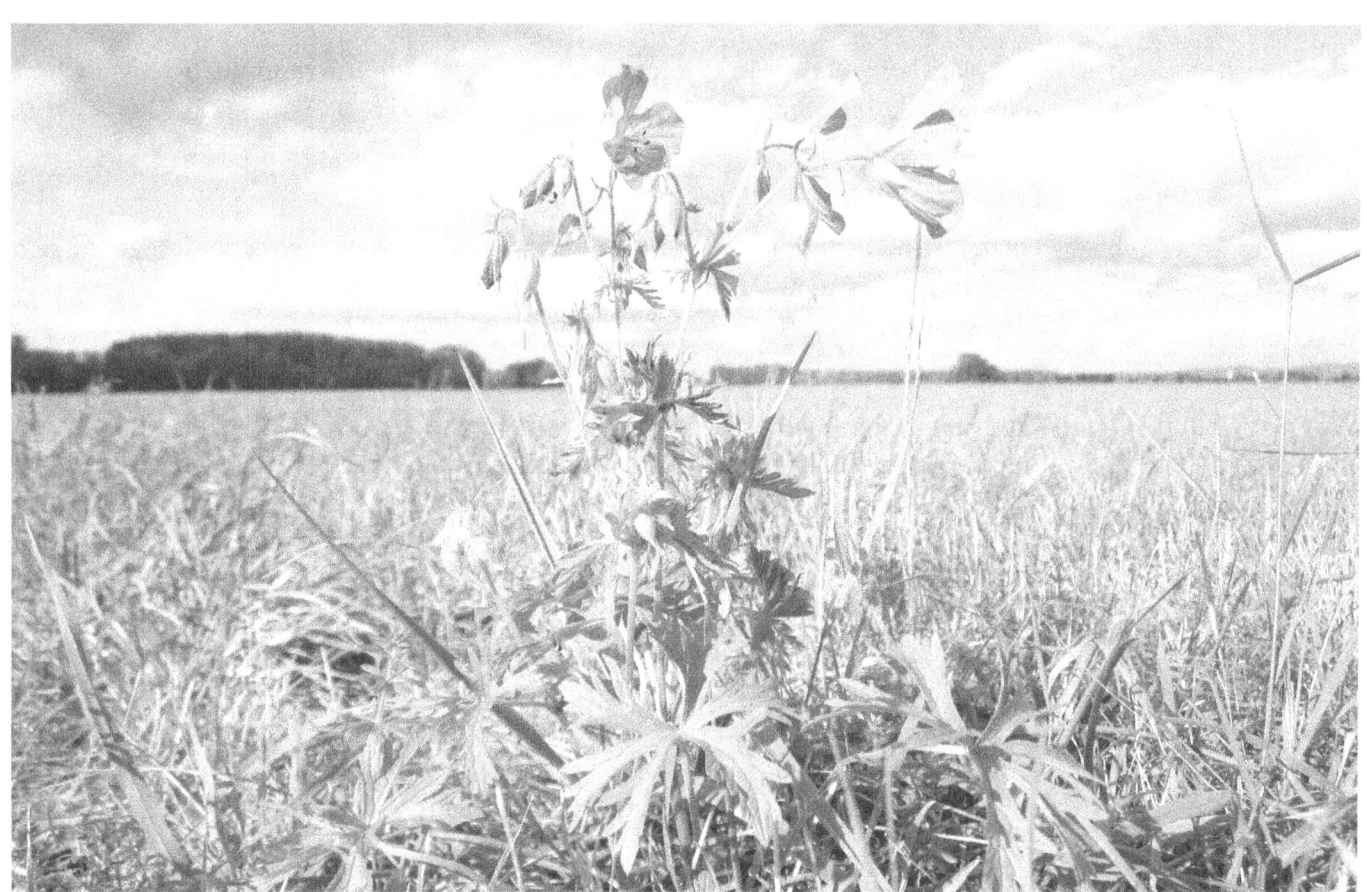

GERANIUM PRATENSE

Alcohol extracts inhibits alpha-amylase activity by greater than 40%, suggesting some possible benefit in reducing the availability of starches and sugars. Kobayashi K et al, *Biol Pharm Bull* 2003 26(7):1045-8.

Meadow Geranium (*G. pratense*) has been studied by Myagmar and Aniya *Phytomedicine* 2000 7:3 and showed strong free radical scavenging effect both *in vitro* and *in vivo*; similar to Blood Red Geranium. Sokmen et al, *Life Sci* 2005 76:25.

Carolina Crane's Bill extracts show activity against hepatitis B virus. Li J et al, *Antiviral Research* 2008 79(2):114-20. Hyperin and geraniin are most probably the active substances. Li J et al, *Biol Pharm Bull* 2008 31(4):743-7.

Blood Red Geranium (*G. sanguineum*) is considered a medicinal plant in Bulgaria, where it grows wild and is also cultivated.

A study in the *Chemistry of Natural Compounds* 1995 31:2 found various catechins and proanthocyanidins from the root exhibited high interferon inducing, as well as anti-viral and anti-tumour activity. The compounds exhibited low toxicity both in vitro and in vivo.

Work by Sokmen et al, *Life Sci* 2005 76:25 suggests the plant contains polyphenols with antioxidant and radical scavenging properties, as well as anti-viral activity. Murzakhmeto et al, *Phytother Res* 2008 22:6 confirmed the anti-oxidant activity in both normal and viral induced animal models.

Polyphenol rich extracts of the herb have been shown to have a favorable effect on protease inhibition. Serkedjieva et al, *Antivir Chem Chemother* 78:2.

The same author noted anti-viral activity against influenza when used nasally. *Antivir Chem Chemother* 2007 8:2.

Work by Serkedjieva at the Institute of Microbiology in Sofia, Bulgaria 1997 has confirmed many of the folkloric uses of the plant.

Alcohol extracts of the whole plant were shown in laboratory studies to inhibit the reproduction of a whole range of viruses including influenza, herpes simplex 1 & 2, vaccinia, and HIV-I.

The anti-influenza effect was very pronounced, in various virus strains in vitro, and in protecting mice from experimental influenza infection.

Follow up work, published in the *Journal of Ethnopharm* 1999 64:1 showed that water extracts of the roots, rich in polyphenols, inhibits herpes simplex virus and is the least toxic for cell cultures.

Recent work by Serkedjieva et al, *Pharmazie* 2008 63:2 found aerosol sprays the most effective transport of activity against influenza infection.

Work by Manolov et al, *Dokl Bolg Akad Nauk* 30:11 published in Bulgaria in 1977, indicates that alcohol extraction of Zdravetz (*G. macrorrhizum*) foliage shows central nervous system depressive, or sedative effect.

Zdravetz leaves and rhizomes have been extracted, and found in clinical research to possess hypotensive properties.

It is very astringent, like its cousins, and useful in diarrhea, skin inflammation, and nose bleeds. The extracts were found to inhibit, *in vitro*, growth of *Staphylococcus aureus* and *Candida albicans*.

Water extracts of the leaves also revealed activity against both gram positive and negative bacteria. Big Root and *G. sanguineum* showed a strong increase in survival rate in mice infected with *Klebsiella pneumoniae*. Ivancheva S et al, *Basic Life Sci* 1992 59:717-28.

Big Root leaves stimulate immune function. Work by Jurkstiene V et al, *Medicina (Kaunas)* 2007 43(1):60-4 found a 10% extract of leaves for four weeks significantly increased both T and B lymphocyte production.

Both *G. sanguineum* and *G. pratense* show activity against *Bacillus cereus*, *E. coli*, and *Pseudomonas aeruginosa*.

Work by Kobayashi et al, *Bio Pharm Bull* 2003 26:7 found methanol extracts of *G. pratense* inhibited alpha amylase activity in mouse plasma.

The aerial parts extracted with water exhibit anti-inflammatory properties. Küpeli et al, J *Ethnopharm* 2007 114:2.

The related *G. sibiricum* inhibits xanthine oxidase, suggestive of benefit in gout. Wu et al, *J Ag Food Chem* 2010 58(8):4737-43. It has been used for diarrhea and cancer in Bulgaria, Peru and Korea. It appears to promote hair growth to a greater degree than minoxidil. Boisvert WA et al, *BMC Complement Altern Med* 2017 17(1):109.

Ethanol extracts decrease gene expression of interleukin 1beta and COX-2, suggestive of anti-inflammatory activity. Shim JU et al, *J Ethnopharm* 2009 126(1):90-5.

Extracts inhibit the occurrence of liver metastases, associated with colon cancer. Huang GD et al, *Zhong Yao Cai* 2009 32(1):97-9.

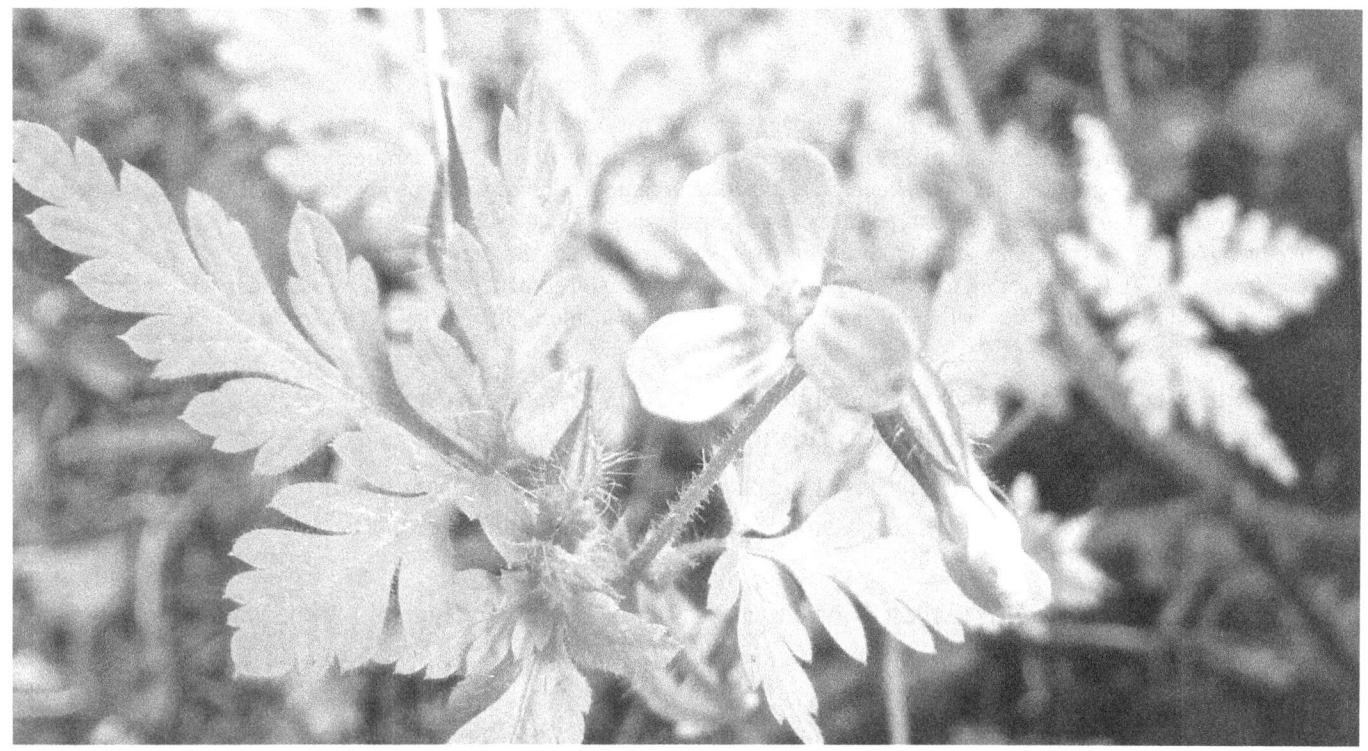

CAROLINA GERANIUM

HOMEOPATHY

Geranium robertianum has astringent action and is used in chronic enteritis, bloody stools and diarrhea. It is also used in gastro-enteritits and as an external astringent in wounds, ulcers, fistulas, eczema; and in gout, rheumatism, calculi, and jaundice.

Beneficial results are also seen in glandular illness, enlargement of the tonsils, swelling of the cervical glands and umbilical colic in children. A proving was conducted in the summer and fall of 1994, by Dr. David Riley.

The following is a concise materia medica from his proving.

Mind- great anxiety, sadness, irritability and restlessness. Vivid dreams remembered in great detail. Rapid pulse, increased energy.

Itching eyes, white coating on tongue, painful swollen gums.

Stomach- nausea is worse in afternoon and evening, particularly after eating. Distention and belching. Low grade pain in the stomach and abdomen. Increased flatulence, constipation and diarrhea.

Chest has burning pain upon inhalation. Perspiration on the chest.

Back- Aching back pain, with pinching under right scapula.

Aching in extremities, eruptions and itching all over the body.

DOSE- Mother tincture to third potency as general rule. The mother tincture is prepared from the fresh plant in flower.

It is worth noting that the older Boericke's Materia Medica uses Cranesbill (*Geranium maculatum*). They are interchangeable.

Geraniin (extracted from above) is used for constant hawking and spitting up in elderly.

DOSE- same as above

ESSENTIAL OIL

CONSTITUENTS- zdravetz aerial parts- germacrone (55%) and germazone (a novel sesquiterpene ketone- 8%), quercitin 3,7,3',4'-tetramethyl ether, tricosane (up to 50%), p-cymene, borneol, dipentene, alpha-phellandrene, gamma terpene, alpha and beta-elemen/elemenone; geraniol, gamma-selinene, terpinolene, curcumene, elemol, guaiazulene, alpha-satalene, beta-eudesmol, junenol, limonene, delta-cadinene, germazol, germazane, andgermazene, 4,5- and 1,10 epoxygermancrones.
concrete- geraniol, germacrol, mono- and bicyclic sesquiterpenes, n-triacontane and free fatty acids.
Yields vary from 0.27-1.44% for leaves, to 0.23-0.34% for roots. Maximum oil content is recorded spring and fall; lesser during flowering and seed formation. Work by the Russian Andreeva showed that among 30 forms of *G. macrorrhizum* the highest yield was from cultivar 11444-1.

The first Zdravetz essential oil was produced in Bulgaria in 1926. Soil can affect the essential oil composition, with calcium rich soils resulting in higher azulene content.

The volatile oil from the above ground parts of the plant possesses a very pleasant odour reminiscent of clary sage, orrisroot, tobacco, broom and particularly rose. Because of the rose-like scent, it is often used in adulteration of costly rose essential oil.

Some data in commercial leaflets suggest Zdravetz can play a role in reducing high blood sugar and blood pressure.

It also acts as an effective anti-microbial, and anti-catarrhal for a variety of respiratory conditions including bronchitis, and asthma.

Unpublished commercial data allude to both anti-tumour activity, as well as helping to dissolve gallstones. None of this has been proven in any laboratory or published in clinical journals this author has seen.

Germacrone, its main component, is very rare, and formerly called Germacrol. It is very faint, sweet woody, somewhat herbaceous, but with extraordinary tenacity. It is produced by isolated, or freezing Zdravetz oil, and could be used as a modifying fixative in Ambre, Chypre, and mossy fragrance types of perfume.

It is used in spicy oriental perfumes, such as Cinnabar by Estee Lauder.

It is obvious the oil has strong anti-microbial properties, and would be a good general antiseptic.

4,5- and 1,10 epoxygermacrones show potent activity against two bacterium, *Bacillus subtilis* and *Pseudomonas aeruginosa*. Radulovic NS et al, *Chem Biodivers* 2014 11(4): 542-50.

Concretes, and their absolutes are also produced from the plant; having a much milder, fuller and longer lasting scent.

The oil is neurotoxic and abortifacient, and should not be used with children or during pregnancy.

Essential oils from *G. robertianum*, along with clove bud and lavender, form a combination called Lamigex. When this product was compared with 0.3% ciprofloxacin on seventy patients with acute external otitis, both groups had similar reductions in tenderness, itching, erythema, edema and discharge. Panahi Y et al, *J Microbiol Immunol Infect* 2014 47(3):211-6.

HYDROSOLS

Zdravetz hydrosols are available commercially, and may be useful, in milder form, for some of the health concerns mentioned above. This is worthy of exploration, as the oil and water can be easily produced on the prairies.

The distilled water of Cranesbill, taken in three or four loth doses before breakfast will dissolve clotted blood in the body, promote urine, and operate against sand in the bladder, as well as sand and stones in the kidneys. It is a certain remedy for scurvy and great heat in the mouth during fevers. If the tongue becomes extended and fully split due to heat, soften a few quince seeds in cranesbill water so that it creates a thin mucusy liquid.

SAUER

Herb Robert water is distilled from the leaf and stalk in June. It is good for the eating sores on privates of women; reduces piles, and congealed blood under the skin is removed inwardly. It helps paralysis in back or legs, and relieves women's breasts when swollen, red and painful.

BRUNSCHWIG

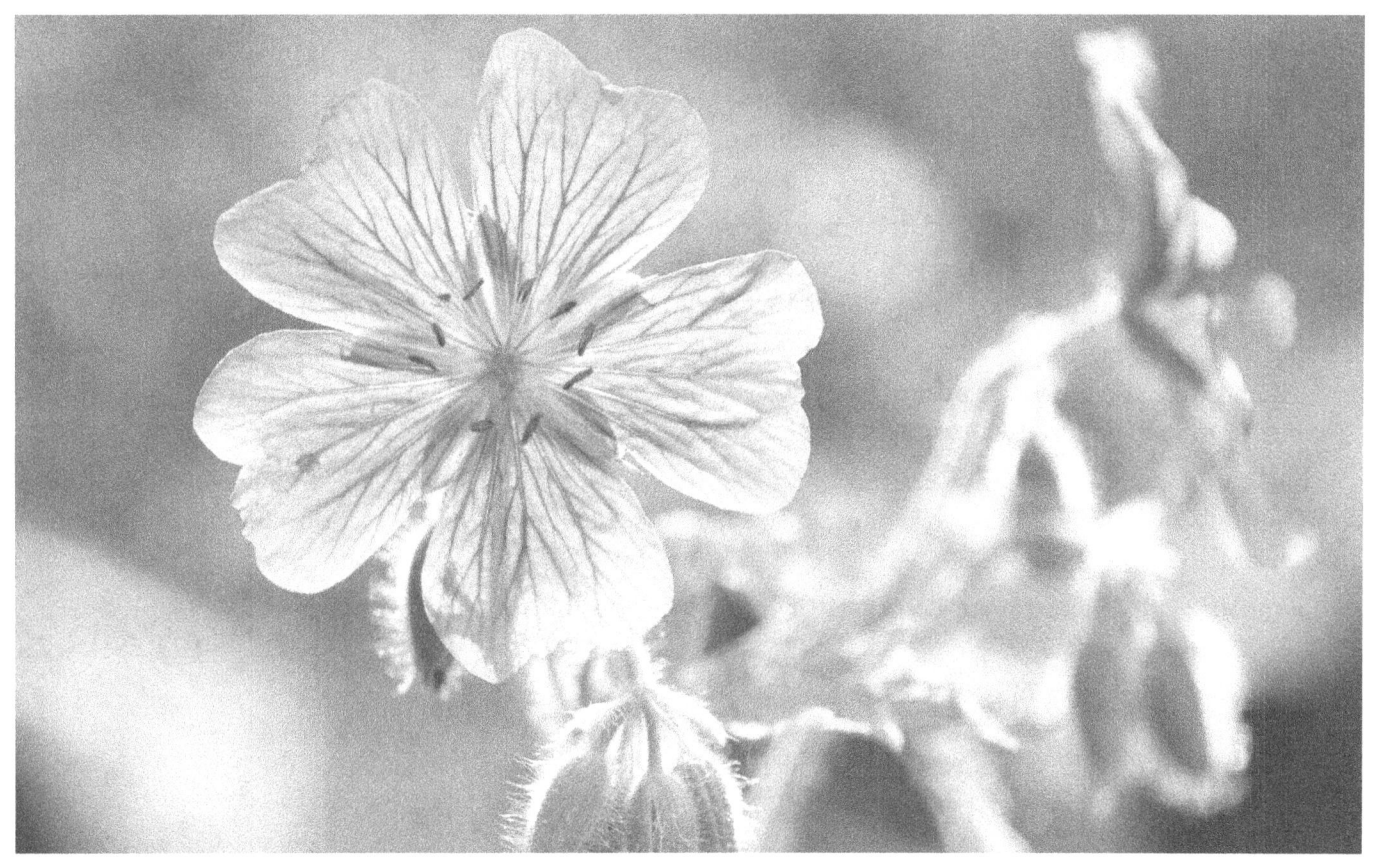

BLOODY GERANIUM

SEED OIL

The seed oil of *G. sanguineum* contains petroselinic and vernolic acid. These fatty acids are usually confined to members of the *Umbelliferae* family.

FLOWER ESSENCES

Sticky Geranium flower essence is for those individuals who need to get unstuck. It helps support decisive and focused action, and helps one move beyond previous stages of growth.

ALASKA

Sticky Purple Geranium essence helps people who do not enjoy, but must attend group social functions.

ROCKY MTN

Spotted Geranium as a flower essence is fabulous for sensitive individuals who are adversely affected by negativity. This essence will allow their negativity to pass straight through the body-like Teflon for your energy field! Geranium can also be very effective on those affected by mass hysteria associated with fear.   **OLIVE**

Herb Robert flower essence helps heal connections to group when no longer appropriate. It helps one free themselves from ties to groups.   **BRYNAHERB**

Meadow Cranesbill (*G. pratense*) essence helps prevent premature and emotionally driven decisions.
                                                                                                                                MIRIANA

MYTHS AND LEGENDS

Herb Robert is connected with animal spirits and healing through the plant.

In the past, it was used in veterinary medicine, especially the treatment of blood in the urine and infectious disease.

An old German name **BISWURM** was the old name for anthrax. Eventually the old beneficial pagan spirits that worked their influence through plants, were replaced by Christian saints.

Orvales, those sprites of the water and air that have the power to heal disease, have long been replaced with Saint Ruprecht or Robert, an archbishop of Salzburg. According to legend, he healed his ulcers and canker sores with the herb.

A guardian of the Celtic underworld, the crane represented great knowledge and was associated with longevity. Aoife, wife of Mannanann Mac Lir, god of the Sea, was turned into a crane for giving humans knowledge. Far from stopping her teaching, this change meant that she could fly over the whole world in crane form, spreading wisdom.   **EASON**

The ancients were also impressed by the beauty and stamina of the Crane, its migrations and spring reappearances, its complex mating dance, its voice and its contemplative stance at rest.

The bird was linked in China with immortality, in Africa with the gift of speech, and widely with the ability to communicate with the gods. Its cyclic return also suggests regeneration, a resurrection symbolism sometimes used in Christianity.

It personifies Vigilance in Western art. In Egypt, the double-headed crane represented prosperity.
                                                                                                                            J TRESIDDER

PERSONALITY TRAITS

The Geranium is like those who suffer from melancholy, a charming plant that...flies the light of day, but its delicious perfume delights those who cultivate it.

Dark and simple in appearance.   **POWELL**

The Cranesbill flower spirit invites you to honor your own expansive nature and to feel the depths of liberation and joy that living a life through love will bring. This exquisite, celestial flower appears to be floating above the earth, as it represents expansion.   **ECLARE**

American Cranesbill is for people who have lost a part of their essence; people who depend on prescription or recreational drugs to function and have lost the ability to function on their own; people in recovery from drug addiction. It helps to separate people who have been closely connected after the failure of a marriage, relationship or friendship.   **WOOD**

American Cranesbill helps mothers separate themselves from children.   **JULIA GRAVES**

When the seeds of *Geranium maculatum* L. (Geraniaceae, cranesbill) are ripe, they are held by five looping carpels, "hooks", attached to the peduncle; it is this plant (occasionally varying species of the genus) which have appeared on the cover.

These hooks provide the logic for using the roots of this plant, along with the others in the category, for cold sores, the sores of venereal disease, and for healing the navel of a newborn. A pharmacologist might attribute any effectiveness of cranesbill in these uses to the fact that the roots contain significant quantities of the astringent tannin. The Iroquois, however, were not aware of the existence of tannin, just as most pharmacologists are unaware of the hooklike and ensnaring quality of cranesbill, ust the sort of thing to apply to an everted, running, escaping thing like a cold sore (at least if you are an Iroquois). A number of these "sticky plants" are used, by the Iroquois as "Love medicines". Typically, these formulations are designed to bring back (to recapture, to ensnare) a wandering wife or an unfaithful husband. These can also be used as "basket medicines," or "peddler medicines". If you sprinkle the root tea on the baskets or other items you are trying to sell, it will hook a buyer.

DANIEL E. MOERMAN

RECIPES

COLD INFUSION- Take 2 tsp. of dried herb to one cup of cold water, and let sit overnight. Drink 1-4 cups as needed. Do not add milk, as the protein will bind with tannins. Warm to body temperature, strain and use as vaginal douche.

TINCTURE- 20-30 drops as needed. Make the tincture at 1:5 of the dried root at 50% alcohol. Michael Moore suggests adding 10% glycerin, for plants high in both tannins and essential oils/alkaloids, to keep the former from precipitating the latter. Good idea.

American Cranesbill tincture- For stomach cancer use 3-4 ml every hour until bleeding stops.

POWDERED ROOT- as a snuff for excessive catarrh and for bleeding from the nose.

INSECTICIDE- The whole, dried plants are powdered and used for dusting insects.

For ringworm and other fungal skin problems on cattle, combine three parts elder leaf, one part cranesbill and one part garlic in a slow decoction, and bathe affected areas frequently.

COUCH GRASS
QUACK GRASS
DOG GRASS
(*Elymus repens* [L.] Gould)
(*Triticum repens* L.)
(*Agropyron repens* [L.] Beauv.) not accepted
BLUEBUNCH WHEATGRASS
BUNCHGRASS
A. spicatum [Pursh.] Scribn. & Smith) not accepted
(*Pseudoroegneria spicata* [Pursh] A. Love)
SQUIRREL TAIL
(*E. elymoides* [Raf.] Swezey)- not accepted
(*X Elyhordeum elymoides* [Hack.] J. H. Hunz. & Xifreda)
WESTERN WHEAT GRASS
(*A. smithii* Rydb.)
(*Pascopyrum smithii* [Rydb.] Barkworth & D.R. Dewey)
PARTS USED- rhizomes, flowers, leaves

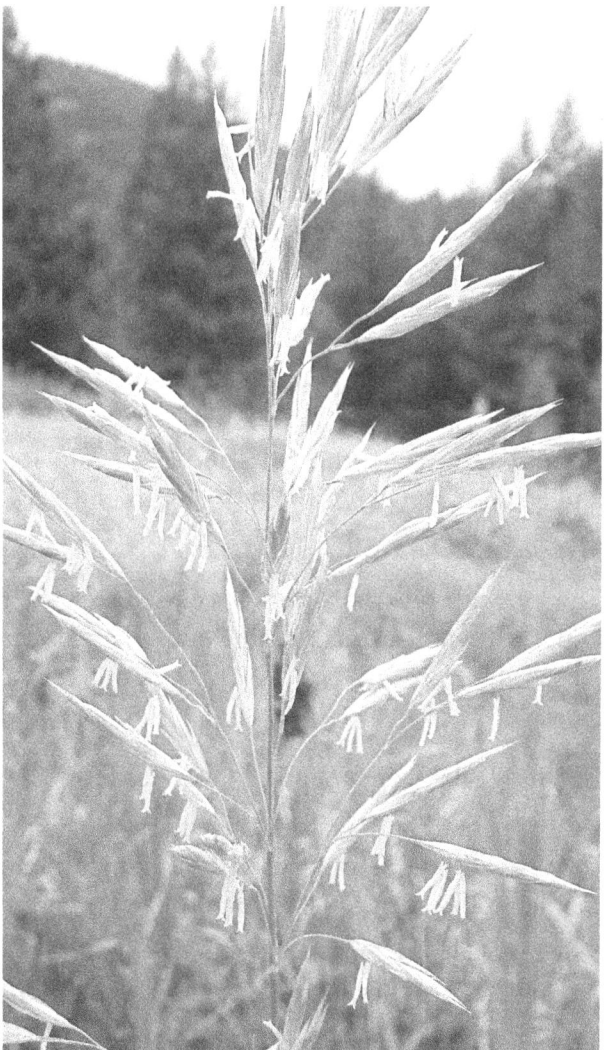

COUCHGRASS IN FLOWER

When a dog barks at the moon, then it is religion;
But when he barks at strangers, it is patriotism!   **DAVID STARR JORDAN**

AGRO is Latin meaning a field, earth or soil and **PYROS** is Greek for fire. Some believe it is from the Greek **PUROS** meaning wheat, and **REPENS** for creeping; which also makes sense. It is commonly known as quack or dog grass. *Elytrigia repens* is a new taxonomic designation, but why, I have no idea!

The Russian name **PIREY POLZUTCHY** quite literally means "field of fire".

Couch is possibly from the Anglo-Saxon **CWICE** for quick or lively, or **CIVICE** meaning "vivacious" in reference to its tenacious growing habits. Some believe the word Couch is from the Anglo-Saxon meaning "holding on to life". Couch is a variation of Quitch, Squitch, Twitch, Whick and Quack.

Quackgrass is from the German **QUECKE** meaning "to live" in honour of the plant's tenacity. Dog grass may originate from ingestion by canines as an emetic.

Cursed and despised by farmers and gardeners, couch grass or dog grass, is extremely stubborn and therefore placed under Saturn/Mars. In the language of flowers, couch grass is related to war and death.

The Scottish word for the plant, Kett, means filth, while Yawl, from the Old Cornish dyawl means devil.

It has an enormous rhizome system and this is where the strength of the plant lies. A single plant can produce over 400 feet of rhizomes per year. The interlocking roots help stabilize slopes and the plant is used in Holland to reinforce new dikes.

Many grasses are called quack grass, but a close look at the leaf will help identification. Each leaf blade looks like it has been pinched with a fingernail about two to four inches from the tip. Once identified, never forgotten. Ruth Yanor, noted herbalist, says the fresh root tips taste like dried watermelon, and I have to agree. Very sweet!

New studies from Michigan indicate that couch grass is effective at reclaiming nutrients from sewage effluent sprays. Couch grass is an indication of soil with a calcium deficiency. Foxtail Barley growth also indicates this mineral imbalance.

Methanol extracts have been used to control mosquito larvae and could be combined with Shepherd's Purse seed (*Mosquito News* 34).

Dogs and cats will seek it out as a purgative to rid the body of parasites. They prefer smooth grasses as an emetic.

Vomiting stimulates the vagus nerve and in turn the digestive and respiratory tracts are cleared. Food poisoning and colds are quickly treated by dogs themselves, when they have access to dog grass.

The seeds may be gathered for bird feed, as well as making bread and beers.

The long, fibrous roots were once used to make brooms. In fact, couch grass is a cleanser and sweeper of the entire uro-genital tract, putting out inflamed, fiery conditions in the water system.

Dioscorides, a Greek physician of the 1st century, recommended decocted rhizomes for gallstones, and reducing fever.

In ancient Babylon, a type of mead was fermented from couch grass rhizomes, juniper, honey and yeast.

Culpepper, an herbalist of 16th century England, proclaimed one acre of couch grass was worth ten acres of carrots. Certainly not taste wise, although the roots are mucilaginous and sugary. The roots were dried and made into bread and the roasted roots were brewed as a coffee substitute.

Culpepper wrote that couch grass "is the most medicinal of all the quick grasses. Being boiled and drunk it openeth obstructions of the liver and gall, and the stoppings of urine, and easeth the griping pains of the belly, and inflammations…the seed doth more powerfully expel urine, and stayeth laxes and vomiting."

Various tribes made use of the roots, for their diuretic and urinary toning effect. The Cherokee, for example, decocted the plant to wash swollen legs, and drank infusions for "gravel" in the urine and for "incontinence and bedwetting". The Iroquois used the plant as a worm remedy, in an unspecified manner, and combined **ER-HAR ENA-WI-RA** rhizomes with alder twigs for thick urine.

Dr. Ellingwood, one of my favorite Eclectics, wrote the herb increased "the flow of the water portion of the urine without to the same extent influencing the actual renal secretion."

During World War I, the US Surgeon General praised couch grass for its diuretic effect on wound and burn victims. African healers chewed the plant and applied it to poison arrow wounds, after sucking out the poison.

Today, the flavour industry uses couch grass extract in baked goods, pastries, ice cream, beers, spirits, and non-alcoholic drinks in 2-6 parts per million.

Many farmers may grimace at this, but research conducted by Christen et al, October 1990 *Journal of Animal Science*, found the nutritive value of quack grass hay similar to that of timothy.

Research by Grela et al, *J of Animal and Feed Sciences* 1998 7 found that supplementing nettle herb, garlic bulb, and couch grass rhizomes to 96 pigs improved daily gains by 5% and feed utilization by 10% over controls. Antibiotic additives also improved performance, but only by half as much.

Bluebunch Wheat Grass was used by various Natives of the interior of British Columbia as tinder for starting fires, insulating footwear in winter and babies' bedding.

The straws were inserted into newly pierced ears to keep the tissue from sealing back in.

Some widows of the Thompson tribe wore breech-cloths of dry bunchgrass for several days after bereavement so "that the ghost of the husband should not have connection with her."

Saskatoon berries were often dried on mats of the grass.

The Secwepemc would use the versatile and handy grass to line root-cooking pits.

Couch grass can be made into a garden spray for mildew and fungus, especially in greenhouses. Planting tomatoes, also known as wolf peaches, will inhibit couch grass, as the roots release enzymes that restrict the "weed".

Ironically, dog grass appears to cause atopic dermatitis in up to 15% of canines. Mueller et al, *Aust Vet J* 2000 78.

When grown in rows for commercial harvest, it is important to mow the plants close to the ground first, and rake all this matter away. Then turn over soil using a simple blade and pick through. Fresh rhizome tincture is best.

An accession of couch grass collected in Turkey and later work in Utah has produced a strain with excellent salinity tolerance along with drought resistance.

The related Western Wheat Grass has been found in studies by McCutcheon & Schmoor 2003 to enhance degradation of toxic TPH and PAHs in soil.

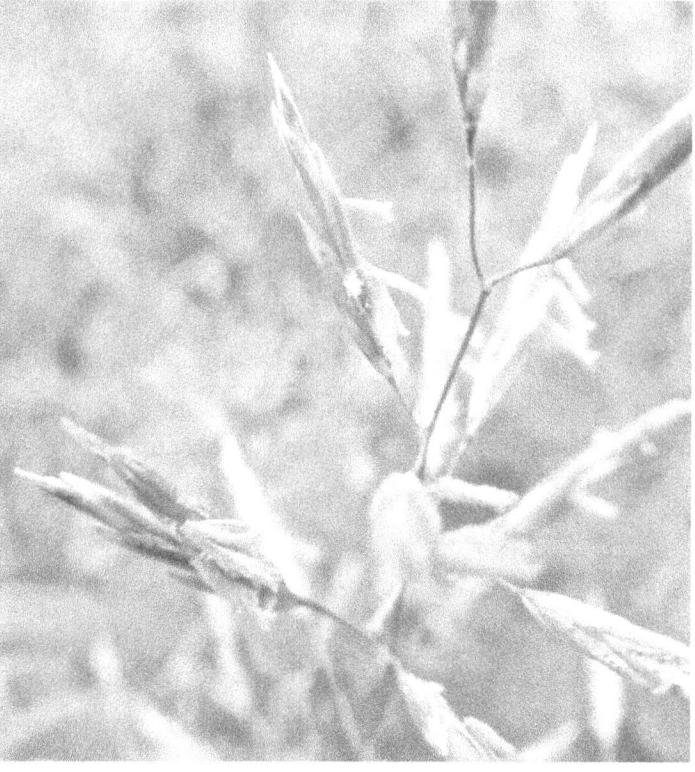

COUCHGRASS- CLOSE UP OF FLOWERS

MEDICINAL

CONSTITUENTS- leaves-mannitol, iron, triticin (polyfructosan up to 7%) tricin, agropyrene, inositol, avenin, amygdalin, an anti-microbal acetylenic carbide, p-hydroxycinnamic acids, vanilloside, silicic acid, potassium (5.65%), pectins, and Vit A and B. rhizomes- 5-hydroxyindole-3-acetic acid (5-HIAA), 5-hydroxy-tryptamine, tetrahydro-B-carboline, and indole-3-acetic acid. Also contains 3-10% fructans (triticin), inositol, mannitol, dormin, abscisic acid, various sugar alcohols, volatile oils (0.05%) vanillin glucoside, quercitin and luteolin glycosides, silicon, potassium, iron, vitamins A and B, fixed oils, and mucilage.
Trace amounts of mammalian steroids have been detected: estrogen (120nanogram/gram), androstenone (120ng/g) progesterone (250ng/g) and androgens (3ng/g). Simons and Grinwich, *Can J Botany* 1989 67.

Couch grass is perhaps our most versatile urinary plant remedy. It is a urinary demulcent that soothes, with its sweet, cool, moist properties, all inflammations of the urethra.

For chronic urinary irritations, such as the passing of kidney stones and gravel, it combines well with yarrow and pipsissewa and can be used as a substitute for job's tear seeds or woolly grass root.

Work by Grases et al, *J Ethnopharm* 1995 45:3 found couch grass decreased citraturia when combined with a high carbohydrate diet; with an increase in calciuria and decrease in magnesiuria.

In an open study, 313 patients suffering from cystitis, prostatitis, urethritis or irritable bladder ingested 50-60 drops three times daily for 12 days of a 1:1 60% fluid extract of the rhizome. Some patients were on antibiotics (23%).

Urological symptoms declined by 69-91% during the course of therapy, with physicians' global assessment of efficacy at good to very good in 84% of cases. Hautmann & Scheithe, *Z Phytotherapie* 2000 21.

Dog grass is useful in prostatitis or enlarged, benign enlargement of the prostate gland, making it one of man's best plant friends. It combines well with aspen poplar and nettle root for this purpose.

For uric-acid related gout, combine couch grass, pipsissewa and dandelion root for best results, and drink cool.

Acute inflammation, or interstitial cystitis is soothed. Dog grass combines best with birch leaf, goldenrod, uva ursi, and other cold antiseptic herbs for this purpose.

Chronically swollen lymphatic glands, with dry or suppurative eczema, respond to couch grass, combining well with mullein leaf, cleavers and plantain.

In all cases, it helps dilate renal capillaries and assists in the passage of more water, what a German herbalist would call an aquaretic.

It does not make the kidneys work harder but opens the tubules to increase water flow. In this manner, various sand and gravel particles can pass more easily.

Mannitol is believed to play a key role in the medicinal value of this plant. It helps to dilute the urine, helping to flush out sites of infection and inflammation, and thus reduce the chance of calculi formation.

Mannitol is soothing to the mucosa; combined with organic silica assists in healing and tissue repair, and saponins and vanillin that further increase urine flow.

Mannitol is a sugar absorbed whole from the gut, and excreted by the kidney tubules, causing extra water to be retained to maintain osmotic pressure at the same level.

Mannitol reduces kidney toxicity in patients treated with cisplatin. Williams RP Jr et al, *J Oncol Pharm Pract* 2016 June 27.

Organic silica helps strengthen the urinary tract and nervous systems.

Triticin is a polysaccharide obtained from the hydrolysis of inulin.

Studies have shown couch grass helps lower blood cholesterol, reduces arteriosclerosis, and relieves fatty liver. The root juice is very effective in treating jaundice and other liver complaints.

Skin problems like chronic eczema (wet or dry), muscular rheumatism, and high blood sugar all benefit from this invaluable plant. If not so common, it would certainly command higher respect.

An older recipe for recent late-onset diabetes is equal parts of couch grass, marshmallow root, uva ursi, poplar bark and pine needles.

Work by Maghrani et al, *Journal of Ethnopharmacology* 2004 90:2 found water extracts of the rhizome lower both body weight and lipid levels in lab-induced diabetic rats. More recent work in same journal 101:1-3 by Eddouks et al, found couch grass rhizomes lower blood sugar levels independent of insulin secretion.

Tincture of the rhizome identified anti-adhesive effects on uropathogenic *Escherichia coli* (*E. coli*). Cornsilk, nettle leaf and birch leaf also were effective. Rafsanjany N et al, *J Ethnopharm* 2013 145(2):591-7.

Recent work found a hexadecyl coumaric acid ester responsible for the inhibition of uropathogenic *E. coli*. Beydokhti SS et al, *Fitoterapia* 2016 117:22-27.

An animal study found a combination of couchgrass, horsetail, black elderberry and *Herniaria glabra* prevent deposit of calcium oxalate crystal formation. Crescenti A et al, *Arch Esp Urol* 2015 68(10):739-49.

The German Commission E recommends couch grass for various respiratory problems such as laryngitis, bronchitis, colds and coughs. It may be used to advantage in asthma due to calcium antagonism. Many herbs that are good for kidney stones are good for asthma and bronchitis, due to balancing the body's metabolism of electrolytes away from calcium ion influx, or calcium antagonist.

The large amount of mucilage helps stubborn cases of constipation.

French herbalists make use of the leaves, the bitter principles stimulating the liver and gallbladder function. A good springtime cleanse for chronic catarrh due to constipation and lymphatic congestion is to drink 1-2 cups of leaf decoction three times daily before meals for two weeks. Infusions of cough grass root have shown sedative effect in mice and activity against gram-positive bacteria.

Couch grass seed is used in Germany as a hot and moist pack applied to the stomach to soothe peptic ulcer pain.

Today, in Japan, the leaves are harvested and sold as a functional food or nutraceutical supplement like wheatgrass or barley grass.

Like rye, and other grasses, couch grass seed is susceptible to ergot infestation. Work by Munch found that ergot from quack grass was 1-3 times as potent in physiological activity as required to meet the minimum standards for ergot of rye.

Couch grass contains the flavonoid tricin. Kuwabara et al, *J Nat Prod* 2003 66:9 found tricin to possess potent anti-histamine activity.

Tricin targets tumor antiogenesis, and may be useful in preventing tumor growth and metastasis. Han JM et al, *Int J Oncol* 2016 49(4):1497-504.

HOMEOPATHY

Triticum-agropyrum repens is an excellent remedy for excessive irritability of the bladder; and relieving prostate inflammation.

Urination is frequent, painful and difficult. There may be gravel or mucous in the urine, with a constant desire to urinate.

One symptom that can help differentiate the use of couch grass from similar herbs is observing the patient always blowing their nose.

DOSE- Mother tincture or infusion. The mother tincture is made from the fresh roots.

ESSENTIAL OIL

The decaying roots of Couch grass release essential oils that help inhibit the growth of cultivated plants.

Couchgrass essential oil contains 61 known compounds, with carvacrol (11%), trans-anethole (6.8%), carvone (5.5%), thymol (4.3%), menthol (3.5%), methane, para-cymene and agropyrene (1-phenyl-2,4-hexadiyne) being of most interest.

The yield from the rhizomes is about 0.05%. Agropyrene has generated much interest for its antibiotic properties, and requires further investigation.

HYDROSOL

The distilled water of Dog Grass, or Couch grass, as some call it, cleanses the reins gallantly, and provokes urine, opens obstructions of the liver and spleen, and kills worms.   **CULPEPPER**

FLOWER ESSENCES

Dog grass is the flower essence for those who find themselves tenaciously holding on to old belief systems. Stubborn to a fault, they will twist their fear of change into a battle of egos. Then comes the lower back pains, and frequent urination that accompanies resistance to change.   **PRAIRIE DEVA**

I highly recommend Couch Grass essence when you need to slow down, take things easy, and recover because it swiftly reduces energy flowing through the valves… It is recommended to help you take steps forward and for alcoholics.   **OLIVE**

Quack grass essence helps in situations where one has behaved badly and others have had to "clean up".   **MIRIANA**

SPIRITUAL PROPERTIES

The feathery, weightless form of the Squirrel tail Grass flower brings with it a message of lightness of spirit and heart. No matter how much is going on in our lives, it is important that we remain lighthearted and playful.   **ECLARE**

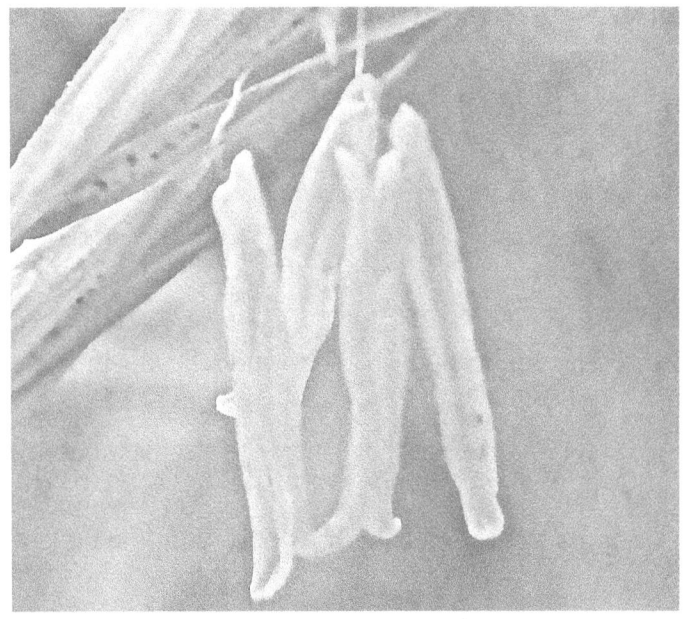

COUCHGRASS FLOWERS

PERSONALITY TRAITS

As every one knows, the quickest way to get rid of a bad dose of quack grass is to plow the land deep in the fall and sell the farm before spring... It is now generally believed that the reason Old MacDonald had a farm, and evidently hasn't got one now, is that the 'quack, quack here and a quack, quack there', referred not to ducks, as the writer of the immortal song appears to have believed, but to patches of quack grass.
COUNTRY GUIDE JULY 1931

RECIPES

INFUSION EXTRACT is made by simmering two ounces of dried rhizomes in quart of water and reducing to pint. Take in four divided doses over 24 hours.

DECOCTION- Take two teaspoons of the cut rhizome to one cup of water. Bring to a boil and simmer for ten minutes.

DOSE- One cup three times daily.

Another recipe is to combine equal parts couch grass rhizomes and parsley root in a decoction. Remove from heat and add a handful of rose petals. Steep, strain and drink lukewarm throughout day for kidney infection or stones.

TINCTURE- 3-6 ml up to three times daily. The fresh root tincture is made 1:2, the dried rhizome at 1:5, both at 40% alcohol.

FLUID EXTRACT- 10-30 drops up to five times daily. Made 1:1 at 25%.

JUICE- Crush the fresh rhizomes with a mortar and express through cheesecloth; or use a wheat grass juicer. Preserve with 25% vodka, or freeze in ice cube trays.

COFFEE- Combine equal parts roasted and ground couch grass roots, dandelion roots and barley grains. It is diuretic so better as morning drink than before bedtime.

CAUTION: German health authorities warn that extra fluids be taken with couch grass. They also advise not to use couch grass in cases of edema caused by heart or kidney insufficiency. The use of couch grass with bloody urine is not advised.

CROWBERRY
MOSSBERRY
***(Empetrum nigrum* L.)**
(***E. nigrum* ssp. *hermaphroditum*** [Lange ex Hagerup] Böcher) not accepted
PARTS USED- berries, leaves

I'm part wood nymph. I require mountains and warm, dense patches of moss to thrive.   **VERA FARMIGA**

The tundra glowed in the mellow sunshine with the colors of the ripe foliage of vaccinium, empetrum, arctostaphylos and dwarf birch: red, purple and yellow, in pure bright tones.   **JOHN MUIR**

Crowberry is named either for the black coloured fruit, or the crows that feed on them.

It also may come from the Old Norse **CRAKE**, meaning crow. Empetrum is from the Greek **EN PETROS**, meaning "on rock", in reference to its rocky, muskeg, arctic, and alpine preference. Nigrum means black. Mossberry alludes to its preference for mossy areas.

The subspecies hermaphroditum is a tetraploid. Taxonomists no longer recognize the binomial.

Crowberry is a low, evergreen shrub with blackish-purple fruit (drupes) that look a lot like juniper. The leaves are needle-like, the flowers dark purple and inconspicuous. The blossoms are early, sometimes seen breaking their way through frozen snow crusts.

Not only crows like the berries. They are also a favourite of bears and humans, as well. They are juicy, but have little taste, beyond their slightly acidic, bitter and astringent nature.

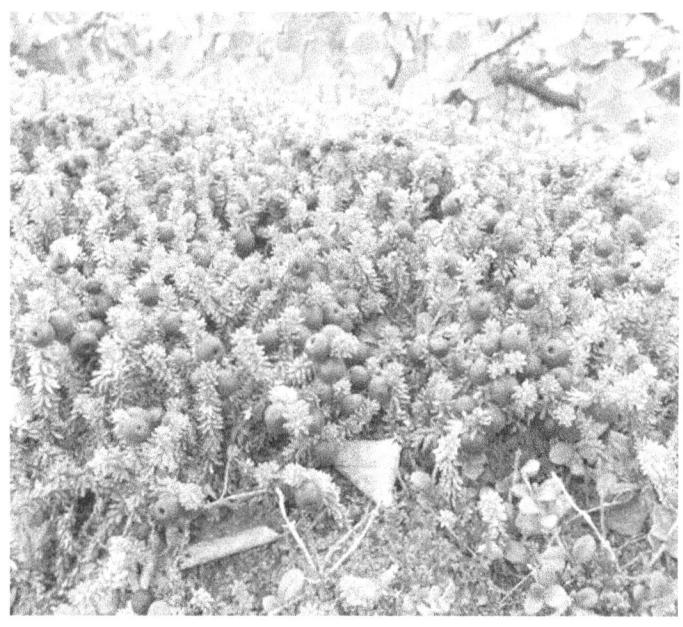

CROWBERRY

They can be eaten raw (not very good), or cooked into jams, jellies, pies, and wine in a similar manner to blueberries, or saskatoons. In Iceland, the berry is made into an alcoholic drink.

Tingaulik is a favorite dish of the Inupiat of Alaska. It is a blend of trout or tommy cod livers and crowberries. Other native people enjoy the berries with seal oil. Traditionally, the berries were mixed with the oil for winter use.

Janice Schofield, in her excellent Discovering Wild Plants, says that the Kobuk River Eskimos use crowberry juice in sore eyes caused by snow blindness. Decoctions of the root and branch bark have also been used for sore eyes and cataracts.

The berry juice is said to be good for relieving kidney trouble.

The Gwich'in of the Mackenzie delta mix crowberry or blackberry, known as **DINEECH'UH**, with bog cranberry to make **IT'SUH**, a dessert prepared with pounded dry fish.

The Inuit of Baffin Island call the berries **PAURNGAIT** because they are black like soot, or **PAUG**. They are said to be constipating if taken in excess, and fattening if mixed with seal fat. What isn't?

Traditionally, the berries have been used for cystitis, nephritis and urethritis, in Korea. Park SY et al, *J Food Biochem* 2012 36:675-682.

The branches with needles attached are used to clean gun barrels, or to make sleeping mattresses.

The Woods Cree boiled the branches into a tea to increase urination, or simply chewed on a branch for same effect.

The roots are boiled with other plants to treat coughs. The leafy branches are chewed, or decocted and mixed with grease and applied externally to treat fevers, especially in children.

The Cree name is **ASKIMINASIHT**, while the Chipewyan call the berry **TSANLHT'ETH**. The Slave call them watery berries, or **DZHIA TETHE**.

Pine bark and crowberry branches are often combined in the Yukon for relieving colds. The northern Dene brewed the branches/roots for mouth infections, and the branches as part of steams, similar to the way juniper branches are used further south.

The Dena'ina of Alaska call it berry black or mountain berry. The leaves and stems were boiled for diarrhea and stomach problems, while the berry juice was good for kidney trouble. The root was boiled and the eyes were washed with the strained tea after it has cooled.

The Bella Coola decocted the green leaves as a purgative, while the Haida decocted the branches, with other plants to treat tuberculosis. The latter also enjoyed the berries, but they believed that eating too many would cause hemorrhaging.

Recent work by Gordieu et al, *Phytother Res* 2009 Oct 13 found the plant active against *Mycobacterium tuberculosis*.

The branches can also be boiled and added to baths for relief of joint and rheumatic pains.

The explorer Samuel Hearne, wrote in his late 18th century journal that the berries around Churchill, Manitoba "are in some years so plentiful, that it is impossible to walk to many places without treading on thousands and millions of them". Natives of this region called them Grey Goose berries, **NISHCA MINNICK**, because the birds found them a favourite food.

In Iceland, the fruit juice is mixed with milk to make a popular beverage, while in northern Norway and Finland, crowberry wine is produced at the local level.

In Germany the name **RAUSCHBEERE**, or inebriating berry, is given to both bog bilberry and crowberry. Today, countries along the North Sea where the plant is common, the berry is considered to cause inebriation or hallucinations without narcotic effect.

When crowberry juice is mixed with black currant, the combination has a higher anti-oxidant level compared to red grape wines. It improves the color and intensity by about 35%.

In Kamchatka, a pudding is made from combining crowberry with Fritillaria bulbs. The berries are sweeter after the first frost. The trouble is that snow may soon follow, so pick anytime in late autumn.

In the Inner Hebrides, the herb was boiled in water and applied to the head and temples for insomnia. The leaf juice was applied to festering sores.

The roots are used in the Shetland Islands as a durable rope protected under thatch.

MEDICINAL

CONSTITUENTS- leaf branches- quercitin 3-arabinoside, quercitin 3-galactoside, quercitin 3-rutinoside, gossypetin 3-galactoside, methylated flavonol, three bibenzyls, alkanes, cycloalkanes, aliphatic esters, chalcone derivatives, empetroxepins A & B, and a 9,10-dihydrophenanthrene derivative. Phenolic content of leaves is higher than berries.
fruit- flavonols, flavan-3-ols, various anthocyanins including delphinidine-3-galactoside (50.3%), malvidine-3-galactoside (20.1%), of cyanidine-3-glucoside and arabinoside, delphinidine-3-arabinoside, quercitin, rutin, myricetin, naringin, morin, kaempferol. The total anthocyanin content is similar to bilberry. Compared to other berry crops, the content of petunidin-3-galactoside is relatively high.
Endophyte- peptide (En-AP1)

Crowberry leaves are used in Russian folk medicine to treat liver and kidney ailments, and exhibit diuretic, anti-spasmodic, anti-bacterial and anti-fungal activity. Crowberry extract is part of a homeopathic drug for the treatment of epilepsy in that country, under the name Empetrin. Ermilova EV et al, *Pharma Chem Journal* 2011 35:610-12.

Research conducted at the University of British Columbia found the branches of crowberry to exhibit strong anti-fungal and anti-bacterial activity against all nine and seven species respectively. McCutcheon et al, *Journal of Ethnopharm* 1992 37 and 1994 44(3):157-69. Of note is moderate activity against methicillin-resistant *Staphylococcus aureus*, MRSA, and inhibition of *Mycobacterium tuberculosis*.

Nearly 60 years ago, Bishop and MacDonald, *Can J Botany* 29, found alcohol ether and acetone extracts effective against *Staphylococcus aureus*.

Kahkonen et al, *Journal of Agricultural and Food Chemistry* 1999 47:10 researched the anti-oxidant activity of 92 various plant materials. Crowberry showed remarkable high antioxidant activity.

Willow bark, spruce needles, pine bark and birch phloem all rated high as well; as did red potato and beet root peels.

The leaves contain flavonoids that inhibit alpha glucosidase, and reduce inflammation. Hyun TK et al, *Saudi Journal Biol Sci* 2016 23:181-88.

Ethanol extracts inhibit angiogenesis, both in vitro and in vivo. This suggests potential use in the prevention and treatment of angiogenesis-dependent human disease. Bae HS et al, *Nat Prod Commun* 2016 11(14):503-6.

Work by Kananykhina and Pilipenko, *Chemistry of Natural Compounds* 2000 36:2 found Crowberry fruit is higher in anthocyanins than bilberry, black elderberry, black currant, cherry or high bush cranberry.

The fruit showed strong inhibition of *Bacillus cereus* in one study, and moderate in another. The latter study found inhibition of *S. aureus, S. epidermis* and *E. coli*. Liisa JN et al, *Nutr Cancer* 2006 54:18-32; Rauha JP et al, *Int J Food Microbiol* 2000 56:3-12.

A study of 51 plants in Russia, found crowberry and *Cassiope tetragona* displayed strong inhibition of *S. aureus* and moderate activity against *Candida albicans*. Paudel A et al, *Journal Antibiot* 2014 2014 67:663-67.

The juice showed inhibition of *Streptococcus pneumoniae* in work by Huttunen S et al, *Phytotherapy Research* 2011 25:122-7.

In addition, specific studies concerning *Mycobacterium tuberculosis and M. avium,* also showed the plant extracts very effective in inhibiting the growth of these pathogens. Gordien AY et al, *Phytotherapy Research* 2010 24:692-8. Juniper roots, aerial parts of heather and roots and stems of *Myrica gale* were also effective, in this Scottish study.

The organism associated with meningitis, *Neisseria meningitides*, has been found to be inhibited in adherence to tissue at rate of 63%. Tolvanen et al, *Phytother Res* 2011 25:6. Lingonberry was 57% effective in same study.

Study by Moss R and Parkinson JA, *British Journal of Nutrition* 1975 33(2):197-206 on crowberries reveal something interesting.

Although they were studying the feeding habits of ptarmigan; they found that crowberries provided sodium, but were short of nitrogen and phosphorus. Blueberries, which were often eaten together with crowberries by native people, were rich in nitrogen and phosphorus, but deficient in sodium.

Ptarmigan does not have a gall bladder in the wild, but when domesticated and fed a fatty diet, will create one. Interesting.

An extract of alpine blueberry and crowberry reduced lipid accumulation in mouse adipocytes. Kellogg J et al, *J Agric Food Chem* 2010 58:3884-3900.

Crowberries, used to fortify black currant juice, elicited slightly attenuated and sustained blood plasma glucose and insulin response, in healthy subjects. Törrönen R et al, *Journal of Functional Foods* 2012 4:746-56. This mixture of juices improved post-prandial glycemic response of a 36 gram dose of sucrose, due to increased bioavailability of polyphenols. *Handbook of Functional Beverages and Human Health*. Shaddi F & Alasavar C (Eds.) CRC Press Boca Raton, FL 2016 page 860.

Fifty-one healthy volunteers were given two grams of powdered fruit daily for four weeks. This resulted in a significant increase in total anti-oxidant status and SOD (super oxide dismutase). Levels of total cholesterol and LDL significantly decreased, as did levels of homocysteine, catalase and triglycerides. Park SY et al, *J Food Biochem* 2012 36:675-82.

The lipophilic fraction of crowberry possesses anti-convulsive activity. It is composed mainly of un-branched aliphatic esters, seven of which with equal alkyl substituents from C24 to C30 making up 90%. The remaining five esters (10%) differ by one methylene group. More information is available from Ermilova et al, *Chemistry of Natural Compounds* 1993-4.

Crowberry reduces intracellular cAMP and inhibits protein kinase A, in work by Moskaug et al, *Eur J Nutr* 2008 Oct 24.

Extracts of the fruit appear to protect skin against UVB and gamma radiation via various mechanisms. Kim KC et al, *Evid Based Complement Altern Med* 2013:983609; and *American Journal Chinese Medicine* 2011 39:161-70.

Crowberry is plentiful in the arctic regions, where twenty-four hour sunshine is present during summer months.

Crowberry juice and its anthocyanins are unstable and require low storage temperatures and removal of oxygen. Twelve weeks at 4 degrees Celsius is a good result.

All of this suggests crowberries are an important bioregional food that could represent a commercial opportunity for the functional food and nutraceutical industry.

An endophyte has been discovered that shows anti-bacterial activity against *S. aureus*. Tejesvi MV et al, *Appl Microbiol Biotechnol* 2016 100(21):9283-93.

Crowberries are used in homeopathic form as part of a compound called Empetrin, for the treatment of epilepsy in Russia. Ermilova EV et al, *Pharma Chem* 2011 35: 610-12.

SEED OIL

The seeds of Crowberry contain fatty acids, composed mainly of oleic, linoleic and alpha linolenic acids. There is no connection between seed size and oil content which ranges from 9-12%.

FLOWER ESSENCES

Crowberry flower essence stimulates awareness of cycles of light and darkness, internally and externally; enables us to hold these variations with respect and gratitude, rather than with attachment or aversion.   **ALASKA**

Crowberry essence is for youthful exuberance and enthusiasm.   **ROCKY MTN**

MYTHS AND LEGENDS

In Norway, the juice of the drunken berry or inebriating berry was used to make wine. King Sverre (12th century) attempted to use such native wines to drive out the foreign wine that German merchants were importing. In 1203, Bishop Jon taught the Icelanders how to make a wine like the one that King Sverre had taught him about. It was apparently this wine or another that was prepared from berries that was involved when the Norweigian and Icelandic clergy asked Pope Gregory IX for permission to use domestic wine during mass because true wine was not available in the country. Although the pope did not give his permission, tradition says that such inebriating berry wine was used in Iceland for Holy Communion.   **HARTWICH**

Crows were sacred to Athena, Greek goddess of Wisdom, but she did not permit crows to perch on the Acropolis in Athens because that was regarded as a bad omen. Apollo, however, seems not to have been well disposed towards crows. Corvus, or crow, was sent by Apollo to fetch a cup of water from a sacred spring. But Corvus wasted time eating figs on the way. When he realized how late he was, he caught Hydra, a water snake and claimed it had blocked the stream.

In his fury, Apollo cast the crow into the skies, along with Hydra and Crater the Cup. The constellation Corvus may be seen in the southern hemisphere close to Virgo. The crow cannot reach the water, and that is why he croaks.   **EASON**

Some forms of the Goddess which were seen, as crows are Coronis, Badb Catha, and the Danish Goddess Krake. This is a good choice for a croning name or for those who seek wisdom of age.   **MCFARLAND**

RECIPES

Crowberry liqueur- Take three pounds of berries, six cups sugar, three cups of water, and a 26 oz. of vodka.

On day one, blend the berries with little water and let stand.

One day two, add the vodka.

On day three, strain through cheesecloth.

In cooking pain combine sugar and water. Bring to boil for 5 minutes. Cool and add strained berry mixture. Let age 6 weeks or more.   **JANICE SCHOFIELD**

Jelly- Two cups water, and three cups of berries. Cook and strain. Then add one cup honey for each cup of juice, and use pectin as directed on box. Unusual, but interesting accent to wild venison.

ABOUT THE AUTHOR

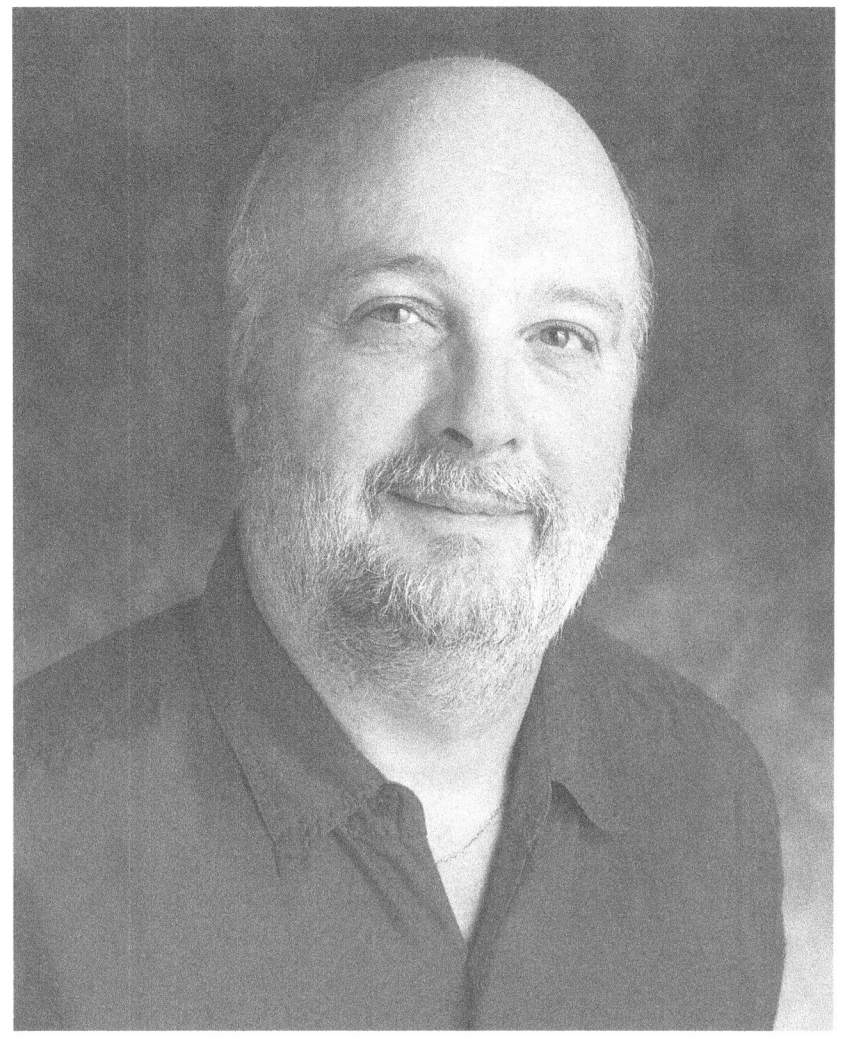

Robert Dale Rogers has been an herbalist for over forty-five years. He has a Bachelor of Science from the University of Alberta, where he is an assistant clinical professor in Family Medicine. He teaches plant medicine, including herbology and flower essences in the Earth Spirit Medicine Program at the Northern Star College of Mystical Studies in Edmonton, Alberta, Canada.

Robert is past chair of the Alberta Natural Health Agricultural Network and Community Health Council of Capital Health. He is a Fellow of the International College of Nutrition, past chair of the medicinal mushroom committee of the North American Mycological Association and on the editorial board of the International Journal of Medicinal Mushrooms. He writes occasional article for Fungi magazine.

Robert co-hosts The Alberta Herb Gathering held every second year (www.albertaherbgathering.com)

He lives on Millcreek Ravine in Edmonton with his beautiful and talented wife, Laurie Szott–Rogers and out of control cat Ceres.

You can email him at scents@telusplanet.net
or visit
www.selfhealdistributing.com

BIBLIOGRAPHY

Abbe, Elfriede, *The Fern Herbal,* Cornell University Press, Ithaca, 1981

Acorn, J. Bugs of Alberta, Lone Pine Publishing, Edmonton, AB, 2000.

Adams, J. *Les Plantes Medicinales.* Bulletin 23, Agriculture Canada. 1916

Adams, Jean. *Insect Potpourri, Adventures in Entomology.* Sandhill Crane Press, FL. 1992

Aggarwal, Bharat. Healing Spices. Sterling Pub. New York 2011.

Albert-Puleo, Michael. *Economic Botany, 32, Jan-Mar, 1978.*

Allaby, Michael. *Temperate Forests.* Facts on File. New York. 1999.

Allen, D & Hatfield, G. *Medicinal Plants in Folk Tradition.* Timber Press, Portland. 2004

Allen,E, Morrison,D, &Wallis,G. *Common Tree Diseases of B.C. Canada Forest Service,* '96

Allende, Isabel. *Aphrodite- A Memoir of the Senses.* Harper Flamingo. New York. 1998.

Alstat, Ed. *Electic Dispensatory of Botanical Therapeutics.* Ecl Med. Oregon. 1989.

Anderson, Anne, *Some Native Herbal Remedies,* Pub 8A, Devonian Botanical Gardens 1980
_____*Plants in Cree.* Duval House Pub. Edmonton AB 2000.

Anderson, C.&Tischer,T. *Poinsettias, the December Flower,* Waters Edge Press, CA, 1997

Andoh, Anthony. *The Science & Romance of Selected Herbs used in Medicine and Religious Ceremony.* North Scale Institute. San Francisco. 1986.

Andre, Alestine & Fehr, Alan. *Gwich'in Ethnobotany.* Gwich'in Social and Cultural Institute, Box 46, Tsiigehtchie, NWT, X0E 0B0, fax 1867-953-3820.

Andrews, Tamra. Nectar and Ambrosia. ABC-CLIO Box 1911 Santa Barbara CA. 2000.

Andrews, Ted. *Animal Speak- The Spiritual and Magical Powers,* Llewellyn. Minn. 1996.
_____*Animal Wise,* DragonHawk, Jackson, TN, 1999.

Antol, Marie. *The Incredible Secrets of Mustard.* Avery Pub. New York. 1999.

Aronson J K Ed. Meyler's Side Effects of Herbal Medicines. Elsevier Amsterdam. 2009.

Arrowsmith, Nancy. Essential Herbal Wisdom. Llewellyn Pub. Woodbury, Minn. 2009.

Arsdall, Anne Van. *Medieval Herbal Remedies.* Routledge, New York. 2002.

Arvigo & Balick, *Rainforest Remedies,* Lotus Press, Twin Lakes, WI. 1993

Arvigo & Epstein. *Rainforest Home Remedies,* Harper SanFrancisco, 2001.

Assiniwi, Bernard. *La Medecine des Indiens d' Amerique,* Guerin Literature, 1988

Atal C.K. & Kapur B. *Cultivation and Utilization of Medicinal Plants,* Jammu-Tawi, 1982

Attenborough, David. *The Private Life of Plants.* Princeton U Press. Princeton NJ 1995.

Ausubel, K. *Seeds of Change The Living Treasure.* HarperSanFrancisco, 1994.

Aversano, Laura. *The Divine Nature of Plants.* Swan•Raven & Co. Columbus, NC, 2002.

Ayensu, Edward,S. *Medicinal Plants of the West Indies,* Reference Publications, 1981

Baïracli Levy, Juliette *Herbal Handbook for Farm and Stable,* Faber&Faber, London, 1952

Baker, Phil. The Dedalus Book of Absinthe. Dedalus 2001.

Barl, Branka et al, *Saskatchewan Herb Database,* U. of Sask. Saskatoon, 1996.

Barlow, Max. *From the Shepherd's Purse.* 1990

Barnes J, Anderson L, &Phillipson J. *Herbal Medicines, A guide for healthcare professionals.* Pharmaceutical Press, London, 2002.

Barnett, Robert A. *Tonics,* Harper Collins, New York, N.Y. 1997

Bartram, Thomas. *Bartram's Encyl. of Herbal Medicine,* Robinson Pub. London, 1998.

Bascom, Angella. *Incorporating Herbal Medicine into Clinical Practice.* F. Davis Co. 2002

Beals, Katherine, M. *Flower Lore and Legend,* Henry Holt, 1917

Beers, Susan-Jane. *Jamu The ancient Indonesian Art of Herbal Healing,* Periplus, 2001.

Belcourt, Christi. Medicines to Help Us. Gabriel Dumont Instit. Saskatoon, SK 2007.

Béliveau, R & Gingras,D. *Foods That Fight Cancer.* McClelland & Stewart Toronto. 2006.

Belsinger S & Dille C. *Cooking with Herbs.* CBI- Van Nostrand Reinhold, N.Y. 1984.

Benjamin, D.R. *Mushrooms: Poisons and Panaceas.* WH Freeman, San Francisco, 1995.

Bennet, Doug & Tiner, Tim. *Up North.* Reed Books Canada. Markham, Ont. 1993.

_____*Up North Again.* McClelland and Stewart. Toronto, 1997.

Bennet, J & Rowley S. *Uqalurait An Oral History of Nunavut.* McGill Queens, Mont. 2004

Benyus, Janine. *Biomimicry Innovation Inspired by Nature.* William Morrow. 1997.

Berenbaum,May R. *Buzzwords, A Scientists Muses on Sex, Bugs and Rock N Roll,* Joseph Henry Press, Washington, D.C. 2000.

_____*Bugs in the System.* Helix Books, Addison-Wesley Pub. 1995.

Beresford-Kroeger, Diana. The Global Forest. Viking Penguin. 2010.

_____Arboretum Borealis. U Michigan Press. 2010.

Berliocchi,Luigi. *The Orchid in Lore and Legend.* Timber Press, Portland Oregon, 2000.

Berlund B & Bolsby C. *The Edible Wild* Pagurian Press, Toronto, Ont. 1971.

Berkowsky, Bruce. *Mount Julius Flower Remedies. Mt. Vernon Washington, 1986*

Bermejo, J & Leon,J. *Neglected Crops-1492 ...* FAO Series 26, United Nations, Rome, 1994.

Bernhardt, P. *The Rose's Kiss, A Natural History of Flowers* . Island Press, Covelo CA 1999

Bianchi, Ivo. *Geriatrics and Homotoxicology.* Aurelia-Verlag GmbH, Baden Baden, 1994.

Bianchini, F. *The Complete Book of Health Plants.* Crescent Books, New York, 1975.

Biship, Carol. *The Book of Home Remedies &Herbal Cures,* Jonathan-James, Toronto, 1979.

Bisset, Norman G. *Herbal Drugs and Phytopharmaceuticals.* 2nd Ed. CRC Press, 2001.

Blackburn, Thomas. *December's Child: A Book of Chumash Oral Narratives* , U of California Press, Berkeley, 1975.

Blanchan, Neltje. *Nature's Garden.* Doubleday, Page&Co. New York, 1900.

Bland, John. *Forests of Liliput.* Prentice Hall, Englewood Cliffs, New Jersey, 1971.

Bliss, Anne. *Rocky Mountain Dye Plants.* Juniper House, Boulder, Colorado, 1976

Blouin, Glen. *Weeds of the Woods.* Goose Lane, Fredericton, New Brunswick 1992.

_____*An Eclectic Guide to Trees, east of the Rockies.* Boston Mills, 2001.

Boas, F. *Ethnology of the Kwakiutl.* Bureau of Am. Ethnology, 35th annual report, 1921.

Boericke, Wm. *Materia Medica with Repetory.* B. Jain Publishers. 1976

Boik, John. *Natural Compunds in Cancer Therapy.* Oregon Med Press, Princeton,Minn 2001

Boland, Bridget. *Gardener's Magic &Other Old Wives' Lore.* The Bodley Head, London, 77.

Bolton, Brett L. *The Secret Powers of Plants.* Berkley Pub Co. New York. 1974.

Bolton, J.L. *Alfalfa, Botany, Cultivation &Utilization.* Interscience Pub, New York, 1962.

Bone, Kerry. *A Clinical Guide to Blending Liquid Herbs.* Churchill Livingstone. 2003

Borrel, Marie. *Healing Plants.* Cassell & Co. Wellington House, London. 2001.

Bouchardon, Patrice. *The Healing Energies of Trees.* Journey Editions, Boston, 1999.

Bossenmaier, Eugene. *Mushrooms of the Boreal Forest.* U. of Saskatchewan Press, 1997

Boulos, Loutfy. *Medicinal Plants of North Africa,* Reference Pub. Algonac, Mich. 1983

Bowles, E. Joy. *The Chemistry of Aromatherapeutic Oils.* Allen & Unwin, Crow's Nest, Australia, 2003.

Bowman, Daria. *Hydrangeas.* Friedman/Fairfax Pub. New York. 1999.

Bradley, Peter. British Herbal Compendium Vol 2 Brit Herb Med Assoc. Bournemouth 2006.

Brahmachari, Goutam Ed. Natural Products, Alpha Sci Int Ltd. Oxford UK 2009.

Brandeis, Gayle. *Fruitflesh.* Harper Collins, San Francisco. 2002.

Brennan, M. *Complete Holistic Care & Healing for Horses*. Trafalgar Sq. Pub. VT. 2001.

Bringhurst, Robert. *A Story as Sharp as a Knife*. Douglas&McIntyre Vancouver, 1999.

Brinker, Francis N.D. *Herb Contraindications and Drug Interactions*. Third Edition
Eclectic Medical Publications, Sandy, Oregon, 2001

_____ *The Toxicology of Botanical Medicines*, revised 2nd. Eclectic Med, Oregon, 1996.

_____ *Eclectic Dispensatory of Botanical Therapeutics*, Vol 2, Ecl. Med . Oregon, 1995.

Brodo, Irwin & Sharnoff. *Lichens of North America*. Yale University Press, 2001.

Brown, Deni. *Encyclopedia of Herbs and Their Uses*. Reader's Digest Press, Que. 1995.

Bruneton, J *Pharmacognosy, Phtyochemistry, Medicinal Plants,* Lavoisier Pub. Paris, 1995

_____ *Toxic Plants Dangerous to Humans and Animals*. Editions TEC&Doc, Paris, '99.

Brunschwig, Hieronymus. *Book of Distillation*. Johnson Reprint Co No. 79. New York, 1971.

Brynaherb Essences 29, Kells Meend Berry Hill, Gloucestershire GL16 7AD

Bubar, Carol et al. *Weeds of the Prairies*. Alberta Agriculture Pub. Edmonton, 2000.

Buchanan, Carol. *Brothers Crow, Sister Corn*. Ten Speed Press, Berkeley, 1997.

Buckle, Jane. *Clinical Aromatherapy. 2nd ed.* Churchill Livingstone, Toronto, 2003.

Buhner, Stephen H. *Sacred and Herbal Healing Beers,* Siris Books, Boulder, Co, 1998

_____ *Sacred Plant Medicine*. Robert Rinehart, Boulder, Co. 1996.

_____ Herbal Antibiotics. Storey Books, Vermont, 1999.

_____ *The Lost Language of Plants*. Chelsea Green Pub. White River, Vt. 2002

_____ Secret Teachings of Plants. Bear & Co. Rochester, Vt. 2004.

_____ The Natural Testosterone Plan. Healing Arts Press, Rochester VT. 2007

Burbridge, Joan. *Wildflowers of the Southern Interior of B.C.* U. of B.C. Press, 1989.

Burger, W. Flowers- *How they changed the world. Prometheus Books.* Amherst NY 2006.

Burgess, Isla. *Weeds Heal.* Viriditas Pub Group. Cambridge NZ 1998.

Burlando, Bruno et al, Herbal Principles in Cosmetics. CRC Press Boca Raton 2010.

Caius, Rev. Fr. Jean F., *The Medicinal and Poisonous Plants of India,* Scientific Pub, 1986.

Cameron, Elizabeth. *A Floral ABC.* John Wiley and Sons. Toronto. 1980.

Carpenter D. Snr Pub. *Nursing Herbal Medicine Handbook,* Springhouse Corp. 2001.

Carpinella, Maria et al. Novel Therapeutic Agents from Plants. Sci Pub. Enfield NJ 2009.

Carr, Emily. *Wild Flowers.* Royal BC Museum, Victoria, B.C, 2006

Carroll, Roisin. *The Crane Bag Celtic Tree Ogam Oils* , Feasibility Pub. Dublin

Carter, Bernard F. *The Floral Birthday Book.* Bloomsbury Books, London. 1990.

Casselman, Bill. *Canadian Garden Words.* Little, Brown & Co. Toronto, 1997.

Castleman, Michael. *The Healing Herbs.* Bantam Books. 1995.

Castro, Miranda. *The Complete Homeopathy Handbook.* MacMillan, 1990

Catty, Suzanne. *Hydrosols the next Aromatherapy,* Healing Arts Press, Vermont, 2001.

Cavers, Paul ed, *The* Biology *of Canadian Weeds* 62-83,Ag Institute of Canada, Ottawa, 1995

_____ 84-102 Ag Inst. of Canada, Ottawa, 2000.

_____ 103-129 Ag Inst. of Canada, Ottawa 2005

Ceres. *Herbal Teas for Health and Healing.* Healing Arts Press, Rochester, Vermont, 1984.

Chan, K, and Cheung L. *Interactions between Chincese Herbal Medicinal Products and Orthodox Drugs.*
        Harwood Academic Publishers, Canada, 2000.

Chandler, F. *Herbs-Everyday Reference for Health Professionals,* Can. Pharm Assoc. 2000

Chang & But. *Pharmacology &Applications of Chinese Materia Medica,* World Scientific, 86

Chang Chao-liang et al, *Vegetables as Medicine,* Pelanduk Pub, Malaysia, 1999.

Chappell, P. Emotional Healing with Homeopathy. North Atlantic Books. Berkeley, 2003.

Charissa's Cauldron. www.charissacauldron.com

Chase, Pamela & Pawlik, J. *Newcastle Trees for Healing*, Newcastle Pub. Van Nuys,1991

Chatroux, Sylvia. *Botanica Poetica*. Poetica Press 2004 1-877-POETICA.

_____*Materica Poetica*. Poetica Press 1998.

Chen, John K & Chen, Tina T. Chinese Medical Herbology & Pharmacology. Art of Medicine Press, City of Industry, CA 2004.

Chevalllier, Andrew. *The Encyclopedia of Medicinal Plants*. Reader's Digest, 1996.

Chishti, Hakim. *The Traditional Healer*, Healing Arts Press, Vermont,1988.

Christchurch Flower Essences. www.christchurchfloweressences.com

Clark, Ella E. *Indian Legends of Canada*. McClelland & Stewart. Toronto, 1960.

Coats, Peter. *Flowers in History*. Weidenfeld and Nicolson, London. 1970.

Coffey, Timothy.*The History and Folklore of North American Wildflowers,* Houghton-Mifflin, 1993.

Cohen, Kenneth. *Honoring the Medicine*. Random House, Toronto. 2003.

Conrad, Chris, *Hemp for Health*, Healing Arts Press, Rochester, Vermont, 1997.

Cook, Wm.H. *The Physio-Medical Dispensatory*. 1869. Reprinted by Eclectic Medical Publications, Portland, Oregon, 1985.

_____A compendium of the new Materia medica together with additional descriptions of some old remedies. Wm. Cook Publisher, Chicago, 1896.

Cooper, J.C. *Dictionary of Symbolic & Mythological Animals,* Thorsons, London, 1992.

Cormack, R.G.H. *Wild Flowers of Alberta*. Hurtig Publishers, 1977

Coupland, Francois. *The Encyclopedia of Edible Plants of N. America*. Keats Pub. 1998.

Cousin, Pierre J. *Eat Well, Be Well*. Thorsons, London. 2001.

Cowan, Eliot. *Plant Spirit Medicine*. Swan Raven & Co. Box 726 Newberg, Oregon, 1995.

Cowan, Thomas. The Fourfold Path to Healing. New Trends Pub. Washington DC 2007.

Crane, Eva. *Honey- A Comprhensive Survey* , Heinemann Pub. London 1975.

Craydon D. & Bellows W. Floral Acupuncture. The Crossing Press Berkeley CA 2005.

Creekmore, H. *Daffodils are Dangerous*. Walker and Co. New York. 1966.

Crow, Tis Mal. *Native Plants, Native Healing*. Native Voices Book Pub. Box 99 Summertown, Tennessee, 2001 1-888-260-8458.

Crowell, Robert L. *The Lore & Legends of Flowers*. Thomas Crowell, New York, 1982.

Crowfoot & Baldensperger. *From Cedar to Hyssop*. Sheldon Press, London, 1932.

Cruden, Loren. Medicine Grove. Destiny Books. Inner Traditions Vermont. 1997.

Cummings, S. and Ullman, Dana. *Everyone's Guide to Homeopathic Medicines,* St. Martins

Cupp, Melanie. *Toxicology and Clinical Pharmacology of Herbal Products*. Humana P. 1999

Curtin, LSM. *Healing Herbs of the Upper Rio Grande*. SouthWest Museum, Los Angeles 1965

Cutler & Cutler Eds. Biologically Active Natural Products: Agrochemicals, CRC Press 1999.

Dai Yin-fang&Liu Cheng-jun. *Fruit As Medicine*. Rams Skull Press, Kuranda, Aust. 1987

Dalton, David. Stars of the Meadow. Lindisfarne Books. Great Barrington, Mass. 2006.

D'Amelio Sr. Frank. *Botanicals A Phytocosmetic Desk Reference* CRC Press, Boca Raton, 99

Darby,Wm et al. *Food: The Gift of Osiris,* Vol 1. Academic Press, San Francisco, 1977

Darwin, Tess. The Scots Herbal, the Plant Lore of Scotland. Birlinn Ltd, Edinburgh 2008

Davidow, Joie. *Infusions of Healing, A Treasury of Mexican-American Herbal Remedies,* Fireside Books, New York, 1999.

Davis,W. *El Gringo, New Mexico and Her People*. Harpers, New York, 1857.

Demargaux, N. *Phytotherapy*. Herbal Health Publishers Ltd. 1989

De Bairacli Levy, Juliette. *Herbal Handbook for Farm and Stable,* Faber and Faber 1952

Deer Lame, J & Erdoes, R. *Lame Deer Seeker of Visions.* Washington Sq Press, 1976.

Deer, Thea Summer. Wisdom of the Plant Devas. Bear&Company Vermont 2011.

Delta Gardens Flower Essences. www.deltagardens.com

De Smet et al. *Adverse Effects of Herbal Drugs.* Springer-Verlag, Berlin. 1997.

Der Marderosian, Ara & Liberti L. *Natural Product Medicine,* George Stickley Co, Philadel.

DeRios, Marlene D. *Hallucinogens: Cross Cultural Perspectives.* U. New Mexico Press, 1984

DeSmet, P. et al. *Adverse Effects of Herbal Drugs. vol 2* Springer-Verlag

Devi, Lila. The Essential Flower Essence Handbook. Crystal Clarity Pub. Nevada City 2007.

Dewey, Laurel. *Plant Power- revised.* Safe Goods/New Century Pub, Markham Ont, 2001.

Dewick, Paul M. *Medicinal Natural Products.*3rd Ed John Wiley and Sons, West Sussex, 2009.

Diederichsen, Axel. *Coriander.* Int. Plant Genetic Resources Institute. Rome, Italy. 1996.

Dixon, Bernard.*Power Unseen, How Microbes Rule the World.* W.H. Freeman, Oxford, 1994

Dow, Elaine. *Simples and Worts.* Historical Presentations, Topsfield, MA. 1982.

Duke, James. *Handbook of Medicinal Herbs.* CRC Press, Boca Raton, Florida, 1985

_____*Handbook of Edible Weeds.* CRC Press. 1992

_____*The Green Pharmacy,* Rodale Press, Emmaus, Pennsylvania, 1997.

_____*The Green Pharmacy Herbal Handbook,* Rodale Press, 2000.

_____*Anti-aging Prescriptions.* Rodale Press. 2001.

Dumas, Anne. Book of Plants and Symbols. English Ed. Octopus Pub. London 2004.

Dymock,Wm. *Pharmacographia Indica, Vol 2*, Kegan Paul, Trench, Trubner and Co. 1891

Earle, Liz. *Vital Oils*, Ebury Press, London, 1991.

Eason, Cassandra. Fabulous Creatures, Mythical Monsters… Greenwood Press, CT. 2008.

Eastman, John. *The Book of Swamp and Bog...* Stackpole Books, Mechanicsburg, Penn, 1995

Ebadi, M. *Pharmacodynamic Basis of Herbal Medicine,* CRC Press, Boca Raton. 2002.

Eckey, E.W. *Vegetable Fats and Oils,* Rheingold Publishing Co, New York, 1954.

Eclare, Melanie. *Flower Spirit Cards.* Quadrille Publishing, London, England, 2004.

Edwards, Lawrence. *The Vortex of Life.* Floris Books. Edinburgh 2nd Ed. 2006.

Eisner T et al. *Secret Weapons.* Belknap Press, Harvard U Press. Cambridge & London 2005.

Ellingwood F. *American Materia Medica,* Eclectic Med. Pub. Portand, Oregon, reprint, 1983

Elliot, Douglas B. *Roots* . Chatham Press, Old Greenwich Conneticut.

Ellis, Hattie. *Sweetness & Light.* Hodder and Stoughton, London, 2004.

Erdoes & Ortiz. *American Indian Myths and Legends,* Pantethon Books, New York, 1984.

Erichsen-Brown,Charlotte. *Use of Plants for the Past 500 Years,* Breezy Creeks Press, 1979

_____*Medicinal and Other Uses of North American Plants,* General Pub, 1979.

Erickson, David, Wai Kit Nip *Food uses of whole oil and protein seeds,* Amer. Oil Chemists Society, 1989.

Eskin, N. A. Michael, Tamir, S. *Dictionary of Nutraceuticals and Functional Foods.* CRC Press, 2006.

Etkin, Nina. Edible Medicines, An Ethnopharmacology of Food. U Arizona Press. 2006.

Evans, W.C. *Trease and Evans' Pharmacognosy.* WB Saunders Co. Toronto, 2000.

Fang Jing Pei, Dr. *Natural Remedies from the Chinese Cupboard.* Weatherhill, 1998.

Farmer-Knowles,Helen. *The Healing Garden.* Sterling Publishing, New York, 1998.

Fielder, Mildred. *Plant Medicne and Folklore,* Winchester Press, New York, 1975.

Felter, Harvery and Lloyd, John. *King's American Dispensatory* . 1898. Reprinted by Eclectic Medical Publications, Portland Oregon, 1983.

Ferguson, Gary. *Spirits of the Wild.* Clarkson Potter/Random New York, 1996.

Fernie, W.T. Dr. *Old Fashioned Herbal Remedies.* Coles Pub. Toronto, 1980. Reprint.

Fingerman M. et al editors. *Bioremediation of Aquatic and Terresrial Ecosytems.* Sci Pub. Enfield NH 2005.

Fischer-Rizzi, S. *Complete Aromatherapy Handbook,* Sterling Pub. New York. 1990.

_____*The Complete Incense Book,* Sterling Pub. New York. 1998.

_____*Medicine of the Earth,* Rudra Press, Portland, Oregon, 1996

Florey, H.W. et al. Antibiotics vol 1. Oxford University Press. London 1949.

Ford, Gillian. *Plant Names Explained.* Friends of the Devonian Botanic Garden, #16, 1984

Foster, Steven. *Herbal Renaissance,* Gibbs Smith Pub. Salt Lake City

_____& Yue Chongxi. *Herbal Emissaries,* Healing Arts Press, Vermont, 1992

_____& Johnson R. *Desk Reference to Nature's Medicine.* Nat Geographic. Washington, D.C.

Fox, H. M. Gardening with Herbs. Macmillan Pub. New York 1933.

Freeman, D. & Mongeau D. Nettles and More…Vol One. Self published 2nd printing 2009.

Freeman, Lyn. *Mosby's Complementary & Alternative Medicine.*3rd Ed. Mosby Elsevier 2009

Friedman, Sara Ann, *Celebrating the Wild Mushroom,* Dodd, Mead & Co. New York, 1986

Friend, Tim. The Third Domain: the Untold Story of Archaea. Joseph Henry Press. 2007.

Fugh-Berman, Adriane. *The 5-minute Herb &Dietary Supplement Consult.* Lippincott Williams &Wilkins, Philadelphia 2003.

Gaertner, Erika. *Reap without Sowing.* General Store Publishing, Burnstown, Ont. 1995

Galun, Margalith. *Handbook of Lichenology,* CRC Press, 1988

Garran, Thomas. *Western herbs according to Traditional Chinese Medicine.* Healing Arts Press. 2008.

Garrett, J.T. *The Cherokee Herbal.* Bear&Company, Rochester, Vermont. 2003.

Genders, Roy. *Floral Scents of the World* . St. Martin's Press, London, 1977

Geuter, *Herbs in Nutrition.* Bio-Dynamic Agricultural Assoc. London. 1978.

Gildemeister, E. *The Volatile Oils.* John Wiley and Sons, New York. 1916

Gifford, Jane. The Wisdom of Trees. Sterling Pub. New York 2000.

Gill S. & Sullivan I. *Dictionary of Native American Mythology.* Oxford U Press 1992.

Gilmore, M.R. Uses of Plants by Indians of the Missouri river region. 33rd Annual Report Bureau American Ethnology, 1911-12, Washington D.C. 1919.

Gladstar R & Hirsch P. *Planting the Future.* Healing Arts Press, Rochester, Vt. 2000.

Gladstar, Rosemary. *Family Herbal.* Storey Books, North Adams, Mass. 2001.

Glasby, J.S. *Dictionary of Plants Containing Secondary Metabolites,* Taylor & Francis, London 1991.

Godfrey, A & Saunders P. Principles and Practices of Naturopathic Botanical Medicine, Vol 1, CCNM Press Toronto ON 2010.

Goodrick-Clarke, Clare. Alchemical Medicine for the 21st Century. Healing Arts Press. 2010.

Gordon, David G. *The Compleat Cockroach.* Ten Speed Press, Berkeley, CA. 1996.

Gordon, Lesley. The Mystery and Magic of Trees & Flowers. Grange Books. London 1993.

Gottesfeld, Leslie M. Johnson. *Plants, Land and People, A Study of Wet'suwet'en Ethnobotany.*U of A, 1993.

Grae, Ida. *Nature's Colors, Dyes From Plants.* Macmillan Pub. New York, 1974.

Graham, Frances K. *Plant lore of an Alaskan Island.* Alaska Northwest Pub. 1985

Grandparents of the Forest flower essences. www.grandparentsoftheforest.com

Grange, Michael etal, *Handbook of Plants with Pest Control Properties,* J. Wiley& Son 1988

Gray, Bev. The Boreal Herbal. Wild Food & Medicine Plants of the North. Aroma Borealis Press 2011

Green, James. *The Male Herbal* . Crossing Press, Freedom, California, 1991.

_____*The Herbal Medicine-Maker's Handbook.* Crossing Press, Freedom CA 2000

Green, Jonathan. *Consuming Passions.* Sphere Books, London, 1985.

Grey Wolf. *Earth Signs,* Raincoast Books, Vancouver, B.C. 1998.

Grieve, M. *A Modern Herbal.* Jonathan Cape. 1931

Griffiths, Deirdre. *Elk Island National Park.* U. of Alberta Press, 1979.

Grigson, Geoffrey. *A Herbal of All Sorts*. Phoenix House, London

Grimaud, Baptiste,Paul. *TAROT DES FLEURS*, France Cartes, France 1989

Grimshaw, John. *The Gardener's Atlas*. Firefly Books, Willowdale, Ont. 2002.

Grohmann,Gerbert. *The Plant Vol 2,* Bio-Dynamic Farming & Gardening Assoc. 1989.

Gruenwald et al, Ed. PDR for Herbal Medicines. 4th Ed. Thomson Pub. 2007.

Guillet, Alma. *Make Friends of Trees and Shrubs.* Doubleday & Co. New York, 1962.

Gumbel, Dietrich. *Principles of Holistic Skin Therapy with Herb Essences.* Haug Pub. Heidelberg 1986.

Gurudas. *The Spiritual Properties of Herbs* , Cassandra Press, 1988

_____*Flower Essences and Vibrational Healing,* Cassandra Press, 1983

Hageneder, Fred. The Spirit of Trees. Continuum. NY and London. 2005.

Hale, Mason. *The Biology of Lichens.* Edward Arnold Pub. London, 1967.

Hall, Dorothy. *Creating Your Herbal Profile* , Keats, 1988

Hallworth, B & Chinnappa CC. *Plants of the Kananaskis Country* U of A Press 1997.

Hanchuk, Rena. *The Word and Wax.* Can Inst of Ukrainian Studies Press, Edmonton, 1999.

Hanson, J, & Morrison D. *Of Kinkajous, Capybaras, Horned Beetles...*Harper Collins, NY '91

Harbourne & Baxter. *The Handbook of Natural Flavonoids Vol 1&2.* John Wiley & Sons, 1999

_____*Phytochemical Dictionary.* Taylor & Francis 1993.

Harrington, Geri. *Growing Your Own Chinese Vegetables,* MacMillan, N.Y. 1978.

Harrington, H.D. *Edible Native Plants of the Rocky Mtns.* U. of New Mexico Press, 1967.

Harris, Ben C. *Eat the Weeds,* Keats Pub. New Cannan, Conneticut 1973.

_____*Make Use of Your Garden Plants.* General Pub. New York. 1978.

Harris, Marjorie. *Botanica North America.* Harper Collins, New York, 2003.

Harrison, Nora. *Flower Remedy Rhymes* , self published, England, 1990.

Hart, Jeff. *Montana Native Plants and Early Peoples,* Montana Historical Society Press. '92

_____The Ethnobotany of the Northern Cheyenne Indians of Montana. Journal of Ethnopharmacology 1981 4.

Hartung, Tammi. *Growing 101 Herbs That Heal.* Storey Books, Pownal, Vt. 2000.

Hartwell, Jonathan, *Plants Used Against Cancer.* Quarterman Pub. 1982

Hartzell, Jr. H. *The Yew Tree A Thousand Whispers.* Hulogosi, Box 1188, Eugene, OR 1991.

Harvey, C & Cochrane A. *The Healing Spirit of Plants.* Godsfield Press, Sterling Pr N.Y. 1999

Harvey Clare. The New Encyclopedia of Flower Remedies. Watkins Pub. London 2007.

Hatfield, Gabrielle. *Encyclopedia of Folk Medicine.* ABC CLIO Santa Barbara. 2004.

Haughton, Claire. *Green Immigrants.* Harcourt Brace Jovanovich. New York and London.

Hawksworth, Frank & Wiens, D. Dwarf Mistletoes, Ag Handbook 709, USDA, Wash, DC, '96

Health Canada, Native Foods and Nutrition. Medical Services Branch, 1995.

Heatherington, M. and Steck,W. *Natural Chemicals from Northern Prairie Plants,* Ag West Biotech Publishers, Saskatoon, Canada. 1997.

Heilmeyer, Marina. The Language of Flowers-Symbols & Myths. Prestel Pub. Munich 2001.

Heinerman, John. *Encyclopedia of Nuts, Berries and Seeds,* Parker Publishing, 1995.

_____*Encyclopedia of Healing Herbs & Spices.* Parker Pub. N.Y. 1996.

Heinrich, Bernd. *Winter World The Ingenuity of animal survival.* HarperCollins. NY 2003.

Heinrich, Clark. *Magic Mushrooms in Religion and Alchemy.* Park St. Press, VT. 2002.

Heiser, Charles B. Jr. *Of Plants and People.* U. of Oklahoma Press, 1985.

Hellson, John C, *Ethnobotany of the Blackfoot Indians* No. 19, National Museums of Canada, Ottawa 1974.

Henderson, Robert K. *The Neighborhood Forager.* Key Porter Books, Toronto, 2000.

Hendrickson, Robert. *Encycl of Word and Phrase Origins.* Facts on File Inc. NewYork, 1997.

Hendry, G. *Natural Food Colorants* , Blackie and Son, Glasgow Scotland, 1992.

Henry, J. David. *Canada's Boreal Forest*. Smithsonian Institute. 2002.

Hilarion. *Wildflowers, Their Occult Gifts*. Marcus Books, Queensville, Ont. 1982.

Hobbs, Christopher. *Usnea : The Herbal Antibiotic*. Botanica Press. 1986.

_____*Medicinal Mushrooms*, Botanica Press, Santa Cruz, 1995.

Hoffman, David. *The Holistic Herbal*. Findhorn Press, 1983.

_____*Welsh Herbal Medicine*. Abercastle Publications, Dyfed, 1978.

_____*Medical Herbalism*. Healing Arts Press, Rochester, VT, 2003.

Hole, Lois. *Favorite Trees and Shrubs*. Lone Pine Pub. Edmonton Alta. 1997.

_____*Perennial Favorites*. Lone Pine Pub. 1995.

Holm, LeRoy G. *World Weeds*, John Wiley and Sons, 1997.

Holmes, Peter. *The Energetics of Western Herbs, Vol 1 and 2,* Artemis Press, 1989.

_____*Jade Remedies, Vol 1 and 2,* Snow Lotus Press, Boulder 1996.

Hopman, Ellen. *A Druid's Herbal*, Destiny Books, Rochester, Vermont. 1995.

Howarth, D& Kahlee Keane. *Wild Medicines of the Prairies* Self Published, 1995.

_____*Native Medecines* Self Published , 1995

Hozeski, Bruce. *Hildegard's Healing Plants*. Beacon Press. Boston, Mass. 2001.

Hsu, Hong-Yen. *Oriental Materia Medica*, Keats Publishing,Connecticut, 1986.

Huang, Kee Chang. *The Pharmacolocy of Chinese Herbs*. 2nd Edition, CRC Press, 1999.

Hu-Nan. *A Barefoot Doctor's Manual*. Running Press, Philadelphia, 1977.

Hudson, James B. *Antiviral Compounds from Plants*, CRC Press, Florida, 1990

Hudson, Rick. *A Field Guide to Gold, Gemstone and Mineral Sites*. Orca Pub, Victoria, 1999

Hurley, Judith. *The Good Herb* Wm. Morrow and Co. New York, 1995.

Hutchens, Alma. *Indian Herbology of North America*. Merco. 1969

Ingram, Cass. *Supermarket Remedies*. Knowledge House, Buffalo Grove, Ill. 1998.

Injoynow essences.

Inkpen W & Van Eyk, R. *Guide to the Common Native Trees and Shrubs of Alberta*, Government of Alberta, Environmental Protection, 1995.

James & Keeler, *Poisonous Plants- 3rd Int. Symposium*, Iowa State U. Press, 1992.

Jason, Dan & Nancy. *Some Useful Wild Plants*, Talon Books, Vancouver, 1972.

Jiao Shu-De. *Ten Lectures on the Use of Medicinals*. Paradigm Pub. Brookline, Mass. 2003.

Johnson, Kershaw, MacKinnon & Pojar *Plants of the Western Boreal Forest and Aspen Parkland*, Lone Pine Press, Edmonton, Alberta 1995.

Johnson, L. *Tending the Earth A Gardener's Manifesto*. Penguin Books, Toronto, 2002.

Johnson, Leslie. Journal of Ethnobotany and Ethnomedicine. 2006 2:29.

_____*Health, Wholeness & the Land: Gitksan Traditional Plant Use and Healing*. U of Alberta 1997.

Jones, Alison. *Larousse Dictionary of World Folklore*. Larousse, New York, 1995.

Jones, Pamela. *Just Weed, History, Myths and Uses*. Prentice Hall Press, Toronto, 1991.

Kamm, Minnie W. *Old Time Herbs for Northern Gardens* Little Brown & Co. 1938.

Kane, Charles W. Herbal Medicine of the American Southwest. Lincoln Town Press. 2007.

_____Herbal Medicine: trends and traditions. Lincoln Town Press 2009.

Kapoor, L.D. *CRC Handbook of Ayurvedic Medicinal Plants,* CRC Press, Boca Raton, 1990.

Kari, Priscilla. *Tanaina Plantlore*. National Park Service, Alaska Region 1987.

Kaur, Sat Dharam. *The Complete Natural Medicine Guide to Breast Cancer*. Robert Rose Inc Toronto, 2003.

Kavash E, Barrie & Barr K, *American Indian Healing Arts*. Bantam Books, Toronto 1999.

_____*The Medicine Wheel Garden*. Bantam Books, N.Y. 2002.

Kay, Margarita Artschwager. *Healing with Plants in the American and Mexican West,* The University of Arizona Press, Tucson. 1996

Kays, S & Nottingham S. Biology and Chemistry of Jerusalem Artichoke. CRC Press 2008.

Keane, Kahlee & Howarth,D. *The Standing People.* Saskatoon, Saskatchewan. 2003.

Kee Chang Huang, *The Pharmacology of Chinese Herbs,* 2nd Edition, CRC Press, 1999.

Kemp, Cynthia. *Cactus and Company.* Desert Alchemy, Tucson, Arizona, 1993.

Kenner D &Requena Y. *Botanical Medicine:* .Paradigm Pub. Brookline, Mass, 1996.

Kerik, Joan. *Living with the Land:Use of Plants by the Native People of Alberta,* Alberta Culture, Circulating Exhibits Program, National Museums of Canada Fund, 1981.

Kershaw, Linda. Edible & Medicinal Plants of the Rockies, Lone Pine, Edmonton 2000.

_____*Alberta Wayside Wildflowers.* Lone Pine, Edmonton, 2003.

_____*Saskatchewan Wayside Wildflowers.* Lone Pine, Edmonton, 2003.

_____*Manitoba Wayside Wildflowers.* Lone Pine, Edmonton, 2003.

Kershaw, L. et al. *Rare Vascular Plants of Alberta.* U. of Alberta Press, Edmonton, 2001.

Kershaw, MacKinnon & Pojar. *Plants of the Rocky Mountains.* Lone Pine, Edmonton 1998.

Keys, John. D. *Chinese Herbs,* Charles E. Tuttle Co. 1976.

Kimmerer,Robin. *Gathering Moss.* Oregon State University Press, Corvallis, 2003.

Kindscher, Kelly. *Medicnal Wild Plants of the Prairies.* Univ. Press of Kansas. 1987.

King, Francis X. *Rudolf Steiner and Holistic Medicine.* Rider & Co. England, 1986.

Klein, Carol. Plant Personalities. Timber Press, Portland, Oregon. 2005.

Klein, Richard. *The Green World.* 2nd edition. Harper Collins, 1987.

Kloss, Jethro. *Back to Eden.* Woodbridge Press Pub.Co. Santa Barbara, Ca. 1975.

Knab, Sophie H. *Polish Herbs, Flowers and Folk Medicine.* Hippocrene Books, N.Y. 1999.

Knowles, Hugh. *Woody Ornamentals for the Prairies.* U. of Alberta , 1995.

Knudtson,P & Suzuki D. Wisdom of the Elders. Greystone Books. Vancouver BC 2006.

Kraft, K & Hobbs C. *Pocket Guide to Herbal Medicine.* Thieme, N.Y. 2004.

Kranich, Ernst M. Planetary Influences Upon Plants. Bio-Dynamic Lit. Wyoming RI 1984.

Krymow, V. Healing Plants of the Bible. Wild Goose Pub. Glasgow, UK 2002.

Kuhnlein, Harriet and Turner, Nancy. *Traditional Plant Foods of Canadian Indigenous Peoples.* Gordon and Breach Science Publishers. 1991.

Kuijt, Job. *The Biology of Parasitic Flowering Plants,* U. of California Press, 1969

Kunkele, U. & Lohmeyer, T. *Herbs for Healthy Living.* Parragon Pub. Bath UK 2007.

Lacey, Laurie. *Micmac Medicines Remedies and Recollections.* Nimbus Pub. Halifax, 1993.

Lahring, Heinjo. *Water and Wetland Plants of the Prairie Provinces,* Can Plains Research Center, U. of Regina, 2003

Lambert, Grant. *Falling Leaf Essences.* Healing Arts Press, Rochester Vermont, 2002.

Lamont, SM. *The Fisherman Lake Slave and their environment: a story of floral and faunal resources.* Master's thesis. U. of Saskatchewan, Saskatoon, 1977.

Langenheim, Jean. *Medicinal Plant Resins.* Timber Press Portland Oregon 2003.

Larsen,Henning. *An Old Icelandic Medical Miscellany,* Norske Akademi, Oslo, Norway '31

Lavabre, Marcel. *Aromatherapy Workbook.* Healing Arts Press, Vermont. 1990.

Lawless, Julia, *The Encyclopedia of Essential Oils ,* Element Books, 1992.

LeClaire,N &Cardinal,G. *Alberta Elders' Cree Dictionary,* U of Alberta Press, 1998.

Leduc, M.A. *The Explorers Guide to Boreal Forest Plants,* Hwy Book Shop, Cobalt, Ont. 1997

Leighton, Anna L. *Wild Plant Use by the Woods Cree (NIHITHAWAK) of East-Central Saskatchewan .* Paper no. 101, National Museums of Canada, Ottawa, 1985

Lepore, Donald. *The Ultimate Healing System.* Woodland Books, Provo, Utah, 1988.

Le Strange, Richard, *A History of Herbal Plants.* Arco Pub. New York. 1977.

Leung, Albert. *Chinese Herbal Remedies.* Universe Books, New York, 1984.

Leung & Foster, *Encyclopedia of Common Natural Ingredients,* J. Wiley&Sons, N.Y. 1996.

Levey,M. *The Medical Formulary or Aqrabadhin of Al-Kindi* U of Wisconsin Press, 1966

Leyel, C.F. *Elixirs of Life,* Faber and Faber, London.1948

Li, Thomas. *Medicinal Plants, Culture, Utilization & Phytopharmacology.* Technomic Publishing, Lancaster, Pennsylvania, 2000.

Li, Thomas. *Chinese and related North American Herbs.* CRC Press, Boca Raton, 2002.

Libster, Martha. *Delmar's Integrative Herb Guide for Nurses.* Delmar, 2002.

Lininger et al. *The Natural Pharmacy.* Healthnotes, Prima Pub. Rocklin Ca, 1999.

L'Orange Darlena, *Herbal Healing Secrets of the Orient.* Prentice Hall, New Jersey, 1998.

Lock, Carolyn. *Country Colours.* Nova Scotia Museum. 1981

Lovejoy, Sharon. *Sunflower Houses.* Workman Pub Co. New York 2001.

Lu, Henry. *Using Foods to Stay Young,* Sterling Press, New York, 1996.

_____*Chinese Natural Cures.* Black Dog & Leventhal Pub. New York, 1994

Luetjohann, Sylvia. *The Healing Power of Black Cumin.* Lotus Light, Twin Lakes, WI, 1998

Lyle, Katie Letcher. *The Wild Berry Book,* NorthWord Press, Minocqua, WI, 1994.

Mabey, Richard. *Plantcraft.* Universe Books. 1978.

MacKinnon, Pojar, Coupe. *Plants of Northern British Columbia.* Lone Pine Press, 1992.

Mailhebiau, Philippe. *Portraits in Oils.* C.W. Daniel Company, Essex, England, 1995.

Malmud, René. *The Amazon Problem,* trans by M. Stein, Spring Pub. Dallas TX, 1980.

Maloof, Joan. *Teaching the Trees, Lessons from the Forest.* U Georgia Pr, Athena GA. 2005.

Manandhar, N.P. *Plants and People of Nepal.* Timber Press, Portland, Oregon, 2002.

Maple, Eric. *The Secret Lore of Plants and Flowers.* Robert Hale Ltd. London 1980.

March, Kathryn & Andrew. *The Wild Plant Companion.* Meridian Hill Pub. 1986.

Marles, Robin. *The Ethnobotany of the Chipewyan of Northern Saskatchewan,* 1984. Thesis.

_____et al. *Aboriginal Plant Use in Canada's Northwest Boreal Forest.* UBC Press, Vancouver, and Natural Resources Canada, 2000

McBride, L.R. *Practical Folk Medicine of Hawaii.* Petroglyph Press, Hilo,Hawaii, 1975.

McCune B. & Geiser L. *Macrolichens of the Pacific Northwest.* Oregon State U. Press, 1997

McFarland, Phoenix. *The Complete Book of Magical Names.* Llewellyn Pub. St Paul 1996

McGrath, Judy. *Dyes from Lichens and Plants.* Van Nostrand Rheinhold, 1977.

McGuffin, Nancy. *Spectrum: dye plants of Ontario.* Burr House Spinner, Richmond Hill '86

McIntyre, Anne. *The Complete Woman's Herbal,* Henry Holt, New York, 1995.

Mears, R & Hillman,G. Wild Food. Hodder and Stoughton

MELODY. *Love is in the Earth, A Kaleidoscope of Crystals.* Earth Love Pub. Col. 1995.

Mercatante, A. S. The Facts on File Encyclopedia of World Mythology. New York 1988

Merriam, C. Hart. *Dawn of the World, Weird Tales of Mewan Indians.* Arthur H. Clark, Cleveland, 1910

Meyer, George et al. *Folk Medicine and Herbal Healing,* Charles Thomas, Springfield, 1981

Meyerowitz,Steve. *Sprout It!* The Sprout House, Box 1100,Great Barrington, MA, 1993.

Meyers, Edward C. *Basic Bush Survival,* Hancock House, Surrey, B.C. 1997.

Miller, L &Murray,W. *Herbal Medicinals A Clinician's Guide.* Hawthorn Press, N.Y. 1998.

Miller, Sandra. Editor Echinacea- Medicinal and Aromatic Plants. CRC Press, 2004.

Mills S. & Bone,K. *Principles and Practice of Phytotherapy.* Churchill Livingstone, 2000.

_____*The Essential Guide to Herbal Safety.* Churchill Livingstone, 2005.

Mills, Simon. *Out of the Earth.* Viking Penquin Books, Toronto. 1991.

Millsbaugh, Charles. *American Medicinal Plants,* Dover Pub. New York, 1974

Milne, Courtney. *Visions of the Goddess*, Penguin Studio, Toronto, 1998

Minnis & Elisens. *Biodiversity and Native America.* U. Oklahoma Press, 2000.

Mitchel, Jr. Wm. *Plant Medicine in Practice.* Churchill Livingstone, St. Louis, 2003.

Moerman, Daniel, *Medicinal Plants of Native America.* U of Michigan No. 19, 1986

Mohammed, G. *Catnip & Kerosene Grass* Candlenut Books, Sault Ste. Marie, Ont, 2002.

Montgomery, Pam. *Plant Spirit Healing.* Bear and Company, Rochester, VT 2008.

Moore, Michael. *Los Remedios.* Red Crane Books, 1990

_____*Medicinal Plants of the Desert and Canyon West.* Museum of New Mexico Press 1989

_____*Medicinal Plants of the Mountain West,* Museum of New Mexico Press '79

_____Med Plants of the Mountain West. Revised, expanded. 2003

_____*Medicinal Plants of the Pacific West,* Red Crane Books, 1993

More, Daphne. *The Bee Book,* Universe Books, New York, 1976.

Morelli, I. et al. *Selected Medicinal Plants.* University of Pisa. FAO 53/1

Morton, Julia. *Major Medicinal Plants* . Charles Thomas, Springfield, Illinois 1977

_____*Atlas of Medicinal Plants of Middle America, Bahamas to Yucatan.* 1981

Moss, E.H. *Flora of Alberta.* University of Toronto Press. 1983

Mother, The. *Flowers and their Messages.* Sri Aurobindo Ashram Trust, India 1979.

Mourning Dove. Coyote Stories. Caxton Press Caldwell Idaho. 1933.

Mowrey, Daniel. *The Scientific Validation of Herbal Medicine.* Cormorant Books, 1986.

Mucz, Michael. *Baba's Kitchen Medicines.* U of Alberta Press, Edmonton, 2012.

Mulders, Evelyn. *Western Herbs for Eastern Meridian & 5 Element Theory. Self publ. 2006.*

Mulligan, G editor *The biology of Canadian Weeds,* 1-32 Pub. 1693 Ag Canada 1979

_____33-61 Pub. 1765 Ag Canada 1984

Murphy, Cristine Editor, *Practical Home Care Medicine,* Lantern Books, New York, 2001

Murray, Michael. *The Pill Book Guide to Natural Medicines.* Bantam Books, April, 2002.

_____& Pizzorno, J. The condensed Encycl of Healing Foods. Pocket Books NY 2005.

Naegele, Thomas A. *Edible and Medicinal Plants of the Great Lakes Region,* Wilderness Adventure Books, Davisburg, Michigan. 1996.

Naiman, Ingrid. *Cancer Salves, A Botanical Approach to Treatment.* N. Atlantic Books, 99.

Nesse R & Williams G. *Why We Get Sick.* Vintage Books/Random House, New York, 1996.

Neuwinger H.D. *African Traditional Medicine.* Medpharm Sci. Pub. Stuttgart 2000.

_____African Ethnobotany, Poisons and Drugs. Chapman & Hall, London 1996.

Newcombe C.F. unpub notes on Haida plants. Dept of Anthro. Am Mus Nat Hist. NY 1897

_____unpublished papers. Prov Archives B.C. Victoria. 1898-1913.

Nicander. *The Poems and Poetical Fragments.* Cambridge U. Press, New York, 1953.

Norman,Howard. *Northern Tales.* Pantheon Books, New York, 1990.

Northcote, Rosalind. *The Book of Herbs.* John Lane: The Bodley Head, London, 1912.

Null, Gary. *The Clinician's Handbook of Natural Healing.* Kensington Books, N.Y. 1997.

Olive, Barbara. *The Flower Healer.* Cico Books, London and New York. 2007.

Ollsin, Don. *Herbal Healing Journey-Playful Workbook.* Aquiline Comm, Victoria,BC 1998.

Ootoova I. et al. *Interviewing Inuit Elders, Perspectives on Traditional Health.* Vol 5, Nunavut Arctic College, Box 600, Iqaluit, Nunavut X0Z 0H0.

Page, George. *Inside the Animal Mind.* Doubleday, New York, 1999.

Pallasdowney, Rhonda. *The Complete Book of Flower Essences.* New World Library, 2002.

Pappalardo, Joe. Sunflowers (the secret history). The Overlook Press. Woodstock NY 2008.

Parish, Coupé & Lloyd. *Plants of S. Interior British Columbia*. Lone Pine Edmonton 1996

Park, Willard Z. *Ethnographic Notes on the Norhern Paiute of Western Nevada, 1933-40* compiled by Catherine Fowler, U. of Utah, Salt Lake City, 1989.

Parvati, J. *Hygieia, A Woman's Herbal*. Freestone Collective. 1978

Paturi, Felix *Nature, Mother of Invention*. Harper and Row Pub. New York. 1976.

Peirce,Andrea. *Practical Guide to Natural Medicines*. Stonesong Press. 1999.

Pelikan, W. Healing Plants. Mercury Press, Spring Valley NY 1997.

Pellowski, Anne. *Hidden Stories in Plants*. MacMillan Pub. New York. 1990.

Penoel,Daniel & Franchomme, P. *L'Aromatherapie Exactement* , Roger Jollois, France, 1990

Peneol, Daniel. *Medecine Aromatique, Medecine Planetaire*. Roger Jollois France 1991.

_____& Peneol, Rose-Marie. *Natural Home Health Care Using Essential Oils*. Osmobiose Pub. 1998.

People of 'Ksan, The. *Gathering What the Great Nature Provided*. Douglas & McIntyre. Vancouver, B.C. 1980.

Peters, Josephine & Ortiz B. After the First Full Moon in April. Left Coast Press. Walnut Creek CA, 2010.

Pettitt,Sabina. Energy Medicine, Healing from the Kingdoms of Nature, Pacific Essences, Box 8317, Victoria, B.C. V8W 3R9 Canada, 1999

Phaneuf, Holly. Herbs Demystified. Marlowe and Company, New York. 2005

Pielou, E.C. *The Naturalist's Guide to the Arctic*. U. of Chicago Press. 1994.

Pieroni, A & Price L. Eating and Healing, Trad Food as Medicine. Haworth Press. N.Y. 2006.

Pfeiffer E. *The Earth's Face and Human Destiny,* Rodale Press, Emmaus, Pa. 1947.

Plotkin, Mark. *Medicine Quest*. Viking Penguin Books, New York, 2000.

Pojar, J & MacKinnon, A. *Plants of Coastal British Columbia* Lone Pine Edmonton 1994.

Pollock, L. With Faith and Physic: the life of a tudor gentlewoman. Collins & Brown,1993.

Polya, Gideon. *Biochemical Targets of Plant Bioactive Comp.* CRC Press, Boca Raton 2003

Pond, Barbara, *A Sampler of Wayside Herbs,* Chatham Press, Riverside, Conn.

Pressor, Arthur, *Pharmacist's Guide to Medicinal Herbs,* Smart Pub. Petaluma, CA,2000

Price, Len & Shirley. *Understanding Hydrolats*. Churchill Livingstone, Toronto, 2004.

_____Aromatherapy for Health Professionals. Churchill Livingstone 1995.

Purvis, William. *Lichens*. Smithsonian Institution Press. Washington D.C. 2000

Quin, Frederick F. *The Flora Homoeopathica*. B. Jain Pub. New Delhi, India. 1997.

Radin, Paul. *The Winnebago Tribe,* Bur of Am Ethnology, Smithsonian Inst. 37th. 1923.

Rätsch, C. *Plants of Love, The History of Aphrodisiacs.* Ten Speed Press, Berkeley,1997.

_____The Dictionary of Sacred & Magical Plants. ABC-CLIO St Barbara 1992.

_____The Encyclopedia of Psychoactive Plants. Park St Press. 2005.

Raven Essences. www.ravenessences.com

Ravenworks flower essences. www.ravenworksministries.weebly.com

Reaume, Tom. 620 Wild Plants of North America. Nature Manitoba. Canadian Plains Research Center, U of Regina, U of Toronto Press. 2009.

Reckeweg, Hans-Heinrich, *Materia Medica, Vol 1. Aurelia-Verlag GmbH, Baden Baden* 1996.

Reich, Lee. *Uncommon Fruits Worthy of Attention,* Addison-Wesley Pub. 1991.

Reid, Daniel, *A handbook of Chinese Healing Herbs,* Shambala, Boston, 1995

Rhode, David. Native Plants of Southern Nevada. U of Utah Press. 2002.

Richards B & Kanecko A. *Japanese Plants- Know Them &Use Them.* Shufunotomo, Tokyo 1995

Richardson, David. *The Vanishing Lichens*. David and Charles, Vancouver, BC, 1975

Riddle, John M. *Eve's Herbs*. Harvard U Press. Cambridge Mass. 1997.

_____Goddesses, Elixirs and Witches. Palgrave MacMillan. England 2010.

Rister, Robert. *Healing Without Medication.* Basic Health Pub. N. Bergen, N.J. 2003.

Roberts, Jonathan. *The Origins of Fruit and Vegetables.* Universe Pub. New York. 2001.

Robicsek, F. *The Smoking God: Tobacco....*Norman: U. of Oklahoma Press, 1978.

Robinson, Peggy. *Profiles of Northwest Plants.* Far West Book Service. Portland, OR 1979

Rogers, Dilwyn. *Edible, Medicinal, Useful & Poisonous Wild Plants of the Northern Great Plains —South Dakota Region.* Buechel Memorial Lakota Museum, St. Francis,SD, 1980.

Rogers, Pattiann. *Firekeeper:New & Selected Poems.* Milkweed Editions, 1994.

Rogers, Robert Dale. *Sundew Moonwort Vols-1-7, self-published.* Edmonton 1995-present.

_____Rogers' Herbal Manual. Karamat Wilderness Ways, Edmonton, 2000.

_____& Capital Health, Herbal Drug Interactions. Mediscript Comm. 2003.

_____The Fungal Pharmacy, The Complete Guide to Medicinal Mushrooms and Lichens of North America, North Atlantic Books 2011.

Rombi, Max. *Phytotherapy.* Herbal Health Publishers. U.K. 1990.

Rosengarten,Jr. F. *The Book of Edible Nuts.* Walker and Co. New York. 1984.

Ross, Gary. *Nature's Guide to Healing.* Freedom Press, Topanga, Ca. 2000.

Ross, Ivan. *Medicinal Plants of the World.* Vol 1 Humana Press, Totowa, New Jersey. 1999.

_____ Vol 2 Humana Press, Totowa, N. J. 2002.

Rotella, Rev. Alexis. *The Essence of Flowers,* Jade Mountain Press, N.J. 1991.

Royer F. & Dickinson R. *Plants of Alberta.* Lone Pine Pub. Edmonton, AB. 2007.

Rudginsky, Marlene *The Flower Speaks.* U.S. Games Systems, Stamford, Conn. 1999.

Rupp, Rebecca. *Red Oaks and Black Birches* , Storey Comm. Garden Way Publishing. 1990

Russell, Sharman Apt. *Anatomy of a Rose.* Perseus Pub. Cambridge, Mass. 2001.

_____An Obsession with Butterflies. Perseus Publishing 2003.

Ryan, J et al, *Traditional Dene Medicine.* Lac La Martre NWT, 1993.

Ryden, Hope. *Wildflowers around the year.* Clarion Books, New York. 2001.

Ryrie, Charlie. Garden Folklore That Works. Reader's Digest. Pleasantville, NY 2001.

Sagadic O. & Ozcan M. *Food Control* 2003 14.

Salmon, Wm. *Botanologia: The English Herbal.* London: I. Dawkes, 1710.

Sandberg & Corrigan. *Natural Remedies, their origins and uses.* Taylor & Francis 2001.

Sanders, Jack. *The Secrets of Wildflowers.* The Lyons Press, Guilford, CT, 2003.

Sapolsky, Robert. *The Trouble with Testosterone.* Scribner, New York. 1997.

Sauer, Johann Christopher, Compendious Herbal-see Weaver below.

Savage, Candace. Bees, Nature's Little Wonders. Greystone Books. Vancouver 2008.

Schalkwijk-Barendsen, Helene. *Mushrooms of Western Canada* . Lone Pine Pub. 1991.

Schar, Douglas. *The Backyard Medicine Chest.* Elliott&Clark Pub. Washington, DC. 1995.

Scheffer, Mechthild, *Bach Flower Therapy, Theory and Practice,* Healing Arts Press, 1988

Schenk, George. *Moss Gardening.* Timber Press, Portland Oregon. 1997.

Schnaubelt, Kurt. *Medical Aromatherapy.* Frog Ltd. Berkeley CA. 1999.

Schneider, Anny. *Wild Medicinal Plants.* Key Porter Books, Toronto. 2002.

Schnell, Donald. *Carnivorous Plants.* 2nd Ed. Timber Press, Portland, Oregon, 2002.

Schofield, Janice. *Discovering Wild Plants.* Alaska Northwest Books. 1989.

_____Nettles. Keats Publishing, New Canaan, Conneticut, 1998.

Schulman, Robert. *Solve It With Supplements.* Rodale Press. New York. 2007.

Shapiro, R & Rapkins J. Awakening to the Plant Kingdom, Cassandra Press 1991.

Shauenberg, Paul and Paris. *Guide to Medicinal Plants.* Keats Publishing, 1977.

Shook, Edward Dr. *Advanced Treatise on Herbology* . Reprint Health Research.

Shosteck,Robert. *Flowers and Plants.* Quadrangle/The New York Times Book Co. 1974.

Siegfried, EV. Masters Thesis, Ethnobotany of the Northern Cree of Wabasca/Desmarais. U of Calgary, Alberta. 1994.

Silverman, Maida. *A City Herbal.* David R. Godine , 1990.

Silvertown, Jonathan. An Orchard Invisible. U of Chicago Press. 2009.

Simonot, Danielle. *Bio-Manufacturing in Saskatchewan-* Assessment of the Manufacturing Potential of Select Saskatchewan Plants, Sask. Nutraceutical Network, Saskatoon, 2000

Simpson, Brenan, M. *Flowers At My Feet,* Hancock House, Surrey, B.C. 1996.

Sionneau, P. *An Introduction to the Use of Processed Chinese Medicinals.* Blue Poppy Press, Second Printing 2003, Translated by Bob Flaws.

Smagghe, Guy Ed. Ecdysone: Structures and Functions. Springer Sci 2009.

Small, E & Catling, P. *Canadian Medicinal Crops,* NRC Research Press, Ottawa 1999.

Small, Ernest. *Culinary Herbs, Second Ed.* NRC Research Press, Ottawa, 2006.

_____*Medicinal Herbs,* NRC Research Press, Ottawa, 2000.

_____Top 100 Food Plants. NRC Press, Ottawa. 2009.

Smith, Andrew. *Strangers in the Garden, the Secret Lives of Our Favorite Flowers.*McClelland & Stewart 2004.

Smith, Annie Lorrain. *Lichens,* Cambridge at the University Press, 1921.

Smith, Harlan, *Ethnobotany of the Gitksan Indians of B.C.* Edited by B. Compton, B. Rigsby, and M.L. Tarpent, Mercury Series, Can Ethno Service, Paper 132, Can Mus of Civil. 1997.

Smith, Huron H. Manataka American Indian Council. www.manataka.org.

Snell, Alma Hogan. A Taste of Heritage. Crow Indian Recipes and Herbal Medicines. University of Nebraska Press 2006.

Soule, Deb. *The Roots of Healing, A Woman's Book of Herbs.* Citadel Press, 1995.

Spencer, Kate. *The Magic of Green Buckwheat ,*Richard Clay, England, 1987.

Spinella, Marcello. *The Psychopharmacology of Herbal Medicine.* MIT Press, 2001.

Steedman, E.V. *The Ethnobotany of the Thompson Indians of British Columbia.* 1930.

Stein, Sara. *My Weeds, A Gardener's Botany.* Harper and Row, 1988.

Stern, Gai. *Australian Weeds.* Harper and Row, Australia 1986

Stern Wm. *Stern's Dictionary of Plant Names for Gardeners.* Cassell Pub, London, 1972

Stewart, Hilary. *CEDAR.* Douglas & McIntyre. Vancouver/Toronto, 1984.

Storl, Wolf D. Healing Lyme Disease Naturally. NorthAtlantic Books, Berkeley, CA 2010.

Strehlow,W & Hertzka,G. *Hildegard of Bingen's Medicine* Bear & Co. Santa Fe 1988

Stuart, David. *Dangerous Garden.* Harvard University Press, Cambridge, Mass. 2004

Sturdivant L.&Blakley,T. *Medicinal Herbs in the Garden, Field and Marketplace* Bootstrap Guide, San Juan Naturals, Friday Harbor,WA, 1999.

Sumner, Judith. *The Natural History of Medicinal Plants.* Timber Press, Oregon, 2000.

Sun Bear & Wabun, *The Medicine Wheel* Prentice Hall, NJ 1980.

Swanton, J.R. *Haida Texts and Myths.* Bureau Am Ethnol, Bull #29. Smithsonian Inst. Washington, D.C. 1905.

_____*Bureau of Am Ethno 26th Ann Report.* Smithsonian Inst. Washington, 1908.

Szczeklik, Andrzej. Kore: On Sickness, the Sick and the Search for the Soul of Medicine. Counterpoint Berkeley 2012.

Tainter, D& Grenis A, *Spices and Seasonings ,* VCH Pubishers, New York, 1993.

Talalaj,S.& Czechowicz,A S. *Herbal Remedies,* Hill of Content Press, Melbourne, 1989

Taylor, Wm &Farnsworth,N. The Vinca Alkaloids, Marcel Dekker, New York, 1973.

Teeguarden, Ron. *The Ancient Wisdom of the Chinese Tonic Herbs.* Warner Bros. 1998.

Telesco, Patricia. *The Victorian Flower Oracle,* Llewellyn Pub. St. Paul 1994

Temple, Robert. *The Genius of China*. Simon and Schuster. New York. 1986.

Thompson, Gerry, *Astral Sex to Zen Teabags*. Findhorn Press, 1994.

Thoreau, Henry David. *Wild Fruits*. W. W. Norton & Co. New York, 2000.

Throop, Priscilla. *Hildegard von Bingen's Physica*. Healing Arts Press, Vt. 1998.

Tick, Edward. *The Practice of Dream Healing*. Quest Books Wheaton, Illinois, 2001.

Tierra, Michael. *The Way of Herbs- revised Pocket Rooks*, New York, 1998.

Tigner, Daniel. *Canadian Forest Tree Essences,* self published,1998. ISBN 0968365809

Tilford, Gregory. *Edible and Medicinal Plants of the West*. Mountain Press, Missoula 1997.

Timbrook, Jan. Chumash Ethnobotany. St. Barbara Mus, Heyday Books, Berkeley Ca 2007.

Traill, E.C. *Studies of Plant Life in Canada*. A. S. Woodburn, Ottawa, 1885.

Traill, C. P. *The Backwoods of Canada*. McClelland and Stewart. Toronto. 1846.

Tobyn, G., Denham, A., Whitelegg, M. The Western Herbal Tradition. 2000 years of medicinal herbal knowledge. Churchill Livingstone Toronto 2011.

Toop, Edgar W & Williams, Sara. *Perennials for the Prairies*. U of A&Saskatchewan. 1991.

Treben, Maria. *Health Through God's Pharmacy*. Wilhelm Ennsthaler. 1982.

Tresidder, Jack. Symbols and Their Meaning. Friedman/Fairfax Pub. 2007.

Tucker A. & DeBaggio,T. *The Big Book of Herbs*. Interweave Press. Loveland CO. 2000.

_____The Encylcopedia of Herbs. Timber Press, Portland. 2009.

Turkington, Carol. *The Home Health Guide to Poisons and Antidotes,* Facts on File 1994

Turner, Nancy J. *Food Plants of Interior First Peoples*. UBC Press, Vancouver, 1997.

_____*Food Plants of Coastal First Peoples*. UBC Press, Vancouver, 1995.

_____*Plant Technology of First Peoples in B.C.* UBC Press, Vancouver, 1998.

_____et al. *Thompson Ethnobotany*. Memoir #3, Royal B.C. Museum, 1996.

_____*Plants of Haida Gwaii*. Sononis Press, Winlaw, B.C. 2004.

_____The Earth's Blanket. Douglas & McIntyre. Vancouver. 2005.

Turner, N & von Aderkas, P. Common Poisonous Plants and Mushrooms. Timber Press 2009

Turner, W.B. *Fungal Metabolites,* Academic Press, London and New York, 1971.

Twitchell, Paul. *Herbs The Magic Healers*. Eckankar, Box 3100 Menlo Park, CA, 1986.

Vermeulen, Nico. *Encyclopedia of Herbs*. Whitecap Books, Vancouver B.C. 1998.

Viereck, Eleanor, G. *Alaska's Wilderness Medicines*. Alaska Northwest Pub. 1987

Vitt, Marsh and Bovey, *Mosses, Lichens, and Ferns,* Lone Pine Press, 1988.

Vogel, A. *Swiss Nature Doctor*. A. Vogel, Switzerland. 1952

_____*Nature-Your Guide to Healthy Living*. Verlag A. Vogel, Teufen, Switzerland 1986.

Vogel, Virgil. *American Indian Medicine,* U. of Oklahoma Press, Norman, 1970

Vortex Essences (Mt. Shasta Essences) www.vortexessences.com

Walker, Barbara. *The Woman's Dictionary of Symbols&Sacred Objects*. Csstle Books, 1988.

Walker, Marilyn. Wild Plants of Eastern Canada. Nimbus Pub. Halifax NS. 2008.

Ward, Bobby J. The Plant Hunter's Garden. Timber Press, Portland. 2004.

Ward-Harris, Joan.*More Than Meets the Eye, The Life and Lore of Western Wildflowers* Oxford University Press, Toronto, 1983

Watanabe & Shibuya. *Pharmacological Research on Traditional Herbal Medicines*. Harwood Academic Publishers, 1999.

Watt, John, and Breyer-Brandwijk, Maria *The Medicinal and Poisonous Plants of Southern and Eastern Africa* . E and S. Livingstone. Edinburgh and London. 1962.

Watts, Donald. Elsevier's Dictionary of Plant Lore. Elsevier. 2007.

Waugh, F.W. *Iroquois Foods and Food Preparation* #12 Anthropological Series, Ottawa. 1916. Reprinted by Iroqrafts, RR #2, Ohsweken, Ontario N0A 1M0, 1991.

Weaver, Wm. *100 Vegetables & Where They Came From*. Workman Pub. New York, 2000.

_____*Sauer's Herbal Cures America's First Book of Botanic Healing 1762-1778,* Routledge, New York, 2001.

Weed, Susan. *Menopausal Years, The Wise Woman Way*. Ash Tree Pub. Woodstock NY, 1992

Weigle, Marta. *Spiders and Spinsters*. U. of New Mexico Press, Albuquerque, 1982.

Weiner, M. *The People's Herbal, A family guide*. Putnam Publishing, New York, 1984.

Weiss, Rudolf. *Herbal Medicine*. Beaconsfield Publishers, 1988.

_____*Herbal Medicine* 2nd Edition. Thieme, Stuttgart, New York, 2000.

Wells, Diana.*100 Flowers and How They Got Their Names,* Algonquin Books, Chapel Hill,97

Westcott, Frank. *The Beaver Nature's Master Builder*. Hounslow Press, Willowdale, ON '89.

Westrich, LoLo, *California Herbal Remedies,* Gulf Pub Co. Houston, TX, 1989.

Wetzel, Suzanne et al. Bioproducts from Canada's Forests. Springer Netherlands 2006.

WHO monographs on selected medicinal plants, vol 1, 1999; vol 2, 2002.

White, Ian. *Australian Bush Flower Essences*. Bantam Books, 1991

White, Florence. *Flowers as Food* . Jonathan Cape. 1934

Whitmont, Edward. *Psyche and Substance*. North Atlantic Books. 1980

Wilkinson, Kathleen. *Trees and Shrubs of Alberta*. Lone Pine Books, Edmonton 1990.

_____*Wildflowers of Alberta*. U of A/Lone Pine Books, Edmonton 1999.

Williams, Jude. *Nature's Gentle Cures*. Sterling Publishing. New York. 1997.

Williamson, Darcy. 130 Medicinal Plant Monographs of the NW. self pub. E-book. 2011.

Williamson, E. *Major Herbs of Ayurveda*. Churchill Livingstone, Elsevier Science, 2002.

FLOWER ESSENCE RESOURCES

Aditi Himalaya Flower Essences, 15,Jaybharat Society, 3rd Road, Khar (W), Bombay 400 052, India.

Alaskan Flower Essence Project, P.O. Box. 1369, Homer, Alaska USA 99603-1369. www.alaskanessences.com.

Australian Bush Flower Essences. Australia. www.ausflowers.com.au.

Bach- Healing Herbs English Flower Essences- in Canada by Self Heal Distributing, Box 95008, Whyte Postal Outlet, Edmonton, AB T6E 0E5, 1800-593-5956 or www.selfhealdistributing.com Also www.healingherbs.co.uk or www.fesflowers.com

Bailey Flower Essences, 8 Neslon Road, Ilkley, West Yorkshire England, LS298HN. www.flowervr.com

Bloesem Remedies. Netherlands. www.bloesem-remedies.com

BrynaHerb Essences. www.brynaherbessences.uk

Canadian Forest Essences, PO Box 29128,1996 W. Broadway, Vancouver, BC V6J 1Z0

Canadian Forest Tree Essences. Ottawa. www.essences.ca. 613-725-9764.

Choming Flower Essences. www.mkprojects.com

Clear Path Essences. www.clearpathessences.com

Dancing Light Orchid Essences. Fairbanks, Alaska. www.orchidessences.com

Desert Alchemy, PO Box 44189, Tucson, Arizona, USA 85733. www.desert-alchemy.com.

Deva Flower Essences BP3 38880, Autrans, France. www.lab-deva.com

Eastern Flower Herbal Essences. julied@hfx.eastlink.ca.

Falling Leaf Essences. Box 78, Kallista, Victoria 3791, Australia. www.advancedalchemy.com.au.

Findhorn Flower Essences, Morayshire, Scotland IV36 0TY. www.findhornessences.com

Florais des Minas, Rua Albita, 194-Sala 408, Cruziero, CEP 30310-160,BH, MG, BRAZIL

FlorAlive˚, Brent Davis. Contact info@floralive.com

FES Flower Essence Society, PO Box 1769, Nevada City, California, USA, 95959. www.fesflowers.com Canadian Distributor- Self Heal Distributing, Box 95008, Whyte Postal Outlet, Edmonton, AB T6E 0E5 – www.selfhealdistributing.com

Green Hope Farm Flower Essences, PO Box 125, Meriden, New Hampshire USA 03770

Green Man Tree Essences. www.greenmantrees.demon.co.uk.

Habundia Flower Essences. c/o Peter Aziz. PO Box 90, Totnes, Devon, England TQ11 0YG.

Harebell Remedies. Scotland. ellie@harebellremedies.co.uk.

Hawaiian Gaia Flower Essences. www.gaiaessences.com

High Sierra Flower Essences. PO. Box 4275 Truclee, CA 96160. holly.hsb@highoctavehealing.com

Horus Flower Essences- horus@floweressences.de.

Hummingbird Remedies, PO Box 50161, Eugene, Oregon, USA 97405

Icelandic Flower Essences. www.kristbjorb.is.

Jade Mountain Flower Essences, Box 125, Mountain Lakes, New Jersey USA 07046-0125

Korte Phi. www.PHIessences.com

Light Heart Essences. England. www.lightheartessences.co.uk.

Light Mountain Flower Essences, Michael A. Vertolli, 1-800-667-HERB.

Living Essences of Australia, Box 355, Scarborough, 6019, Perth, Australia. www.livingessences.com.au

Living Flower Essences, www.livingfloweressences.com . Rhonda Pallasdowney.

Master's Flower Essences, 14618 Tyler Foote Rd Nevada City, California, USA, 95959. www.masteressences.com

Miriana fortem Flower Essences. www.mirianaflowers.com and info@miraflowers.com.

NaturaSacredplay, PO Box 32, Buckhorn, New Mexico, 88025, (505-535-2255).

New Millenium Flower Essences of New Zealand. info@nmessences.com.

New Zealand New Perception Flower Essences, PO Box 60-127,Titirangi, Auckland 7, NZ

Pacific Essences, Box 8317, Victoria, B.C. V8W 3R9. www.pacificessences.com.

Pegasus Products, PO Box 228, Boulder, Colorado, USA 80306-0228. 1-800- 527-6104.

Perelandra, Box 3603, Warrenton, VA. 22186. www.perelandra-ltd.com

Petite Fleur Essence, 8524 Whispering Creek Trail, Fort Worth, Texas, USA 76134. www.aromahealthtexas.com

Prairie Deva Flower Essences, Box 95008, Whyte Postal Outlet, Edmonton, AB T6E 0E5 1-(780) 433-7882. www.selfhealdistributing.com

Ravenworks- joni@ravenworksministries.org

Running Fox Farm PO Box 381,Worthington, Maryland USA 01098

Star Peruvian Flower Essences. Santa Barbara. www.starfloweressences.com

Stars of the Meadow, David Dalton, Lindisfarne Books, Mass. 2006.

Sun Essences. Norfolk, England. www.sunessence.co.uk

Sweetwater Sanctuary Essences. www.plantspirithealing.com

Tree Frog Farm Flower Essences. www.treefrogfarm.com

Whole Energy Essences, PO Box 285, Concord, Mass. 01742

Wild Rose Essences. www.wildrose.com

Woodland Essence, PO Box 206, Cold Brook, New York, USA 13324.